OKU

D0619684

3

Orthopaedic Knowledge Update:

Musculoskeletal Tumors

AAOS

AMERICAN ACADEMY OF
ORTHOPAEDIC SURGEONS

OKU 3

Orthopaedic Knowledge Update:

Musculoskeletal Tumors

EDITOR

J. Sybil Biermann, MD
Professor
Associate Chair for Education and
*   Residency Program Director*
Department of Orthopaedic Surgery
University of Michigan
Ann Arbor, Michigan

DEVELOPED BY
THE MUSCULOSKELETAL TUMOR SOCIETY

MSTS

AAOS
AMERICAN ACADEMY OF
ORTHOPAEDIC SURGEONS

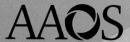

AMERICAN ACADEMY OF ORTHOPAEDIC SURGEONS

Published 2014 by the
American Academy of Orthopaedic Surgeons
6300 North River Road
Rosemont, IL 60018

Library of Congress Control Number:
2013955806

ISBN
978-0-89203-968-5

Printed in the USA

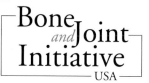

Acknowledgments

Editorial Board, Orthopaedic Knowledge Update: Musculoskeletal Tumors 3

J. Sybil Biermann, MD
Professor
Associate Chair for Education and Residency
Program Director
Department of Orthopaedic Surgery
University of Michigan
Ann Arbor, Michigan

Albert J. Aboulafia, MD, FACS, MBA
Director, Sarcoma Services, Cancer Institute
Sinai Hospital
Assistant Clinical Professor, University of
Maryland
Baltimore, Maryland

Joseph Benevenia, MD
Professor and Chair
Department of Orthopaedics
Rutgers New Jersey Medical School
Newark, New Jersey

Ginger E. Holt, MD
Associate Professor
Department of Musculoskeletal Oncology
Vanderbilt Orthopaedic Institute
Nashville, Tennessee

Patrick P. Lin, MD
Associate Professor
Department of Orthopaedic Oncology
University of Texas
MD Anderson Cancer Center
Houston, Texas

Carol D. Morris, MD, MS
Associate Professor
Department of Orthopaedic Surgery
Weill Cornell School of Medicine
Memorial Sloan-Kettering Cancer Center
New York, New York

R. Lor Randall, MD
Professor
Department of Orthopaedics
Huntsman Cancer Institute at the University
of Utah
Salt Lake City, Utah

Board of Directors, Musculoskeletal Tumor Society

Kristy L. Weber, MD, *President*

Richard M. Terek, MD, *President-Elect*

Ted W. Parsons, MD, FACS, *Secretary*

Robert H. Quinn, MD, *Treasurer*

John H. Healey, MD, FACS, *Immediate Past President*

Edward Y. Cheng, MD, *Past President*

Joseph Benevenia, MD, *Education Committee Chair*

R. Lor Randall, MD, FACS, *Research Committee Chair*

Douglas J. McDonald, MD, *Membership Committee Chair*

Contributors

John A. Abraham, MD
Chief, Orthopedic Oncology
Department of Orthopedic Surgery
Rothman Institute
Philadelphia, Pennsylvania

Raffi S. Avedian, MD
Assistant Professor
Department of Orthopaedic Surgery
Stanford University Medical Center
Palo Alto, California

Elizabeth H. Baldini, MD, MPH
Associate Professor of Radiation Oncology
Dana-Farber Cancer Institute
Brigham and Women's Hospital
Harvard Medical School
Boston, Massachusetts

Kathleen S. Beebe, MD
Assistant Professor
Department of Orthopaedics
Rutgers New Jersey Medical School
Newark, New Jersey

Justin E. Bird, MD
Assistant Professor
Department of Orthopaedic Oncology
University of Texas
MD Anderson Cancer Center
Houston, Texas

Patrick J. Boland, MD
Attending Orthopaedic Surgeon
Orthopaedic Service, Department of Surgery
Memorial Sloan-Kettering Cancer Center
New York, New York

Shahram Bozorgnia, MD
Assistant Professor, Musculoskeletal Oncologist
Department of Orthopaedic Surgery
Georgia Health Sciences University
Augusta, Georgia

Emily E. Carmody Soni, MD
Clinical Instructor
Department of Orthopaedic Oncology
MedStar Georgetown Orthopaedic Institute
Washington, DC

Saad B. Chaudhary, MD, MBA
Assistant Professor
Department of Orthopaedic Surgery
Rutgers New Jersey Medical School
Newark, New Jersey

David Cheong, MD
Associate Professor of Orthopedics
Sarcoma Program
Moffitt Cancer Center
Tampa, Florida

Alexander J. Chou, MD
Department of Pediatrics
Memorial Sloan-Kettering Cancer Center
New York, New York

Warren A. Chow, MD, FACP
Associate Professor
Department of Medical Oncology
City of Hope Medical Center
Duarte, California

Ernest U. Conrad III, MD
Professor/Director
Department of Orthopedics and Sports
  Medicine
Seattle Children's Hospital
Seattle, Washington

Judd E. Cummings, MD
Clinical Assistant Professor
Department of Orthopaedic Surgery
University of Arizona
Tucson, Arizona

Yee-Cheen Doung, MD
Assistant Professor
Department of Orthopaedics and Rehabilitation
Oregon Health and Science University
Portland, Oregon

Janet F. Eary, MD
Professor
Department of Radiology
University of Washington
Seattle, Washington

Kirsten Ecklund, MD
Division Chief of Musculoskeletal Imaging
Department of Radiology
Boston Children's Hospital
Boston, Massachusetts

Robert J. Esther, MD
Assistant Professor of Orthopaedics
Department of Orthopaedics
University of North Carolina
Chapel Hill, North Carolina

Peter C. Ferguson, MD, FRCSC
Associate Professor
Department of Surgery
Mount Sinai Hospital
University of Toronto
Toronto, Ontario, Canada

Valerie A. Fitzhugh, MD
Assistant Professor
Department of Pathology and Laboratory
  Medicine
Rutgers, The State University of New Jersey
New Jersey Medical School
Newark, New Jersey

Spencer J. Frink, MD
Orthopedic Oncologist
Department of Orthopedics
Surgical Oncology Associates of South Texas
San Antonio, Texas

Michelle Ghert, MD, FRCSC
Associate Professor
Department of Surgery
McMaster University
Hamilton, Ontario, Canada

Howard J. Goodman, MD
Director of Musculoskeletal Oncology
Department of Orthopaedic Surgery
Maimonides Medical Center
Brooklyn, New York

Mark A. Goodman, MD
Visiting Associate Professor
Department of Orthopaedic Surgery
University of Pittsburgh Medical School
Pittsburgh, Pennsylvania

Jennifer L. Halpern, MD
Assistant Professor
Department of Orthopaedics and Rehabilitation
Vanderbilt University Medical Center
Nashville, Tennessee

Robert K. Heck Jr MD
Associate Professor
Department of Orthopaedic Surgery
University of Tennessee – Campbell Clinic
Memphis, Tennessee

Robert Mikael Henshaw, MD
Director
Department of Orthopaedic Oncology
MedStar Georgetown University
  Medical Center
Washington, DC

Kelly C. Homlar, MD
Assistant Professor
Department of Orthopaedics
Medical College of Georgia at
  Georgia Health Sciences University
Augusta, Georgia

Kevin B. Jones, MD
Assistant Professor
Department of Orthopaedics
University of Utah
Salt Lake City, Utah

Satoshi Kawaguchi, MD
Fellow
Department of Orthopaedic Oncology
University of Texas
MD Anderson Cancer Center
Houston, Texas

Jeffrey E. Krygier, MD
Orthopaedic Oncologist
Department of Orthopaedic Surgery
Santa Clara Valley Medical Center
San Jose, California

G. Douglas Letson, MD
Professor of Surgery, Radiology, Orthopedics
Sarcoma Program
Moffitt Cancer Center
Tampa, Florida

Adam S. Levin, MD
Assistant Professor, Orthopaedic Surgery
Department of Orthopaedic Surgery
North Shore/Long Island Jewish Medical Center
Great Neck, New York

Valerae O. Lewis, MD
Associate Professor
Department of Orthopaedic Oncology
University of Texas
MD Anderson Cancer Center
Houston, Texas

Antoinette W. Lindberg, MD
Acting Assistant Professor
Department of Orthopedics and Sports Medicine
Seattle Children's Hospital
Seattle, Washington

Farbod Malek, MD
Fellow
Department of Orthopedic Surgery
Memorial Sloan-Kettering Cancer Center
New York, New York

Joel L. Mayerson, MD
Associate Professor, Chief, Division of
*   Orthopaedic Oncology*
Department of Orthopaedic Surgery
The Ohio State University
Wexner Medical Center
Columbus, Ohio

Sean V. McGarry, MD
Assistant Professor
Department of Orthopaedics,
*   Orthopaedic Oncology*
University of Nebraska Medical Center
Omaha, Nebraska

Richard L. McGough III, MD
Chief, Division of Musculoskeletal Oncology
Departments of Orthopaedic and
*   General Surgery*
University of Pittsburgh
Pittsburgh, Pennsylvania

David McKeown, MD
Orthopaedic Research Fellow
Department of Surgery
Memorial Sloan-Kettering Cancer Center
New York, New York

Bryan S. Moon, MD
Assistant Professor
Department of Orthopaedic Oncology
University of Texas
MD Anderson Cancer Center
Houston, Texas

Christian M. Ogilvie, MD
Associate Professor
Department of Orthopaedic Surgery
University of Minnesota
Minneapolis, Minnesota

William M. Parrish, MD
Section Chief, Orthopedics
Department of Surgery
Lancaster Regional Medical Center
Lancaster, Pennsylvania

Francis R. Patterson, MD
Associate Professor
Department of Orthopedics
Rutgers-New Jersey Medical School
Newark, New Jersey

Theresa Pazionis, MD, MA
PGY 4 Orthopaedic Surgery
Department of Orthopaedic Surgery
McMaster University
Hamilton, Ontario, Canada

Stephanie E. W. Punt, BS
Research Assistant
Department of Orthopaedics and
*   Sports Medicine*
University of Washington
Seattle, Washington

Robert H. Quinn, MD
Chair, Professor, Residency Program Director
Department of Orthopaedic Surgery
University of Texas
Health Science Center San Antonio
San Antonio, Texas

Rajiv Rajani, MD
Assistant Professor
Department of Orthopaedic Surgery
University of Texas
Health Science Center San Antonio
San Antonio, Texas

Kevin A. Raskin, MD
Assistant Professor of Orthopaedic Surgery
Department of Orthopaedic Surgery
Massachusetts General Hospital
Boston, Massachusetts

Bruce Rougraff, MD
Orthopaedic Surgeon
OrthoIndy
Indianapolis, Indiana

Robert L. Satcher Jr, MD, PhD
Assistant Professor
Department of Orthopaedic Oncology
University of Texas
MD Anderson Cancer Center
Houston, Texas

Adam J. Schwartz, MD
Assistant Professor
Department of Orthopedic Surgery
Mayo Clinic
Phoenix, Arizona

Herbert S. Schwartz, MD
Professor and Chairman
Department of Orthopaedics and Rehabilitation
Vanderbilt University Medical Center
Nashville, Tennessee

Matthew J. Seidel, MD
Clinical Assistant Professor of
*   Orthopaedic Surgery*
University of Arizona
Orthopaedic Surgical Oncology of Arizona
Scottsdale, Arizona

Matthew R. Steensma, MD
Assistant Professor
Department of Surgery
Spectrum Health/Michigan State University
*   College of Human Medicine*
Van Andel Institute
Grand Rapids, Michigan

Patrick C. Toy, MD
Instructor
Department of Orthopaedic Surgery
University of Tennessee – Campbell Clinic
Memphis, Tennessee

Wakenda K. Tyler, MD, MPH
Assistant Professor
Department of Orthopaedics
University of Rochester Medical Center
Rochester, New York

Michael J. Vives, MD
Associate Professor, Department of
*   Orthopaedics*
Chief, Spine Division
Rutgers New Jersey Medical School
Newark, New Jersey

Nicholas P. Webber, MD
Director, Orthopaedic Oncology
Aurora Advanced Orthopaedics
Aurora Cancer Care
Milwaukee, Wisconsin

Kurt R. Weiss, MD
Assistant Professor
Department of Orthopaedic Surgery
Division of Musculoskeletal Oncology
University of Pittsburgh
Pittsburgh, Pennsylvania

Jennifer Wright, MD
Assistant Professor, Pediatrics
Adjunct Assistant Professor, Internal Medicine
University of Utah
Salt Lake City, Utah

Preface

This book would not be possible without the diligence, hard work, and perseverance of the members of the Musculoskeletal Tumor Society. With a long tradition of educational excellence, members of this society brought forth this book as yet another example of its unwavering commitment to education. Despite the society's small size, it has throughout its history gladly shouldered the responsibility of educating fellow orthopaedic surgeons and the medical community as a whole on the importance of recognizing and treating this collection of esoteric but sometimes devastating disorders.

We collectively owe the greatest debt to our patients, who not only entrust to us their care, but also who allow us to use the information garnered to better the care of those who follow. We thank the referring physicians, who selflessly refer the patients with these often unusual maladies to us, along with our colleagues in pathology, radiology, medical and pediatric oncology, and radiation oncology. As time goes on, the data mounts to show that it is not the expertise of a single physician that makes the difference, but rather the collaborative environment of a dedicated group of specialized health professionals in which most of these patients will have the best outcomes.

I thank the MSTS and the American Academy of Orthopaedic Surgeons for their faith in entrusting me the important task of editing this volume. Lisa Moore and Rachel Winokur from the AAOS deserve special mention. On a personal note, I thank my family— Victoria Sylvia, Ellena, Anne, and David—for their unfailing support, which truly makes anything and everything possible.

This current volume amasses extensively illustrated chapters with updated clinical, radiographic, histologic, and surgical information, as well as updates in the contemporary understanding of the molecular basis of these diseases. We hope this volume empowers physicians to care for patients, and to diagnose, treat, and refer as needed.

Thank you!

J. Sybil Biermann, MD
Editor

Table of Contents

General Evaluation and Treatment of Musculoskeletal Tumors

SECTION EDITOR:

R. Lor Randall, MD

Chapter 1

Clinical Presentation and Staging of Bone Tumors

Judd E. Cummings, MD   Matthew J. Seidel, MD

Introduction

The clinical presentation of bone tumors varies greatly. Patients may have an asymptomatic lesion detected incidentally. Bone abnormalities may alternatively be associated with fracture, soft-tissue mass, or swelling. Conditions such as fibrous dysplasia may cause limb deformity. Nonetheless, because both benign and malignant conditions have such a broad array of clinical findings and features, thoughtful and deliberate analysis is required. Misdiagnosis and inappropriate treatment of bone lesions can have serious implications. Patients may be subjected to unnecessary, expensive, and morbid testing or treatments when simple observation and follow-up are warranted. Conversely, aggressive or malignant lesions can cause limb- or life-threatening conditions if misdiagnosed and the appropriate treatment is not rendered. A careful and systematic approach using a detailed history and physical examination with appropriate plain radiographs are the mainstay of the initial evaluation, which should lead to an accurate and brief differential diagnosis. The initial evaluation can then be used to guide an efficient workup, eventually resulting in a definitive radiographic diagnosis or a definitive and safe plan for biopsy. Referral to a musculoskeletal oncologist should be considered if a biopsy is needed to establish a diagnosis or for ongoing treatment of patients with benign and malignant conditions.

Clinical Presentation

Benign Lesions

Benign conditions are much more common than primary bone malignancies. Orthopaedic surgeons from all subspecialties encounter patients with common benign lesions such as enchondroma, osteochondroma, degenerative cysts, simple bone cysts, and nonossifying fibromas. Patient evaluation should begin with a de-

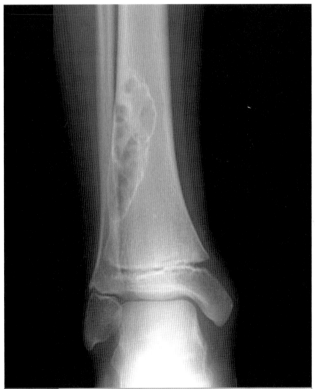

Figure 1   A 12-year-old boy had a 6-month history of ankle pain while running. The pain was relieved with over-the-counter NSAIDs. An AP radiograph of the right distal tibia shows a geographic lesion with sharp transition and sclerotic borders, eccentrically located. Clinical and radiographic features were consistent with nonossifying fibroma.

Dr. Seidel or an immediate family member is a member of a speakers' bureau or has made paid presentations on behalf of Biomet, and serves as a paid consultant to or is an employee of Wright Medical Technology. Neither Dr. Cummings nor any immediate family member has received anything of value from or has stock or stock options held in a commercial company or institution related directly or indirectly to the subject of this chapter.

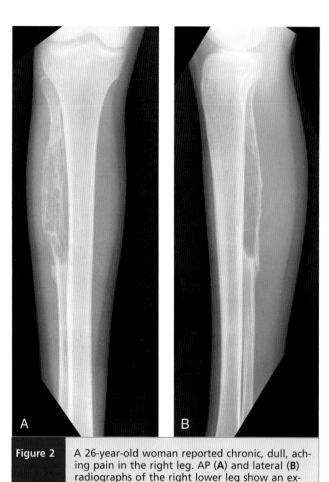

Figure 2 A 26-year-old woman reported chronic, dull, aching pain in the right leg. AP (**A**) and lateral (**B**) radiographs of the right lower leg show an expansile bone lesion with associated pathologic fracture of the right fibula. Biopsy revealed desmoplastic fibroma.

Table 1

Common Diagnoses by Location

Site	Benign	Malignant
Pelvis	ABC	Chondrosarcoma
	SBC	MBD
Spine (anterior)	Infection	MBD
	Hemangioma	Lymphoma
	Histiocytosis	Ewing sarcoma
Spine (posterior)	ABC	MBD
	Osteoid osteoma	
	Osteoblastoma	
Long bones		
Diaphyseal	Fibrous dysplasia	Ewing sarcoma
	Histiocytosis	Adamantinoma
	Osteoid osteoma	Lymphoma
		MBD
Metaphyseal	Nonossifying fibroma	Osteosarcoma
	ABC	Chondrosarcoma
	SBC	MBD
	Enchondroma	
	Osteochondroma	
Epiphyseal	Chondroblastoma	Clear cell chondrosarcoma
	Giant cell tumor	MBD
	ABC	
	Infection	

ABC = aneurysmal bone cyst, MBD = metastic bone disease, SBC = simple bone cyst.

tailed history and physical examination. Mild pain relieved with over-the-counter medication is generally consistent with a benign condition. Pain associated with benign lesions is generally slow in onset and may be related to activity or trauma. Some benign conditions such as osteoid osteoma have characteristic symptomatology such as night pain that is very responsive to NSAIDs or aspirin. Additionally, many benign lesions such as nonossifying fibroma, osteoid osteoma, and unicameral bone cysts have classic radiographic appearances and require no further workup (**Figure 1**). Generally, most benign lesions do not cause systemic complaints or laboratory abnormalities, with the exception of Langerhans cell histiocytosis, which may be associated with elevated inflammatory markers, low-grade fever, rash, or headache. Active or aggressive benign lesions may be painful depending on size and location. Pathologic fractures may be seen in association with a benign condition following a single traumatic event or after repetitive trauma (**Figure 2**). Knowledge of any antecedent pain or symptoms is particularly useful in this scenario to help guide further workup if a malignant diagnosis is suspected.

If a patient has no pain or symptoms, and a lesion is detected incidentally on imaging studies, a benign condition is likely. Variables such as patient age, location of the lesion within the bone, and plain radiograph characteristics can help confirm the diagnosis as benign or requiring prompt additional workup (**Tables 1** and **2**). Radiographic evaluation should commence with plain radiographs of the entire bone containing the lesion. Benign tumors typically are defined by a geographic radiological margin with a narrow zone of transition and sclerotic border. Endosteal thinning can be seen with benign tumors (**Figure 3**). Cortical violation is rarely seen. CT scans provide three-dimensional characterization of the lesion and surrounding bone. Information regarding matrix formation, endosteal erosion, cortical thinning or violation, and zone of transition are important determinants of a lesion's biologic potential. CT scans can also provide information to help the surgeon evaluate the bone for potential weakness or propensity for fracture. MRI helps in the assessment of soft-tissue extension, pattern of contrast enhancement, associated bone marrow edema, and signal characteristics of the lesion. Reactive bone marrow edema is usually absent or minimal with varied degrees and patterns of contrast enhancement (**Figure 4**). Soft-tissue extension or periosteal reaction is uncommon. Bone scintigraphy or technetium bone scanning is useful as a screening tool to assess for multiple sites of bone involvement such as may occur in polyostotic fibrous dysplasia, multiple enchondromatosis, or histiocytosis. The presence of abnormal radiotracer uptake does not accurately characterize a lesion as benign or malignant. A negative or cold bone scan may indicate a latent or quiescent lesion. Notable exceptions include multiple myeloma or some types of metastatic carcinoma such as renal cell carcinoma. Conversely, many benign conditions such as giant cell tumor or enchondroma may indeed show abnormal radiotracer activity. Thus, the routine use of technetium bone scans is not recommended to evaluate a suspected benign bone lesion. It rarely provides diagnostic information and subjects patients to unnecessary and expensive testing that may ultimately delay an accurate diagnosis. The importance of a complete and detailed history and physical examination coupled with appropriate plain radiographs cannot be overstated. Patients who have pain, deformity, swelling, mass, or pathologic fracture may

Table 2		
Common Diagnoses by Age		
Age	**Benign**	**Malignant**
0–5 years	Histiocytosis	Metastatic neuroblastoma
	Infection	
5–20 years	Nonossifying fibroma	Osteosarcoma
	Aneurysmal bone cyst	Ewing sarcoma
	Simple bone cyst	
	Osteoid osteoma	
	Osteochondroma	
20–40 years	Giant cell tumor	Lymphoma
	Fibrous dysplasia	Ewing sarcoma
	Enchondroma	
> 40 years	Enchondroma	Metastatic carcinoma
	Bone infarct	Lymphoma
	Infection	Multiple myeloma
		Chondrosarcoma

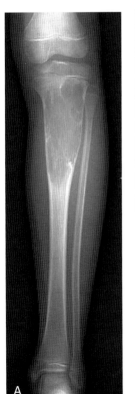
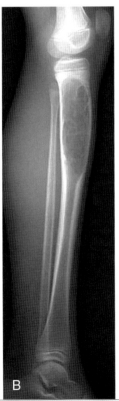
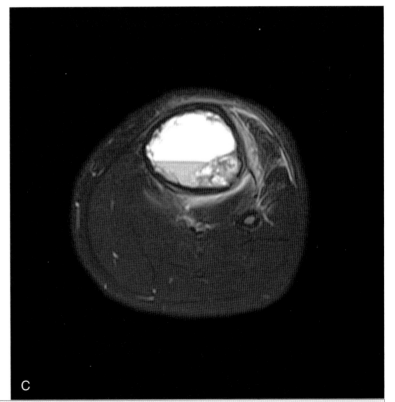

Figure 3   An 8-year-old girl had mild leg pain. AP (**A**) and lateral (**B**) radiographs of the left lower leg show a concentrically located geographic bone lesion with cortical expansion in the tibial metaphysis. **C,** Axial T2 fat-suppressed, non-contrasted MRI (**C**) of the proximal tibia shows a fluid-fluid level and no soft-tissue mass. Biopsy revealed aneurysmal bone cyst.

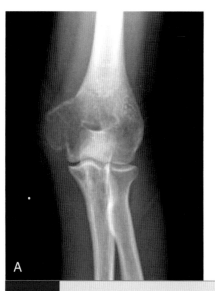
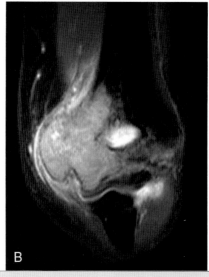
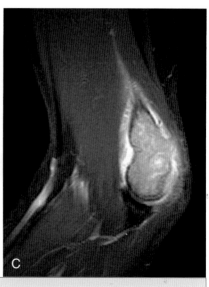

Figure 4 A 33-year-old woman had chronic, mild elbow pain. **A,** AP radiograph of the left elbow shows a lucent lesion within the medial condyle and trochlea causing cortical expansion without obvious cortical disruption. Coronal (**B**) and sagittal (**C**) T1 fat-suppressed contrast MRI show the tumor extent with minimal adjacent marrow edema. Biopsy revealed giant cell tumor.

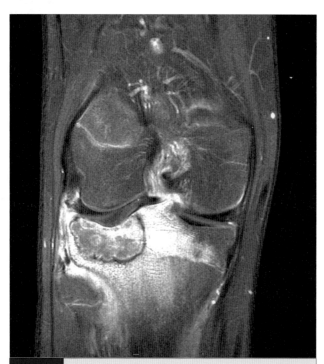

Figure 5 A 17-year-old boy had chronic left knee pain and swelling. Coronal T2 fat-suppressed MRI of the left knee shows a well-demarcated, epiphyseal lesion involving the lateral condyle with mild joint surface irregularity. Biopsy revealed chondroblastoma.

also have a benign diagnosis. Lesions in juxta-articular locations must be carefully assessed to rule out other common causes of pain, such as degenerative joint disease or overuse conditions (**Figure 5**). Lesions that demonstrate radiographic features of concern, such as cortical disruption, permeative growth, or periosteal reaction, require additional imaging. If the diagnosis remains uncertain after advanced imaging such as CT or MRI, then biopsy should be considered.

Following establishment of a benign diagnosis, appropriate treatment can be initiated. This may include observation and repeat imaging after an appropriate interval, usually 3 to 6 months, to ensure radiographic stability. Alternatively, surgical intervention may be warranted to limit bone destruction, stabilize a pathologic fracture or impending pathologic injury, and/or prevent deformity.

Malignant Lesions

Unlike their benign counterparts, malignant lesions are rarely asymptomatic and are commonly characterized by pain of varying amount, duration, and character that is generally more severe and less often relieved with over-the-counter medications. Symptoms may include dull or deep ache both with activity and rest, depending on the amount of structural compromise of the host bone and the amount of surrounding muscular edema (**Figure 6**). Pain can be acute or sudden when lesions are associated with pathologic fracture. These patients often experience antecedent pain of varying duration before fracture. Neurologic symptoms including paresthesias or bowel and bladder dysfunction can accompany spinal or sacral tumors. An associated soft-tissue mass and/or swelling is often seen, especially for extremity lesions. Systemic symptoms such as fatigue, malaise, and fever may be present. Laboratory abnormalities such as hypercalcemia, elevated alkaline phosphatase, or anemia may also be encountered.

A complete history and physical examination with appropriate plain radiographs are fundamental. Per-

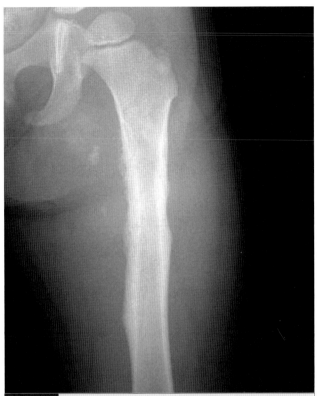

Figure 6 A 4-year-old boy had a painful limp; a large, deep painful thigh mass; limited hip motion; and inguinal adenopathy. AP radiograph of the left proximal femur shows an ill-defined, meta-diaphyseal lesion with cortical irregularity, periosteal reaction, and permeative growth pattern. Biopsy revealed Ewing sarcoma.

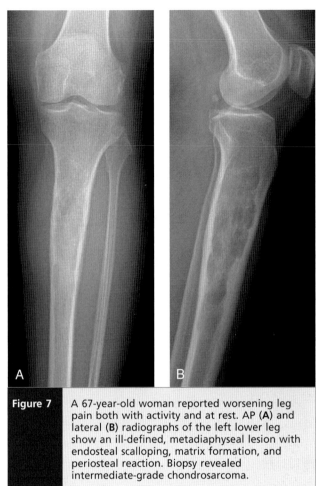

Figure 7 A 67-year-old woman reported worsening leg pain both with activity and at rest. AP (**A**) and lateral (**B**) radiographs of the left lower leg show an ill-defined, metadiaphyseal lesion with endosteal scalloping, matrix formation, and periosteal reaction. Biopsy revealed intermediate-grade chondrosarcoma.

sonal or family history of cancer or bone malignancy should be considered. Conditions such as retinoblastoma, Li-Fraumeni syndrome, and Rothmund-Thompson syndrome are known to predispose patients to primary bone malignancies such as osteosarcoma. Malignant transformation of benign conditions such as multiple enchondromatosis has been described. Finally, bone malignancies are known to occur in the setting of Paget disease, prior irradiation, chronic osteomyelitis, or bone infarct.

Patient age and the location of the bone lesion (epiphyseal, metaphyseal, diaphyseal) are factors that help establish a differential diagnosis. Lesions demonstrating aggressive features clinically and/or radiographically require further workup (**Figure 7**). Advanced three-dimensional imaging (either CT or MRI) is used to better define and characterize the lesion (**Figure 8**). If malignancy is suspected, a biopsy of the lesion should be obtained to establish a tissue diagnosis. Strong consideration for orthopaedic oncology referral should be given before biopsy to ensure that appropriate techniques are used and to minimize subsequent surgical challenges or complications resulting in suboptimal outcome.[1,2] If a primary bone malignancy is diagnosed, the patient will require appropriate staging studies.

Historically, whole-body bone scans and chest CT have been recommended. Recently, positron emission tomography (PET) and CT both have gained popularity in the assessment of both skeletal and nonskeletal sites of metastatic disease. Patients older than 40 years who have a malignant bone lesion most commonly have metastatic carcinoma, multiple myeloma, or lymphoma. Appropriate clinical examination findings, including a breast or prostate examination, should be documented. Additional laboratory studies such as serum or urine protein electrophoresis should be obtained.

The treatment of malignant bone lesions typically involves multidisciplinary input and cooperation. Referral to an established orthopaedic oncology center is recommended. Adjuvant or neoadjuvant therapies including chemotherapy or radiation therapy may be coordinated with surgical intervention as deemed appropriate. Ongoing surveillance is indicated to assess for local recurrence and/or the presence of distant disease.

Staging of Bone Tumors

Bone tumor staging provides a framework for patient evaluation, may help direct treatment, and stratifies risk or prognosis. An ideal staging system should be

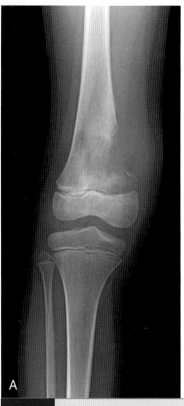
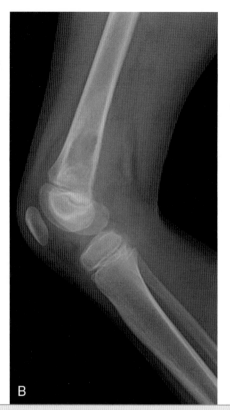
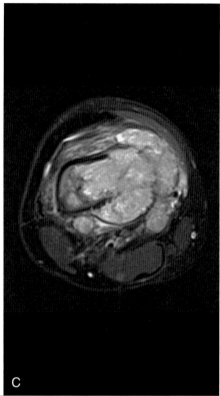

| Figure 8 | A 9-year-old boy had atraumatic right knee pain, stiffness, and intermittent swelling. AP (**A**) and lateral (**B**) radiographs of the right knee show a lytic metaphyseal lesion with cortical disruption and knee effusion. **C**, Axial T2 fat-suppressed MRI with contrast shows obvious cortical violation and soft-tissue extension of the tumor. Biopsy revealed osteosarcoma. |

Table 3

Enneking Staging System for Benign Bone Lesions

Stage	Definition	Behavior
1	Latent	Remains static or heals spontaneously
2	Active	Progressive growth, limited by natural barriers
3	Aggressive	Progressive growth, not limited by natural barriers

practical and reproducible, and is important for disease control in individual patients and for the population at large. As defined by the International Union Against Cancer,[3] the objectives of cancer staging are as follows:

1. To aid in planning the course of treatment
2. To provide insight into the prognosis
3. To assist in evaluating the results of treatment
4. To facilitate effective interinstitutional communication
5. To contribute to continuing investigation of human malignancies

Staging systems for both benign and malignant conditions are described in the following sections.

Benign Tumors

Enneking proposed a simple and commonly used system for benign conditions using Arabic numerals.[4] Stage 1 lesions are defined as inactive or latent, stage 2 lesions as active, and stage 3 lesions as aggressive (Table 3). Biopsy is not required and is often not useful in assigning a stage to a benign lesion. Rather, clinical and radiographic features are used to critically assess tumor behavior and characteristics. Serial imaging is often needed to accurately stage a benign lesion. A tumor initially thought to be inactive or latent may later merit classification as active or aggressive based on changing growth patterns and clinical behavior. Conversely, lesions initially assigned to higher stages may ultimately become inactive as growth slows during skeletal maturity.

Stage 1

These lesions are usually detected incidentally and cause minimal, if any, symptoms. Radiographs demonstrate well-defined borders often with sclerotic edges. Cortical disruption, permeative growth, and periosteal reaction are not seen. Stage 1 lesions remain within the host bone without causing expansion or deformity.

They demonstrate little or no growth over time and rarely require surgical treatment. Pathologic fracture can occur but is infrequent. Common examples of stage 1 (inactive or latent) lesions include nonossifying fibromas, enchondromas, and ostoechondromas.

Stage 2

Active bone lesions cover a broad spectrum of conditions and presentations. Clinically, patients may have variable amounts of pain and deformity. Pathologic fracture can occur and may be the initial presenting complaint. Plain radiographs may demonstrate varying amounts of bone destruction or cortical thinning. Despite their biologic activity, active lesions remain confined and limited by anatomic barriers (joint surface, bone cortex). These lesions commonly require surgical intervention to limit bone destruction, give prophylactic support to the host bone, and provide pain relief. Osteoid osteoma, chondromyxoid fibroma, and unicameral bone cysts are common examples of active bone lesions.

Stage 3

Aggressive lesions, although benign, can cause significant local bone destruction and morbidity. Patients almost always experience pain and demonstrate tenderness or swelling on examination. These lesions may exhibit significant growth, causing expansion or deformity of the host bone. Cortical violation and soft-tissue extension can occur, causing structural compromise. Pathologic fracture is a common occurrence with stage 3 lesions. Consequently, surgical intervention is indicated to reduce patient morbidity and preserve limb function. Recurrence following local curettage can be as high as 20% to 30%. Occasionally, en bloc resection with allograft or endoprosthetic reconstruction is required. Despite a benign histology, the pulmonary spread of giant cell tumor and chondroblastoma has been described. Other examples of aggressive benign lesions include aneurysmal bone cyst and osteoblastoma.

Malignant Tumors

Enneking described a staging system for malignant lesions in 1980.[5] This system was subsequently adopted by the Musculoskeletal Tumor Society. Variables used to assign stage include tumor grade based on histology, extent of tumor, and presence or absence of metastatic disease based on appropriate imaging studies. Low-grade lesions are designated G1, and high-grade tumors, G2. Lesions that remain within an anatomic compartment (intraosseous for bone tumors) are designated T1, and lesions extending through or beyond the host cortex are labeled T2. The final criterion is the presence or absence of metastasis. Nonmetastatic lesions are M0, whereas tumors with regional or distant metastasis are M1 (Table 4). This system continues to be an easy and reproducible system for the assessment of malignant bone tumors.

The American Joint Committee on Cancer (AJCC) proposed a slightly different and more thorough system

Table 4

Enneking Surgical Staging System for Musculoskeletal Sarcoma

Stage	Grade	Site
IA	Low (G1)	Intracompartmental (T1)
IB	Low (G1)	Extracompartmental (T2)
IIA	High (G2)	Intracompartmental (T1)
IIB	High (G2)	Extracompartmental (T2)
III	Any (G) plus	Any (T); regional or distant metastasis (M1)

in 1983.[6] Four variables are used to assign stages using the AJCC system: tumor size, histologic grade, the presence or absence of regional (nodal) metastasis, and the presence or absence of distant metastasis. Tumors are assigned a stage (IA, IB, IIA, IIB, III, IVA, IVB) based on the combined assessment of these variables (Table 5). The AJCC system for bone tumors, which does not account for primary malignant lymphoma of bone and multiple myeloma, has undergone small changes and refinements over the past 29 years. Currently, tumors smaller than 8 cm in greatest dimension are designated T1, and larger tumors are designated T2 (previously, until 2003, the extent of the tumor was defined as contained or not contained within the host bone). Low-grade tumors are designated G1 or G2 based on the extent of differentiation, and high-grade tumors are assigned G3 or G4 based on the extent of differentiation. In cases in which a tumor grade cannot be assessed, a GX designation is given. The presence and absence of regional (nodal) metastasis are designated N1 and N0, respectively. Beginning in 2003 with the sixth edition of the AFCC system, distant metastasis now receives a subclassification based on the site of involvement.[7] Pulmonary distant metastasis is designated M1a, whereas nonpulmonary distant metastasis is designated M1b. The seventh and most recent edition of the AJCC system was released in January, 2010.[8] The only update from the sixth edition involves stage III lesions. This stage is now reserved for noncontiguous G3 and G4 tumors (high-grade, poorly differentiated tumors, and high-grade, undifferentiated tumors, respectively).

Determining tumor size, histologic grade, and the presence of metastatic disease requires a combination of clinical assessment, imaging studies, and tissue sampling. Lymphatic involvement by primary bone sarcoma is rare but can occur. Thus, a careful clinical assessment of the lymphatic system is warranted in any patient with a suspected primary bone sarcoma. Imaging of the tumor should begin with plain radiographs of the entire host bone, allowing the clinician to characterize the lesion as likely benign or malignant and to determine the risk of pathologic fracture. MRI is recommended to accurately define the extent of the tumor and assess for noncontiguous tumor (skip metastasis)

Table 5

American Joint Committee on Cancer (AJCC) Staging System for Bone Sarcoma

Stage	Primary Tumor (T)[a]	Regional Lymph Nodes (N)[b]	Distant Metastasis (M)[c]	Histologic Grade (G)[d]
Stage IA	T1	N0	M0	G1, G2 (low grades); GX
Stage IB	T2, T3	N0	M0	G1, G2 (low grades); GX
Stage IIA	T1	N0	M0	G3, G4 (high grades)
Stage IIB	T2	N0	M0	G3, G4 (high grades)
Stage III	T3	N0	M0	G3, G4 (high grades)
Stage IVA	Any T	N0	M1a	Any G
Stage IVB	Any T	N1	Any M	Any G
	Any T	Any N	M1b	Any G

[a] TX, primary tumor cannot be assessed; T0, no evidence of primary tumor; T1, tumor 8 cm or less in greatest dimension; T2, tumor more than 8 cm in greatest dimension; T3, discontinuous tumors in the primary bone.
[b] NX, regional lymph nodes cannot be assessed; N0, no regional lymph node metastasis; N1, regional lymph node metastasis.
[c] M0, no distant metastasis; M1, distant metastasis; M1a, lung; M1b, other distant sites.
[d] GX, grade cannot be assessed; G1, well differentiated, low grade; G2, moderately differentiated, low grade; G3, poorly differentiated; G4, undifferentiated.

within the host bone. Consequently, at least one series of sagittal and coronal MRI studies of the entire host bone is needed. Bone scintigraphy is used to screen for osseous metastasis (M1b). Finally, CT of the chest is performed to screen for pulmonary disease (M1a).

PET, used alone or in conjunction with CT, has generated interest as a tool to screen for both osseous and nonosseous sites of metastasis, including the lymphatic system. PET is thought to be particularly useful for cases in which the detection of bone destruction is primarily osteoclast-mediated, because conventional bone scintigraphy relies on the detection of osteoblastic activity (as opposed to osteoclastic activity). In a prospective multicenter study[9] of 46 pediatric patients with proven sarcomas (23 with Ewing sarcoma), the authors compared the effectiveness of conventional imaging modalities (MRI, CT, bone scintigraphy) with that of fluorodeoxyglucose (FDG) PET in tumor staging and therapeutic planning. Both FDG PET and conventional imaging helped detect 100% of primary tumors. However, FDG PET was superior in the detection of bone metastases (90% versus 57% sensitivity) and lymphatic metastases (90% versus 25% sensitivity). In patients with Ewing sarcoma, the superiority of FDG PET to bone scintigraphy in detecting osseous metastases was significant (88% versus 37% sensitivity). Similarly, the authors of a 2006 study[10] found in a series of primary bone sarcomas that FDG PET was able to detect bone metastasis not seen with conventional bone scintigraphy in 18% of patients. These patients had subsequent changes in staging and the resultant treatment recommendations.

However, FDG PET has clear limitations. It has been shown to be less sensitive than conventional CT for the detection of pulmonary metastasis. In a 2007 study,[11] the authors found that hybrid PET/CT is a more accurate tool for the detection and localization of pulmonary disease than standard FDG PET alone. Thus, consideration may be given to using whole-body hybrid PET/CT in lieu of bone scintigraphy. Evidence- and consensus-based guidelines published by the National Comprehensive Cancer Network, an alliance of 23 major academic cancer centers, indicate either bone scan or PET scan may be used in the staging of malignant bone tumors, in addition to MRI/CT of the primary site, chest CT, laboratory studies, and biopsy.[12]

Summary

The proper initial evaluation of bone tumors is critical to ensure accurate diagnosis, staging, and treatment. A thorough history and physical examination with appropriate plain radiographs are paramount. This approach should allow the surgeon to generate an accurate differential diagnosis from which further workup can be directed. Asymptomatic or incidentally noted lesions are commonly benign. Larger or more active lesions may be mildly symptomatic and require further advanced three-dimensional imaging. If the diagnosis is uncertain, referral to a musculoskeletal oncologist and biopsy should be considered. Confirmed benign lesions are staged according to the Enneking system (1, latent; 2, active; 3, aggressive). Observation with radiographic follow-up or surgical intervention may be required.

Bone lesions that cause significant pain or demonstrate radiographic features of concern should be evaluated by a musculoskeletal oncologist using advanced imaging. A carefully planned biopsy is often required to establish a definitive diagnosis. Appropriate imaging studies including MRI of the entire host bone, chest CT, bone scan, or PET scan are needed for accurate staging. Commonly used staging systems include the AJCC and Enneking systems. Appropriate management requires multifaceted input from surgical and medical disciplines including oncology, radiology, and pathology.

Annotated References

1. Simon MA: Biopsy of musculoskeletal tumors. *J Bone Joint Surg Am* 1982;64(8):1253-1257.

2. Mankin HJ, Mankin CJ, Simon MA; Members of the Musculoskeletal Tumor Society: The hazards of the biopsy, revisited. *J Bone Joint Surg Am* 1996;78(5): 656-663.

3. Gospodarowicz M, Benedet L, Hutter RV, Fleming I, Henson DE, Sobin LH: History and international developments in cancer staging. *Cancer Prev Control* 1998;2(6):262-268.

4. Enneking WF: Staging tumors, in Enneking WF (ed): *Musculoskeletal Tumor Surgery*. New York, NY: Churchill Livingstone, 1983, pp. 87-88.

5. Enneking WF, Spanier SS, Goodman MA: A system for the surgical staging of musculoskeletal sarcoma. *Clin Orthop Relat Res* 1980;153:106-120.

6. American Joint Committee on Cancer: Bone, in Fleming ID, Cooper JS, Henson DE, et al (eds): *AJCC Cancer Staging Manual*. Philadelphia, PA, Lippincott-Raven, 1997, pp 143-147.

7. American Joint Committee on Cancer: Bone, in Fleming ID, Cooper JS, Henson DE, et al (eds): *AJCC Cancer Staging Manual*. New York, NY, Springer-Verlag, 2002, pp 213-219.

8. American Joint Committee on Cancer: Musculoskeletal, in Edge SB, Byrd DR, Compton CC, et al (eds): *AJCC Cancer Staging Manual*. New York, NY, Springer-Verlag, 2010, pp 279-290.

   This is the seventh edition of the AJCC cancer staging manual. Applicable changes and highlights pertaining to orthopaedic oncology are discussed in the chapter.

9. Völker T, Denecke T, Steffen I, et al: Positron emission tomography for staging of pediatric sarcoma patients: Results of a prospective multicenter trial. *J Clin Oncol* 2007;25(34):5435-5441.

   The authors conducted a prospective multicenter trial of 46 patients with sarcoma comparing the effectiveness of conventional imaging to FDG PET for staging purposes. PET was superior to conventional imaging for the detection of lymph node involvement and bone manifestations, whereas CT was more reliable than FDG PET in the depiction of lung metastases.

10. Kneisl JS, Patt JC, Johnson JC, Zuger JH: Is PET useful in detecting occult nonpulmonary metastases in pediatric bone sarcomas? *Clin Orthop Relat Res* 2006; 450:101-104.

11. Gerth HU, Juergens KU, Dirksen U, Gerss J, Schober O, Franzius C: Significant benefit of multimodal imaging: PET/CT compared with PET alone in staging and follow-up of patients with Ewing tumors. *J Nucl Med* 2007;48(12):1932-1939.

    A total of 163 ^{18}F-FDG PET/CT studies performed in 53 patients with confirmed Ewing tumor were evaluated retrospectively. PET and CT data were assessed independently. PET/CT was significantly more accurate than PET alone for the detection and localization of lesions and improves staging for patients with Ewing tumor.

12. Biermann JS, Adkins DR, Aguinik M, et al : Bone Cancer. *J Natl Compr Canc Netw* 2013;11:688-723.

    This article summarizes recommended diagnostic and treatment algorithms for malignant bone tumors, combining evidence-based and consensus-based guidelines.

1: General Evaluation and Treatment of Musculoskeletal Tumors

Chapter 2

Imaging of Musculoskeletal Tumors: Updates and Current Practice

Kirsten Ecklund, MD

Introduction

Diagnosis and treatment of musculoskeletal tumors depends upon high-quality imaging for evaluation and surveillance. The modalities involved—radiography, ultrasonography, CT, MRI, and nuclear scintigraphy—have remained constant for many years. The goals of imaging assessment, however, have evolved from anatomic, morphologic assessment to tissue characterization. In recent years, advances especially in MRI, CT, and nuclear medicine have improved the ability to define lesions at diagnosis, assess response to therapy, and conduct surveillance with increased accuracy and far lower irradiation exposure. High-field-strength MRI, diffusion-weighted and perfusion-based MRI, whole-body MRI, and combined positron emission tomography (PET) and CT (PET-CT) have dramatically enhanced the capability to detect ever-smaller lesions and predict tumor necrosis.

Imaging Assessment at Diagnosis

Despite advances of the past decade, conventional radiography remains the mainstay of initial imaging of primary bone and soft-tissue tumors. Regardless of the location of the lesion or the age of the patient, imaging evaluation should begin with radiographs. For primary bone tumors, the classic teaching that patient age and radiographic appearance of the lesion most closely predict the pathologic diagnosis remains true. Lesion location, matrix, periosteal reaction, associated soft-tissue mass and calcification, and pathologic fracture all are adequately assessed with routine radiographs properly centered and coned to the area of abnormality.[1] Most important, radiographs direct subsequent imaging.

They also may eliminate nonneoplastic causes of musculoskeletal complaints, such as occult fracture.

Soft-tissue masses without bone involvement are often next evaluated ultrasonographically. With the advent of higher-frequency linear transducers, ultrasonography has become increasingly important for assessment of musculoskeletal pathology. Ultrasonography quickly differentiates between solid and cystic lesions and assesses perfusion without ionizing irradiation, an especially desirable feature for pediatric patients. Features such as fluid-fluid levels and intravascular calcifications can indicate a venous malformation, which often needs no further imaging (**Figure 1**). Ultrasonography is also the modality most frequently used for image-guided percutaneous biopsy of soft-tissue masses.[2]

Following radiographic evaluation, most primary osseous and soft-tissue neoplasms require further evaluation with MRI, which provides unparalleled soft-tissue, cartilaginous, and bone marrow detail. Standard MRI techniques are especially important at presentation, and unless there are medical contraindications, all MRI scans to evaluate musculoskeletal tumors should be completed with intravenous contrast. Fast spin-echo sequences with T1, intermediate proton density, and T2 weighting provide high-resolution anatomic detail and exquisite lesion conspicuity (**Figure 2**). Postcontrast images differentiate between solid and cystic regions within a lesion. High-field-strength MRI scanners, specifically 3 T and even 7 T, have become increasingly available. The enhanced signal-to-noise ratio at higher field strengths can be used to increase spatial and temporal resolution. High-resolution images can be obtained at large fields of view (**Figure 3**). Magnetic resonance angiography acquisition speeds now allow accurate tumoral vascular assessment that rivals conventional angiography.

In recent years, advanced MRI techniques have been developed that allow for tissue characterization not possible with standard sequences. In contrast to standard MRI sequences, diffusion-weighted imaging (DWI) depends on the microscopic, brownian motion

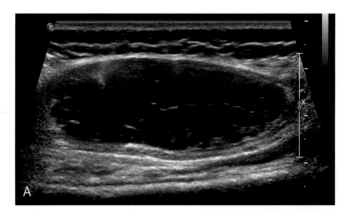

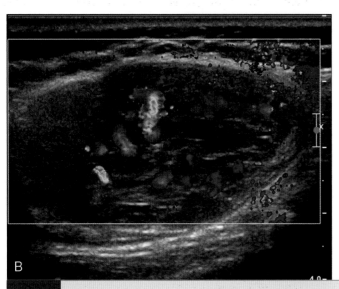

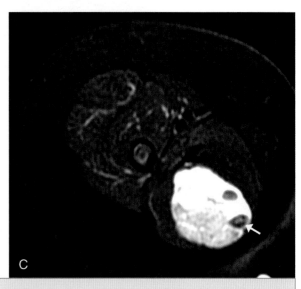

Figure 1 Imaging studies of a 9-year-old boy with a right posterior thigh mass. Grayscale (**A**) and color Doppler (**B**) ultrasonography of this intramuscular lesion reveals multilocular cystic components with diffuse, low-velocity vascular flow. Axial T2-weighted fat-suppressed-MRI (**C**) demonstrates a fluid-fluid level and phleboliths (arrow), confirming a venous malformation rather than a cystic, hypervascular neoplasm.

of water molecules within tissues.[3] Developed for brain imaging, DWI has only recently become useful in the skeleton as technologic improvements have overcome the artifacts previously associated with the imaging of bones and their adjacent tissues. The advantage of DWI is its capacity to suggest tissue structure, especially cellularity. Diffusion of water molecules becomes restricted when there is a decrease in extracellular space, as occurs with edema, or an increase in the number or size of cells, as occurs in tumors and fibrosis. Free diffusion of water molecules increases when there is an increase in cell membrane permeability, as with ischemia, or when there is a decrease in cell number, such as in cysts and areas of tumor necrosis. DWI can be assessed both qualitatively and quantitatively. Visually, areas of restricted diffusion appear bright on DWI. Unfortunately, areas of high T2 signal intensity, like fluid, may still appear bright even if water diffusion is increased. The phenomenon is referred to as "T2 shine-through" and is common with cysts and necrotic foci. To overcome this problem, apparent diffusion coefficient

(ADC) maps, generated from several DWI datasets, should be reviewed in conjunction with DWI. ADC maps are less susceptible to T2 effects, and thus are more valuable for musculoskeletal lesions (**Figure 4**). Lesions with restricted diffusion lose signal on ADC maps, whereas areas of increased diffusion are higher in signal intensity. Because of modifications used to overcome the limited marrow water content and susceptibility artifacts that occur at bone-tissue interfaces, DWI and ADC images have inherently lower resolution than standard MRI scans. ADC values are easily obtained within a lesion and have been used to predict histologic diagnosis. Low ADC values, indicating restricted diffusion, tend to correlate with high cellularity, often seen in malignant neoplasms. High ADC values, indicating increased diffusion, suggest benign or necrotic neoplasms.[4] High ADC values are also typically seen in benign tumorlike masses such as hematomas, infection, and vascular malformations (**Figure 5**). Unfortunately, factors other than cellularity, such as perfusion and myxoid content, can influence the ADC

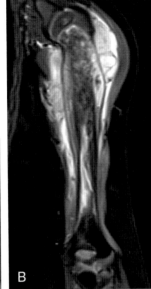

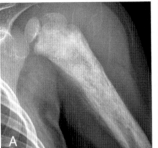

Figure 2 Imaging studies of a 2-year-old girl with left upper arm swelling and pain. **A,** The frontal radiograph shows a permeative, aggressive lesion within the metaphysis and diaphysis. **B,** Coronal inversion recovery MRI obtained at 3 T defines the intramedullary tumor, better demonstrates the periosteal elevation, and reveals the associated large soft-tissue mass in this child with Ewing sarcoma. Imaging at 3 T with a dedicated surface coil allows high resolution at faster image acquisition times than imaging at 1.5 T.

value.[5] Many authors, however, think that there is too much overlap between benign and malignant lesions for quantitative ADC values to be of use.[6] In current practice, most radiologists view the DWI and ADC images as complementary to the standard morphologic imaging sequences when arriving at a differential diagnosis for a particular lesion.

Another advanced MRI technique that is being used with increasing frequency in the evaluation of musculoskeletal tumors is dynamic contrast-enhanced (DCE) imaging. This perfusion sequence monitors tumor enhancement over several minutes following the intravenous administration of a gadolinium-based contrast agent. Previously somewhat limited, this method now has high temporal resolution as a result of the development of faster gradient echo sequences and parallel imaging techniques.[7] Like DWI, DCE offers both qualitative and quantitative assessment. At the time of diagnosis, DCE images depict tumor vascularity and often delineate tumor margins, essential for staging and surgical planning, better than any other MRI sequence. These images are also extremely helpful for biopsy guidance because the most highly vascular tumor regions are more likely to yield definitive results. Quantitative DCE assessment requires generation of time versus signal intensity curves for regions within the tumor. Rapid slope rates (percentage of signal intensity in-

crease per minute) are thought to correlate with increased likelihood of malignancy.[8]

Newly diagnosed bone and soft-tissue masses rarely require CT for evaluation of the primary lesion. In an effort to limit irradiation exposure, CT should be avoided in favor of MRI. Specific exceptions to this guideline are osteoid osteoma and myositis ossificans. In these lesions, the MRI appearance tends to be misleadingly aggressive because of the associated inflammatory response. The CT features, however, are so characteristic that the benefits of the examination outweigh the risk of irradiation exposure (**Figure 6**). Because of the high risk of pulmonary metastases, patients with a diagnosis of osteosarcoma or Ewing sarcoma continue to undergo chest CT at the time of diagnosis. In all instances where CT is necessary, use of the lowest possible irradiation dose technique with indication-based imaging protocols should be emphasized. Many medical centers are now replacing existing CT scanners with new dual-energy units capable of iterative reconstruction to achieve high-resolution images at significantly lower irradiation doses.

Diagnostic assessment of new musculoskeletal tumors also often relies on nuclear scintigraphy. Currently, most patients with new bone lesions that elicit high suspicion of primary malignancy undergo bone scintigraphy with technetium Tc-99 methylene diphosphonate (^{99}Tc MDP) to assess the primary mass and to look for additional bone lesions including metastases or synchronous sites of disease. These bone scans, however, do not detect soft-tissue lesions or lesions exclusively involving bone marrow. Fluorodeoxyglucose (FDG) PET identifies abnormalities in glucose metabolism and can reveal associated marrow and soft-tissue masses. The use of PET at the time of diagnosis for the most common bone tumors, including osteosarcoma, Ewing sarcoma, and multiple myeloma remains controversial. In many institutions, PET is replacing bone scanning for initial staging of bone tumors. PET has been most widely advocated for Ewing sarcoma, which has a fairly high (approximately 25%) incidence of metastases at diagnosis. In addition to metastatic survey, PET can provide physiologic information with regard to the primary tumor.[9] FDG PET is widely used for the evaluation of soft-tissue lesions, with high degrees of FDG avidity seen in several malignant lesions such as synovial sarcoma. PET has been especially useful in differentiating malignant peripheral nerve sheath tumors in patients with neurofibromatosis type 1 (**Figure 7**).[10] A 2010 study of 40 peripheral nerve sheath tumors found that a cutoff maximum standardized uptake value (SUV) of 6.1 g/mL separated the benign lesions from the malignant ones.[11] The SUV can provide a quantitative measure of metabolic activity, with malignant tumors generally having higher SUVs. The degree of overlap, however, between benign and malignant lesions, as well as inherent technical bias, prevents the use of a reliable threshold value. Most centers interpret FDG PET information on the basis of visual in-

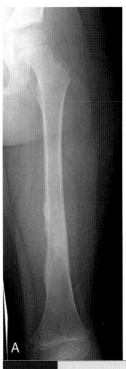
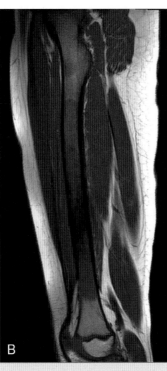

Figure 3 Imaging studies of a 13-year-old boy with osteosarcoma of the femur. **A**, AP radiograph reveals the sclerotic diaphyseal lesion with medial cortical destruction and periosteal reaction. **B**, Sagittal T1-weighted MRI is a composite of two sequences obtained for high resolution of both the proximal and distal femur. Postprocessing composition allows accurate measurements of the entire tumor relative to anatomic landmarks in preparation for limb salvage surgery with an intercalary allograft. Low signal intensity tumor margins are easily distinguished from the high signal intensity, normal fatty marrow, proximally and distally.

spection of the images and do not report SUV measurements.

Imaging Assessment of Therapeutic Response

Radiographs play a limited role in assessing response to therapy in patients with malignant bone and soft-tissue tumors. Bone tumors often reveal increased density and even increased size after the initiation of chemotherapy as a result of osseous remodeling and healing. CT is used primarily to assess change in size or number of pulmonary metastases and is not valuable for primary tumor assessment.

During therapy, MRI is the most helpful imaging study to assess the morphologic and physiologic tumor response. Standard high-resolution sequences allow for accurate measurement of tumor size and assessment of change in signal characteristics. The previously mentioned DWI and DCE techniques have their greatest value in the assessment of treatment response. Both

methods can help when the anatomic images show an overall increase in size that could reflect tumor growth or response to therapy. DWI and ADC images show facilitated diffusion in areas of necrosis, ischemia, and hemorrhage. Several studies have shown increasing ADC values in musculoskeletal tumors over time as diffusion improves with treatment.[12] In contrast, residual or recurrent tumor will demonstrate restricted diffusion. This finding can be especially important in telangiectatic osteosarcoma with cystic, hemorrhagic areas that may increase or regress during therapy (**Figure 8**). DCE images with time versus intensity curves tend to show diminished overall perfusion and flattened slopes with treatment. Recurrent tumor manifests as areas of increased perfusion. DCE also provides high-resolution angiographic imaging, which can be helpful for planning of limb salvage surgery, especially when vascularized fibular grafts are used.

Finally, FDG PET has been shown to be highly effective in the assessment of physiologic changes associated with therapy. Like DWI and DCE MRI, PET and PET-CT can help differentiate between treatment-associated change and tumor growth when anatomic imaging is inconclusive. FDG PET is a measure of tissue metabolic activity and reflects the histology within the lesion. The two most common primary bone tumors, Ewing sarcoma and osteosarcoma, respond quite differently to chemotherapy, and this response is apparent on FDG PET images. Ewing sarcoma typically has greater volume reduction during therapy due to the large extraosseous component and lack of calcified matrix. Osteosarcoma shows less volume reduction largely because of the osteoid matrix, which requires active resorption. Overall FDG avidity and SUV may not accurately reflect response to therapy in patients with osteosarcoma. Some institutions have advocated the use of a metabolic tumor volume, obtained by calculating the number of voxels with increased SUV within the entire tumor volume, as a better surrogate for histologic response.[13] In general, however, FDG PET plays an important role in Ewing sarcoma for staging and chemotherapy efficacy assessment but has a limited role in osteosarcoma.

Surveillance Imaging

The mainstay of surveillance imaging for local recurrence following primary bone tumor resection remains standard radiography. Artifact associated with metallic hardware following skeletal reconstruction limits the utility of routine CT and MRI. Recent advances in MRI metallic susceptibility artifact reduction are promising and may offer high-quality local imaging follow-up in the near future.[14] CT can be extremely helpful for postsurgical assessment following limb salvage surgery. Allograft union and fibular graft incorporation are well demonstrated with CT multiplanar reconstructions and volume-rendered techniques.[15] In

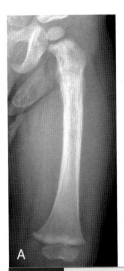
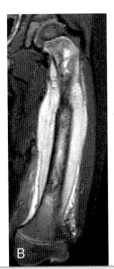
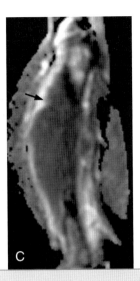
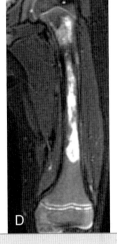
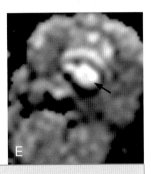

Figure 4 Imaging studies of an 18-month-old boy with Ewing sarcoma of the left femur. **A**, AP radiograph demonstrates the mixed permeative, sclerotic lesion within the metaphysis and diaphysis, with associated periosteal reaction and a suggestion of a soft-tissue mass. Coronal inversion recovery MRI (**B**) and sagittal ADC map (**C**) MRI scans at diagnosis show the large metaphyseal/diaphyseal tumor and associated soft-tissue mass. Restricted diffusion of water is seen as low signal intensity throughout the lesion (**C**), indicating high cellularity. This finding can be differentiated from the higher signal intensity perilesional edema, which demonstrates increased diffusion at the periphery (**C**, arrow). Following two cycles of chemotherapy, the coronal inversion recovery image (**D**) shows a dramatic decrease in size of the soft-tissue mass, and resolution of the surrounding edema, but persistent intramedullary high signal intensity. The corresponding axial ADC map also shows intramedullary high signal intensity (**E**, arrow), indicating increased diffusion and response to therapy. At resection, there was no viable tumor in the specimen.

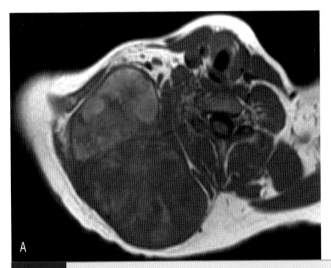
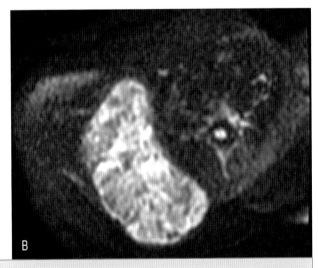

Figure 5 Imaging studies of an adolescent girl with a right shoulder mass. The axial T1-weighted MRI (**A**) shows a large soft-tissue mass with regions of mixed high and low signal intensity. The high signal intensity regions followed fat on all pulse sequences. The axial ADC map (**B**) also demonstrates a mixed pattern of increased and restricted diffusion. Biopsy revealed liposarcoma with the myxoid components accounting for the increased diffusion not typically seen in malignant tumors.

contrast to bone tumor recurrence, soft-tissue tumor recurrence is well demonstrated with a combination of morphologic and DWI MRI.

Long-term surveillance imaging for distant metastases is an area of significant development in the last decade. Although detection of metastases was previously limited to identification of osseous metastasis by technetium scintigraphy, and pulmonary metastasis with chest radiographs or chest CT, the advent of FDG PET, PET-CT, and whole-body MRI has enabled much broader and earlier detection of recurrences. Hybrid PET-CT has been shown to have higher sensitivity and specificity than FDG PET alone for the detection of occult metastases.[16,17] The ability to localize areas of increased FDG avidity to anatomic correlates has decreased the false-positive rates associated with PET

1: General Evaluation and Treatment of Musculoskeletal Tumors

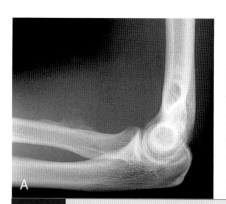
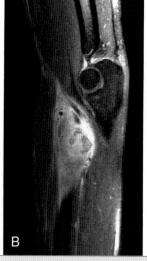
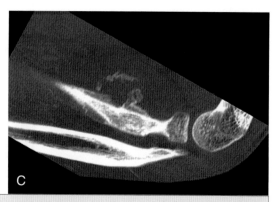

Figure 6 Imaging studies of a 25-year-old man with an elbow mass. Lateral radiograph of the elbow (**A**) shows periosteal calcification along the anterior margin of the distal radius. The sagittal contrast-enhanced, T1-weighted, fat-suppressed MRI (**B**) confirms the hypervascular soft-tissue mass and bone marrow edema within the proximal radius (not shown). Sagittal reformatted image from the axially acquired CT scan (**C**) obtained 4 weeks after the radiograph shows characteristic peripheral calcification extending from the periosteum, typical of myositis ossificans. This lesion has a typically aggressive, masslike appearance on MRI. High-resolution CT differentiates myositis ossificans from surface lesions that should cause more concern.

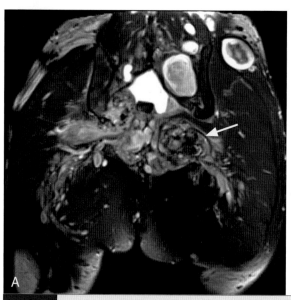
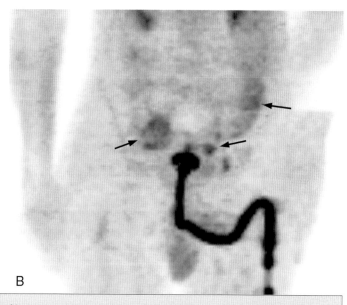

Figure 7 Imaging studies of a 27-year-old man with neurofibromatosis type 1. Coronal T2-weighted, fat-suppressed MRI scan of the pelvis (**A**) demonstrates extensive plexiform neurofibromas throughout the deep pelvis and gluteal regions. The left parasacral mass (**A**, arrow) is more complex and heterogeneous than the others, eliciting suspicion of malignancy. The accompanying FDG PET scan (**B**), however, shows three areas of avidity—bilateral parasacral regions (**B**, arrows) and left gluteal (**B**, arrowhead, partially obscured by bowel activity but confirmed on axial images). All three of these FDG-avid lesions proved to be malignant peripheral nerve-sheath tumor upon biopsy.

imaging alone. For Ewing sarcoma, FDG PET-CT has been shown to be more sensitive than bone scanning for the detection of local and distant recurrence, and many experts advocate elimination of dedicated bone scintigraphy in this patient population.[18] Technical advances in MRI including coil development, table mobility, and faster image acquisition have permitted whole-body scanning within a reasonable period with high image quality. Whole-body MRI has been used for several years to detect osseous metastases in patients with breast and lung cancer and is now being applied to musculoskeletal tumors with success. The technique es-

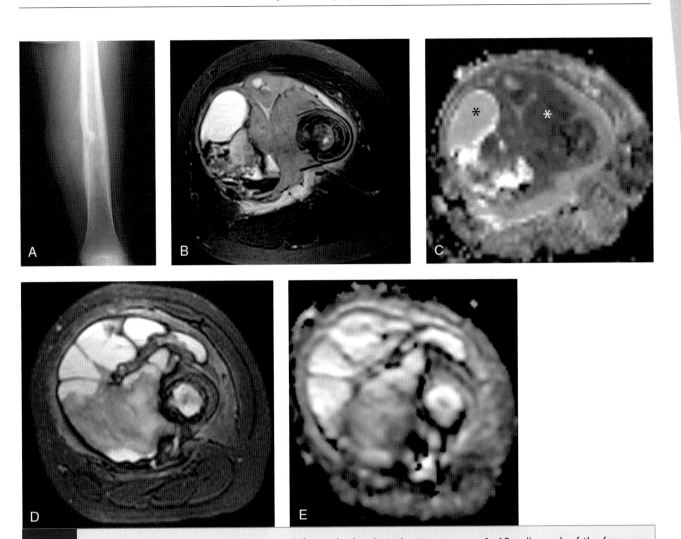

Figure 8 Imaging studies of an 18-year-old man with femoral telangiectatic osteosarcoma. **A,** AP radiograph of the femur reveals an aggressive lesion with starburst periosteal reaction and a soft-tissue mass. In addition to the typical osseous changes, the axial T2-weighted, fat-suppressed MRI (**B**) at diagnosis shows numerous cystic areas within the soft-tissue mass. Hemosiderin and fluid levels indicate hemorrhage. The accompanying ADC map (**C**) shows restricted diffusion in the solid portions of the tumor (white asterisk) and increased diffusion within the cystic components (black asterisk). Following chemotherapy, the axial T2-weighted, fat-suppressed morphologic MRI sequence (**D**) shows overall enlargement of the mass with increased size and complexity of the cystic regions. In telangiectatic osteosarcoma, this finding could reflect either tumor growth or necrosis with increased hemorrhage. The posttherapy ADC map (**E**) confirms increased diffusion compared with the pretreatment scan. Greater than 90% necrosis was confirmed at resection.

sentially involves wrapping the patient within multiple overlapping coils and performing pulse sequences at multiple stages to cover the entire body. Typically, T1 and fluid-sensitive sequences are obtained in the coronal and axial planes. On water-sensitive images, most soft-tissue and osseous metastatic lesions have high signal intensity relative to surrounding normal tissues (**Figure 9**). The addition of diffusion-weighted sequences to the whole-body MRI examination to increase lesion conspicuity is a current investigational technique that is likely to be clinically useful.[19] Several studies comparing whole-body MRI to PET-CT for metastatic disease tend to show similar sensitivities and specificities, each with their own advantages and limitations. Whole-body MRI may be more sensitive to visceral lesions, whereas PET-CT may be more useful for

lymph node and soft-tissue abnormalities.[20] The lack of ionizing irradiation with whole-body MRI is an important advantage, especially in young patients and those with malignancy predisposition syndromes. In addition to metastatic surveillance in patients with malignant musculoskeletal tumors, whole-body MRI is extremely useful for evaluation of multifocal diseases of bone such as Langerhans cell histiocytosis, chronic recurrent multifocal osteomyelitis, and neurofibromatosis.

Summary

Imaging continues to play an important role in the diagnosis and management of musculoskeletal neoplasms. Although radiography remains essential for many lesions, physicians increasingly rely upon new technologies. The past decade has seen a shift toward tissue characterization imaging in addition to high-resolution anatomic imaging. Diffusion-weighted MRI, DCE perfusion MRI, whole-body MRI, and FDG PET-CT are now in routine clinical use and have enhanced the assessment of response to therapy and long-term surveillance. Unprecedented image resolution is now achievable at faster acquisition times. The emphasis on irradiation exposure reduction is also an important advancement that should lead to overall improved outcomes for patients with malignancies.

Annotated References

1. Nichols RE, Dixon LB: Radiographic analysis of solitary bone lesions. *Radiol Clin North Am* 2011;49(6): 1095-1114, v.

   This article is a general review of the radiographic manifestations of common and less common primary bone tumors and lesions.

2. Torriani M, Etchebehere M, Amstalden E: Sonographically guided core needle biopsy of bone and soft tissue tumors. *J Ultrasound Med* 2002;21(3):275-281.

3. Bley TA, Wieben O, Uhl M: Diffusion-weighted MR imaging in musculoskeletal radiology: Applications in trauma, tumors, and inflammation. *Magn Reson Imaging Clin N Am* 2009;17(2):263-275.

   The authors reviewed the principles and techniques of diffusion-weighted MRI as applied to musculoskeletal pathology. DWI in various bone and soft-tissue tumors is discussed.

4. van Rijswijk CS, Kunz P, Hogendoorn PC, Taminiau AH, Doornbos J, Bloem JL: Diffusion-weighted MRI in the characterization of soft-tissue tumors. *J Magn Reson Imaging* 2002;15(3):302-307.

5. Maeda M, Matsumine A, Kato H, et al: Soft-tissue tumors evaluated by line-scan diffusion-weighted imaging: Influence of myxoid matrix on the apparent diffusion coefficient. *J Magn Reson Imaging* 2007;25(6): 1199-1204.

   This article describes a prospective study of DWI in 44 soft-tissue tumors. Those with myxoid content had significantly higher ADC values, regardless of benign or malignant nature.

6. Humphries PD, Sebire NJ, Siegel MJ, Olsen OE: Tumors in pediatric patients at diffusion-weighted MR imaging: Apparent diffusion coefficient and tumor cellularity. *Radiology* 2007;245(3):848-854.

   Prospective comparison of malignant and benign extracranial pediatric tumors revealed an inverse relationship between ADC and tumor cellularity but no significant difference in ADC between benign and malignant lesions. This study suggests that cellularity is not the sole determinant of ADC.

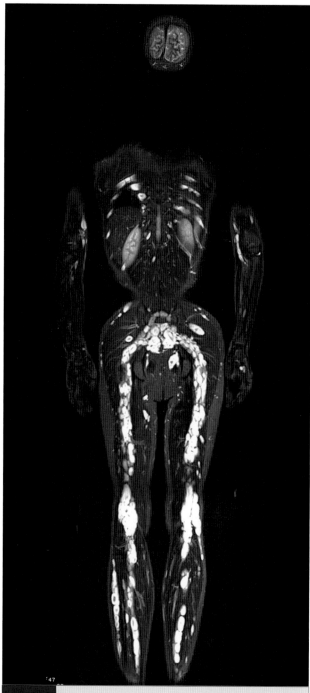

Figure 9 Imaging studies of a 9-year-old boy with neurofibromatosis type 1 and prior history of malignant peripheral nerve sheath tumor resection. Coronal inversion recovery whole-body MRI posteriorly shows extensive plexiform neurofibromas involving the intercostal, brachial, lumbosacral, sciatic, and lower extremity nerve roots. All of the lesions have typical "target sign" morphology and show no interval increase in size or change in signal characteristics. Serial whole-body MRI is performed every 6 months in this patient to avoid irradiation associated with FDG PET.

7. Guo JY, Reddick WE: DCE-MRI pixel-by-pixel quantitative curve pattern analysis and its application to osteosarcoma. *J Magn Reson Imaging* 2009;30(1):177-184.

    This prospective study describes methods used for DCE MRI analysis, including a new pattern analysis technique that is shown to be more reproducible.

8. Costa FM, Canella C, Gasparetto E: Advanced magnetic resonance imaging techniques in the evaluation of musculoskeletal tumors. *Radiol Clin North Am* 2011;49(6):1325-1358, vii-viii.

    The authors provided an extensive review of advanced MRI techniques including DWI, DCE perfusion imaging, and spectroscopy and their applications for musculoskeletal tumor imaging.

9. Bestic JM, Peterson JJ, Bancroft LW: Pediatric FDG PET/CT: Physiologic uptake, normal variants, and benign conditions [corrected]. *Radiographics* 2009; 29(5):1487-1500.

    This review article describes the use of FDG PET in the evaluation of Ewing sarcoma. PET has higher sensitivity than bone scintigraphy in detection of osseous metastases. PET allows assessment of therapeutic response when morphologic changes are minimal or confusing.

10. Bredella MA, Torriani M, Hornicek F, et al: Value of PET in the assessment of patients with neurofibromatosis type 1. *AJR Am J Roentgenol* 2007;189(4):928-935.

    This study is a retrospective review of PET evaluation of 45 patients with tumors related to neurofibromatosis type 1. PET was highly sensitive (95%) but less specific (72%) for the detection of malignant peripheral nerve sheath tumors. The addition of carbon methionine PET improved specificity.

11. Benz MR, Czernin J, Dry SM, et al: Quantitative F18-fluorodeoxyglucose positron emission tomography accurately characterizes peripheral nerve sheath tumors as malignant or benign. *Cancer* 2010;116(2):451-458.

    This study is a retrospective review of FDG PET-CT in 34 patients with peripheral nerve sheath tumors. Significantly higher SUVs were found in malignant peripheral nerve sheath tumors compared with neurofibromas. Malignant peripheral nerve sheath tumors and schwannomas were less reliably distinguished.

12. Costa FM, Ferreira EC, Vianna EM: Diffusion-weighted magnetic resonance imaging for the evaluation of musculoskeletal tumors. *Magn Reson Imaging Clin N Am* 2011;19(1):159-180.

    The authors provide a detailed review of diffusion-weighted MRI assessment of musculoskeletal tumors. Technical aspects, tumor characterization, and response to therapy are discussed.

13. Gaston LL, Di Bella C, Slavin J, Hicks RJ, Choong PF: 18F-FDG PET response to neoadjuvant chemotherapy for Ewing sarcoma and osteosarcoma are different. *Skeletal Radiol* 2011;40(8):1007-1015.

    This study is a retrospective comparison of the FDG PET imaging features of Ewing sarcoma and osteosarcoma. The predictive value of SUVs and metabolic tumor volume measurements as assessments of therapy response varied between the two histologies.

14. Ai T, Padua A, Goerner F, et al: SEMAC-VAT and MSVAT-SPACE sequence strategies for metal artifact reduction in 1.5T magnetic resonance imaging. *Invest Radiol* 2012;47(5):267-276.

    This phantom and volunteer study of two new imaging sequences was aimed at metallic artifact mitigation. Qualitative and quantitative measurements of artifact volume in these sequences were compared to those in standard sequences. The novel techniques achieved a 49% to 72% reduction in metallic artifact.

15. Fritz J, Fishman EK, Corl F, Carrino JA, Weber KL, Fayad LM: Imaging of limb salvage surgery. *AJR Am J Roentgenol* 2012;198(3):647-660.

    This review article illustrates the imaging findings associated with current complex surgical techniques designed to reconstruct limbs following tumor resection. Expected appearances and complications are reviewed.

16. Treglia G, Salsano M, Stefanelli A, Mattoli MV, Giordano A, Bonomo L: Diagnostic accuracy of ¹⁸F-FDG-PET and PET/CT in patients with Ewing sarcoma family tumours: A systematic review and a meta-analysis. *Skeletal Radiol* 2012;41(3):249-256.

    This diagnostic accuracy meta-analysis of 13 studies, including a total of 342 patients with Ewing sarcoma who underwent FDG PET or PET-CT, revealed a pooled sensitivity of 96% and pooled specificity of 92%.

17. Gerth HU, Juergens KU, Dirksen U, Gerss J, Schober O, Franzius C: Significant benefit of multimodal imaging: PET/CT compared with PET alone in staging and follow-up of patients with Ewing tumors. *J Nucl Med* 2007;48(12):1932-1939.

    This retrospective review compared PET-CT to PET alone in the evaluation of Ewing sarcoma. PET-CT was significantly more accurate in terms of lesion detection and location.

18. Walter F, Czernin J, Hall T, et al: Is there a need for dedicated bone imaging in addition to 18F-FDG PET/CT imaging in pediatric sarcoma patients? *J Pediatr Hematol Oncol* 2012;34(2):131-136.

    A retrospective review of 39 paired ⁹⁹Tc MDP bone and ¹⁸F-FDG PET-CT scans in 29 pediatric patients with bone or soft-tissue sarcoma is presented. ⁹⁹Tc MDP bone scans had significantly lower accuracy, and the authors concluded that ⁹⁹Tc MDP bone scanning provides no additional value.

19. Padhani AR, Koh DM, Collins DJ: Whole-body diffusion-weighted MR imaging in cancer: Current status and research directions. *Radiology* 2011;261(3): 700-718.

    This state-of-the-art update describes the technical aspects of whole-body, diffusion-weighted MRI data ac-

1: General Evaluation and Treatment of Musculoskeletal Tumors

quisition and image analysis. Advantages of this technique include lesion conspicuity, especially in bone marrow, and the ability to obtain quantitative ADC data. The technique is now readily available through most vendors.

20. Jaramillo D: Whole-body MR imaging, bone diffusion imaging: How and why? *Pediatr Radiol* 2010;40(6): 978-984.

This study reviewed the technical aspects and imaging assessment of whole-body MRI and DWI of the musculoskeletal system. Indications, imaging features, pitfalls, and future trends are discussed.

Chapter 3

Biopsy

Nicholas P. Webber, MD

Introduction

One of the most important procedures in the diagnosis and preliminary staging of musculoskeletal neoplasms is the biopsy. An appropriately planned and performed biopsy is imperative for obtaining definitive diagnostic tissue in bone and soft-tissue tumors. The method, location, and approach are paramount for directing further treatment and minimizing morbidity when definitive surgical intervention is appropriate. This chapter describes the principles, indications, techniques, and outcomes of the biopsy of musculoskeletal neoplasms on the basis of historical data, practice among sarcoma surgeons, and recent literature.

Principles of Biopsy

Several key principles of the biopsy of musculoskeletal neoplasms, when followed appropriately, can optimize the diagnosis and subsequent treatment. Although some of these principles are based on biology and technology, others have been developed with the goal of avoiding historically common pitfalls that can affect the diagnosis, definitive treatment, and outcome. Each of the principles shares a common goal of minimizing morbidity and contamination, and maximizing diagnostic accuracy to allow for optimal definitive treatment, while remaining economically prudent.

The most commonly practiced principles include (1) assembling a skilled and experienced team for prebiopsy evaluation, (2) obtaining adequate radiographic imaging before biopsy, (3) using appropriate techniques when obtaining tissue, and (4) having experienced physicians to interpret and handle the tissue in question.[1-4] When these principles are followed, biopsy of bone and soft-tissue tumors can achieve the goals of minimizing morbidity to the patient and obtaining the correct diagnosis so that staging and treatment can be performed in an expeditious and appropriate manner.

The first principle is that the biopsy should be performed by a team that is familiar with the diagnosis and treatment of musculoskeletal tumors.[2,3] It is widely accepted among sarcoma surgeons that the biopsy of suspected musculoskeletal neoplasms should be done at an institution where the physicians are familiar with such lesions. Furthermore, the institution should be equipped to carry out the definitive procedure if resection is recommended. Although it is much more common for a patient to have a benign rather than a malignant tumor, it is important that each lesion be examined closely. Any soft-tissue or bone lesion that cannot be diagnosed as a benign lesion clinically and radiographically by a primary care physician, general orthopaedic surgeon, or general surgeon should be referred to a center in which the physicians are familiar with these lesions. Although different tertiary centers have different preferred staging and advanced imaging modalities, when biopsy is considered, it is most appropriately done at the treating center.

It is unclear in the literature whether the particular individual performing the biopsy should be a surgeon, a radiologist, or another clinician. However, having a skilled team familiar with musculoskeletal neoplasms allows for several advantages.[5] First, biopsy is done only when it is deemed necessary and appropriate. Although the question of when to biopsy a soft-tissue or bone lesion is an often underused reason for referral, referring the patient to an experienced team for this decision can be advantageous to the patient and economically prudent. Given the wide range of benign and malignant musculoskeletal tumors and the fact that many lesions can be diagnosed and followed clinically and/or radiographically, deciding when to biopsy a lesion is a sophisticated skill. Particular lesions that may not necessitate a biopsy include some chondroid lesions, fibro-osseous lesions with characteristic radiographic findings, and small, superficial soft-tissue masses. A select group of masses, even when large and deep, can also be treated without biopsy when characteristic findings are recognized on advanced imaging, such as in the case of some lipomatous and vascular lesions (**Figure 1**). On the contrary, many lesions that are inaccurately assumed to be benign lipomas or posttraumatic hematomas can cause marked contamination and complicate definitive treatment and outcomes if they are resected before appropriate imaging (**Figure 2**). To avoid these pitfalls, some basic guidelines indicate when a biopsy is most likely to be the definitive method of diagnosis. A biopsy is generally indicated in tumors in which a de-

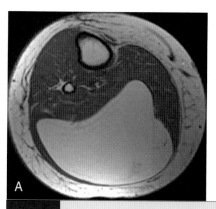
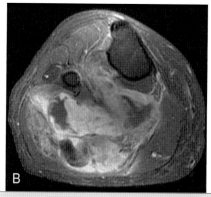
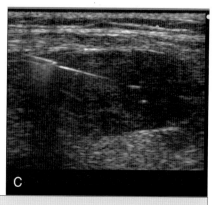

| Figure 1 | Imaging studies from a 50-year-old woman who had a painless mass in the posterior musculature of the leg. **A**, The mass was removed without biopsy given its MRI characteristics indicating a lipoma or well-differentiated liposarcoma (intramuscular atypical lipoma). **B**, A painless heterogeneous mass necessitating biopsy is shown. **C**, Ultrasound-guided biopsy revealed a high-grade pleomorphic sarcoma. |

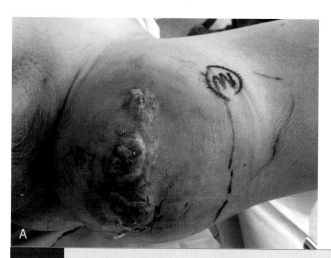
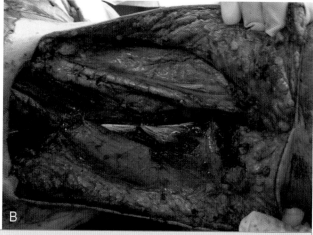

| Figure 2 | **A**, Progression of tumor through transverse, open excisional biopsy is shown. The tumor was initially thought to be a hematoma. Local control was complicated by preoperative sepsis; a complex, infected wound; and the inability to receive neoadjuvant local therapy. **B**, After resection, the tumor site with large soft-tissue defect is shown. |

finitive diagnosis cannot be made on the basis of clinical examination and imaging, soft-tissue masses in any location that are larger than 5 cm, masses that reach the depth of the muscular fascia, and bone lesions having characteristics that are not universally benign (excluding previously diagnosed metastatic disease). Although these features can help guide the need for biopsy, there is no substitute for experience with these complex lesions.

Diagnostic Imaging

When evaluating a lesion and planning a biopsy, obtaining appropriate imaging to optimize the differential diagnosis is critical. A wide range of imaging studies is available to clinicians. Imaging can be as simple as plain radiography and as complicated as combined positron emission tomography and CT scanning (PET-CT) or functional MRI. The choice of the imaging study in

diagnosis depends on the familiarity/experience with treating the lesion and the relationship of the radiologists, the pathologists, and the surgeons performing the biopsies. Usually, a plain radiograph is the initial study of choice when evaluating a tumor, whether of soft tissue or of bone. Often, a plain radiograph is sufficient for the diagnosis of benign bone lesions, and can often be second only to the biopsy in the diagnosis of many malignant neoplasms. The plain radiograph can also be extremely helpful in diagnosing some soft-tissue tumors, such as hemangiomas, myositis ossificans, and chondrosarcomas, which are apparent on plain radiographs with their calcific patterns.

MRI is often the advanced imaging modality of choice. Contrast-enhanced MRI with high-field, consistent magnets allows for highly accurate definition of the extent of both bone and soft-tissue components of the tumor. MRI can also allow for appropriate localization of viable and necrotic portions of the tumor, and can demonstrate diagnostic enhancement patterns, especially

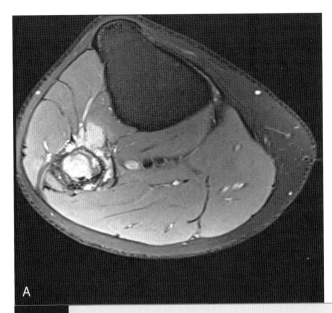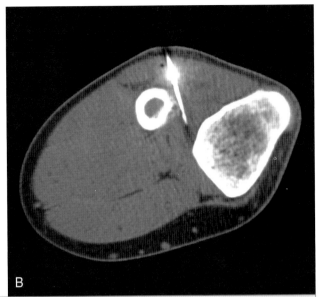

Figure 3 **A**, MRI of the fibula of a 20-year-old patient shows a destructive mass. **B**, Core biopsy using a coaxial biopsy system under CT guidance established the diagnosis of Ewing sarcoma.

when interpreted by radiologists familiar with these lesions (**Figure 3**). A thorough overview of MRI is provided in chapter 2, Imaging of Musculoskeletal Tissues.

Other modalities that can aid in diagnosis and planning of the biopsy include ultrasound, CT scan, PET-CT, and angiography. These modalities are used variably at different institutions. There is no definitive standard as to which lesions require which imaging modality for biopsy. Although these imaging modalities have a very different role in staging, their role in biopsy can be simplified to attaining the most diagnostic study in order to fine-tune the clinical suspicion that will lead to the highest chance of obtaining diagnostic tissue while limiting morbidity. Finally, appropriate imaging before the biopsy can allow for examination of the tissue in its prebiopsy state analyzing and planning for appropriate definitive local control.

Performing the Biopsy

There are no definitive data on who is the most appropriate person to perform the biopsy. However, no matter who physically performs the procedure, the goals and principles remain the same. First, the biopsy method used remains the decision of the multidisciplinary team. When choosing the method, it is important that the biopsy, whether it involves a small core needle tract or a true surgical incision, be placed so that the biopsy approach is amenable to resection at the time of definitive local treatment. Second, when deciding the approach to the tumor, it is important to minimize contamination of tissues and morbidity to the patient. This is accomplished by directing the biopsy through one compartment, and ensuring that tissue

planes are not violated, so that the tumor does not spread along fascial planes. Furthermore, hemostasis throughout the biopsy is necessary, and, when not respected, can compromise local control. Although there is often discussion of whether the needle tract needs to be resected at the time of definitive resection, the incision from an open biopsy is routinely excised. For this reason, it is important to use a longitudinal incision that can be excised en bloc with the final specimen. In so doing, the physician who does the biopsy can optimize the conditions for the surgeon to obtain successful soft-tissue coverage, healing, and the ability to perform longitudinal extension as indicated. Furthermore, an appropriate incision can decrease the need for unnecessary free tissue coverage and can improve the ability to perform limb salvage surgery.

The type of biopsy that should be done to obtain an accurate diagnosis is a matter of debate. Open or incisional biopsy with on-site histologic examination is considered by some to be the preferred method and is usually performed by the surgeon who would ultimately perform the definitive resection. This technique is thought to reduce the problems of other techniques with regard to sampling error, histologic heterogeneity, and necrosis. However, many physicians argue that other modalities of biopsy are as appropriate. With the increasing popularity of the image-guided percutaneous biopsy, radiologists, pathologists, and surgeons skilled in using MRI, CT, and ultrasound are moving toward performing percutaneous biopsies using image-guided techniques. In a study comparing the accuracy of the three biopsy techniques, the authors found that "all three modalities are acceptable biopsy techniques for soft tissue masses."[5] This statement is based on the authors' findings that whatever biopsy method is chosen,

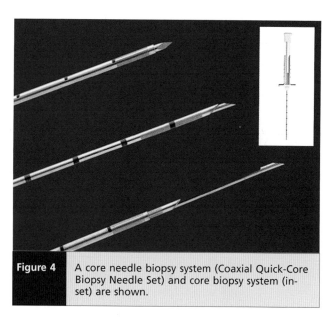

Figure 4 A core needle biopsy system (Coaxial Quick-Core Biopsy Needle Set) and core biopsy system (inset) are shown.

it should be performed in conjunction with a frozen section to ensure that diagnostic tissue is obtained. Historically, the most accurate method of obtaining diagnostic tissue was thought to be the open biopsy, followed by core biopsy and fine-needle aspiration (FNA) biopsy.[6-8] However, results are variable, and if the biopsy is performed by an experienced team with on-site histologic tissue evaluation, all three techniques have strong proponents in the sarcoma community and an increasing amount of supporting literature. When deciding on the type of biopsy, the team must also take into account what form of biopsy has the most acceptable morbidity for the patient, yields the highest likelihood of obtaining a sufficient sample of diagnostic tissue, and is the most economically efficient manner, keeping in mind the implications of a poorly performed biopsy.

Percutaneous Techniques

Many tumors can be biopsied using percutaneous techniques. These techniques can be applied in the clinical setting using ultrasound or palpation when appropriate,[9] in the radiology suite using imaging modalities in coordination with or by interventional radiologists, and in the operating room under fluoroscopy or intraoperative advanced imaging. Although the technique and imaging modality used for localization of the tumor depends on the experience and preferences of the team, the goal of obtaining highly accurate results while limiting morbidity remains the same.

Fine-Needle Aspiration Biopsy

FNA biopsy is a technique in which tissue is obtained by placing a needle (20-gauge or smaller) into the mass and aspirating tissue into the needle. FNA biopsy has widespread utility in diagnostic oncology, but opinions vary regarding its diagnostic accuracy in musculoskeletal oncology. The needle can be placed under ultra-

sound, fluoroscopy, CT, and other methods of guidance that can improve the accuracy of obtaining diagnostic tissue from the portion of the tumor desired. This technique can, theoretically, result in the least contamination of tissue, with minimal morbidity, and can usually be done with the use of local anesthesia, eliminating the risk of general or regional anesthesia often necessary in an incisional biopsy. It is imperative that a cytopathologist be available at the time of biopsy to decide whether an adequate amount of diagnostic tissue has been obtained. Similarly, a pathologist skilled in examining and interpreting tissue obtained in this manner must be available to make the diagnosis accurately. Although historically regarded as the least diagnostic of the three modalities, FNA biopsy is commonly used for both bone and soft-tissue neoplasms in some reputable institutions, and in several recent studies, the diagnostic accuracy was approximately 90%.[10,11] Data suggest that masses that contain myxoid or round cell neoplastic tissue, masses accompanied by infection, and masses in paraspinal anatomic locations have the lowest diagnostic accuracy with FNA biopsy.[12,13] Although it is beyond the scope of this chapter, discussion as to the ability and necessity of the biopsy to accurately determine the subtype of sarcoma is ongoing. In summary, the use of FNA biopsy as a technique in sarcoma diagnosis must be evaluated very closely. Although many sarcoma specialists argue that this technique has a limited role, others who are very familiar with FNA biopsy can use it with accuracy.[14,15] Although FNA biopsy for primary diagnosis of sarcoma may be controversial, it clearly has a role in the diagnosis of local recurrence and of metastatic carcinoma in the musculoskeletal system.

Core Biopsy

Core or trocar biopsy involves obtaining tissue from a bone or soft-tissue mass, either directly or with radiographic guidance, using a large-bore needle (commonly 14-gauge or larger). This type of biopsy has the advantages of FNA biopsy and avoids the morbidity of incisional biopsy while obtaining tissue that approaches the diagnostic accuracy of an incisional biopsy. Core biopsy is performed with different instruments, depending on whether bone or soft tissue is to be biopsied. Coaxial bone biopsy systems that allow for controlled drilling are often used in bone, and variations thereof are often used in soft tissue (**Figure 4**). The diagnostic accuracy in percutaneous core biopsy of bone lesion, based on several studies, is from 75% to 95%, with most studies reporting greater than 90% accuracy.[16-20] In core biopsy of soft tissue, the diagnostic accuracy is generally higher, with most studies showing 90% to 94% accuracy. CT guidance is often used to allow for better visualization of small lesions, to enable identification of compartmental anatomy to localize the biopsy to nonnecrotic areas, and to allow for identification of deep lesions that would otherwise not be identified on ultrasound (**Figure 5**). However, studies

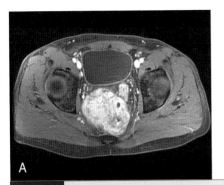
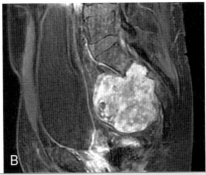
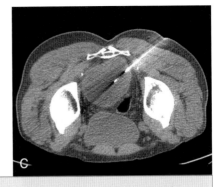

Figure 5   Axial (**A**) and sagittal (**B**) MRIs show a large presacral soft-tissue mass. **C**, CT-guided core biopsy demonstrated schwannoma.

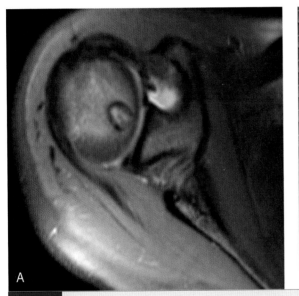
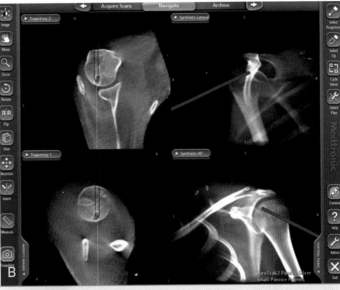

Figure 6   **A**, MRI of the proximal humerus in an 11-year-old girl shows a proximal humeral lesion (chondroblastoma). **B**, Intra-operative CT navigation used to biopsy the lesion with a Craig core needle biopsy system confirmed the diagnosis of chondroblastoma. (Panel B courtesy of Medtronic, Minneapolis, MN.)

with contrast-enhanced ultrasound show similar rates of diagnostic accuracy.[21]

Some centers also use techniques aimed at furthering the accuracy of obtaining diagnostic tissue. Intraoperative navigation is gaining acceptance for several indications in orthopaedics and is being used more commonly for localizing lesions to obtain tissue in anatomically difficult locations (**Figure 6**).

Incisional Biopsy

An incisional biopsy is a method of obtaining tissue from a bone or soft-tissue mass by making an incision into the skin directly into the lesion, without raising flaps, violating multiple compartments, or using standard internervous planes, to obtain a portion of the tissue in question for diagnostic sampling. Historically, incisional biopsy has been considered the preferred method for biopsy, yielding diagnostic accuracy of 94% to 98%. However, with data showing that percutane-

ous techniques are nearly as accurate when performed with immediate cytologic evaluation, other techniques are increasing in popularity. The incisional, or open, biopsy is usually performed under general anesthesia, or monitored anesthesia care with local or regional anesthetic supplementation, and generally necessitates an operating room. This technique, more than any other reviewed in this chapter, should be performed by or in coordination with the surgeon to plan for the definitive surgery. The incision should be in line with the proposed surgical incision if wide resection is anticipated or considered possible. It should be longitudinal on the extremities, and complete hemostasis must be attained to decrease the risk of contamination. Disadvantages include the possibility of contamination and the need for a more expensive and potentially morbid procedure for the patient. The major advantages to an open biopsy are the ability to obtain a large amount of tissue and the ability to obtain a wedge-shaped specimen that

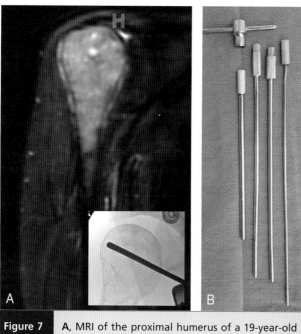

Figure 7 **A,** MRI of the proximal humerus of a 19-year-old woman. A coaxial core biopsy was performed on a destructive, uniform lesion (giant cell tumor). **B,** A Craig needle biopsy set is shown.

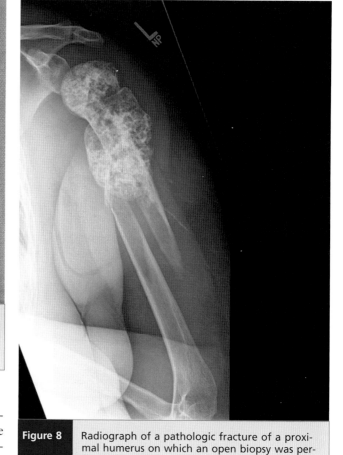

Figure 8 Radiograph of a pathologic fracture of a proximal humerus on which an open biopsy was performed through a chondroid lesion to maintain architecture for pathologic diagnosis (dedifferentiated chondrosarcoma).

retains the architecture of the tissue (**Figures 7** and **8**).

With the increasing availability of intraoperative imaging, including CT, MRI, and ultrasound, it is possible to attempt a percutaneous biopsy using these modalities, send a frozen section for pathologic analysis, and, if the percutaneous biopsy is unsuccessful, do an open biopsy in the same setting. Incisional biopsies are commonly used when evaluating a suspected benign, locally aggressive lesion (aneurysmal bone cyst, giant cell tumor). If the suspected diagnosis is verified at the time of biopsy, these lesions can be definitively treated if proper planning has been completed.

Excisional Biopsy
Excisional biopsy refers to an open technique in which the tumor is removed without having a pathologic diagnosis before the surgery. This technique is usually limited to lesions that have diagnostic characteristics on imaging, including intramuscular lipomas and small, superficial lesions that can be completely excised with little morbidity and using oncologic principles.

Tissue Handling
The well-known adage "biopsy everything you culture, and culture everything you biopsy" has taken on new scope and breadth in the evolving era of molecular genetics, chemosensitivity testing, biorepositiories, and the increasing need for information on rare neoplasms. In addition, the type of biopsy is also predicated on the clinical suspicion of the neoplasm in question. Meaningful information can be obtained by a correct biopsy and can preclude the necessity for repeat biopsy (**Figure 7**). The question of whether to send a specimen in formalin or fresh, although seemingly simple, is actually a complex decision based on the preoperative differential diagnosis, and, in an operating room or interventional suite, can become a source of confusion when the team doing the biopsy is not familiar with the expectations. Intraoperatively, the role of the pathologist is to interpret the frozen section, or a portion of the tissue from the specimen, to determine if diagnostic tissue is present in the sample. No matter what method of biopsy is chosen, it is extremely helpful to have a skilled pathologist present to verify that diagnostic tissue is sampled. In a recent study, percutaneous needle biopsies had much higher accuracy when performed with immediate cytologic evaluation.[22,23] This evaluation is especially helpful in tumors that are extensively necrotic, in which there is a high likelihood of having nondiagnostic tissue, especially if the tissue is from the center of a large necrotic tumor.

When the pathologist has determined that the frozen section contains diagnostic tissue, the physician doing the biopsy and the pathologist must rely on both their clinical suspicion and their preoperative evaluation. For example, if lymphoma or myeloma is suspected, it is important that fresh tissue that has not been placed in formalin be separated for flow cytometry. Similarly, if tissue is to be sent for chemosensitivity testing, or the patient has consented to have some of the tissue evaluated in a study that requires fresh tissue, then the need for fresh tissue must be clearly stated to the staff.[24] Many sarcoma surgeons clearly state at the beginning of the case the specific plans for the specimen so that there is no question as to its fate. Furthermore, the adage "biopsy everything you culture, and culture everything you biopsy" continues to be a reasonable rule of thumb. Given the complex patients often seen in tertiary care centers, with many sources of infection as well as complex medical histories, even a team with decades of experience can make a misdiagnosis. It is imperative to have a reasonable differential diagnosis and be able to evaluate each of the plausible diagnoses while being economically conservative.

Summary

A properly planned and executed biopsy is imperative to diagnosing and treating musculoskeletal neoplasms. Obtaining diagnostic tissue for evaluation of bone and soft-tissue tumors can be relatively straightforward if the principles and techniques are followed and used appropriately. Although debate regarding some specifics of this process continues, sarcoma surgeons strive to achieve the most reliable, accurate, safe, and cost-efficient way to treat these potentially complex lesions. Further studies aim to help improve techniques, decrease morbidity, improve accuracy, and optimize knowledge of these complex neoplasms.

Annotated References

1. Liu K, Layfield LJ, Coogan AC, Ballo MS, Bentz JS, Dodge RK: Diagnostic accuracy in fine-needle aspiration of soft tissue and bone lesions: Influence of clinical history and experience. *Am J Clin Pathol* 1999;111(5):632-640.

2. Mankin HJ, Mankin CJ, Simon MA; Members of the Musculoskeletal Tumor Society: The hazards of the biopsy, revisited. *J Bone Joint Surg Am* 1996;78(5):656-663.

3. Markel DC, Neumann KU, Steinau HU: Appropriate techniques for musculoskeletal tumor biopsy. *Orthop Rev* 1994;23(2):176-180.

4. Bickels J, Jelinek JS, Shmookler BM, Neff RS, Malawer MM: Biopsy of musculoskeletal tumors: Current concepts. *Clin Orthop Relat Res* 1999;368:212-219.

5. Rougraff BT, Aboulafia A, Biermann JS, Healey J: Biopsy of soft tissue masses: Evidence-based medicine for the musculoskeletal tumor society. *Clin Orthop Relat Res* 2009;467(11):2783-2791.

This review of the literature by a subcommittee of the Musculoskeletal Tumor Society concluded that open biopsy has the highest diagnostic accuracy, frozen section at the time of biopsy may improve diagnostic accuracy, and myxoid and round cell neoplasms, infections, and tumors in the paraspinal region can present difficulty. Level of evidence: III.

6. Yeow KM, Tan CF, Chen JS, Hsueh C: Diagnostic sensitivity of ultrasound-guided needle biopsy in soft tissue masses about superficial bone lesions. *J Ultrasound Med* 2000;19(12):849-855.

7. Yang YJ, Damron TA: Comparison of needle core biopsy and fine-needle aspiration for diagnostic accuracy in musculoskeletal lesions. *Arch Pathol Lab Med* 2004;128(7):759-764.

8. Smith TJ, Safaii H, Foster EA, Reinhold RB: Accuracy and cost-effectiveness of fine needle aspiration biopsy. *Am J Surg* 1985;149(4):540-545.

9. Adams SC, Potter BK, Pitcher DJ, Temple HT: Office-based core needle biopsy of bone and soft tissue malignancies: An accurate alternative to open biopsy with infrequent complications. *Clin Orthop Relat Res* 2010;468(10):2774-2780.

The authors retrospectively reviewed 233 office-based core biopsies and found 91% to be diagnostic of malignancy with 3% major error, defined as benign diagnosis in malignant tumor. The authors concluded that this procedure has high diagnostic and accuracy rates. Level of evidence: II.

10. Kilpatrick SE, Cappellari JO, Bos GD, Gold SH, Ward WG: Is fine-needle aspiration biopsy a practical alternative to open biopsy for the primary diagnosis of sarcoma? Experience with 140 patients. *Am J Clin Pathol* 2001;115(1):59-68.

11. Fleshman R, Mayerson J, Wakely PE Jr: Fine-needle aspiration biopsy of high-grade sarcoma: A report of 107 cases. *Cancer* 2007;111(6):491-498.

The authors retrospectively reviewed FNA biopsy data for high-grade sarcoma in 107 specimens from 98 patients and found diagnosis to be accurate in 91% of specimens.

12. Hau A, Kim I, Kattapuram S, et al: Accuracy of CT-guided biopsies in 359 patients with musculoskeletal lesions. *Skeletal Radiol* 2002;31(6):349-353.

13. Ogilvie CM, Torbert JT, Finstein JL, Fox EJ, Lackman RD: Clinical utility of percutaneous biopsies of musculoskeletal tumors. *Clin Orthop Relat Res* 2006;450:95-100.

14. Cormier JN, Pollock RE: Soft tissue sarcomas. *CA Cancer J Clin* 2004;54(2):94-109.

15. Geisinger KR, Ward WG, Levine EA: Soft-tissue sarcoma [letter]. *N Engl J Med* 2005;353(21):2303-2304, author reply 2303-2304.

16. Hryhorczuk AL, Strouse PJ, Biermann JS: Accuracy of CT-guided percutaneous core needle biopsy for assessment of pediatric musculoskeletal lesions. *Pediatr Radiol* 2011;41(7):848-857.

   The authors reviewed 63 CT-guided biopsies in 61 children and found accurate diagnostic information in 84% of biopsies.

17. Heslin MJ, Lewis JJ, Woodruff JM, Brennan MF: Core needle biopsy for diagnosis of extremity soft tissue sarcoma. *Ann Surg Oncol* 1997;4(5):425-431.

18. Shin HJ, Amaral JG, Armstrong D, et al: Image-guided percutaneous biopsy of musculoskeletal lesions in children. *Pediatr Radiol* 2007;37(4):362-369.

   The authors reviewed 127 percutaneous core biopsies in children and found that the diagnostic success was 76% overall and 92% in primary malignant tumors.

19. Domanski HA, Akerman M, Carlén B, et al: Core-needle biopsy performed by the cytopathologist: A technique to complement fine-needle aspiration of soft tissue and bone lesions. *Cancer* 2005;105(4):229-239.

20. Rimondi E, Staals EL, Errani C, et al: Percutaneous CT-guided biopsy of the spine: Results of 430 biopsies. *Eur Spine J* 2008;17(7):975-981.

   The authors reviewed 430 biopsies and found that a correct diagnosis was made in 401 (93.3%). The authors concluded that percutaneous CT-guided biopsy of the spine should be the preferred method.

21. De Marchi A, Brach del Prever EM, Linari A, et al: Accuracy of core-needle biopsy after contrast-enhanced ultrasound in soft-tissue tumours. *Eur Radiol* 2010; 20(11):2740-2748.

   This study examined 115 soft-tissue masses biopsied using contrast-enhanced ultrasound and found that 94.8% were adequate for diagnosis.

22. Virayavanich W, Ringler MD, Chin CT, et al: CT-guided biopsy of bone and soft-tissue lesions: Role of on-site immediate cytologic evaluation. *J Vasc Interv Radiol* 2011;22(7):1024-1030.

   The authors reviewed 299 CT-guided percutaneous biopsies and found that biopsies performed with immediate cytologic assessment had a greater success rate.

23. Azabdaftari G, Goldberg SN, Wang HH: Efficacy of on-site specimen adequacy evaluation of image-guided fine and core needle biopsies. *Acta Cytol* 2010;54(2): 132-137.

   The authors found that on-site evaluation of specimens improved the percentage of definite positive diagnoses of malignant lesions but had no effect on diagnostic yield of benign lesions.

24. Rubin BP, Cooper K, Fletcher CD, et al; Members of the Cancer Committee, College of American Pathologists: Protocol for the examination of specimens from patients with tumors of soft tissue. *Arch Pathol Lab Med* 2010;134(4):e31-e39.

   This College of American Pathologists protocol assists pathologists in providing clinically useful information on soft-tissue sarcomas in teenagers and adults.

Chapter 4

The Molecular Biology of Musculoskeletal Neoplasia

Kevin B. Jones, MD

1: General Evaluation and Treatment of Musculoskeletal Tumors

Introduction

Molecular biology once focused almost entirely on genes and the proteins they produce. The central dogma of molecular biology was that the DNA of genes was transcribed into RNA, which was translated into amino acid sequences, which folded into proteins. It was long thought that this process worked only in that direction. The first clue that the central dogma could be defined differently came from study of HIV and other retroviruses, which proved the capacity of certain natural enzymes to engage in reverse transcription, generating DNA from RNA.

A key finding of the Human Genome Project is the realization that there appear to be only approximately 20,000 genes in humans; much of the DNA in the genome codes for no recognizable purpose (junk DNA). This new knowledge produced one immediate question: how did the complexity of human biology arise from a paltry 20,000 genes? Their regulation had to be much more complex than immediately known. The place to look for the answer to this question was in the junk DNA between and around the gene coding sequences.

Molecular biology subsequently broadened to include the study of many new fields as new classes of molecules and new modes of regulation were discovered. The field of cancer biology has undergone parallel expansion.

Making a Cancer Diagnosis

When a mass is referred to as a cancer, it is part of a group of entities with the capacity to destructively spread to distant sites. Categorizing a particular tumor in a given patient under a certain diagnosis does not mean the tumor will or has metastasized. The heterogeneity in behavior observed among all the masses assigned any specific cancer diagnosis suggests the existence of heterogeneity on the molecular level that, once identified, may offer more specific diagnoses, treatments, and prognostic information.

Much has been learned in recent years about the heterogeneity of the cells that comprise a single malignancy.[1] Further, heterogeneity among the human hosts of any cancer type also affect each malignancy's behavior and biologic potential. The molecular biology of cancer therefore works to bring into focus both the molecular underpinnings of oncogenesis and the heterogeneity in the malignancies it produces.

Cancer cells use the same tools as normal cells to regulate their biology. Some fundamental differences in the products of that regulation (or goals, although intent seems a tough-to-resolve concept for a cell) have been dubbed the hallmarks of cancer.[2,3] The hallmarks are, essentially, the characteristics by which cancer cells are distinguished from their noncancerous counterparts.

The first hallmark is self-sufficiency in growth. Normal cells depend on signals from their environment, including neighboring cells, the extracellular matrix, and factors diffusing from local sources or from the vasculature after delivery from distant, systemic sources. Cancer cells achieve independence from external growth signals by aberrant expression of both the ligand and the receptor of some growth-signaling pathway, by expression of a mutated growth receptor that activates the downstream pathway without the need for a signal from the ligand binding, or by overexpression—or normal expression of an overactive variant—of one of the downstream factors of that growth pathway.

Normal cells stop growing either by senescence (permanent exit from the cell cycle) or apoptosis (programmed cell death). Cancer cells evade internal and external signals that otherwise prompt senescence or apoptosis. It is impossible to distinguish these capacities entirely from the self-sufficiency of growth, because many of the involved pathways overlap. These pathways include evasion of contact inhibition, loss of organizing polarity, and silencing of both immune-mediated and intrinsic apoptosis in response to genetic or chromosomal instability.

Even if induced to grow independently from external

signals and free from signals prompting senescence or apoptosis, most cells can only copy or replicate their DNA (a critical portion of the cell cycle) so many times before the telomeres, or caps on the ends of chromosomes, have been shortened to a length that no longer permits stability and continued growth. Some very aggressive malignancies manage to silence apoptotic responses to the instability derived from critically shortened telomeres, but most other malignancies must activate some mechanism of lengthening the telomeres to continue limitless growth.

Another hallmark is that the metabolism of cancer cells can differ markedly from that of other cells. For example, many use inefficient glycolysis alone, rather than the full Krebs cycle and the mitochondrial electron transport chain to generate energy in the form of adenosine triphosphate. Nonetheless, even metabolically abnormal cancer cells require a constant supply of nutrients and removal of waste products. Because many cancer cells inefficiently burn through glucose much faster than other cells, they are even more dependent than other cells on an excellent blood supply. To address this need, the cells of most solid tumors induce and encourage angiogenesis, the ingrowth of blood vessels.

Invasion is another hallmark of cancer cells. The invasion of basement membranes or other tissue planes defines many malignancies on a histopathologic basis. Before a cell can spread to a distant site and begin growing, it must free itself from the physical constraints of its initial environment and enter the bloodstream.

The final capacity to metastasize formally depends on additional abilities to survive in the bloodstream, cross another basement membrane after landing somewhere else, and then grow in the new, unfamiliar environment. The last requirement may be the most stringent and most rarely attained.

The original article on the hallmarks of cancer was published in 2000, but an update in 2011 emphasized a new hallmark, immune evasion.[2,3] Of course, consideration of musculoskeletal neoplasia more generally than sarcoma alone must include entities that acquire only one or a few of these hallmarks.

The Molecular Biology of Malignancies

The 2011 report on the hallmarks of cancer also emphasized certain molecular tools by which malignancies achieve their phenotypic hallmarks. Specifically noted were genomic instability, inflammation, reprogramming of metabolism, and interactions with the microenvironment.

Each cancer cell's capacities result from two principal inputs: the cell of origin and the transformation process that changes that cell into a malignant cell. Any cellular phenotype or differentiation characteristic discernible in a cancer cell was once presumed necessary

to reflect the cell of origin alone, and the transformation to achieve the hallmarks of cancer was considered an entirely separate or even dedifferentiating series of events. Any malignant cell producing bone matrix was assumed to derive originally from an osteoblast; any cell producing cartilaginous matrix, from a chondrocyte; any cell staining for smooth muscle markers, from a smooth muscle myocyte; and any cell expressing keratins, from an epithelial cell.

Researchers have recently become aware that transformation may powerfully affect the differentiation phenotype of the resultant malignancy. For example, synovial sarcomas are not thought to arise from epithelial cells, yet most of them express cytokeratins.

Innate capacities of certain cells of origin may contribute to the hallmarks themselves. Because most human malignancies are—and an even greater proportion of most human cancer biologists study—carcinomas, or cancers of epithelial tissues, generalized philosophical considerations such as these hallmarks may not fully apply to cancers derived from mesenchymal cells. Many normal mesenchymal cells innately bear the capacity to move through basement membranes or even survive in the bloodstream or other tissues. A popular theory in the study of epithelial cancers is that they must become more like mesenchymal tissues in the process of gaining metastatic potential. The innate mesenchymal characteristics do not necessarily eliminate the difficulties of full-fledged cell transformation, but may make the process easier.

This chapter reviews the molecular biology related to cells undergoing malignant transformation. The central dogma serves as a foundation for the discussion, and examples from musculoskeletal neoplasia are discussed.

Changes at the DNA Level

At the level of the genetic code in some malignancies, some genes are simply missing or deleted. These changes may arise from the loss of an entire chromosome or the start site or critical coding section of a gene. Large sections of chromosomal loss or gain have been detectable for decades using formal cytogenetics. Newer technologies using hybridization, or the adherence of complementary DNA sequences to each other on a microscale (single-nucleotide polymorphism arrays) or macroscale (fluorescent in situ hybridization), or direct sequencing of partial or entire genomes have revealed much more than was previously known about important smaller losses and gains in the copy number of genes.

The loss of some genes grants new capacities to some malignancies; such genes are called tumor suppressors because their native suppression must be lost for a tumor to develop. A cell must lose both copies of most tumor suppressors to gain any related cancer hallmark, but the loss of even one copy of other genes will

Table 1

Oncogenes and Tumor Suppressors

Neoplasm	Tumor Suppressor Genes	Oncogenes
Atypical lipomatous tumor (well-differentiated liposarcoma, lipoma-like liposarcoma)		MDM2, TSPAN31, CDK4, HMGA2 (formerly HMGIC)
Desmoid-type fibromatosis	APC	β-catenin
Undifferentiated pleomorphic sarcoma (malignant fibrous histiocytoma)	TP53, RB1, CDKN2A	TSPAN31, MDM2, CDK4, CHOP, HMGA2 (formerly HMGIC)
Embryonal rhabdomyosarcoma	IGF2, H19, CDKN1C, TP53, CDKN2A	RAS family
Alveolar rhabdomyosarcoma		GLI1, CDK4, MDM2, MYCN
Synovial sarcoma	PTEN	BCL2, β-catenin
Osteosarcoma	RB1, TP53, INK4A	CDK4, CCND1, MDM2, MYC, FOS, ERBB2, MET
Parosteal osteosarcoma		CDK4, TSPAN31, MDM2
Osteochondroma	EXT1, EXT2	
Peripheral chondrosarcoma	EXT1, EXT2, CKDN2A	
Ewing sarcoma	KCMF1, CDKN2A, IGFBP3	STAT3, GLI1, NKX2-2, NR0B1, GSTM4
Fibrous dysplasia		GNAS (formerly GNAS1)

lead to haploinsufficiency, which can enable new cell behaviors (**Table 1**).

Musculoskeletal neoplasia, although it comprises less than 1% of all malignancies, actually played a major role in identification of the two most important tumor suppressor genes, *RB1* and *TP53*.[4] Osteosarcoma, the most common bone sarcoma, and undifferentiated pleomorphic sarcoma (previously called malignant fibrous histiocytoma), the most common soft-tissue sarcoma, are both characterized by *TP53* and *RB1* dysfunction.[5] Osteosarcoma is the second most common malignancy in patients with hereditary retinoblastoma. Although these patients inherit one mutated copy of *RB1*, a critical portion of their remaining functional copy is often lost or deleted in the process of osteosarcomagenesis. Both *TP53* and *RB1* are cell-cycle checkpoint regulators, which means that their loss can enable growth independent from external signals and free the cells from the senescent or apoptotic signals that would normally result from DNA damage.

After these two genes, the next most frequent genetic locus lost in malignancies is *CDKN2A*, which contains two overlapping genes, *INK4A* and *ARF*. Interestingly, these also disrupt the *RB1* and *TP53* checkpoints, respectively. *CDKN2A* also is the most common locus lost in the peripheral chondrosarcomas that arise secondary to osteochondromas.[6]

PTEN is another tumor suppressor gene commonly deleted in sarcomas. Unlike *TP53*, *RB1*, and *CDKN2A*, loss of only one allele of *PTEN* can contribute to oncogenesis by shifting apoptosis pathways and blunting growth signals. *PTEN* is a common site of copy number loss in synovial sarcomas.[7]

Additional copies of other genes contribute to transformation in other malignancies. These oncogenes require no mutations or alterations to make them dangerous, only additional gene copies. Two groups of musculoskeletal neoplasms are characterized by amplification of almost the same region of chromosome 12, usually appearing as an extra ring or rod chromosome.[8] Although recently sequenced to identify all elements contained therein, three genes—*CDK4*, *TSPAN31* (formerly *SAS*), and *MDM2*—have long been recognized to have extra copies on these extra chromosomes. Excess *CDK4* silences *RB1*; excess *MDM2* silences *TP53*. The two tumor types are atypical lipomatous tumors (also called well-differentiated liposarcoma or lipoma-like liposarcoma) and parosteal osteosarcoma.

Although copy number losses and gains at certain genes or chromosomal regions characterize different musculoskeletal neoplasms (**Table 2**), they can be generally grouped into genomically stable neoplasms, which have few copy number variations, and genomically complex and unstable neoplasms, which have rampant copy number variations and significant heterogeneity among cells within each tumor. Osteosarcoma is the typical prototype of genetically complex and unstable neoplasms.[9]

Other genes whose activation or inactivation contributes to oncogenesis not only show an increase or decrease in copy number but must undergo some change to their coding sequence. Mutations can affect genes in a variety of ways. They can change nothing and remain functionally silent mutations (generally

Table 2		

Chromosomal Gains and Losses

Neoplasm	Chromosomal Losses	Chromosomal Gains
Atypical lipomatous tumor (well-differentiated liposarcoma, lipoma-like liposarcoma)		12q14-15
Dedifferentiated liposarcoma		12q14-15
Undifferentiated pleomorphic sarcoma (malignant fibrous histiocytoma)	2p24-pter, 2q32-qter, 11, 13, 16	7p15-pter, 7q32, 1p31
Leiomyosarcoma	3p21-23, 8p21-pter, 13q12-13, 13q32-qter, 1q, 2, 4q, 9p, 10, 11q, 13q, 16	1q21-31, 5p14-pter, 12q13-15, 13q31, 15, 17p11, 19, 20q13, 22, X
Embryonal rhabdomyosarcoma	11p15, 16	2, 8, 13
Alveolar rhabdomyosarcoma		12q13-15, 2p24
Synovial sarcoma	3	7, 8, 12
Osteosarcoma	3q, 4q32-q34, 6q, 13q, 15q, 17p, 18q	1q21-23, 3q26, 4q12-13, 5p13-14, 6p, 7q31-32, 8q21-23, 12q12-15, 17p11-12, 19q12-q13
Parosteal osteosarcoma		12q13-q15
Chondrosarcoma	1p13.3-p33, 4q13.1, 6p12.1-qter, 9p13.1-pter, 10p11.1-pter, 11p13-p15.2, 13q11-q34, 14q21.1-q21.2, 17p12-pter	5p15.2-pter, 5p13.2-p13.3, 5q31.1, 5q34-qter, 12p13.31-pter, 19p13.11-p13.12, 19q12-qter, 20pter-q13.11, 21q22.11-q22.3, 22q11.23-q12.1

called polymorphisms), either because the changed DNA code is just an alternate codon for the same amino acid or because the amino acid change does not affect the protein's function. A mutation can introduce a translational stop codon, yielding a truncated protein with no function or a different function; or a missense mutation can introduce a new amino acid that abrogates or changes the function of the protein. Missense mutations near the catalytic site of an enzyme can completely silence the enzyme's function. This is the case in many inherited silent alleles of *EXT1* and *EXT2*, which lead to multiple osteochondromas.[10] Such silencing missense mutations are less common in transcription factors, but exostosin-1 and exostosin-2 (products of *EXT1* and *EXT2*) are enzymes.

Activating mutations are common in receptor tyrosine kinases (RTKs), such as those active in gastrointestinal stromal tumors.[11] The mutations each essentially make a specific RTK activation independent from ligand binding and therefore constitutively active.

Other genes are afforded new and oncogenic functions by the addition of pieces of other genes. Balanced chromosomal translocations with breakpoints between in-frame exons produce fusion genes, some of which have new functions different from those of either contributing gene. Some of these are as simple as those associated with pigmented villonodular synovitis or tenosynovial giant cell tumor, which simply move an intact macrophage colony-stimulating factor (M-CSF) gene to

a position under the control of a highly expressed promoter, such as the collagen VI gene.[12] Others produce entirely novel proteins, usually combining the functions of the ends of the parent genes. Those that produce novel proteins generally have one end that attaches to DNA or some transcriptional cluster of proteins and another end that has a powerful activator or repressor function. Approximately one third of sarcomas associate with such fusion oncogenes (**Table 3**). Although only *PAX3-FOXO1* (formerly *PAX3-FKHR*), *SS18-SSX2* (formerly *SYT-SSX2*), *EWS-ATF1*, and *FUS-DDIT3* (formerly *FUS-CHOP*) have proved capable of in vivo transformation in mouse models, similar function is expected from the others. Other genes, such as *EWS-FLI1*, have proved to be master regulators of gene transcription.

Changes in Transcription

Even without changes in sequence or copy number, tumor suppressors can be silenced or oncogenes overexpressed by changes in transcriptional activity at a given gene or locus. One means by which cells turn off a gene during development or differentiation is by methylation of the gene's promoter, making it difficult for transcriptional protein complexes to recognize the sequences and bind to initiated transcription. Anywhere a cytosine is adjacent to a guanine residue in the DNA, an en-

Table 3		

Sarcoma Chromosomal Translocations and Fusion Gene Products

Neoplasm	Translocation	Fusion Gene
Alveolar rhabdomyosarcoma	t(2;13)(q35;q14)	*PAX3-FOXO1*
	t(1;13)(q36;q14)	*PAX7-FOXO1*
	t(2;2)(q35;p23)	*PAX3-NCOA1*
Alveolar soft-part sarcoma	t(X;17)(p11;q25)	*ASPSCR1-TFE3*
Aneurysmal bone cyst	17p3 rearrangement	*USP6* increase
Clear-cell sarcoma	t(12;22)(q13;q12)	*EWS-ATF1*
	t(2;22)(q32;q12)	*EWS-CREB1*
Congenital fibrosarcoma	t(12;15)(p13;q25)	*ETV6-NTRK3*
Dermatofibrosarcoma protuberans	t(17;22)(q22;q13)	*COL1A1-PDGFB*
Desmoplastic small round cell tumor	t(11;22)(p13;q11)	*EWS-WT1*
Extraskeletal myxoid chondrosarcoma	t(9;22)(q22;q12)	*EWS-CHN1*
	t(9;17)(q22;q11)	*TAF2N-CHN1*
Ewing sarcoma family of tumors	t(11;22)(q24;q12)	*EWS-FLI1*
	t(21;22)(q22;q12)	*EWS-ERG*
	t(7;22)(p22;q12)	*EWS-ETV1*
	t(2;22)(q33;q12)	*EWS-E1AF*
	t(17;22)(q12;q12)	*EWS-FEV*
Fibromyxoid sarcoma, low grade	t(7;16)(q33;p11)	*FUS-CREB3L2*
	t(11;16)(p11;p11)	*FUS-CREB3L1*
Inflammatory myofibroblastic tumor	t(1;2)(q22;p23)	*TPM3-ALK*
	t(2;19)(p23;p13)	*TPM4-ALK*
Myxoid liposarcoma	t(12;16)(q13;p11)	*FUS-DDIT3*
	t(12;22)(q13;q12)	*EWS-DDIT3*
Pigmented villonodular synovitis	5q33 rearrangement	*CSF1* increase
Synovial sarcoma	t(X;18)(p11;q11)	*SS18-SSX1*
		SS18-SSX2
Undifferentiated bone and soft-tissue sarcomas	t(6;22)(p21;q12)	*SS18-SSX4*
		EWS-OCT4

zyme can add a methyl group to the cytosine residue. Methylated cytosines are copied as such during replication, meaning that these methylated promoters will be maintained in daughter cells. Some cancer cells manage to activate machinery both to increase methylation of the promoters of tumor suppressor genes and to remove methylation of the promoters of oncogenes. In radiation-induced sarcomas, unsilencing of some old viral oncogenes, buried and inactive in the genome before transformation, has been shown. Ewing sarcoma has been found to change transcription of several genes upon administration of 5-aza-2'-deoxycytidine, which removes promoter methylation and unsilences some important tumor suppressors. *RASSF1A* is a gene that has been shown to be silenced by promoter methylation in osteosarcoma, Ewing sarcoma, and synovial sarcoma. Reexpression of the gene by the administration of 5-aza-2'-deoxycytidine explains some of the antitumor effects of this drug in culture conditions.[13-15]

Another method of adjusting gene transcription down is by altering the histone packaging of the DNA. In cells, most DNA is not available to the transcription factors floating around the nucleus. Rather, it is tightly wrapped around histone proteins. How firmly those histones bind and keep unavailable any genomic locus has much to do with the level of histone acetylation. Some malignancies activate histone deacetylase (HDAC) to remove acetyl groups and bind DNA more firmly, making it unavailable for transcription. This is the primary mode of transcriptional control by SS18-SSX proteins in synovial sarcoma.[16] The fusion oncogene *SS18-SSX* creates a bridge between factors that bind the DNA of certain promoters, such as the tumor suppressor *EGR1*, and a repressor complex that activates HDACs to make the *EGR1* promoter less available to transcription.

1: General Evaluation and Treatment of Musculoskeletal Tumors

Microsatellites as a means of changing transcription of genes has received attention in a study of Ewing sarcoma.[17] Microsatellites are regions upstream of the formal promoters of certain genes that are characterized by repetitive sequences; they were previously thought to be junk DNA. Recently, *EWS-FLI1*, the dominant fusion oncogene active in Ewing sarcoma, was noted to primarily bind to these microsatellites near target genes, thus activating the genes.

Changes in Translation

Another level at which gene expression can be regulated is the messenger RNA (mRNA) level, at which transcript longevity and access to translational machinery can be altered for specific genes. The initial product of transcription must be spliced to remove introns and link exons into purely coding sequences, ready for translation. The final mRNA sequences can then be more or less stable, influencing the quantity of polypeptides translated from each. One new area of research has been focused on microRNAs (miRNAs), which are short nucleotide sequences that are never intended to be translated. miRNAs bind to complementary sequences, generally in the 3' untranslated region of mRNA, marking some specific transcripts for degradation. Others are simply blocked from translation. miRNAs can also have a tumor suppressive or oncogenic function, usually by blocking the opposite class of formal genes. In musculoskeletal neoplasia, a few specific entities have had miRNAs profiled using microarray technology.

Synovial sarcomas have upregulation of *miR-99B* and *Let7B*, the blockade of which results in reduced proliferation and survival, suggesting that they are important to the cell's function.[18] Osteosarcomas have reduced expression of *miR-16* family members, the reintroduction of which results in blunted growth.[19] Although the effect is only beginning to be sorted out, the powerful role of miRNAs in development may play a prominent role in the differentiation state of cancer cells.[20]

Changes in Posttranslational Modifications

After proteins are translated, those headed for the cell surface or the extracellular matrix are processed in the Golgi apparatus and coated with a variety of sugar moieties. Here is another level at which a cell may alter its oncogenic potential. Osteochondromas arise after chondrocytes in the growth plate lose both copies of *EXT1* or *EXT2*, which normally function in the Golgi apparatus to add heparan sulfate, a specific sugar moiety.[21] The loss of heparan sulfate at the cell surface and extracellular matrix grants the cell new capacities. Several signaling pathways depend on the presence of heparan sulfate to function properly. Thus, loss of a glycosylation enzyme significantly alters cell signaling.

Changes in Final Protein Stability

Proteins that stay within the cell, functioning in the cytoplasm or nucleus, do not generally receive glycosylation modifications. Nonetheless, a protein's stability and longevity in the cell can be changed. By increasing the stability or longevity of a protein, a cell effectively increases the amount of that protein around at any given time, even without additional expression. Such is the case with β-catenin. Normal β-catenin has a site that can be phosphorylated by an enzyme complex in the cytoplasm. This complex contains the adenomatous polyposis coli (APC) gene, *APC*, commonly silenced in colon cancer. A mutation common in non–*APC*-related colon cancers is in the region that codes for the phosphorylation site in β-catenin itself. Mutations in this region block the phosphorylation that would otherwise target β-catenin for degradation. Such stabilizing mutations in β-catenin do not noticeably change its function, but they significantly lengthen its longevity and therefore increase its prevalence in the cell and its activity. This pathway has been identified in a minority of synovial sarcomas as well as in many desmoid-type fibromatoses.[22-24]

Altered Signaling Pathways

Ultimately, an increase or decrease in the presence or activity of any protein, resulting from changes at the DNA level, in the transcriptional, translational, or posttranslational efficiency, or in the stability of the final product, has various effects on the cell's behavior. In many cases, researchers have identified the important aberrant pathways for a given tumor but do not yet know at what level these pathways are deranged. Malignancies in general, and musculoskeletal neoplasms in particular, harness several developmental pathways that are otherwise silent in fully developed tissues.

One of the most popular topics in the study of carcinomas is the epithelial-mesenchymal transition, in which an epithelial cell loses some of its epithelial characteristics and behaves, temporarily, more like mesenchymal tissues as it moves through tissue planes, invades basement membranes, and metastasizes.[25] The transforming growth factor-beta (TGF-β) superfamily of signaling molecules is thought to be very important in epithelial-mesenchymal transition. Of course, the epithelial-mesenchymal transition cannot occur in existing mesenchymal cells in a sarcoma, but TGF-β signaling may be important for maintaining a dedifferentiated mesenchymal phenotype. Wnt signaling pathways, which lead to β-catenin stabilization and other effects on a cell, have also been implicated in epithelial-mesenchymal transition. The pathways are similarly important in empowering some mesenchymal tumors, although they do not make them more mesenchymal.

In addition, osteosarcomas in which Wnt signaling has been blunted can attain an almost epithelial phenotype and lose their metastatic potential.[26] Although these findings each derive from a rather artificial, albeit elegant, experimental setting, they suggest that the importance of Wnt signaling and even something like the epithelial-mesenchymal transition may apply to musculoskeletal neoplasia.

Hedgehog signaling is another pathway overactive in several musculoskeletal neoplasms, probably through derangements at a variety of levels. Hedgehog signaling was specifically identified as overactive in the cartilaginous lesions of Ollier disease. What is interesting is that the gene mutation that was transferred to mice and led to the discovery of the pathway is specifically mutated in a small number of cases.[27] Nonetheless, an important pathway was discovered.[28]

Summary

Malignancies complicate normal biologic process by repurposing pathways that lead to abnormal conditions. As the understanding of human biology on a cellular and organismic level continues to increase, so will the understanding of the molecular underpinnings of neoplasia. Reciprocally, as cancer pathways are elucidated, normal molecular biology will be clarified.

Annotated References

1. Shackleton M, Quintana E, Fearon ER, Morrison SJ: Heterogeneity in cancer: Cancer stem cells versus clonal evolution. *Cell* 2009;138(5):822-829.

   The authors of this science review article discussed the ongoing debate about the source of the heterogeneity observed within any given tumor.

2. Hanahan D, Weinberg RA: The hallmarks of cancer. *Cell* 2000;100(1):57-70.

3. Hanahan D, Weinberg RA: Hallmarks of cancer: The next generation. *Cell* 2011;144(5):646-674.

   The authors updated the classic "hallmarks of cancer" article from 2000 with consideration of inflammation, microenvironment, and alternate cellular metabolism to the prior list of characteristics and capacities that identify a tumor as malignant.

4. Ito M, Barys L, O'Reilly T, et al: Comprehensive mapping of p53 pathway alterations reveals an apparent role for both SNP309 and MDM2 amplification in sarcomagenesis. *Clin Cancer Res* 2011;17(3):416-426.

   TP53 is the most important single cancer gene generally in the study of oncology. The authors of this article dissect its pathway, specifically regarding sarcomas and some of the alternate means of disrupting the p53 pathway.

5. Walkley CR, Qudsi R, Sankaran VG, et al: Conditional mouse osteosarcoma, dependent on p53 loss and potentiated by loss of Rb, mimics the human disease. *Genes Dev* 2008;22(12):1662-1676.

   The authors reported on a mouse model and highlight the power of disrupting both the p53 and Rb pathways in the generation of osteosarcomas.

6. Hallor KH, Staaf J, Bovée JV, et al: Genomic profiling of chondrosarcoma: Chromosomal patterns in central and peripheral tumors. *Clin Cancer Res* 2009;15(8): 2685-2694.

   The authors of this article reported on an effort to decipher the chromosomal and genetic aberrations of different types of chondrosarcoma, specifically noting the difference between central and peripheral chondrosarcomas, driven variably by hedgehog signaling and the loss of *CDKN2A*, respectively.

7. Barretina J, Taylor BS, Banerji S, et al: Subtype-specific genomic alterations define new targets for soft-tissue sarcoma therapy. *Nat Genet* 2010;42(8):715-721.

   The authors of this tour-de-force genetic assessment by microarray of a broad group of soft-tissue sarcoma subtypes identified the common genetic aberrations in each type.

8. Garsed DW, Holloway AJ, Thomas DM: Cancer-associated neochromosomes: A novel mechanism of oncogenesis. *Bioessays* 2009;31(11):1191-1200.

   One mechanism of oncogene amplification is adding copies of the gene in a new, distinct chromosome. Such neochromosomes are common in certain sarcoma subtypes.

9. Selvarajah S, Yoshimoto M, Ludkovski O, et al: Genomic signatures of chromosomal instability and osteosarcoma progression detected by high resolution array CGH and interphase FISH. *Cytogenet Genome Res* 2008;122(1):5-15.

   Osteosarcoma is the prototype complex-genetic sarcoma, characterized not only by genetic instability on a cellular basis but also by its effects, noted as widespread chromosomal and genetic aberrations that often vary from cell to cell.

10. Pedrini E, Jennes I, Tremosini M, et al: Genotype-phenotype correlation study in 529 patients with multiple hereditary exostoses: Identification of "protective" and "risk" factors. *J Bone Joint Surg Am* 2011; 93(24):2294-2302.

    This is the largest population-based study of the multiple osteochondromas phenotype, with detailed analysis of the effect of genetically defined subgroups.

11. Jones AV, Cross NC: Oncogenic derivatives of platelet-derived growth factor receptors. *Cell Mol Life Sci* 2004;61(23):2912-2923.

12. West RB, Rubin BP, Miller MA, et al: A landscape effect in tenosynovial giant-cell tumor from activation of CSF1 expression by a translocation in a minority of tumor cells. *Proc Natl Acad Sci U S A* 2006;103(3):690-695.

13. Lim S, Yang MH, Park JH, et al: Inactivation of the RASSF1A in osteosarcoma. *Oncol Rep* 2003;10(4):897-901.

14. Numoto K, Yoshida A, Sugihara S, et al: Frequent methylation of RASSF1A in synovial sarcoma and the anti-tumor effects of 5-aza-2'-deoxycytidine against synovial sarcoma cell lines. *J Cancer Res Clin Oncol* 2010;136(1):17-25.

    The authors provide examples of the effect of methylation on the biology of a sarcoma, as well as the power of pharmacologic reversal of that methylation.

15. Avigad S, Shukla S, Naumov I, et al: Aberrant methylation and reduced expression of RASSF1A in Ewing sarcoma. *Pediatr Blood Cancer* 2009;53(6):1023-1028.

    The authors discussed RASSF1A and provided examples of the effect of methylation and its clinical significance in Ewing sarcoma.

16. Su L, Sampaio AV, Jones KB, et al: Deconstruction of the SS18-SSX fusion oncoprotein complex: Insights into disease etiology and therapeutics. *Cancer Cell* 2012;21(3):333-347.

    The authors of this article dissected one of the mechanisms by which the fusion gene product of the t(X;18) translocation in synovial sarcoma exerts influence on gene expression.

17. Gangwal K, Sankar S, Hollenhorst PC, et al: Microsatellites as EWS/FLI response elements in Ewing's sarcoma. *Proc Natl Acad Sci U S A* 2008;105(29):10149-10154.

    The authors of this article explored the biology of the *EWS-FLI1* fusion oncogene of Ewing sarcoma, specifically deciphering how the protein binds to what were considered junk DNA sequences as a means of joining transcriptional complexes and controlling transcription of target genes.

18. Hisaoka M, Matsuyama A, Nagao Y, et al: Identification of altered MicroRNA expression patterns in synovial sarcoma. *Genes Chromosomes Cancer* 2011;50(3):137-145.

    The authors investigated the effect of microRNA expression on the characteristics of different types of sarcoma, both their cancer characteristics and their stunted differentiation.

19. Jones KB, Salah Z, Del Mare S, et al: miRNA signatures associate with pathogenesis and progression of osteosarcoma. *Cancer Res* 2012;72(7):1865-1877.

    The authors identified a microRNA signature associated with pathogenesis of osteosarcoma, along with pretreatment biomarkers for metastasis and therapy response.

20. Danielson LS, Menendez S, Attolini CS, et al: A differentiation-based microRNA signature identifies leiomyosarcoma as a mesenchymal stem cell-related malignancy. *Am J Pathol* 2010;177(2):908-917.

    The authors reported on a microRNA signature associated with smooth muscle differentiation of mesenchymal stem cells.

21. Jones KB: Glycobiology and the growth plate: Current concepts in multiple hereditary exostoses. *J Pediatr Orthop* 2011;31(5):577-586.

    The authors of this article discussed the evolving science of glycobiology and its specific effect on multiple osteochondromas.

22. Subramaniam MM, Calabuig-Fariñas S, Pellin A, Llombart-Bosch A: Mutational analysis of E-cadherin, β-catenin and APC genes in synovial sarcomas. *Histopathology* 2010;57(3):482-486.

    The authors of this study analyzed the application in synovial sarcoma of a pathway well characterized in colorectal carcinoma, and found similar genetic disruptions in both cancers regarding this pathway.

23. Cheon SS, Cheah AY, Turley S, et al: beta-Catenin stabilization dysregulates mesenchymal cell proliferation, motility, and invasiveness and causes aggressive fibromatosis and hyperplastic cutaneous wounds. *Proc Natl Acad Sci U S A* 2002;99(10):6973-6978.

24. Le Guellec S, Soubeyran I, Rochaix P, et al: CTNNB1 mutation analysis is a useful tool for the diagnosis of desmoid tumors: A study of 260 desmoid tumors and 191 potential morphologic mimics. *Mod Pathol* 2012;25(12):1551-1558.

    The authors of this study established the association that led to appreciation for a causative role of mutations in the β-catenin gene in desmoid fibromatoses.

25. Mani SA, Guo W, Liao MJ, et al: The epithelial-mesenchymal transition generates cells with properties of stem cells. *Cell* 2008;133(4):704-715.

    The authors of this landmark article reviewed a hot topic in the current world of cancer biology, in which cancer cells are thought to use certain genetic programs from development to attain characteristics necessary for their function as cancer cells.

26. Guo Y, Rubin EM, Xie J, Zi X, Hoang BH: Dominant negative LRP5 decreases tumorigenicity and metastasis of osteosarcoma in an animal model. *Clin Orthop Relat Res* 2008;466(9):2039-2045.

    This article is one of the first to recognize the importance of a reverse of the so-called epithelial-mesenchymal transition that impairs osteosarcoma in the same manner as with carcinoma cells.

27. Hopyan S, Gokgoz N, Poon R, et al: A mutant PTH/PTHrP type I receptor in enchondromatosis. *Nat Genet* 2002;30(3):306-310.

28. Tiet TD, Hopyan S, Nadesan P, et al: Constitutive hedgehog signaling in chondrosarcoma up-regulates tumor cell proliferation. *Am J Pathol* 2006;168(1):321-330.

Chapter 5

Pseudotumors and Tumorlike Lesions

Raffi S. Avedian, MD

1: General Evaluation and Treatment of Musculoskeletal Tumors

Introduction

Many conditions, ranging from metabolic disease to traumatic injury, can mimic bone tumors and soft-tissue tumors. It is important for clinicians and radiologists to be aware of these entities in order to include them in the differential diagnosis for patients with bone and soft-tissue abnormalities and avoid unnecessary diagnostic tests or invasive procedures. Distinguishing a true neoplastic bone tumor from a pseudotumor may not be straightforward at initial presentation, and requires that the treating physician conduct a thorough history, physical examination, and review of appropriate diagnostic tests. The purpose of this chapter is to review some of the more common musculoskeletal conditions that mimic bone and soft-tissue tumors.

Infection

Osteomyelitis occurs in both adults and children and may be difficult to distinguish from a bone tumor.[1] In children, hematogenous spread of infection is more likely than by direct extension from surrounding tissues, whereas in adults, hematogenous seeding is less common.[2] The clinical presentation and course of osteomyelitis varies greatly and depends on several factors including virulence of the infecting organism, the patient's ability to fight infection, local tissue status, and appropriateness of medical and surgical care.[3,4] Patients with acute osteomyelitis often have bone pain, fever, and at times no clear source of infection. Examination may reveal swelling and tenderness at the site of infection similar to that found with bone sarcomas. Chronic osteomyelitis or subacute osteomyelitis can cause relatively minor symptoms aside from mild discomfort at the site of disease, and physical examination may not be revealing. Depending on the timing and severity of the infection, radiographs may demonstrate

no obvious abnormality or alternatively may demonstrate a geographic or even permeative pattern of bone destruction. A lamellar periosteal reaction similar to that seen in Ewing sarcoma can be present in acute infections, whereas a solid, mature periosteal new bone formation similar to that seen in osteoid osteoma can be encountered with chronic infections (**Figure 1**). The T2-weighted and T1-weighted MRI of infected bone show high and low signal, respectively. This is very similar to the appearance of bone tumors. However, when a bone abscess is present, gadolinium-enhanced MRI typically demonstrates only peripheral enhancement of the lesion rather than internal enhancement, which may help distinguish it from a neoplastic process. Appropriate treatment of osteomyelitis relies on a timely and accurate diagnosis. A thorough history and physical examination should be obtained to identify risk factors such as immune deficiency, poor nutrition, previous trauma, and travel history. Laboratory tests should include erythrocyte sedimentation rate and C-reactive protein, which are typically elevated in cases of bacterial osteomyelitis. However, a minority of patients have normal inflammatory markers in spite of active infection, especially if tested early in the course of the disease or in cases of chronic smoldering infection.[5-7] Once the diagnosis of osteomyelitis is made, treatment should focus on an appropriate course of antibiotics and aggressive surgical débridement of the sequestrum and other devitalized tissues.[8]

Inflammatory Conditions

Sarcoidosis

Sarcoidosis is a disorder of unknown etiology that is characterized by the formation of noncaseating granulomas in tissues without any other identifiable cause. Sarcoidosis may involve any organ system, the most common being the lungs, lymph nodes, skin, and eyes. It is estimated that 5% of patients will have musculoskeletal involvement.[9] Sarcoidosis involving bone classically is described as involving the short tubular bones of the hands and feet, where the diagnosis is straightforward, especially in a patient known to have sarcoidosis.[10,11] However, when lesions are found in other

---

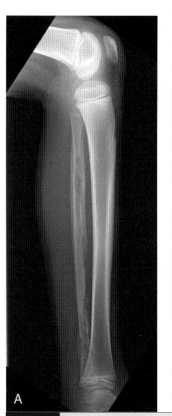
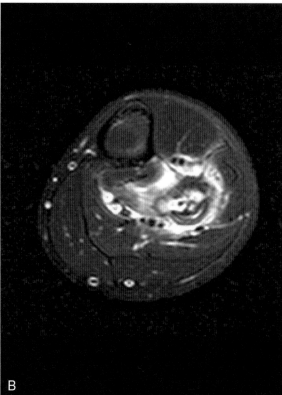
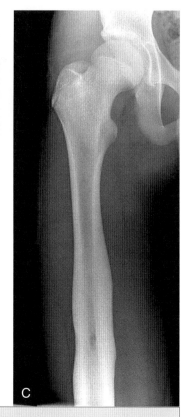

Figure 1 **A,** Lateral tibia-fibula radiograph of a 7-year-old girl shows osteomyelitis of the fibula. Notice the lamellar periosteal reaction, saucerization of the posterior cortex, and permeative bone destruction, which is similar to findings in Ewing sarcoma. **B,** Axial T2-weighted MRI of the lower leg demonstrates cortical disruption of the fibula with an associated large soft-tissue abscess and surrounding edema that can mimic the appearance of a bone sarcoma. **C,** AP radiograph of the femur of a 14-year-old boy shows chronic osteomyelitis. Notice the solid periosteal new bone formation along most of the bone. The small cortical break represents the location of the intramedullary infection breaking out into the soft tissues (better seen on MRI; not shown).

skeletal sites such as the spine, they can appear very similar to metastatic bone disease, and rendering a correct diagnosis on the basis of imaging alone is difficult. Sarcoid lesions in the spine and long bones demonstrate a variable appearance. They may appear as well-defined, round multifocal lesions, diffuse marrow infiltration, or larger, round cannonball-like lesions.[12] However, it is rare to see extensive bone destruction with these lesions. Sarcoid lesions demonstrate variability in signal intensity on T1-weighted, T2-weighted, proton density, and gadolinium-enhanced MRI sequences. Occasionally, lesions have signal characteristics similar to fat, which helps differentiate them from metastatic malignancy (**Figure 2**). In a study evaluating the ability to distinguish metastatic carcinoma from sarcoidosis using MRI, the authors compared 22 patients with metastatic disease with 12 patients with osseous sarcoidosis for a total of 79 lesions. The results showed 97.4% specificity but only 46.3% sensitivity and interobserver concordance of 0.364, indicating a fair agreement among radiologists.[13] The authors concluded that sarcoid lesions of bone could not be reliably distinguished from metastatic disease. The ability to arrive at a correct diagnosis therefore relies on the correlation of information gained from history, imaging, and histology, if available.

Gout

Gout, or monosodium urate crystal deposition disease, is characterized biochemically by extracellular fluid urate saturation. The clinical manifestations include recurrent attacks of acute inflammatory arthritis, chronic arthropathy, accumulation of urate crystals in the form of tophaceous deposits, or uric acid nephrolithiasis. In some cases, chronic uric acid deposition with the associated inflammatory process leads to bone destruction that may be seen as end-stage joint degeneration or the classic "rat bite" eccentric bone defect along the first metatarsal. At times, extensive bone destruction and soft-tissue mineralization can mimic chondrosarcoma (**Figure 3**). As with other inflammatory joint conditions, the diagnosis is based on recognizing that the pathology is joint based, with erosive changes on both sides of the joint, a finding unlikely to be seen with malignant tumors. In addition to osseous manifestations, tophaceous gout deposits can occur within tendons, resulting in joint pain, trigger finger, carpal tunnel syndrome, and rotator cuff impingement.[14-16] Treatment involves collabora-

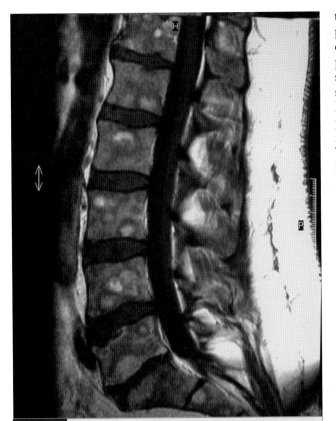

Figure 2 Sagittal T1-weighted MRI shows the lumbar spine in a 38-year-old man with sarcoidosis. Notice the well-marginated round lesions, some of which are high signal, indicating the presence of fat, while others are low to intermediate signal.

tion between the rheumatologist and orthopaedic surgeon with the goal of lowering serum uric acid levels, minimizing gout attacks, and surgically addressing symptoms associated with joint degeneration, painful tophi, and soft-tissue damage from tophaceous deposits.

Metabolic Bone Diseases

Tumoral Calcinosis

Tumoral calcinosis is a rare disorder characterized by periarticular calcium phosphate deposition most commonly into the soft tissues near the hips, shoulders, and elbows.[17] The disease may be classified into three forms; one type is without hyperphosphatemia and is associated with dental anomalies and elevated serum levels of 1,25-dihydroxyvitamin D. Another form occurs in dialysis patients, and the third type is associated with hyperphosphatemia and normal or elevated levels of calcium and 1,25-dihydroxyvitamin D. The latter form is thought to be inherited in an autosomal recessive manner.

Although the exact pathomechanics of tumoral calcinosis are not completely understood, most investiga-

tors think that mutations in genes responsible for phosphate homeostasis are responsible for the development of the familial type of tumoral calcinosis. Endocrine pathways that interconnect the kidneys, intestines, and skeleton tightly regulate serum phosphate levels. Researchers have suggested that disruption in these regulatory pathways results in deposition of calcium phosphate minerals into the soft tissue and is in part responsible for the development of tumoral calcinosis.[18] The clinical presentation of tumoral calcinosis is varied. In severe cases, extensive mineralization leads to significant functional deficits, discomfort, and skin ulcerations. Other patients have few to no symptoms or dysfunction.[19] Radiographs demonstrate periarticular soft-tissue mineralization arranged in a confluent lobular pattern. The size of the mineralization varies, but in some cases it may be extremely large. MRI is not necessary to make the diagnosis, but is helpful in confirming that the tumoral calcinosis is physically distinct from the underlying bone, which helps rule out a juxtacortical osteosarcoma or chondrosarcoma (**Figure 4**).

The treatment of tumoral calcinosis should focus on reversing the underlying metabolic abnormality. In patients with familial high serum phosphate levels, medical treatment with aluminum, phosphate binders, and/or low-phosphate, low-calcium diets may be helpful.[19-21] In dialysis patients, partial or total parathyroidectomy is usually effective.[22] Surgical excision has high recurrence and complication rates, and should be reserved for situations where medical management is not successful or the patient is experiencing significant dysfunction or pain.[21,23] Some authors have reported good results for surgical excision in infants, but these have been only small case series or case reports.[24,25]

Paget Disease of Bone

Paget disease of bone (PDB), also known as osteitis deformans, is a metabolic disorder of bone characterized by increased bone remodeling, resulting in overgrowth of bone at a single site or multiple sites and impaired integrity of affected bone. Commonly affected areas include the skull, spine, pelvis, and long bones of the lower extremities. The majority of patients with PDB are asymptomatic. The diagnosis in such patients is usually made incidentally following a routine chemistry screen showing an elevated serum alkaline phosphatase level of bone origin or an imaging study obtained for some other reason that shows pagetic changes in bone.

PDB is a relatively common finding in older people of European descent, with an estimated prevalence of 2% to 9% in those older than 40 years.[26] The pathophysiology is not entirely clear but is thought to be osteoclast mediated. The rationale for this theory is that osteoclasts from patients with Paget disease are atypical in appearance, are hypersensitive to vitamin D, and have intranuclear inclusion bodies that are not seen in osteoblasts, and patients improve with bisphosphonate therapy.[27,28] Genetic factors influence the development of PDB, and inheritance appears to be autosomal dom-

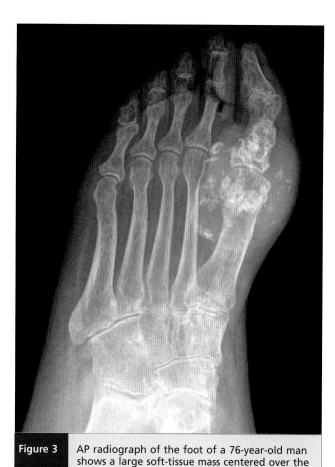

Figure 3 AP radiograph of the foot of a 76-year-old man shows a large soft-tissue mass centered over the first metatarsophalangeal joint with peripheral mineralization reminiscent of a chondrosarcoma. The disease process involved both sides of the joint, suggesting a joint-based process; fluid analysis confirmed the diagnosis of gout.

outer table of the skull. In the long bones, PDB typically extends from one end of the bone into the diaphysis, with the leading edge of the disease process having the appearance of flame-shaped or "blade of grass" osteolysis.[31] The inactive or sclerotic phase of the disease is characterized by cortical thickening, trabecular coarsening, and bone enlargement. In the skull and spine this sclerotic appearance can be mistaken for sclerotic metastasis. Although radiographs are sufficient to make the diagnosis, laboratory tests can be performed to aid in diagnosing and monitoring the disease. The most useful finding is a high serum alkaline phosphatase level, which reflects the high bone turnover rate. Urine tests may reveal collagen type I breakdown products, including pyridinium cross-links.

Treatment of PDB is geared toward alleviating symptoms and minimizing future complications that could occur if the disease were to progress. Treatment therefore must be tailored to the individual on the basis of the patient's symptoms and site of disease. Pain and other problems associated with rapid bone turnover can be alleviated with bisphosphonate therapy.[32] The results of a recent randomized study that examined the difference between intensive bisphosphonate therapy compared to standard bisphosphonate therapy demonstrated no difference between the two groups with respect to quality of life, pain, and audiology outcome measures.[33] Surgical intervention is indicated to treat degenerative joint disease, neural compression from bone hypertrophy, fracture, or unacceptable deformity. Excessive bleeding may be encountered at the time of surgery because of the vascular nature of pagetic bone. Treating patients with bisphosphonates before surgery can help minimize this problem.[34]

Hyperparathyroidism

Lytic bone lesions can occur in patients who have increased levels of parathyroid hormone from either a primary or secondary hyperparathyroidism. Terms used to describe these bone lesions include osteitis fibrosa cystica and brown tumor. Patients may have either single or multiple lesions that have the appearance of lucent bone tumors such as aneurysmal bone cyst, giant cell tumor, myeloma, and metastatic carcinoma (**Figure 5**). Both primary and secondary hyperparathyroidism result in elevated levels of serum parathyroid hormone, a finding that helps differentiate this disease process from hypercalcemia of malignancy. Histologic examination reveals numerous giant cells in a benign-appearing, fibroblast-rich background. Hemosiderin staining of the giant cells led to the term brown tumor of hyperparathyroidism. Because of the appearance rich in giant cells, brown tumors can easily be confused with giant cell tumor of bone and aneurysmal bone cyst. Age of the patient and clinical presentation can help narrow the differential diagnosis. Treatment consists of reversing the endocrine abnormality that is the underlying cause of the elevated hyperparathyroid hormone level. Once this has been accomplished, rapid

inant with variable penetrance. At least seven genetic loci that are associated with PDB have been mapped; the best documented of these is the P392L mutation in the ubiquitin-associated domain of *SQSTM1* (gene map locus 5q35).[29] Earlier theories that viral infection contributes to the pathogenesis of PDB remain controversial.[30]

As noted previously, most patients with PDB are asymptomatic. When patients do become symptomatic, the most common complaint is pain that is due to the pagetic lesion in bone itself or from secondary consequences of bone overgrowth and deformity in affected areas. Problems that patients develop include nerve compression syndromes, hearing loss, arthritis, headache, fractures, and rarely secondary bone sarcoma. Abnormalities in calcium and phosphate balance can also occur.

The diagnosis of PDB is usually made on the basis of radiographic findings, which can vary depending on the phase of the disease. The lytic or active phase of the disease is characterized by osteoporosis circumscripta cranii that appears as a band of lucency deep to the

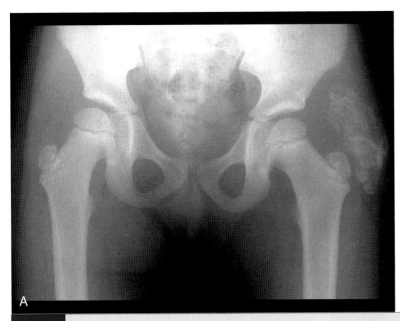

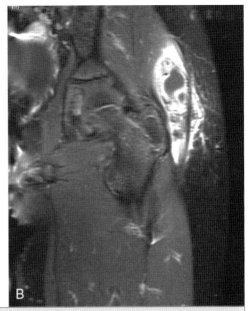

Figure 4 **A,** AP pelvis radiograph of a 3-year-old girl shows a prominent soft-tissue mass along her left lateral hip that her family noted would increase and decrease in size. The lobulated mineralization is typical for tumoral calcinosis, but is reminiscent of low-grade surface osteosarcoma and periosteal chondrosarcoma. **B,** Coronal T1-weighted, fat-suppressed, gadolinium-enhanced MRI reveals the sometimes cystic nature of tumoral calcinosis with associated edema in the surrounding soft tissues. Notice that the mass is distinct from the underlying bone, which helps rule out a periosteal chondrosarcoma or parosteal osteosarcoma. This patient was treated with phosphate binders and a low-phosphate, low-calcium diet, and the most recent radiograph (not shown) showed that the mass had almost disappeared.

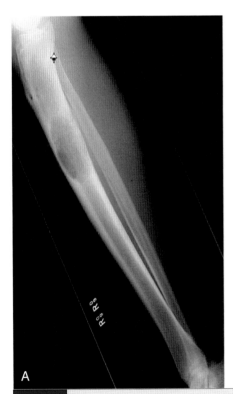

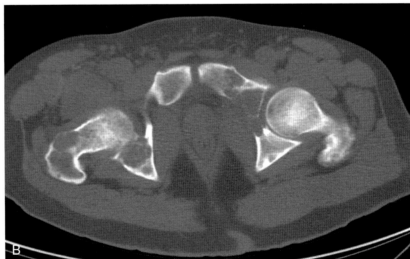

Figure 5 **A,** Lateral tibia-fibula radiograph of a 33-year-old man with end-stage renal disease shows a large lytic bone lesion. The lesion appears very similar to metastatic disease, aneurysmal bone cyst, and myeloma but is a brown tumor resulting from secondary hyperparathyroidism. **B,** Axial pelvic CT scan of the same patient demonstrates multiple lytic bone lesions that can easily be confused with metastatic disease or myeloma.

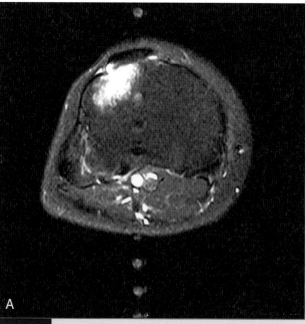
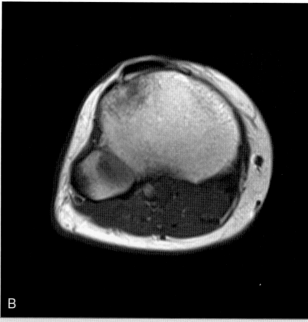

Figure 6 **A,** Axial T2-weighted MRI of a 70-year-old woman with newly diagnosed soft-tissue sarcoma shows a lesion along the proximal tibia that was incidentally noted and caused concern for metastases. **B,** Axial T1-weighted MRI shows bone marrow edema. Note that the lesion is less pronounced than on the T2-weighted images and that normal marrow fat (high signal) is seen interspersed diffusely through the lesion. In spite of the lack of symptoms, a presumed diagnosis of stress reaction was made, and the lesion was no longer evident on repeat imaging 9 weeks later.

healing of the bone lesions is often seen.[35] Orthopaedic surgical intervention is reserved for fractures, impending fractures, or extensive deformity.

Posttraumatic Conditions and Overuse Syndromes

Stress-Reactive Lesions

Stress-reactive lesions include stress fractures, chronic stress periostitis (shin splints), and tendon avulsion injuries. Although more common in athletic individuals, these injuries can occur in any age group and in individuals who have no history of trauma or athletic participation. The most common locations for stress fractures are the tibia, tarsal navicular, metatarsal, fibula, femur, pelvis, and spine.[36,37] Upper extremity stress fractures can occur but are much less common. The radiographic appearance varies from no appreciable abnormality on plain radiographs to extensive periosteal reaction that can mimic benign and malignant bone tumors such as osteoid osteoma or Ewing sarcoma. In most cases MRI can distinguish a stress fracture from a more aggressive process by demonstrating a linear signal abnormality on all sequences, representing a fracture line. Malignancy, on the other hand, is associated with diffuse signal abnormalities and bone destruction.[38] Although most stress-related abnormalities are due to an obvious trauma or overuse type of physical activity, occasionally bone lesions are noted inciden-

tally on imaging studies obtained for unrelated reasons and are not associated with any type of injury. With this type of presentation, the combination of absent trauma history and the nonspecific edema seen on MRI can lead to an incorrect diagnosis of neoplasm. However, most stress-reactive lesions seen on MRI typically have more pronounced edema signal on T2-weighted images than on T1-weighted images and in general are ill defined. Normal marrow fat signal is often present and easily seen interspersed through the edema on T1-weighted images (**Figure 6**). In contrast, neoplasms typically appear as well-defined, marrow-replacing lesions on T1-weighted images.[31]Chronic stress periostitis (shin splints) is seen in runners and can be confused with tumor, but is easily diagnosed on the basis of history. However, atypical presentations of traction periostitis may be confused with tumor.[39]

Myositis Ossificans

Myositis ossificans is a reactive condition characterized by bone formation in the soft tissues commonly as a result of trauma, surgical incisions, and burns. Although the typical presentation is in men aged 20 to 40 years, there are reports of myositis ossificans occurring as early as 10 weeks of age.[40] The radiographic appearance of this lesion can elicit suspicion of malignancy, especially when the patient has no clear history of trauma. The MRI characteristics depend on the maturity of the lesion. In the early phase the lesion will have mixed low signal on T1-weighted images and heteroge-

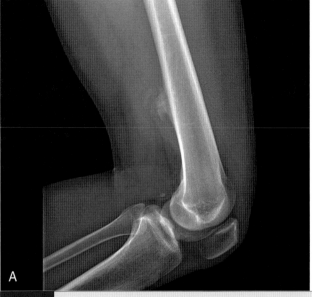
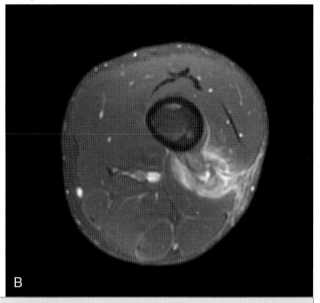

Figure 7 **A,** Lateral radiograph of a 16-year-old boy who was hit in the thigh while playing soccer demonstrates a bone-forming lesion along the posterior distal femur. **B,** Axial T1-weighted, fat-suppressed postgadolinium MRI demonstrates marked enhancement of the lesion. The radiographic and MRI appearance initially elicited suspicion of a parosteal osteosarcoma; however, biopsy was consistent with reactive bone formation, and follow-up imaging demonstrated progressive resolution of the lesion.

neous high signal on T2-weighted images with enhancement after administration of a contrast agent; these findings are very similar to soft-tissue or bone sarcomas (**Figure 7**). In the mature phase, myositis ossificans appears as mature bone with low signal on T2-weighted images and high internal signal on T1-weighted images consistent with normal bone marrow fat. In a recent study, the authors outlined diagnostic clues to help differentiate myositis ossificans from neoplasm.[41] They stressed the importance of understanding the so-called zone phenomenon whereby, on histology, myositis ossificans begins as mesenchymal cells with fibroblasts secreting a myxoid matrix, then in the subacute phase the fibroblasts differentiate into osteoblasts and produce immature bone, and in the chronic phase, as this process matures, bone formation is seen in the periphery of the lesion. This phenomenon is reflected in radiographic studies of myositis ossificans, where mineralization is seen in the periphery, whereas in osteosarcoma bone formation is primarily seen centrally. Parosteal osteosarcoma can appear similar to myositis ossificans, but the former arises from the surface of bone and may have a soft-tissue component along its periphery. These features are not seen with myositis ossificans[31] (**Figure 8**).

Myonecrosis

Calcific myonecrosis is most often a late complication of untreated compartment syndrome characterized by replacement of muscle with a calcified mass. Distinguishing it from a neoplastic process can be difficult because often the responsible traumatic event occurred decades ago, there may be chronic erosions in surrounding bone, and patients will often have new-onset pain indirectly related to the myonecrosis.[42,43] The key to making a correct diagnosis is to elicit a history of trauma and recognize that the calcified mass has a typical fusiform shape and has replaced a muscle group (**Figure 9**). The treatment of myonecrosis involves recognizing that it is a chronic and benign problem and avoiding unnecessary tests or invasive procedures. For symptomatic patients, supportive care is usually sufficient given that most patients' symptoms are indirectly related to the myonecrosis and are self-limited. Aggressive surgical treatment can lead to complications such as wound dehiscence, draining sinus, and excessive bleeding, and in most cases the morbidity outweighs potential benefits.[44]

Avulsive Cortical Irregularity

Avulsive cortical irregularity is a term that describes cortically based bone lesions that occur at sites of tendon insertions and are thought to result from traction or avulsion of the tendon at its insertion site. Variability in the nomenclature of this entity, including cortical desmoid; tug lesion; shin splints; and periosteal, parosteal, and juxtacortical desmoid can lead to confusion regarding the nature of this lesion; however, all of these terms refer to the spectrum of benign bone lesions that occur at tendon insertion sites.[45] These lesions are reactive rather than neoplastic in nature, and occur most often in children and young adults after a minor, often sports-related, injury. The most common locations are the insertion of the gastrocnemius along the posterior medial femoral condyle and the adductor magnus insertion along the medial distal femur. In most cases it is

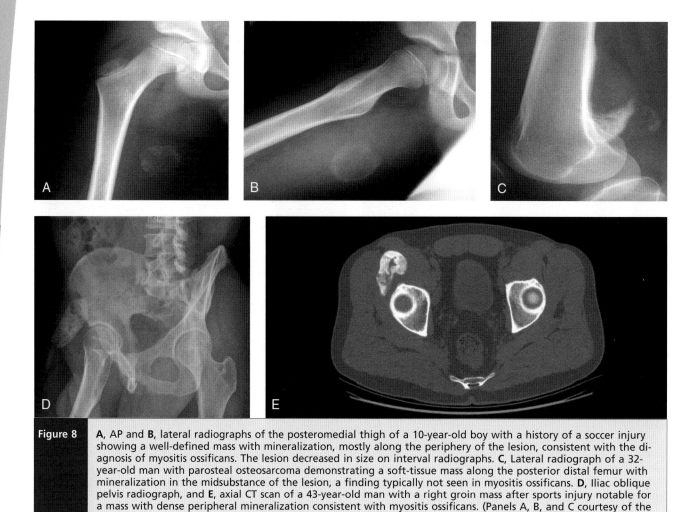

Figure 8 **A**, AP and **B**, lateral radiographs of the posteromedial thigh of a 10-year-old boy with a history of a soccer injury showing a well-defined mass with mineralization, mostly along the periphery of the lesion, consistent with the diagnosis of myositis ossificans. The lesion decreased in size on interval radiographs. **C**, Lateral radiograph of a 32-year-old man with parosteal osteosarcoma demonstrating a soft-tissue mass along the posterior distal femur with mineralization in the midsubstance of the lesion, a finding typically not seen in myositis ossificans. **D**, Iliac oblique pelvis radiograph, and **E**, axial CT scan of a 43-year-old man with a right groin mass after sports injury notable for a mass with dense peripheral mineralization consistent with myositis ossificans. (Panels A, B, and C courtesy of the University of Chicago, Department of Orthopaedic Surgery, Chicago, IL; D and E courtesy of Dr. Kathryn Stevens, Stanford Radiology, Stanford, CA.)

thought that the lesion is the result of chronic traction and is in fact present before it is noticed on radiographs taken at the time of an acute injury (**Figure 10**). The lesion may be mistaken for an aggressive neoplastic process when the patient has had an injury and there is an "acute on chronic" appearance of the lesion, such as edema in the surrounding bone marrow and soft tissues.[46,47] The correct diagnosis can be made, however, by knowing that avulsive cortical irregularities exist and recognizing that the underlying lesion does in fact have a well-marginated benign appearance, often with a sclerotic border. These lesions are self-limited and require no specific treatment.

Bone Infarcts

Bone infarcts, also called osteonecrosis, occur as a result of ischemia to bone and marrow cells resulting in tissue death. The etiology of this disorder is not clear; however, there are well-known associations with sickle cell anemia, chronic steroid use, alcohol abuse, Gaucher disease, dysbarism, lupus, renal transplantation, and other factors. Bone infarcts in the metadiaphysis can appear similar to cartilaginous tumors such as enchondromas, and have a typical pattern of serpentine bands of sclerosis separating the central area of necrosis from the surrounding normal bone. However, early in the natural history of infarcts the lesion appears lucent and mimics a lytic bone tumor. MRI is helpful in distinguishing osteonecrosis from neoplastic processes. On T1-weighted images, infarction appears as a well-defined serpentine rim of low signal intensity. On T2-weighted images, the rim may be low signal or high signal. The presence of parallel bands of low and high signal, called the double line sign, is essentially pathognomonic for bone infarction.[31] Inside the rim the bone appears mostly similar to the surrounding normal fat. On T1-weighted images, the fat signal may be interspersed with poorly defined bands of low to intermediate signal that represent fibrosis or sclerotic bone.

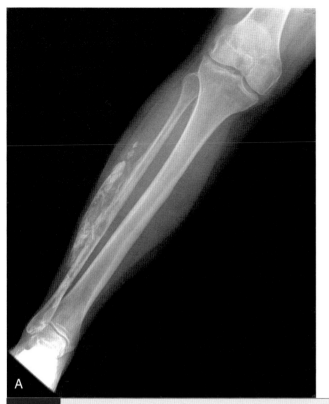

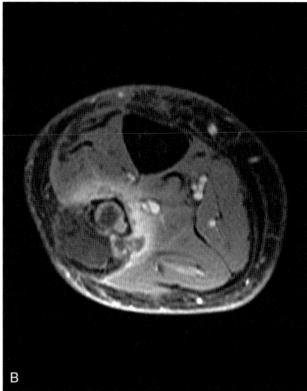

Figure 9 AP radiograph of the leg of a 57-year-old woman with a remote history of trauma that she could not recall in full detail except that she experienced severe swelling and ecchymosis and was under the influence of alcohol when the trauma occurred. She recently developed pain in her leg without any appreciable inciting event. **A,** Calcific mass with lucent lesion that proved to be a fracture that resolved on subsequent imaging is seen. **B,** Axial T1-weighted, fat-suppressed, gadolinium-enhanced MRI demonstrates complete replacement of the lateral compartment of the lower leg with a calcific mass, likely resulting from previous compartment syndrome. Fracture of the fibula with surrounding edema is noted.

Hemorrhagic Disorders

Patients on anticoagulation therapy or patients who have bleeding disorders such as hemophilia can experience repetitive hemorrhage in or around bony structures that results in tumorlike lesions. Bleeding into the soft tissues results in hematoma that can mimic a soft-tissue sarcoma with a hemorrhagic component. Contrast MRI of the hematoma will demonstrate peripheral enhancement with no internal nodularity to suggest neoplasm, and a diagnosis of hematoma can be made. In cases where the MRI characteristics are equivocal, a biopsy may be indicated. Chronic hematomas can enlarge and erode into bone. More recently, the pathophysiology of the lesion has been identified as recurrent hemorrhage into muscle, followed by encapsulation and calcification. The mass can continue to enlarge and erode into adjacent bone. Hemorrhage can also occur directly within bone. Because the pseudotumor is a response of bone to hemorrhage, the radiographic appearance will vary depending on the location and severity of the lesion. In skeletally immature patients,

hematomas canoccur in an intraosseous or subperiosteal location. In the acute or subacute setting, this type of hematoma can resemble an aggressive benign bone tumor or bone sarcoma. Imaging often is not sufficient to distinguish neoplasm from acute hematoma; therefore a biopsy must be performed in most cases to determine the correct diagnosis.

Summary

Nonneoplastic condition such as trauma, metabolic bone disease, inflammatory disease, and repetitive stress can produce bone lesions that have the radiographic appearance of tumors. Incorrect diagnosis can lead to unnecessary tests and procedures that ultimately prolong a patient's suffering and contribute to patient and physician frustration. Clinician awareness of these lesions facilitates an accurate differential diagnosis. A thorough history and physical examination provide the appropriate context to interpret radiographs and are critical to the clinician's ability to render a correct diag-

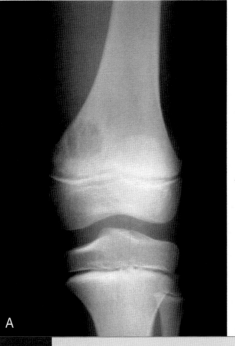
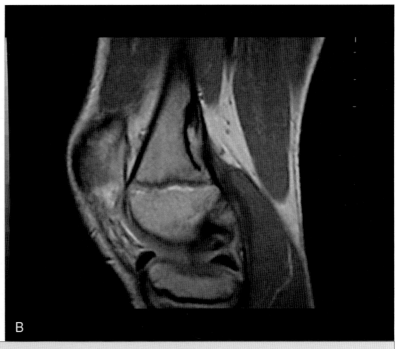

Figure 10   **A,** AP radiograph of the knee of a 10-year-old girl who had anterior knee pain. A well-marginated lesion along the posteromedial metaphysis of the distal femur is seen. **B,** A lateral T1-weighted MRI showing a well-marginated lesion with a sclerotic rim located along the posterior distal femoral metaphysis near the origin of the gastrocnemius. The lesion is high signal intensity, suggesting the presence of normal marrow, a finding indicative of a benign process. The radiographic characteristics, location of the lesion, and clinical symptoms are consistent with a diagnosis of avulsive cortical irregularity.

nosis. In cases where the diagnosis is not clear, multidisciplinary collaboration among the orthopaedic surgeon, radiologist, rheumatologist, and other specialists may be helpful in identifying the diagnosis.

Annotated References

1. Seybold U, Talati NJ, Kizilbash Q, Shah M, Blumberg HM, Franco-Paredes C: Hematogenous osteomyelitis mimicking osteosarcoma due to Community Associated Methicillin-Resistant Staphylococcus aureus. *Infection* 2007;35(3):190-193.

   The authors reported on two patients with thigh pain. Radiographs demonstrated a lytic lesion and acute periosteal reaction and elicited suspicion of osteosarcoma. However, clinical symptoms of fevers, chills, and other sites of infection as well as biopsy indicated osteomyelitis. Level of evidence: IV.

2. Lew DP, Waldvogel FA: Osteomyelitis. *Lancet* 2004; 364(9431):369-379.

3. Ju KL, Zurakowski D, Kocher MS: Differentiating between methicillin-resistant and methicillin-sensitive Staphylococcus aureus osteomyelitis in children: An evidence-based clinical prediction algorithm. *J Bone Joint Surg Am* 2011;93(18):1693-1701.

   This is a retrospective review of 129 children (118 had methicillin-sensitive *Staphylococcus aureus*; 11 had

methicillin-resistant S aureus [MRSA]). Results indicated a 92% predicted probability of having MRSA if the four clinical findings of temperature > 38°C, white blood cells count > 12K, hematocrit level <34%, and C-reactive protein level > 13 mg/L were present. Level of evidence: III.

4. Cierny G III, Mader JT, Penninck JJ: A clinical staging system for adult osteomyelitis. *Clin Orthop Relat Res* 2003;414:7-24.

5. Harris JC, Caesar DH, Davison C, Phibbs R, Than MP: How useful are laboratory investigations in the emergency department evaluation of possible osteomyelitis? *Emerg Med Australas* 2011;23(3):317-330.

   The authors conducted a literature review to determine which laboratory investigations are useful for the emergency department evaluation of osteomyelitis. Thirty-six relevant papers were identified. It was concluded that in adult and pediatric patients with a clinically low level of suspicion of osteomyelitis, an age-adjusted normal erythrocyte sedimentation rate (ESR) and C-reactive protein (CRP) <5 mg/L indicate that no further urgent investigation is required. For patients with risk factors for osteomyelitis or clinically high level of suspicion, a normal ESR or CRP <5 mg/L does not rule out the diagnosis of osteomyelitis, especially in patients with puncture wounds or foot ulcers/infections. In patients suspected of having osteomyelitis and otherwise unexplained ESR >30 mm/h and/or CRP >10-30 mg/L, additional investigation is required.

6. Lammin KA, Taylor J, Zenios M: The usefulness of c reactive protein and erythrocyte sedimentation rate in diagnosing long bone osteomyelitis in children: Are we being falsely reassured? *J Bone Joint Surg Br* 2012;94-B(suppl XXXIX):156.

    The authors conducted a review of all radiologically confirmed cases of long bone osteomyelitis without septic arthritis, joint effusion or abscess, in pediatric patients presenting to one hospital over an 18-month period. The authos found that the initial rise in inflammatory markers due to long bone osteomyelitis is significantly less than that in septic arthritis. A number of patients with osteomyelitis have normal inflammatory markers at presentation. A high index of suspicion is required in diagnosing osteomyelitis. Inflammatory markers are a useful adjunct to monitoring treatment but may offer false reassurance regarding the initial diagnosis.

7. Unkila-Kallio L, Kallio MJ, Eskola J, Peltola H: Serum C-reactive protein, erythrocyte sedimentation rate, and white blood cell count in acute hematogenous osteomyelitis of children. *Pediatrics* 1994;93(1):59-62.

8. Cierny G III: Surgical treatment of osteomyelitis. *Plast Reconstr Surg* 2011;127(suppl 1):190S-204S.

    The author reported his experience with treating 2207 patients with chronic osteomyelitis. He has developed a classification scheme for osteomyelitis based on the location and severity of the infection. Treatment recommendations are driven by the severity of the infection, host comorbidities, disability, and status of the soft tissue. Emphasis is placed on aggressive and complete surgical resection of all devitalized tissue, appropriate adjuvant antibiotic therapy, and robust soft-tissue reconstruction. Level of evidence: III.

9. Sartoris DJ, Resnick D, Resnik C, Yaghmai I: Musculoskeletal manifestations of sarcoidosis. *Semin Roentgenol* 1985;20(4):376-386.

10. Talmi D, Smith S, Mulligan ME: Central skeletal sarcoidosis mimicking metastatic disease. *Skeletal Radiol* 2008;37(8):757-761.

    The authors described an unusual presentation of sarcoidosis in a 48-year-old man with widespread axial and long bone lesions, but no involvement in the lungs, peripheral skeleton, or skin. The lesions were apparent on radiograph, CT, and FDG PET (fluorodeoxyglucose positron emission tomography). Level of evidence: IV.

11. Moore SL, Teirstein A, Golimbu C: MRI of sarcoidosis patients with musculoskeletal symptoms. *AJR Am J Roentgenol* 2005;185(1):154-159.

12. Moore SL, Teirstein AE: Musculoskeletal sarcoidosis: Spectrum of appearances at MR imaging. *Radiographics* 2003;23(6):1389-1399.

13. Moore SL, Kransdorf MJ, Schweitzer ME, Murphey MD, Babb JS: Can sarcoidosis and metastatic bone lesions be reliably differentiated on routine MRI? *AJR Am J Roentgenol* 2012;198(6):1387-1393.

    The purpose of this study was to determine if osseous sarcoidosis lesions could be differentiated from osseous metastases on MRI and to propose and evaluate features distinguishing these entities. MRI scans of 34 subjects with 79 single or multiple bone lesions (40 metastatic, 39 sarcoidal) were reviewed independently by two blinded, experienced musculoskeletal radiologists. Fluid-sensitive and T1-weighted images were viewed separately. Proposed discriminating features were perilesional or intralesional fat, specified border characteristics, and the presence of an extraosseous soft-tissue mass. An additional feature for spinal lesions was posterior element involvement. On the basis of these criteria, the readers provided a binary diagnosis and confidence score. The overall sensitivity for both readers was 46.3% and specificity, 97.4%. The authors concluded that osseous sarcoidosis lesions cannot be reliably distinguished from metastatic lesions on routine MRI studies by readers experienced in evaluating these lesions. Level of evidence: III.

14. Lin YC, Chen CH, Fu YC, Lin GT, Chang JK, Hu ST: Carpal tunnel syndrome and finger movement dysfunction caused by tophaceous gout: A case report. *Kaohsiung J Med Sci* 2009;25(1):34-39.

    The authors presented a case of a middle-aged man with history of gout and who had finger flexor dysfunction and median nerve symptoms. Imaging was consistent with tophaceous gout in the carpal tunnel. Decompression was performed, and resolution of symptoms occurred. Level of evidence: IV.

15. Chang CH, Lu CH, Yu CW, Wu MZ, Hsu CY, Shih TT: Tophaceous gout of the rotator cuff: A case report. *J Bone Joint Surg Am* 2008;90(1):178-182.

    The authors described a 26-year-old man with shoulder pain and no history of gout. T1, T2, and gradient-recalled echo T2 MRI sequences revealed low signal mass under the rotator cuff near the insertion on the humerus. Open decompression alleviated all symptoms.

16. Estrada A, Allen NB: Gouty tophus and tarsal tunnel syndrome. *J Clin Rheumatol* 1999;5(1):42-43, author reply 43.

17. Pakasa NM, Kalengayi RM: Tumoral calcinosis: A clinicopathological study of 111 cases with emphasis on the earliest changes. *Histopathology* 1997;31(1):18-24.

18. Farrow EG, Imel EA, White KE: Miscellaneous non-inflammatory musculoskeletal conditions: Hyperphosphatemic familial tumoral calcinosis (FGF23, GALNT3 and αKlotho). *Best Pract Res Clin Rheumatol* 2011;25(5):735-747.

    The authors reviewed phosphate and calcium homeostasis and pathophysiology of tumoral calcinosis including hyperphosphatemia, increased percent tubular resorption of phosphate, and inappropriately normal or elevated 1,25-dihydroxyvitamin D concentrations. The effect of loss-of-function mutations related to the phosphaturic hormone fibroblast growth factor-23 (FGF23) is discussed. Level of evidence: V.

1: General Evaluation and Treatment of Musculoskeletal Tumors

19. Alkhooly AZ: Medical treatment for tumoral calcinosis with eight years of follow-up: A report of four cases. *J Orthop Surg (Hong Kong)* 2009;17(3):379-382.

   The authors reported on four patients age 13 to 25 years. All had normal serum laboratory data except elevated phosphorus concentration and decreased calcium value. All were treated with diet modification and phosphate binders without complications. Two patients had complete resolution, and two patients had improvement. Level of evidence: IV.

20. Gregosiewicz A, Warda E: Tumoral calcinosis: Successful medical treatment. A case report. *J Bone Joint Surg Am* 1989;71(8):1244-1249.

21. Carmichael KD, Bynum JA, Evans EB: Familial tumoral calcinosis: A forty-year follow-up on one family. *J Bone Joint Surg Am* 2009;91(3):664-671.

   The authors reported the medical history as it pertains to tumoral calcinosis of one family encompassing as long as 40 years. Of the 16 siblings, seven had tumoral calcinosis. A retrospective chart review and interviews with surviving members were conducted. All seven affected children had hyperphosphatemia. Subsequent generations did not have tumoral calcinosis. The seven affected patients were followed for up to 40 years and underwent an average of 21 operations (range, 4 to 36 operations) for the treatment of calcified lesions. The genetic defect has been identified as the *GALNT3* gene, thus leading to the hyperphosphatemic form of the disease. Some members had relatively few lesions and surgical procedures (as few as 4), whereas others had an unrelenting course of lesions, recurrences, and surgical procedures (as many 36, with numerous other procedures). Three patients had multiyear periods with few symptoms—one for 7 years, one for 12 years, and one for 15 years. No effective medical therapy was found to control the lesions, and operations were associated with a high recurrence rate. Level of evidence: IV.

22. Möckel G, Buttgereit F, Labs K, Perka C: Tumoral calcinosis revisited: Pathophysiology and treatment. *Rheumatol Int* 2005;25(1):55-59.

23. King JJ, Brennan KB, Crawford EA, Fox EJ, Ogilvie CM: Surgical complications associated with extensive tumoral calcinosis. *Am J Orthop (Belle Mead NJ)* 2011;40(5):247-252.

   The authors reviewed the presenting features, radiographic appearance, and classification schemes for tumoral calcinosis and present two case examples. The authors concluded that tumoral calcinosis treatment is challenging and requires aggressive medical management. Surgical resection may be helpful in cases where patients are experiencing severe pain; however, complications and recurrence rates are high with surgery alone. Level of evidence: IV.

24. Hammoud S, McCarthy EF, Weber K: Tumoral calcinosis in infants: A report of three cases and review of the literature. *Clin Orthop Relat Res* 2005;436:261-264.

25. Polykandriotis EP, Beutel FK, Horch RE, Grünert J: A case of familial tumoral calcinosis in a neonate and review of the literature. *Arch Orthop Trauma Surg* 2004;124(8):563-567.

26. Altman RD, Bloch DA, Hochberg MC, Murphy WA: Prevalence of pelvic Paget's disease of bone in the United States. *J Bone Miner Res* 2000;15(3):461-465.

27. Harvey L, Gray T, Beneton MN, Douglas DL, Kanis JA, Russell RG: Ultrastructural features of the osteoclasts from Paget's disease of bone in relation to a viral aetiology. *J Clin Pathol* 1982;35(7):771-779.

28. Menaa C, Barsony J, Reddy SV, Cornish J, Cundy T, Roodman GD: 1,25-Dihydroxyvitamin D3 hypersensitivity of osteoclast precursors from patients with Paget's disease. *J Bone Miner Res* 2000;15(2):228-236.

29. Chung PY, Beyens G, Boonen S, et al: The majority of the genetic risk for Paget's disease of bone is explained by genetic variants close to the *CSF1*, *OPTN*, *TM7SF4*, and *TNFRSF11A* genes. *Hum Genet* 2010; 128(6):615-626.

   The authors performed genetic analysis on 247 patients with Paget disease in a Belgian population, 79 patients in a Dutch population, and 350 controls to elucidate the genetic pathomechanism of Paget disease. Their results support the *CSF1*, *OPTN* (optineurin), and *TNFRSF11A* gene regions as being involved in the pathogenesis of Paget disease.

30. Helfrich MH, Hobson RP, Grabowski PS, et al: A negative search for a paramyxoviral etiology of Paget's disease of bone: Molecular, immunological, and ultrastructural studies in UK patients. *J Bone Miner Res* 2000;15(12):2315-2329.

31. Stacy GS, Kapur A: Mimics of bone and soft tissue neoplasms. *Radiol Clin North Am* 2011;49(6):1261-1286, vii.

   The authors provide an extensive review of tumor mimics resulting from anatomic and developmental variants, trauma, infection and inflammation, osteonecrosis and myonecrosis, articular and juxta-articular conditions, and miscellaneous causes. Emphasis is placed on the importance of obtaining a thorough history and having a high level of suspicion for tumor mimics in order to develop an accurate differential diagnosis. Because malignancy cannot always be excluded, patients with a suspected bone or soft-tissue tumor should be referred to specialists at an orthopedic oncology facility. Level of evidence: V.

32. Siris ES, Lyles KW, Singer FR, Meunier PJ: Medical management of Paget's disease of bone: Indications for treatment and review of current therapies. *J Bone Miner Res* 2006;21(suppl 2):94-98.

33. Langston AL, Campbell MK, Fraser WD, et al; PRISM Trial Group: Randomized trial of intensive bisphosphonate treatment versus symptomatic management in Paget's disease of bone. *J Bone Miner Res* 2010;25(1):20-31.

The authors reported the results of a randomized trial that compared the effects of symptomatic treatment with intensive bisphosphonate therapy in a cohort of 1,324 patients with PDB who were followed up for a median of 3 years (range 2 to 5 years). The symptomatic treatment group was treated only if they had pagetic bone pain, for which they were first given analgesics or anti-inflammatory drugs, followed by bisphosphonates if they did not respond. The intensive group received repeat courses of bisphosphonates irrespective of symptoms with the aim of reducing and maintaining serum alkaline phosphatase levels within the normal range. Neither management strategy had a significant beneficial effect on pain or quality of life. Level of evidence: II.

34. Ralston SH, Langston AL, Reid IR: Pathogenesis and management of Paget's disease of bone. *Lancet* 2008; 372(9633):155-163.

The pathogenesis and treatment options for Paget disease are discussed. No firm evidence as yet exists to show that bisphosphonates can prevent the development of complications of Paget disease of bone, and further work is needed to address the effects of treatment on long-term clinical outcomes.

35. Agarwal G, Mishra SK, Kar DK, et al: Recovery pattern of patients with osteitis fibrosa cystica in primary hyperparathyroidism after successful parathyroidectomy. *Surgery* 2002;132(6):1075-1083, discussion 1083-1085.

36. Brukner P, Bradshaw C, Khan KM, White S, Crossley K: Stress fractures: A review of 180 cases. *Clin J Sport Med* 1996;6(2):85-89.

37. Matheson GO, Clement DB, McKenzie DC, Taunton JE, Lloyd-Smith DR, MacIntyre JG: Stress fractures in athletes: A study of 320 cases. *Am J Sports Med* 1987; 15(1):46-58.

38. Gaeta M, Minutoli F, Scribano E, et al: CT and MR imaging findings in athletes with early tibial stress injuries: Comparison with bone scintigraphy findings and emphasis on cortical abnormalities. *Radiology* 2005;235(2):553-561.

39. Reshef N, Guelich DR: Medial tibial stress syndrome. *Clin Sports Med* 2012;31(2):273-290.

The authors reviewed the etiology, prevalence, nomenclature, diagnostic criteria, treatment, and prevention strategies for medial tibial stress syndrome. The authors stated that the exact cause of this condition is unknown. The most important risk factors are thought to be hyperpronation of the foot, female sex, and history of previous medial tibial stress syndrome. Level of evidence: V.

40. Harmon J, Rabe AJ, Nichol KK, Shiels WE: Precervical myositis ossificans in an infant secondary to child abuse. *Pediatr Radiol* 2012;42(7):881-885.

A 10-week-old girl had ultrasound-guided, biopsy-proven myositis ossificans that was a result of nonaccidental trauma. Imaging characteristics including peripheral mineralization rather than central mineralization seen in neoplasms aided in the diagnosis.

41. Lacout A, Jarraya M, Marcy PY, Thariat J, Carlier RY: Myositis ossificans imaging: Keys to successful diagnosis. *Indian J Radiol Imaging* 2012;22(1):35-39.

The authors describe the zone phenomenon associated with myositis ossificans. The first zone is mesenchymal cells in a myxoid matrix, followed by osteoblasts producing immature bone. Finally, mineralization matures and bone formation is seen in the periphery of the lesion.

42. De Carvalho BR: Calcific myonecrosis: A two-patient case series. *Jpn J Radiol* 2012;30(6):517-521.

The authors described two patients with a remote history of trauma who developed calcific myonecrosis. The authors stressed that recognizing that a muscle compartment has been replaced with mineralization is the key to the correct diagnosis.

43. Dhillon M, Davies AM, Benham J, Evans N, Mangham DC, Grimer RJ: Calcific myonecrosis: A report of ten new cases with an emphasis on MR imaging. *Eur Radiol* 2004;14(11):1974-1979.

44. O'Dwyer HM, Al-Nakshabandi NA, Al-Muzahmi K, Ryan A, O'Connell JX, Munk PL: Calcific myonecrosis: Keys to recognition and management. *AJR Am J Roentgenol* 2006;187(1):W67-W76.

45. Hall FM: Cortical desmoid: A misnomer? *AJR Am J Roentgenol* 2011;197(4):1022, author reply 1023.

The author's opinion is that the term desmoid is used incorrectly to describe this completely benign and latent bone lesion. He believes that cortical desmoids are in fact enthesopathies and not neoplastic conditions, and cautions using the term desmoid, which is most commonly understood to mean a locally aggressive soft tissue tumor that can cause severe morbidity and in some cases death. This misuse of terminology may lead to unnecessary testing, treatment, and anxiety regarding an otherwise innocuous bone lesion. Level of evidence: V.

46. Vieira RL, Bencardino JT, Rosenberg ZS, Nomikos G: MRI features of cortical desmoid in acute knee trauma. *AJR Am J Roentgenol* 2011;196(2):424-428.

The authors describe the MRI appearance of "cortical demoids" in 11 patients who had a history of trauma and pain within 4 weeks before an MRI. Size range was 8 to 12 mm; defects were hypointense or isointense on proton density images and hyperintense on T2-weighted fat-suppressed images. Most patients had associated bone marrow edema, periostitis, swelling, and edema at the origin of the medial head of the gastrocnemius tendon. All patients were asymptomatic after conservative treatment.

47. Goodin GS, Shulkin BL, Kaufman RA, McCarville MB: PET/CT characterization of fibroosseous defects in children: 18F-FDG uptake can mimic metastatic disease. *AJR Am J Roentgenol* 2006;187(4):1124-1128.

Chapter 6

Chemotherapy

Jennifer Wright, MD

Introduction

It is an exciting time in the medical management of sarcoma. Although the search for the holy grail of universal cure without major toxicity continues, targeted therapy has recently provided more treatment options for patients with sarcoma. Many diseases for which there was previously no effective chemotherapy now have drug trials in progress.

Over the past decades, chemotherapy for musculoskeletal malignancies has evolved from single- or double-agent therapy to intense multidrug regimens and targeted therapy. For a generation or so, the ruling concept was that if some is good, more is better. With time, it became clear that multidrug therapies are certainly more toxic but not necessarily curative. As late effects emerge in the sarcoma survivor population, more thought has been given to the development of chemotherapy regimens in an attempt to maximize survival and minimize adverse sequelae to the rest of the body.

This chapter briefly reviews the historical and current standard chemotherapy regimens and details the development of emerging therapies for each of the major sarcoma types. The discussion focuses on chemotherapy regimens used with curative intent rather than those used for palliation.

Bone Tumors

Osteosarcoma

Most patients have subclinical metastases at diagnosis, given the high rate of recurrent disease at distant sites in spite of excellent local control (ie, amputation). In the early 1980s, the first multi-institutional, randomized trials of adjuvant chemotherapy for nonmetastatic osteosarcoma were performed. Although only 95 patients were randomized in the two trials, the results were striking: The 2-year relapse-free survival was 17% to 20% in the control groups compared to 55% to

66% in the chemotherapy groups.[1,2] These results became the basis for modern-day therapy. Although specific regimens vary regionally and by cooperative group, the standard agents are some combination of methotrexate, doxorubicin, cisplatin, and ifosfamide.

Only one randomized study has evaluated the timing of chemotherapy initiation. Immediate resection and adjuvant chemotherapy was compared to a period of neoadjuvant chemotherapy followed by resection.[3] This study showed no difference in survival in the two groups, and most current regimens use neoadjuvant chemotherapy before resection. This method also allows for an assessment of chemotherapy response on pathologic review of the resected tumor, which is useful for prognosis. Although an early study has not shown a benefit to changing therapy on the basis of this response,[4] other trials with this goal are ongoing.

Interestingly, chemotherapy-associated toxicity and infection have been shown to be independent predictors of survival in osteosarcoma.[5,6] This observation has led to the use of agents intended to produce an inflammatory response, such as muramyl tripeptide (MTP) and interferon, in addition to traditional chemotherapy for osteosarcoma. To date, the results of studies with these agents have not clearly shown a survival benefit,[7,8] but additional studies with both agents are continuing. Response may also depend on genetic polymorphisms[9] that regulate drug metabolism or toxicity.

The first trial using targeted therapy in osteosarcoma was recently completed. The researchers evaluated the addition of trastuzumab to therapy for metastatic osteosarcoma demonstrating *HER2* positivity; the short-term results unfortunately showed no survival improvement.[10] Agents useful in recurrent disease include etoposide and ifosfamide,[11] gemcitabine and docetaxel,[12] sorafenib,[13] or even rechallenge of first-line chemotherapy. Logical targets to evaluate for possible future drug studies in osteosarcoma are receptor activator of nuclear factor-κB, ligand inhibitors, Wnt pathway inhibition,[14] and modifiers of methylation.[15]

Most treatment regimens for osteosarcoma were developed in the pediatric population and may not be tolerated well by adults with comorbid conditions. Challenges also exist in patients with secondary osteosarcoma and Li-Fraumeni syndrome, because their chemotherapy options may be limited by prior exposures.

Neither Dr. Wright nor any immediate family member has received anything of value from or has stock or stock options held in a commercial company or institution related directly or indirectly to the subject of this chapter.

Ewing Sarcoma

As with osteosarcoma, it is presumed that a significant percentage of patients with Ewing sarcoma have subclinical metastases at diagnosis. Chemotherapy, therefore, is essential for the successful treatment of Ewing sarcoma. Multiagent chemotherapy first came into routine use in Ewing sarcoma in the 1970s. Vincristine and cyclophosphamide have been mainstays of therapy since that time. Several trials, mainly in pediatrics, have evaluated other agents including doxorubicin, dactinomycin, ifosfamide, and etoposide. Current protocols usually include four or five of these drugs in various combinations. Interestingly, two studies have shown that the greatest benefit of increased-intensity regimens occurs in patients without metastatic disease.[16,17]

Ewing sarcoma is the only sarcoma for which the model of dose intensification of chemotherapy has been examined. This method, made possible by the availability of granulocyte colony-stimulating factor (GCSF), administers chemotherapy every 14 days instead of every 21 days in an effort to increase the treatment dose over a given period. Using this compressed pattern of therapy delivery, two research groups found outcomes to be the same as using standard therapy.[18] The schedule is challenging to maintain even with the use of GCSF. Nonetheless, many groups now use this style of therapy routinely, so that more chemotherapy is given before local control and total duration of treatment is shorter.

Because of the chemoresponsiveness of the disease, much research has gone into the use of high-dose chemotherapy and stem cell rescue in patients with high-risk Ewing sarcoma. Debate about which patients are appropriate candidates for this therapy continues, but benefit has been shown for select patient groups.[17,19]

Second-line agents with activity in Ewing sarcoma include topotecan,[20] irinotecan and temozolomide,[21] insulin-like growth factor (IGF) receptor antibodies,[22] and mammalian target of rapamycin (mTOR) inhibitors.[23] Preclinical testing of histone deacetylase inhibitors shows response in Ewing sarcoma.[24] The EWS-FLI1 fusion protein is an interesting potential therapeutic target. Cytarabine was shown to be effective at decreasing EWS-FLI1 protein levels in preclinical studies, but did not lead to clinical response in refractory disease,[25] so research is ongoing.

Chondrosarcoma

Unlike Ewing sarcoma and osteosarcoma, most chondrosarcomas are low to intermediate grade, have been shown to be largely chemotherapy resistant, and are usually managed surgically. High-grade chondrosarcomas, particularly dedifferentiated and mesenchymal chondrosarcoma, have been reported to respond to chemotherapy. Doxorubicin with or without cisplatin is the most commonly used regimen, based on small studies[26,27] and a lack of strong evidence for other effective drugs. Given the rarity of high-grade chondrosarcoma, a large randomized trial comparing the efficacy of multiple agents is unlikely to take place.

Rhabdomyosarcoma

Because of the wide range of presentations and the variability of resectability depending on primary location, a complex staging system has been developed for rhabdomyosarcoma (RMS). A combination of the stage and clinical group determines the risk of recurrence and directs treatment. The combination of vincristine, actinomycin, and cyclophosphamide (VAC) was first used against RMS in 1969. In the intervening decades, research groups have evaluated regimens with additional drugs such as doxorubicin, ifosfamide, etoposide, and topotecan. To date, none of these regimens has shown improvement in outcomes[28-30] in RMS, and VAC remains the standard of care for localized disease. In spite of there being no prior proven benefit, most cooperative groups continue to evaluate multidrug regimens for patients with metastatic RMS because outcomes for these patients are dismal. Aberrancies in anaplastic lymphoma kinase (ALK) have recently been described in relatively high frequency in alveolar RMS and serve as a target for future drug studies.[31]

Nonrhabdomyosarcoma Soft-Tissue Sarcoma

The category of nonrhabdomyosarcoma soft-tissue sarcoma (NRSTS) is made up of multiple heterogeneous diseases. They are clustered together in spite of their diversity for convenience and because of their orphan status and the lack of separate clinical trials.

Several subtypes of NRSTS have traditionally been managed surgically because of their overall lack of response to chemotherapy. These include pleomorphic spindle cell sarcomas, malignant peripheral nerve sheath tumors, angiosarcoma, fibrosarcoma, clear cell sarcoma (CCS), epithelioid sarcoma, and alveolar soft-part sarcoma (ASPS).

Although technically not a sarcoma, and with no metastatic potential, desmoid fibromatosis frequently demonstrates local aggressivity and high local recurrence rates, warranting consideration of systemic therapy. Several chemotherapeutic approaches have been tried in patients with recurrences not amenable to resection or radiation. Reasonable treatment options include imatinib or other tyrosine kinase inhibitors, antiestrogen therapy such as tamoxifen, NSAIDs, methotrexate and vinblastine, or doxorubicin.[32-35] Chemotherapy selection is often selected on the basis of the anticipated tolerability of each regimen and often leads to stabilization of disease, not regression.

Angiosarcomas are aggressive vascular tumors most common in the cutaneous tissue of the scalp or breast. A significant percentage of angiosarcomas develop after exposure to carcinogenic chemicals or therapeutic radiation. These tumors have been proven to be largely chemoresistant, and chemotherapy has been proven not to improve long-term survival in patients with localized disease.[36-38] Chemotherapy can prolong progression-free survival in patients with metastatic disease; the most commonly used agents are doxorubicin[39] and paclitaxel.[40] Reports of response to antiangiogenesis agents, which would logically be an excellent targeted therapy, are quite rare. Dermatofibrosarcoma protuberans is a rare, low-grade cutaneous sarcoma with a natural history of frequent local recurrences. It is characterized by a translocation between chromosomes 17 and 22 leading to upregulation of *PDGFB*, and has been proven to be responsive to imatinib,[41] potentially enabling less morbid resections. The treatment of infantile fibrosarcoma usually requires only local control, given the general lack of metastases and overall good prognosis. However, chemotherapy is sometimes used neoadjuvantly in an attempt to reduce tumor size and enable a less morbid resection. Vincristine and dactinomycin with or without cyclophosphamide have been shown to have some efficacy in infantile fibrosarcoma.[42]

Chemotherapy-resistant sarcomas provide excellent opportunities for the evaluation of targeted therapy. For example, epithelioid sarcoma cell lines have shown synergistic response to mTOR and epidermal growth factor receptor inhibition.[43] There are reports of ASPS responding to sunitinib;[44,45] this response is plausible because the ASPL-TFE3 fusion protein of ASPS transcriptionally activates *MET*, one of sunitinib's targets.

Other subtypes of NRSTS are more commonly responsive to chemotherapy, and their management is usually multimodal. Adjuvant chemotherapy is standard for uterine leiomyosarcoma (LMS). The combination of gemcitabine and docetaxel has recently proven to be quite effective in uterine LMS.[46,47] Trabectedin is active in refractory uterine LMS.[48] Prior to the use of gemcitabine and docetaxel, doxorubicin and ifosfamide were commonly used for the treatment of LMS. Despite their widespread use, the literature on doxorubicin and ifosfamide describes only low percentages of response.[49,50] Nonuterine primary LMS has been less well studied given its rarity, but is usually treated with the same agents as uterine LMS.

The efficacy of chemotherapy in liposarcoma is highly linked to histologic subtype. Myxoid/round cell liposarcomas are often chemotherapy sensitive, whereas well-differentiated and dedifferentiated liposarcomas are often chemotherapy resistant. Neoadjuvant therapy may be given in an attempt to improve surgical outcomes; for example, in retroperitoneal liposarcomas that require extensive resections. Myxoid liposarcomas have most often been treated with doxorubicin and ifosfamide,[51] and recently have been shown to have a good response rate to trabectedin.[52] A recent report notes frequent epigenetic abnormalities in dedifferentiated liposarcomas, which may provide a target for treatment with histone deacetylase inhibition.[53]

Synovial sarcoma is often thought to be more chemotherapy sensitive than most other soft-tissue sarcoma types. Most reports of response are retrospective or from nonrandomized multimodality trials not specific to a single histology. There is also a lack of consistency between studies of adjuvant versus neoadjuvant chemotherapy and metastatic versus nonmetastatic populations. It is therefore difficult to determine the actual role of chemotherapy in the relatively favorable prognosis of this disease. Nevertheless, there are sufficient data to suggest that synovial sarcoma responds to anthracyclines and ifosfamide either alone or in combination,[54-56] although the ideal regimen has not been determined.

Malignant peripheral nerve sheath tumor (MPNST) responds modestly at best to chemotherapy and is most commonly treated with doxorubicin and ifosfamide.[57] Ongoing studies are investigating the response of MPNST to everolimus because of its success in preclinical models. Unfortunately, patients with underlying neurofibromatosis type 1 are less likely to have tumor response to chemotherapy than patients with sporadic MPNST.

Desmoplastic small round cell tumor (DSRCT) is generally chemosensitive yet without many long-term remissions. Because DSRCT is rare, there are no large patient series or trials. However, DSRCT is often treated with regimens similar to those for Ewing sarcoma, sometimes with high-dose cyclophosphamide or even autologous stem cell transplant.[58,59] Because its primary tumor site is usually abdominal, DSRCT is sometimes treated with intraperitoneal chemotherapy, usually cisplatin.[60] Undifferentiated pleomorphic sarcoma (previously called malignant fibrous histiocytoma) is an aggressive tumor often treated with chemotherapy, particularly in the setting of metastatic disease. Results of published studies are difficult to interpret, given that they often include mixed histologies, but pleomorphic sarcoma may be treated with combination agents known to work in other NRSTSs, such as doxorubicin/ifosfamide, gemcitabine/docetaxel, or trabectedin.

The Children's Oncology Group (COG) recently completed a study (ARST0332) of risk-based therapy for NRSTS. This study included patients up to age 30 years who were nonrandomly assigned to resection and observation only, resection and adjuvant radiation, resection and adjuvant chemoradiotherapy, or neoadjuvant chemoradiotherapy with resection based on tumor grade, maximal tumor diameter, margin status, and presence of metastatic disease. Chemotherapy consisted of either 19 or 22 weeks of doxorubicin and ifosfamide, depending on assigned treatment arm. In 5 years, this study accrued 552 eligible patients with more than 30 sarcoma subtypes. The most common diagnoses, accounting for approximately one third of the patients, were synovial sarcoma and MPNST. The results of this study are expected to improve understanding of the chemosensitivity of some of the more common NRSTS subtypes.

Kaposi sarcoma is an HIV-associated malignancy that is rare in the developed world where highly active antiretroviral therapy (HAART) is available. The pres-

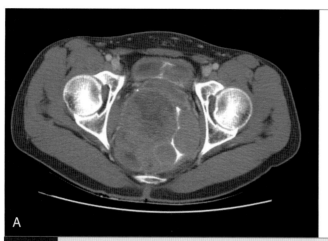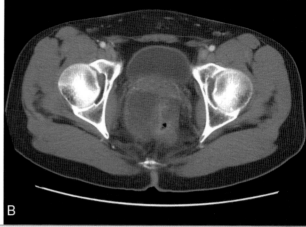

Figure 1 CT scans from a 39-year-old-man with rectal gastrointestinal stromal tumor. **A,** Diagnostic scan. Resection at that time would have required pelvic exenteration. The patient received imatinib therapy for 1 year. **B,** Scan after imatinib therapy. The patient went on to have an uncomplicated resection.

ence of Kaposi sarcoma signals significant immune deficiency and often responds at least in part to the initiation of HAART. Chemotherapy has been used successfully in addition to HAART, with observed responses to vincristine, bleomycin, doxorubicin, etoposide, dexamethasone, and paclitaxel.[61-63] Unfortunately, the administration of these chemotherapeutic agents may be difficult in the social or geographic circumstances that have led to the development of Kaposi sarcoma.

One exception to CCS being unresponsive to chemotherapy is CCS of the kidney in pediatric patients. This tumor variant was shown to be responsive to various combinations of vincristine, doxorubicin, dactinomycin, and cyclophosphamide.[64] Current pediatric protocols also frequently include the use of etoposide. Patients with metastatic CCS of the kidney still have poor outcomes.

Gastrointestinal stromal tumor (GIST) is the first sarcoma type to be successfully treated with targeted therapy. Most GISTs were categorized as LMS before the late 1980s, so care must be exercised when reading older literature. Largely unresponsive to classic chemotherapy agents, most GISTs have an activating mutation of *KIT* or *PDGFRA* that responds to tyrosine kinase inhibition. Imatinib may be used neoadjuvantly or adjuvantly according to prognosis based on risk factors (**Figure 1**). Sunitinib is a second-line tyrosine kinase inhibitor for GIST. Wild-type or mutation-negative GIST is more common in children and young adults and does not respond to imatinib. Studies have revealed that most wild-type GISTs are deficient in succinate dehydrogenase and a significant portion of patients harbor germline mutations related to succinate dehydrogenage.[65] The current standard of care for these patients is symptom management, although trials of sunitinib, vandetanib, and IGF receptor antibodies are ongoing.

Palifosfamide is a newer agent being investigated in sarcomas usually responsive to ifosfamide. It has the advantage of fewer side effects and easier administration compared to ifosfamide.[66]

In addition to previously mentioned uses, trabectedin has been shown to have activity with doxorubicin in recurrent NRSTS.[67] Investigations into the use of trabectedin as upfront therapy in translocation-associated sarcomas are ongoing. Pazopanib[68] is a multitarget kinase inhibitor that has been shown to prolong progression-free survival in metastatic NRSTS. As more is learned about the molecular and biologic features of sarcomas, drug options for their treatment will continue to multiply (**Table 1**).

Late Effects of Sarcoma Chemotherapy

As more patients with sarcoma are surviving, the long-term toxicities of their therapies are becoming apparent. These effects are particularly important in young patients, who have long lives ahead of them. Radiation and surgery cause long-term complications; however, this section focuses on late effects caused by chemotherapy agents[69] used commonly in sarcomas (**Table 2**).

Certainly one of the most tragic late effects is a second malignancy. Etoposide and cyclophosphamide are both used in sarcoma therapy and can lead to secondary leukemia in 1% to 2% of survivors. Etoposide may lead to an 11q23-associated myeloid leukemia, usually occurring within a few years of exposure. Cyclophosphamide may cause myelodysplasia or monosomy 5– or monosomy 7–associated leukemia, usually several years after completion of primary therapy.

Doxorubicin and other anthracyclines are associated with cardiomyopathy. Cardiomyopathy can occur as acute systolic failure, usually associated with doses greater than 500 mg/m² and often occurring during continuing therapy. It can occur as either restrictive or dilated cardiomyopathy, appearing years to decades after therapy. Once cardiomyopathy has developed, a

Table 1

Summary of Chemosensitivities by Subtype

Histologic Subtype	Most Useful Agents
Osteosarcoma	Methotrexate/doxorubicin/cisplatin
	Ifosfamide/etoposide
Chondrosarcoma	Doxorubicin/cisplatin
Ewing sarcoma	Vincristine/doxorubicin/actinomycin-D
	Ifosfamide/cyclophosphamide/ temozolomide
	Etoposide
	Topotecan/irinotecan
Rhabdomyosarcoma	Vincristine/actinomycin-D/ cyclophosphamide
	Irinotecan
	Doxorubicin
Desmoid tumor	Imatinib/sorafenib
	Tamoxifen/sulindac
	Methotrexate/vinblastine
	Doxorubicin
Angiosarcoma	Paclitaxel
	Doxorubicin
	Bevacizumab
Leiomyosarcoma	Gemcitabine/docetaxol
	Trabectedin
	Doxorubicin
Liposarcoma	Doxorubicin/ifosfamide
Synovial sarcoma	Doxorubicin/ifosfamide
MPNST	Doxorubicin/ifosfamide
DSRCT	Vincristine/doxorubicin/ cyclophosphamide
	Ifosfamide/etoposide
	Cisplatin (intraperitoneal)
Pleomorphic spindle cell sarcoma	Doxorubicin/ifosfamide
	Gemcitabine/docetaxol
Kaposi sarcoma	Vincristine/bleomycin/doxorubicin
	Dexamethasone/paclitaxel
GIST	Imatinib/sunitinib

MPNST = malignant peripheral nerve sheath tumor; DSRCT = desmoplastic small round cell tumor; GIST = gastrointestinal stromal tumor.

Table 2

Late Effects of Common Sarcoma Therapies

Therapeutic Modality	Late Effect
Surgery	
Limb salvage surgery	Hardware failure or complications
Amputation/ rotationplasty	Cosmetic concerns Limb length discrepancy
Abdominal resections	Single kidney Infertility/gonadal failure Ostomy Adhesions
Radiation	Limb length discrepancy
	Second malignancy (skin, breast, sarcoma, etc)
	Endocrinopathies
	Infertility/gonadal failure
Chemotherapy	
Doxorubicin	Cardiomyopathy
Ifosfamide/ cyclophosphamide	Infertility/gonadal failure Cystitis/bladder fibrosis
Cisplatin	High-frequency hearing loss
	Renal insufficiency/hypomagnesemia
Methotrexate	Renal insufficiency
Vincristine	Peripheral neuropathy

high percentage of patients progress to require cardiac transplantation. Imatinib has also been associated with cardiotoxicity, but long-term outcomes are unknown.

Alkylating agents are known to cause premature gonadal failure and infertility. This is a dose-associated effect, which is potentiated by local radiation. Cumulative cyclophosphamide doses greater than 8 g/m^2 are associated with ovarian and testicular dysfunction, and ifosfamide doses greater than 60 g/m^2 are associated with testicular failure. Alkylating agents may also lead to hemorrhagic cystitis, bladder fibrosis, bladder malignancy, and dysfunctional voiding, again with patients who receive pelvic radiation having an increased risk.

Platinum therapy, used mainly in osteosarcoma, is associated with high-frequency hearing loss. This risk is higher in younger patients and with cisplatin doses greater than 360 mg/m^2. Cisplatin can also cause renal insufficiency and hypomagnesemia, usually only during drug exposure, but occasionally persisting for years. Osteosarcoma is the only sarcoma treated with high-dose methotrexate. Methotrexate can also cause renal insufficiency.

Chronic peripheral neuropathy may be an issue for patients exposed to multiple doses of vincristine. This situation is most common in patients with RMS who develop neuropathy during treatment. The neuropathy usually improves significantly after the end of therapy, but may persist at a low level for years.

Knowledge of these late effects has led to modifications in current protocols in an effort to decrease morbidity of therapy; for example, the cumulative dose of cyclophosphamide has been decreased in the lowest-risk RMS groups. Only time will tell what late effects are correlated with newer chemotherapy agents, such as inhibitors of angiogenesis, tyrosine kinases, and camptothecins. It will be particularly interesting to see how these drugs affect developing tissues in young patients.

Summary

Along with improved surgical and radiation techniques, chemotherapy has helped improve the outlook for patients with sarcoma over the past decades. For some time, doxorubicin alone or doxorubicin with ifosfamide were the only options for patients with advanced sarcoma. A good range of both intravenous and oral chemotherapy options exist, including traditional cytoreductive agents and drugs that target oncogenic proteins. Innovations in supportive care have allowed patients with previously limiting comorbidities to tolerate more aggressive chemotherapy. Oncologists are starting to prescribe the aggressive therapies first designed for children for their adult patients, and patients up to age 40 or 50 years are eligible for most COG sarcoma studies. With this abundance of chemotherapy options, advanced sarcoma can be converted from a death sentence to chronic disease in many situations. In this time of advanced treatment options, oncologists have the privilege of working with patients to balance technologic advances, quality of life, and risk of late effects, considerations not necessary previously.

Annotated References

1. Link MP, Goorin AM, Miser AW, et al: The effect of adjuvant chemotherapy on relapse-free survival in patients with osteosarcoma of the extremity. *N Engl J Med* 1986;314(25):1600-1606.

2. Eilber F, Giuliano A, Eckardt J, Patterson K, Moseley S, Goodnight J: Adjuvant chemotherapy for osteosarcoma: A randomized prospective trial. *J Clin Oncol* 1987;5(1):21-26.

3. Goorin AM, Schwartzentruber DJ, Devidas M, et al; Pediatric Oncology Group: Presurgical chemotherapy compared with immediate surgery and adjuvant chemotherapy for nonmetastatic osteosarcoma: Pediatric Oncology Group Study POG-8651. *J Clin Oncol* 2003;21(8):1574-1580.

4. Provisor AJ, Ettinger LJ, Nachman JB, et al: Treatment of nonmetastatic osteosarcoma of the extremity with preoperative and postoperative chemotherapy: A report from the Children's Cancer Group. *J Clin Oncol* 1997;15(1):76-84.

5. McTiernan A, Jinks RC, Sydes MR, et al: Presence of chemotherapy-induced toxicity predicts improved survival in patients with localised extremity osteosarcoma treated with doxorubicin and cisplatin: A report from the European Osteosarcoma Intergroup. *Eur J Cancer* 2012;48(5):703-712.

   The authors reported a 20-year retrospective review of toxicity from a European cooperative group's osteosarcoma trials. Multivariate analysis showed that along with distal primary site and good histological response, mucositis, nausea, and thrombocytopenia were predictors of increased survival. Level of evidence: I.

6. Lee JA, Kim MS, Kim DH, et al: Postoperative infection and survival in osteosarcoma patients. *Ann Surg Oncol* 2009;16(1):147-151.

   The authors reported a nonstatistical trend toward increased survival in osteosarcoma patients with a postoperative deep-tissue infection. This study is a retrospective analysis of 13 years of patient data. Level of evidence: II.

7. Meyers PA, Schwartz CL, Krailo MD, et al; Children's Oncology Group: Osteosarcoma: The addition of muramyl tripeptide to chemotherapy improves overall survival—a report from the Children's Oncology Group. *J Clin Oncol* 2008;26(4):633-638.

   This article is a follow-up to the 2005 report of a pediatric osteosarcoma trial of ifosfamide and MTP with standard chemotherapy. The investigators reported a slight improvement in overall survival with MTP, but no change in overall survival with ifosfamide. Neither drug improved event-free survival. Level of evidence: Ib.

8. Strander H, Bauer HC, Brosjö O, et al: Long-term adjuvant interferon treatment of human osteosarcoma: A pilot study. *Acta Oncol* 1995;34(6):877-880.

9. Windsor RE, Strauss SJ, Kallis C, Wood NE, Whelan JS: Germline genetic polymorphisms may influence chemotherapy response and disease outcome in osteosarcoma: A pilot study. *Cancer* 2012;118(7):1856-1867.

   The authors genotyped five different polymorphisms of 60 osteosarcoma patients. The authors found associations between polymorphisms and histologic response as well as between polymorphisms and drug toxicity. Level of evidence: II.

10. Ebb D, Meyers P, Grier H, et al: Phase II trial of trastuzumab in combination with cytotoxic chemotherapy for treatment of metastatic osteosarcoma with human epidermal growth factor receptor 2 overexpression: A report from the children's oncology group. *J Clin Oncol* 2012;30(20):2545-2551.

    The authors reported on results of an osteosarcoma trial. New patients with metastatic osteosarcoma were eligible. Those with tumors that stained *HER2* positive received trastuzumab in addition to standard therapy. Addition of trastuzumab did not improve outcomes. Level of evidence: I.

11. Gentet JC, Brunat-Mentigny M, Demaille MC, et al: Ifosfamide and etoposide in childhood osteosarcoma: A phase II study of the French Society of Paediatric Oncology. *Eur J Cancer* 1997;33(2):232-237.

12. Navid F, Willert JR, McCarville MB, et al: Combination of gemcitabine and docetaxel in the treatment of children and young adults with refractory bone sarcoma. *Cancer* 2008;113(2):419-425.

The authors presented a retrospective case report. Twenty-two patients with refractory sarcoma received 109 courses of gemcitabine and docetaxel. The overall response rate was 29%, with three osteosarcoma patients having partial response. Level of evidence: IV.

13. Grignani G, Palmerini E, Dileo P, et al: A phase II trial of sorafenib in relapsed and unresectable high-grade osteosarcoma after failure of standard multimodal therapy: An Italian Sarcoma Group study. *Ann Oncol* 2012;23(2):508-516.

The authors reported on a nonrandomized trial of sorafenib for recurrent/progressive osteosarcoma from Italy. Of 34 patients, only 8% had a partial response, but 34% had stable disease. Median overall survival was 7 months. Level of evidence: II.

14. McQueen P, Ghaffar S, Guo Y, Rubin EM, Zi X, Hoang BH: The Wnt signaling pathway: Implications for therapy in osteosarcoma. *Expert Rev Anticancer Ther* 2011;11(8):1223-1232.

In this review, the authors described the role of Wnt signaling in osteosarcoma, as well as potential mechanisms to modify Wnt signaling for treatment of osteosarcoma. Level of evidence: V.

15. Cui Q, Jiang W, Guo J, et al: Relationship between hypermethylated MGMT gene and osteosarcoma necrosis rate after chemotherapy. *Pathol Oncol Res* 2011;17(3):587-591.

Investigators evaluated *MGMT* methylation in 51 osteosarcoma tumor samples. They retrospectively identified increased rates of histologic response in patients whose tumors showed *MGMT* methylation. Level of evidence: II.

16. Grier HE, Krailo MD, Tarbell NJ, et al: Addition of ifosfamide and etoposide to standard chemotherapy for Ewing's sarcoma and primitive neuroectodermal tumor of bone. *N Engl J Med* 2003;348(8):694-701.

17. Paulussen M, Craft AW, Lewis I, et al; European Intergroup Cooperative Ewing's Sarcoma Study-92: Results of the EICESS-92 Study: Two randomized trials of Ewing's sarcoma treatment—cyclophosphamide compared with ifosfamide in standard-risk patients and assessment of benefit of etoposide added to standard treatment in high-risk patients. *J Clin Oncol* 2008; 26(27):4385-4393.

The authors reported the results of a pediatric Ewing sarcoma trial. There was no difference in outcomes in standard-risk patients randomized to ifosfamide or cyclophosphamide. High-risk patients were randomized to receive standard chemotherapy with or without etoposide. Etoposide improved outcomes for patients without metastasis but not for patients with metastasis. Level of evidence: I.

18. Granowetter L, Womer R, Devidas M, et al: Dose-intensified compared with standard chemotherapy for nonmetastatic Ewing sarcoma family of tumors: A Children's Oncology Group Study. *J Clin Oncol* 2009; 27(15):2536-2541.

The authors reported the results of a Ewing sarcoma trial. New patients with nonmetastatic Ewing sarcoma were randomized to chemotherapy given over 48 weeks or compressed into 30 weeks. Dose compression did not improve outcomes. Level of evidence: I.

19. Diaz MA, Lassaletta A, Perez A, Sevilla J, Madero L, Gonzalez-Vicent M: High-dose busulfan and melphalan as conditioning regimen for autologous peripheral blood progenitor cell transplantation in high-risk Ewing sarcoma patients: A long-term follow-up single-center study. *Pediatr Hematol Oncol* 2010;27(4):272-282.

The authors reported their institutional experience using busulfan and melphalan as conditioning for autologous stem cell transplant in high-risk Ewing sarcoma. Progression-free survival at 92 months was 56% for the entire group; patients with localized disease fared significantly better than those with metastatic disease. Level of evidence: IV.

20. Hunold A, Weddeling N, Paulussen M, Ranft A, Liebscher C, Jürgens H: Topotecan and cyclophosphamide in patients with refractory or relapsed Ewing tumors. *Pediatr Blood Cancer* 2006;47(6):795-800.

21. Casey DA, Wexler LH, Merchant MS, et al: Irinotecan and temozolomide for Ewing sarcoma: The Memorial Sloan-Kettering experience. *Pediatr Blood Cancer* 2009;53(6):1029-1034.

The authors presented a retrospective case report in which 20 patients with refractory Ewing sarcoma received 154 courses of irinotecan and temozolomide. Twelve patients had a complete or partial response. Level of evidence: IV.

22. Malempati S, Weigel B, Ingle AM, et al: Phase I/II trial and pharmacokinetic study of cixutumumab in pediatric patients with refractory solid tumors and Ewing sarcoma: A report from the Children's Oncology Group. *J Clin Oncol* 2012;30(3):256-262.

The authors reported on the results of a phase 1/phase 2 study of cixutumumab in refractory solid tumors. The maximum tolerated dose was determined. Three patients with Ewing sarcoma had partial response to single-agent cixutumumab. Level of evidence: II.

23. Naing A, LoRusso P, Fu S, et al: Insulin growth factor-receptor (IGF-1R) antibody cixutumumab combined with the mTOR inhibitor temsirolimus in patients with refractory Ewing's sarcoma family tumors. *Clin Cancer Res* 2012;18(9):2625-2631.

The authors reported on the results of a phase 2 study of temsirolimus and cixutumumab in refractory Ewing sarcoma and DSRCT. This combination of agents was determined to be feasible to administer. Seven of 20 patients had stable, partial, or complete response. Level of evidence: II.

24. Sonnemann J, Dreyer L, Hartwig M, et al: Histone deacetylase inhibitors induce cell death and enhance the apoptosis-inducing activity of TRAIL in Ewing's sarcoma cells. *J Cancer Res Clin Oncol* 2007;133(11): 847-858.

Three different histone deacetylase inhibitors (suberyolanilide hydroxamic acid, sodium butyrate, and MS-275) were applied to Ewing sarcoma cell lines, and all led to increased cell death. Level of evidence: V.

25. DuBois SG, Krailo MD, Lessnick SL, et al; Children's Oncology Group: Phase II study of intermediate-dose cytarabine in patients with relapsed or refractory Ewing sarcoma: A report from the Children's Oncology Group. *Pediatr Blood Cancer* 2009;52(3):324-327.

The authors reported on the results of a phase 2 study of cytarabine in relapsed or refractory Ewing sarcoma. The regimen was noted to have significant hematologic toxicity. No patients showed clinical disease response. Level of evidence: II.

26. Nooij MA, Whelan J, Bramwell VH, et al; European Osteosarcoma Intergroup: Doxorubicin and cisplatin chemotherapy in high-grade spindle cell sarcomas of the bone, other than osteosarcoma or malignant fibrous histiocytoma: A European Osteosarcoma Intergroup Study. *Eur J Cancer* 2005;41(2):225-230.

27. Cesari M, Bertoni F, Bacchini P, Mercuri M, Palmerini E, Ferrari S: Mesenchymal chondrosarcoma: An analysis of patients treated at a single institution. *Tumori* 2007;93(5):423-427.

The authors conducted a retrospective review of 26 patients with mesenchymal chondrosarcoma. At 48 months, no patients were alive who had not undergone complete surgical resection. In patients who underwent surgical resection, adjuvant chemotherapy significantly improved 10-year disease-free survival compared to those who did not receive chemotherapy. Level of evidence: IV.

28. Arndt CA, Stoner JA, Hawkins DS, et al: Vincristine, actinomycin, and cyclophosphamide compared with vincristine, actinomycin, and cyclophosphamide alternating with vincristine, topotecan, and cyclophosphamide for intermediate-risk rhabdomyosarcoma: Children's oncology group study D9803. *J Clin Oncol* 2009;27(31):5182-5188.

The authors reported the results of a pediatric RMS trial. There was no difference in outcomes in intermediate-risk patients randomized to VAC compared to VAC alternating with vincristine, topotecan, and cyclophosphamide. Level of evidence: I.

29. Crist W, Gehan EA, Ragab AH, et al: The Third Intergroup Rhabdomyosarcoma Study. *J Clin Oncol* 1995; 13(3):610-630.

30. Crist WM, Anderson JR, Meza JL, et al: Intergroup rhabdomyosarcoma study-IV: Results for patients with nonmetastatic disease. *J Clin Oncol* 2001;19(12): 3091-3102.

31. van Gaal JC, Flucke UE, Roeffen MH, et al: Anaplastic lymphoma kinase aberrations in rhabdomyosarcoma: Clinical and prognostic implications. *J Clin Oncol* 2012;30(3):308-315.

The authors evaluated 189 paraffin-embedded RMS tumor samples. The authors retrospectively identified statistically increased rates of cytoplasmic ALK protein expression and ALK copy number in alveolar RMS samples compared to embryonic RMS samples. Level of evidence: IV.

32. Bocale D, Rotelli MT, Cavallini A, Altomare DF: Antioestrogen therapy in the treatment of desmoid tumours: A systematic review. *Colorectal Dis* 2011; 13(12):e388-e395.

The authors presented a systematic review of 26 years of English-language articles of antiestrogen-based therapy for desmoid tumors. Forty-one articles reported on 168 patients and had an overall 51% response rate of anti-estrogen agents. Level of evidence: II.

33. Chugh R, Wathen JK, Patel SR, et al; Sarcoma Alliance for Research through Collaboration (SARC): Efficacy of imatinib in aggressive fibromatosis: Results of a phase II multicenter Sarcoma Alliance for Research through Collaboration (SARC) trial. *Clin Cancer Res* 2010;16(19):4884-4891.

The authors reported the results of a phase 2 study of imatinib in unresectable aggressive fibromatosis. Only 3 of 51 patients had an objective response, but 66% of patients had stable disease at 1 year. Level of evidence: II.

34. Garbay D, Le Cesne A, Penel N, et al: Chemotherapy in patients with desmoid tumors: A study from the French Sarcoma Group (FSG). *Ann Oncol* 2012;23(1): 182-186.

The authors conducted a retrospective review of 62 patients with desmoid tumor who received chemotherapy. The most common regimen was vinblastine and methotrexate. The highest response rate was for patients who received anthracycline-containing regimens. Level of evidence: IV.

35. Skapek SX, Ferguson WS, Granowetter L, et al; Pediatric Oncology Group: Vinblastine and methotrexate for desmoid fibromatosis in children: Results of a Pediatric Oncology Group Phase II Trial. *J Clin Oncol* 2007;25(5):501-506.

The authors reported the results of a phase 2 trial of methotrexate and vinblastine for desmoid tumors. In 28 patients, 31% showed responsive disease. Sixty-four percent of patients had progressive disease at a mean of 9.1 months. Level of evidence: II.

36. Agulnik M, Yarber JL, Okuno SH, et al: An openlabel, multicenter, phase II study of bevacizumab for the treatment of angiosarcoma and epithelioid hemangioendotheliomas. *Ann Oncol* 2013;24(1):257-263.

37. Ray-Coquard I, Italiano A, Bompas E, et al; French Sarcoma Group (GSF/GETO): Sorafenib for patients with advanced angiosarcoma: A phase II Trial from the

French Sarcoma Group (GSF/GETO). *Oncologist* 2012;17(2):260-266.

38. Italiano A, Cioffi A, Penel N, et al: Comparison of doxorubicin and weekly paclitaxel efficacy in metastatic angiosarcomas. *Cancer* 2012;118(13):3330-3336.

39. Fayette J, Martin E, Piperno-Neumann S, et al: Angiosarcomas, a heterogeneous group of sarcomas with specific behavior depending on primary site: A retrospective study of 161 cases. *Ann Oncol* 2007;18(12): 2030-2036.

    The authors conducted a retrospective review of three institutions' experiences with angiosarcoma over 24 years. The analysis showed that primary tumor sites in nonorgan soft tissue had the best outcomes. Level of evidence: IV.

40. Schlemmer M, Reichardt P, Verweij J, et al: Paclitaxel in patients with advanced angiosarcomas of soft tissue: A retrospective study of the EORTC soft tissue and bone sarcoma group. *Eur J Cancer* 2008;44(16):2433-2436.

    The authors reported the results of a retrospective multicenter review of 32 patients treated with paclitaxel for angiosarcoma. The response rate was 62%. Primary scalp angiosarcomas had the highest rates and longest duration of response. Level of evidence: IV.

41. McArthur GA, Demetri GD, van Oosterom A, et al: Molecular and clinical analysis of locally advanced dermatofibrosarcoma protuberans treated with imatinib: Imatinib Target Exploration Consortium Study B2225. *J Clin Oncol* 2005;23(4):866-873.

42. Kurkchubasche AG, Halvorson EG, Forman EN, Terek RM, Ferguson WS: The role of preoperative chemotherapy in the treatment of infantile fibrosarcoma. *J Pediatr Surg* 2000;35(6):880-883.

43. Xie X, Ghadimi MP, Young ED, et al: Combining EGFR and mTOR blockade for the treatment of epithelioid sarcoma. *Clin Cancer Res* 2011;17(18):5901-5912.

    The investigators evaluated epithelioid sarcoma tumor samples and cell lines. Microarray showed increased EGFR and mTOR expression. In vivo testing of erlotinib and rapamycin on cell lines revealed increased rates of apoptosis both separately and synergistically. Level of evidence: V.

44. Hilbert M, Mary P, Larroquet M, et al: Alveolar soft part sarcoma in childhood: Is Sunitinib-Sutent® treatment an effective approach? *Pediatr Blood Cancer* 2012;58(3):475-476.

    The authors presented a case report of two patients with progressive ASPS. They were treated with sunitinib and had continued regression of disease at 10 and 18 months after starting therapy. Level of evidence: V.

45. Stacchiotti S, Negri T, Zaffaroni N, et al: Sunitinib in advanced alveolar soft part sarcoma: Evidence of a direct antitumor effect. *Ann Oncol* 2011;22(7):1682-1690.

    The authors presented a case report of nine patients with ASPS. They were treated with sunitinib; five had partial response, three had stable disease, and one had progressive disease. Median progression-free survival was 17 months. Level of evidence: IV.

46. Hensley ML, Blessing JA, Mannel R, Rose PG: Fixed-dose rate gemcitabine plus docetaxel as first-line therapy for metastatic uterine leiomyosarcoma: A Gynecologic Oncology Group phase II trial. *Gynecol Oncol* 2008;109(3):329-334.

    The authors reported the results of a trial of gemcitabine and docetaxel for LMS. In 42 patients, the objective response rate was 35.8% with an additional 26.2% having stable disease. Median overall survival was 16 months. Level of evidence: II.

47. Hensley ML, Ishill N, Soslow R, et al: Adjuvant gemcitabine plus docetaxel for completely resected stages I-IV high grade uterine leiomyosarcoma: Results of a prospective study. *Gynecol Oncol* 2009;112(3):563-567.

    The authors reported the results of a trial of adjuvant gemcitabine and docetaxel for resected LMS. Twenty-five patients participated. At a median follow-up of 49 months, progression-free survival was 45%. There was a trend toward increased survival in stage I/II patients. Level of evidence: II.

48. Monk BJ, Blessing JA, Street DG, Muller CY, Burke JJ, Hensley ML: A phase II evaluation of trabectedin in the treatment of advanced, persistent, or recurrent uterine leiomyosarcoma: A gynecologic oncology group study. *Gynecol Oncol* 2012;124(1):48-52.

    The authors reported the results of a phase 2 study of single-agent trabectedin in advanced LMS. Two of 20 patients had an objective response, and 10 patients had stable disease. Overall survival was 26 months, with the median not yet reached. Level of evidence: II.

49. Pearl ML, Inagami M, McCauley DL, Valea FA, Chalas E, Fischer M: Mesna, doxorubicin, ifosfamide, and dacarbazine (MAID) chemotherapy for gynecological sarcomas. *Int J Gynecol Cancer* 2002;12(6):745-748.

50. Sutton G, Blessing JA, Malfetano JH: Ifosfamide and doxorubicin in the treatment of advanced leiomyosarcomas of the uterus: A Gynecologic Oncology Group study. *Gynecol Oncol* 1996;62(2):226-229.

51. Katz D, Boonsirikamchai P, Choi H, et al: Efficacy of first-line doxorubicin and ifosfamide in myxoid liposarcoma. *Clin Sarcoma Res* 2012;2(1):2.

    The authors reported the results of a retrospective review of 9 years of myxoid liposarcoma patients. Thirty-seven patients received doxorubicin and ifosfamide. The response rate was 43.2% by Response Evaluation Criteria in Solid Tumors (RECIST) and 86.5% by Choi criteria. Median overall survival was 31.1 months. Level of evidence: IV.

52. Gronchi A, Bui BN, Bonvalot S, et al: Phase II clinical trial of neoadjuvant trabectedin in patients with advanced localized myxoid liposarcoma. *Ann Oncol* 2012;23(3):771-776.

The authors reported the results of a phase 2 study of neoadjuvant trabectedin in advanced myxoid liposarcoma. The primary end point of this trial was histologic response. Of 23 patients, 1 had complete response, 2 had good response, and 10 had moderate response. Level of evidence: II.

53. Taylor BS, DeCarolis PL, Angeles CV, et al: Frequent alterations and epigenetic silencing of differentiation pathway genes in structurally rearranged liposarcomas. *Cancer Discov* 2011;1(7):587-597.

The investigators performed genome, exome, transcriptome, and cytosine methylome sequencing in dedifferentiated liposarcoma tumor samples. About 8% of samples contained mutations in *HDAC1*. The role of *CEBPA* alteration is also reviewed. Level of evidence: V.

54. Canter RJ, Qin LX, Maki RG, Brennan MF, Ladanyi M, Singer S: A synovial sarcoma-specific preoperative nomogram supports a survival benefit to ifosfamide-based chemotherapy and improves risk stratification for patients. *Clin Cancer Res* 2008;14(24):8191-8197.

The authors conducted a review of a large institution's 24-year experience with synovial sarcoma. Multivariate analysis showed that tumor size and primary site were predictors of disease-related death. The authors provided a nomogram to estimate patient survival. Level of evidence: IV.

55. Dantonello TM, Int-Veen C, Harms D, et al: Cooperative trial CWS-91 for localized soft tissue sarcoma in children, adolescents, and young adults. *J Clin Oncol* 2009;27(9):1446-1455.

The authors reported the results from a trial for young patients with RMS and NRSTS. Although decreased irradiation for lower-risk patients did not worsen outcomes, intensified chemotherapy did not improve outcomes for the highest-risk patients. Level of evidence: II.

56. Eilber FC, Brennan MF, Eilber FR, et al: Chemotherapy is associated with improved survival in adult patients with primary extremity synovial sarcoma. *Ann Surg* 2007;246(1):105-113.

Results of a review of 12 years of synovial sarcoma patients are reported. Of 101 patients, 68 received ifosfamide-containing chemotherapy and 33 received no chemotherapy. Patients who received ifosfamide had significantly improved survival and lower metastatic recurrence, but no difference in local recurrence. Level of evidence: IV.

57. Carli M, Ferrari A, Mattke A, et al: Pediatric malignant peripheral nerve sheath tumor: The Italian and German soft tissue sarcoma cooperative group. *J Clin Oncol* 2005;23(33):8422-8430.

58. Kushner BH, LaQuaglia MP, Wollner N, et al: Desmo-

plastic small round-cell tumor: Prolonged progression-free survival with aggressive multimodality therapy. *J Clin Oncol* 1996;14(5):1526-1531.

59. Cook RJ, Wang Z, Arora M, et al: Clinical outcomes of patients with desmoplastic small round cell tumor of the peritoneum undergoing autologous HCT: A CIBMTR retrospective analysis. *Bone Marrow Transplant* 2012;47(11):1455-1458.

The authors reported the results of a retrospective review of autologous transplant for DSRCT. Median survival was 36 months for those in complete remission compared to 21 months for those not in complete remission. Level of evidence: IV.

60. Aguilera D, Hayes-Jordan A, Anderson P, Woo S, Pearson M, Green H: Outpatient and home chemotherapy with novel local control strategies in desmoplastic small round cell tumor. *Sarcoma* 2008;2008: 261589.

The authors presented a case report of a pediatric patient with DSRCT treated with adjuvant peritoneal perfusion of cisplatin. The patient had a retroperitoneal relapse 18 months after initial therapy that was amenable to secondary treatment. Level of evidence: V.

61. Cianfrocca M, Lee S, Von Roenn J, et al: Pilot study evaluating the interaction between paclitaxel and protease inhibitors in patients with human immunodeficiency virus-associated Kaposi's sarcoma: An Eastern Cooperative Oncology Group (ECOG) and AIDS Malignancy Consortium (AMC) trial. *Cancer Chemother Pharmacol* 2011;68(4):827-833.

This multicenter trial evaluated the pharmacokinetics of paclitaxel in Kaposi sarcoma patients also on protease inhibitors. Although paclitaxel levels were higher in patients on protease inhibitors, outcomes and toxicities were no different than in patients not taking protease inhibitors. Level of evidence: II.

62. Mosam A, Shaik F, Uldrick TS, et al: A randomized controlled trial of highly active antiretroviral therapy versus highly active antiretroviral therapy and chemotherapy in therapy-naive patients with HIV-associated Kaposi sarcoma in South Africa. *J Acquir Immune Defic Syndr* 2012;60(2):150-157.

The authors reported the results of a randomized trial in Africa of chemotherapy and HAART versus HAART alone in patients with Kaposi sarcoma. The chemotherapy and HAART regimen produced higher response rates but no difference in overall survival. Level of evidence: Ib.

63. Zhong DT, Shi CM, Chen Q, Huang JZ, Liang JG, Lin D: Etoposide, vincristine, doxorubicin and dexamethasone (EVAD) combination chemotherapy as second-line treatment for advanced AIDS-related Kaposi's sarcoma. *J Cancer Res Clin Oncol* 2012;138(3):425-430.

The authors presented a retrospective analysis of etoposide, vincristine, doxorubicin, and dexamethasone in progressive Kaposi sarcoma. The response rate was 59.1%, most of which were partial responses. Median overall survival was 14.2 months. Level of evidence: IV.

64. Green DM, Breslow NE, Beckwith JB, Moksness J, Finklestein JZ, D'Angio GJ: Treatment of children with clear-cell sarcoma of the kidney: A report from the National Wilms' Tumor Study Group. *J Clin Oncol* 1994;12(10):2132-2137.

65. Janeway KA, Kim SY, Lodish M, et al; NIH Pediatric and Wild-Type GIST Clinic: Defects in succinate dehydrogenase in gastrointestinal stromal tumors lacking KIT and PDGFRA mutations. *Proc Natl Acad Sci USA* 2011;108(1):314-318.

    The authors reported on wild-type GIST patients who had tumor and underwent germline testing for SDH. Twenty-six who 30 tumors were SDHB negative by immunohistochemistry. Twelve percent of patients who underwent germline analysis were found to have *SDHB, SDHC,* or *SDHD* mutations. Level of evidence: IV.

66. Jung S, Kasper B: Palifosfamide, a bifunctional alkylator for the treatment of sarcomas. *IDrugs* 2010;13(1):38-48.

    The authors presented a review of the pharmacologic features of palifosfamide. Results from initial phase 1 and phase 2 trials were discussed. Level of evidence: IV.

67. Blay JY, von Mehren M, Samuels BL, et al: Phase I combination study of trabectedin and doxorubicin in patients with soft-tissue sarcoma. *Clin Cancer Res* 2008;14(20):6656-6662.

    The authors reported the results of a phase 1 trial of trabectedin and doxorubicin in progressive NRSTS. Forty-one patients participated, and maximum tolerated dose was determined. Five patients had a partial response, and 34 had stable disease. Median progression-free survival was 9.2 months. Level of evidence: IIb.

68. van der Graaf WT, Blay JY, Chawla SP, et al; EORTC Soft Tissue and Bone Sarcoma Group; PALETTE study group: Pazopanib for metastatic soft-tissue sarcoma (PALETTE): A randomised, double-blind, placebo-controlled phase 3 trial. *Lancet* 2012;379(9829):1879-1886.

    The authors reported the results of an international randomized phase 3 trial of pazopanib versus placebo in progressive NRSTS. In 369 patients, pazopanib extended progression-free survival from 1.6 to 4.6 months and extended overall survival from 10.7 to 12.5 months. Level of evidence: Ib.

69. Children's Oncology Group: Long-Term Follow-Up Guidelines for Survivors of Childhood, Adolescent, and Young Adult Cancers. http://survivorshipguidelines.org/pdf/LTFUGuidelines.pdf. Published October 2008. Accessed August 15, 2013.

    This Website contains detailed descriptions of known late effects from chemotherapy agents. It also contains recommendations for screening for these late effects. Detailed references are given for each recommendation.

Chapter 7

Targeted Therapy for Soft-Tissue and Bone Sarcomas

Warren A. Chow, MD, FACP

1: General Evaluation and Treatment of Musculoskeletal Tumors

Introduction

Sarcomas are rare malignant mesenchymal neoplasms that account for less than 1% of all human malignancies. Their significance lies in their demographics. Sarcomas account for approximately 15% of all pediatric malignancies, and are the fourth most common malignancy in young adults (ages 20 to 39 years). The difficulty in studying novel therapeutic agents for these tumors lies in their heterogeneity and relative rarity. Soft-tissue sarcomas (STSs) have more than 50 histologic subtypes, and osseous sarcomas occur at an incidence of approximately one tenth of STSs. Despite these substantial barriers to progress in understanding the biology and therapy of sarcomas, significant strides have been achieved in the last decade on both fronts.

Sarcomas can be broadly classified into those with characteristic chromosomal translocations that create oncogenic fusion proteins that are pathognomonic for the particular sarcoma type (eg, synovial sarcoma, t(X; 18) [SYT-SSX1, SYT-SSX2, SYT-SSX4]; Ewing sarcoma, t(11;22) [EWS-FLI1]; and alveolar rhabdomyosarcomas, t(2;13) [PAX3-FKHR, now known as FOXO1], t(1;13) [PAX7-FKHR]); those with more complex karyotypes (eg, leiomyosarcomas, pleomorphic undifferentiated sarcomas, and osteosarcomas); those with deletion of tumor suppressor genes (eg, rhabdoid tumors); those with a single genetic alteration (for example, well-differentiated or dedifferentiated liposarcomas); and those with tyrosine kinase mutations (for example, gastrointestinal stromal tumors [GISTs]).[1] The development of targeted therapy for sarcomas began with GISTs.

Historical Perspective

GISTs, which are the most common mesenchymal tumor of the gastrointestinal tract, arise from the intersti-

tial cells of Cajal (ICC) of the myenteric plexus, or their precursors. ICC are responsible for generating the electrical impulses necessary for peristalsis. Approximately 95% of GISTs overexpress the type 3 receptor tyrosine kinase KIT (CD117), which is detectable using immunohistochemistry. Pathognomonic for GISTs, single-driver mutations of KIT or the related tyrosine kinase platelet-derived growth factor receptor, alpha polypeptide (PDGFRA) gene (PDGFRA), were identified in Approximately 85% and 5% to 7% of GISTs, respectively.[2,3] These mutations lead to constitutive activation of their respective tyrosine kinase in the absence of their cognate ligand (stem cell factor and platelet-derived growth factor alpha polypeptide [PDGFA] respectively). Constitutive activation of ICC KIT or PDGFRA leads to phosphorylation of downstream substrates, including phosphatidylinositol 3-kinase (PI3K) and the serine/threonine kinase Akt, and results in malignant transformation to a GIST.

In 2001, an exploratory study was reported of a woman with metastatic gastric GIST, which was refractory to chemotherapy and immunotherapy following surgery.[4] She was treated with imatinib mesylate, a small molecule inhibitor of BCR-ABL1, KIT, and PDGFRA. Imatinib inhibits these tyrosine kinases by competitively binding to the adenosine triphosphate binding site and preventing phosphorylation of specific tyrosine residues. The patient experienced a rapid clinical response with disappearance of excess metabolic activity at 4 weeks using ^{18}F fluorodeoxyglucose (FDG) positron emission tomography (PET). A 75% reduction in tumor size was observed at 8-month follow-up, and tumor biopsies showed histologic evidence of myxoid degeneration and absence of mitotic activity. In rapid succession, an international, randomized phase 2 trial of imatinib at 400 mg versus 600 mg reproduced this dramatic result in patients with advanced or metastatic GIST.[5] Overall, 53.7% had a partial response, and 27.9% had stable disease. Two large, international phase 3 trials of imatinib at 400 mg versus 800 mg confirmed the phase 2 results and led to the approval of imatinib by the European Medicines Agency and the FDA in 2002.[6,7] These dramatic results ushered in the era of targeted molecular therapy for sarcomas and other solid tumors. Imatinib became the second

Dr. Chow or an immediate family member is a member of a speakers' bureau or has made paid presentations on behalf of Norvartis, and has received research or institutional support from Pfizer and Merck.

molecularly targeted agent for solid tumors approved by the FDA following approval of trastuzumab for metastatic HER2-positive breast cancer in 1998.

Molecular Pathology of Selected Sarcomas

Translocation-Associated Sarcomas

Chromosomal translocations comprise most of the specific genetic alterations associated with sarcomas. Altogether, translocation-associated sarcomas account for approximately one third of all sarcomas.[8]

Ewing sarcoma and primitive neuroectodermal tumors are characterized by a translocation between chromosomes 11 and 22 in approximately 85% of patients, where an in-frame fusion between the 5' end of the *EWS* gene from chromosome band 22q12 fuses with the 3' portion of the 11q24 *FLI1* gene, a member of the ETS family of transcription factor genes.[9] In 10% to 15% of patients, a variant translocation between chromosomes 21 and 22 fuses *EWS* to a closely related ETS gene, *ERG*, from chromosome band 21q22. The EWS-ETS chimeric transcription factors are required for maintenance of the malignant phenotype in Ewing sarcoma cell lines, and forced expression of EWS-FLI1 in mesenchymal stem cells results in transformation to a phenotype similar to Ewing sarcoma.[10,11] Importantly, EWS-FLI1 inhibits expression of insulinlike growth factor binding protein 3, which binds and transports insulin-like growth factor 1 (IGF1), the cognate ligand for IGF1 receptor (IGF1R), which leads to autocrine growth.[12] IGF1R is a target for drug development.

Desmoplastic small round cell tumor (DSRCT), like Ewing sarcoma, is characterized by a translocation between chromosomes 11 and 22. In this instance, *EWS* is fused to the Wilms tumor gene, *WT1*, at 11p13.[9] The chimeric EWS-WT1 product transactivates the IGF1R promoter and increases receptor expression.[13]

Clear cell sarcoma is distinguished by a translocation between chromosomes 11 and 22 in which *EWS* is fused to the activating transcription factor 1 (ATF1) gene (*ATF1*). ATF1 is a member of the CREB/ATF basic leucine zipper transcription factor family.[9] The fusion protein results in transcriptional activation of the microphthalmia transcription factor (MiT), a melanocyte differentiation factor. Notably, MiT transcriptionally activates the tyrosine kinase MNNG HOS transforming gene (*MET*).[14] *MET* is a target for drug development.

Alveolar rhabdomyosarcoma is characterized by two recurring chromosomal translocations: a translocation between chromosomes 2 and 13 results in *PAX3-FKHR*, and a translocation between chromosomes 1 and 13 results in *PAX7-FKHR*. The fusion proteins combine the DNA-binding domain of either *PAX* gene with the transactivation domain of *FKHR*.[9] The chimeric transcription factors target the IGF1R promoter, increasing receptor expression in these tumors.[15]

Synovial sarcoma is defined by detection of a translocation in which *SYT/SS18* from chromosome 18 joins *SSX1*, *SSX2*, or *SSX4* from the X chromosome.[9] Recent progress has demonstrated that SYT-SSX interacts with the transcriptional corepressor transducin-like enhancer of split 1 (TLE1) to target activating transcription factor 2 (ATF2), while simultaneously recruiting repressive histone deacetylase 1 (HDAC1) and polycomb repressive complex 2 (PRC2) to ATF2 targets.[16] This finding is important because HDAC inhibitors disrupt the interaction between TLE1 and the fusion protein, thus releasing HDAC and PRC2 complexes from ATF2 target promoters and derepressing expression of the target gene. HDAC inhibitors are approved for other oncologic indications.

Dermatofibrosarcoma protuberans (DFSP) is identified by a translocation between chromosomes 17 and 22 that translocates the *COL1A1* promoter to the platelet-derived growth factor beta polypeptide (PDGFB) gene, *PDGFB*.[17] The fusion protein is processed to mature PDGFB and exerts its pathogenic effect on the PDGFB receptor present on the cell surface of DFSP.

Inflammatory myofibroblastic tumor can be recognized by a rearrangement in chromosome band 2p23. Approximately 50% of inflammatory myofibroblastic tumors carry rearrangements of the anaplastic lymphoma kinase (ALK) locus in chromosome band 2p23 (*ALK*), including one that results in TPM3-ALK, which induces transformation in cell lines and animal models.[18] ALK inhibitors are in clinical use for non–small-cell lung cancer.

Alveolar soft part sarcoma (ASPS) is characterized by a translocation between chromosomes X and 17 resulting in the fusion gene *ASPL-TFE3*. Transcription factor E3 (TFE3) is a member of the MiT transcription factor family, and, similar to MiT, TFE3 can transactivate *MET*.[14]

Complex Karyotype Sarcomas

Leiomyosarcoma demonstrates highly complex, unstable karyotypes. Additionally, frequent losses of chromosome bands 13q and 10q, where two tumor suppressor genes, the retinoblastoma gene (*RB1*) and the phosphatase and tensin homolog gene (*PTEN*), reside, are observed.[19] PTEN antagonizes the kinase activity of PI3K, and loss of *PTEN* results in dysregulation of PI3K and hyperactivation of Akt. Akt lies upstream of mammalian target of rapamycin (mTOR), and hyperactivation of mTOR in leiomyosarcoma is common.

Pleomorphic undifferentiated sarcoma also demonstrates frequent loss of *RB1*. In addition, *TP53* mutation rates of approximately 60% are observed.[20]

Sarcomas With Tumor Suppressor Gene Deletion

Rhabdoid tumor is unique in that 85% of rhabdoid tumors demonstrate biallelic inactivation of the tumor suppressor gene *hSNF5/INI1*, now known as

SMARCB1, due to either deletion or mutation.[9] hSNF5/INI1 is a component of a chromatin-remodeling complex that controls expression of certain target genes involved in cell cycle regulation.

Sarcomas With a Single Genetic Alteration

Well-differentiated or dedifferentiated liposarcoma is characterized by amplification of the 12q13-15 chromosomal region that results in murine double minute (MDM2) overexpression, which binds p53 and inactivates it.[1] MDM2 inhibitors are currently in clinical trials.

Tyrosine Kinase Mutation Sarcomas

In GISTs, oncogenic mutations in KIT typically occur in the juxtamembrane domain encoded by exon 11 (71.3%) or the extracellular domain encoded by exon 9 (8.2%). Much less common mutations in PDGFRA were observed in exons 17 (1%) and 18 (1.2%) in a phase 3 study of imatinib in advanced or metastatic GIST; 16.7% of specimens had no identifiable mutation of KIT or PDGFRA (wild-type).[21] Importantly, sensitivity to tyrosine kinase inhibitors appears to depend upon mutation location.

Targeted Agents

Tyrosine Kinase Inhibitors

Imatinib was approved in 2002 by the FDA for advanced and metastatic GIST, and significant insight into its application has been garnered since then (Table 1). The objective response rate for imatinib was significantly higher for KIT exon 11 mutant genotypes (71.7%) compared to KIT exon 9 mutant and wild-type genotypes (44.4%) (P = 0.007) in the previously mentioned phase 3 study.[21] This difference extends to overall survival also (median, 60.0 months versus 38.5 and 49.0 months, respectively). Notably, an improved response rate was found for patients with exon 9 mutant tumors treated with imatinib at 800 mg versus 400 mg (67% versus 17%; P = 0.02), suggesting that higher doses of imatinib can overcome genotype-mediated resistance. Importantly, continuous dosing of imatinib is paramount in the setting of advanced disease. Investigators reported in two randomized, phase 3 trials that discontinuation (with retreatment upon progression) versus continuation of imatinib in patients with advanced GIST in whom the disease is controlled after either 1 year or 3 years led to significantly poorer progression-free survival (PFS) (18.0 months versus 6.1 months after 1 year, P < 0.0001, and 80% 2-year PFS versus 16% after 3 years, P < 0.0001, respectively).[22,23] These seminal studies have significantly influenced the management of advanced GIST.

Given the efficacy of imatinib in advanced GIST, its use in the adjuvant setting was evaluated in two randomized phase 3 trials. The first was a double-blind, placebo-controlled study enrolling 713 patients comparing imatinib at 400 mg daily to a placebo for 1 year.[24] Patients were at least age 18 years with a histologic diagnosis of KIT-positive GIST, had a resected tumor size of 3 cm or greater, and had undergone a complete gross resection within 84 days prior to the start of treatment. The study was terminated after an interim analysis demonstrated 30 recurrence-free survival (RFS) events (8%) in the imatinib group and 70 RFS events (20%) in the placebo group. The RFS rate at 1 year was 98% versus 83%. The hazard ratio in favor of imatinib was 0.398 (95% confidence interval, 0.26-0.61; P < 0.0001). Overall survival results were immature. Subset analysis demonstrated that the improvement in RFS in patients with tumors 3 cm to 10 cm was marginal, but still significant. Most of the benefit occurred in patients with tumors greater than 10 cm. On the basis of these results, the FDA granted approval of imatinib in the adjuvant setting in 2008, although there were no restrictions based on tumor size or length of treatment. The second phase 3 trial evaluated adjuvant imatinib at 400 mg daily for 3 years compared to 1 year in patients with high-risk GIST.[25] This study defined high-risk GIST as tumor diameter greater than 10 cm, mitotic activity of more than 10 mitotic figures per 50 high-power fields, size greater than 5 cm and mitotic activity of more than 5 mitotic figures per 50 high-power fields, or tumor rupture either spontaneously or during surgery. At a median follow-up of 54 months, 50 patients of 198 (25%) receiving 36 months of imatinib experienced recurrence or died, compared to 84 patients of 199 (42%) receiving 12 months of imatinib. These results yielded RFS rates of 86.6% at 3 years and 65.6% at 5 years, respectively, compared to 60.1% and 47.9% with 12 months of treatment (hazard ratio = 0.46; P < 0.0001). Given the efficacy of imatinib on relapse, it was quite unexpected that the secondary objective, overall survival, was also favored by longer treatment. The overall survival was 96.3% at 3 years and 92.0% at 5 years with 36 months of treatment, compared to 94.0% and 81.7%, respectively, with 12 months of imatinib (hazard ratio = 0.45; P = 0.019). These landmark studies were considered practice changing.

Imatinib has been evaluated in other sarcomas. Because DFSP is caused by activation of the PDGFB receptor, a patient with unresectable, metastatic DFSP was treated with 400 mg of imatinib twice daily.[17] The patient's PET scan normalized within 2 weeks of treatment, and the tumor volume shrank by more than 75% during the 4 months of therapy, allowing for resection of the mass. This result was confirmed in a pooled analysis of two phase 2 trials conducted in the United States and Europe, in which 24 patients with advanced DFSP were treated with either 400 mg or 800 mg of imatinib daily.[26] Eleven patients (46%) experienced a partial response, and the median time to progression (TTP) was 1.7 years, confirming significant activity of imatinib in this sarcoma subtype.

Chordomas are rare sarcomas of the notochord remnant that express PDGFB and/or platelet-derived

1: General Evaluation and Treatment of Musculoskeletal Tumors

Table 1

Selected Agents and Their Targets in Soft-Tissue and Bone Sarcomas

Agent(s)	Target(s)	Sarcoma Subtype(s)
Tyrosine Kinase Inhibitors		
Imatinib mesylate	BCR-ABL1, KIT, PDGFRA, PDGFRB	GIST;[4-7,21-25] DFSP [t(17;22)];[17,26] chordoma;[27] desmoid fibromatosis[28-30]
Sunitinib malate	KIT, PDGFRA, PDGFRB, VEGFRs 1 to 3, FLT3, RET, CSF-1	GIST[31]
Sorafenib	KIT, PDGFRB, VEGFRs 1 to 3, B-raf, FLT3	GIST[33]; angiosarcoma[34]
Regorafenib	c-Kit, PDGFRA, PDGFRB, , VEGFRs 2 and 3, B-raf, RET	GIST[36]
Masatinib	c-Kit, PDGFRA, PDGFRB, FGFR3, FAK	GIST[37]
Pazopanib	c-Kit, PDGFRA, PDGFRB, VEGFRs 1 to 3	Anthracycline-refractory soft-tissue sarcomas with exception of liposarcoma[38, 39]
Crizotinib	ALK, MET	Inflammatory myofibroblastic tumor [t(2p23)][18]
Cediranib	VEGFRs 1 to 3	Alveolar soft part sarcoma [t(X;17)][40]
Tivantinib (ARQ 197)	MET	Clear cell sarcoma [t(12;22)];[41] alveolar soft part sarcoma [t(X;17)][41]
Monoclonal Antibodies		
Bevacizumab	VEGF	Angiosarcoma;[43] hemangiopericytoma;[44] malignant solitary fibrous tumor[44]
R1507, ganitumab (AMG 479)	IGF1R	Ewing sarcoma [t(11;22), t(21;22)];[46] desmoplastic small round cell tumor [t(11;22)];[46, 47] alveolar rhabdomyosarcoma [t(2;13), t(1;13)][15]
Denosumab	RANKL	Giant cell tumor of bone;[55] pigmented villonodular synovitis[55]
Other Small Molecule Inhibitors		
Ridaforolimus (AP23573)	mTOR	Unselected soft-tissue and bone sarcomas[48, 49]
SB939	Histone deacetylase	Synovial sarcoma [t(X;18)][50]
RG7112 (RO5045337, Nutlin-3)	MDM2	Well-differentiated/dedifferentiated liposarcoma [amplification of 12q13-15][51]
PD0332991	CDK4/cyclin D1	Liposarcoma[52]
IPI-504, AT13387	HSP90	GIST[53, 54]
Vismodegib (GDC-0449)	Hedgehog	Unselected soft-tissue sarcomas[58]
RO4929097	γ-secretase/Notch	Unselected soft-tissue sarcomas[58]
Oncolytic Viruses		
Reolysin	double-stranded-RNA–activated protein kinase	Unselected soft-tissue and bone sarcomas[59]
Adoptive Immunotherapy		
Genetically engineered lymphocytes	NY-ESO-1	Synovial sarcoma [t(X;18)][60]

ALK = anaplastic lymphoma kinase, B-raf = B-rapidly accelerated fibrosarcoma kinase, CDK4 = cyclin-dependent kinase 4, CSF-1 = colony-stimulating factor 1 kinase, DFSP = dermatofibrosarcoma protuberans, FAK = focal adhesion kinase, FGFR3 = fibroblast growth factor receptor 3, FLT3 = Fms-like tyrosine kinase 3, GIST = gastrointestinal stromal tumor, HSP90 = heat shock protein 90, IGF1R = insulin-like growth factor 1 receptor, MDM2 = murine double minute, MET = MNNG HOS transforming receptor, mTOR = mammalian target of rapamycin, NY-ESO-1 = New York ESO-1 cancer/testis antigen, PDGFR = platelet-derived growth factor receptor, RANKL = receptor activator of nuclear factor-κ B ligand, RET = rearranged during transfection kinase, VEGF = vascular endothelial growth factor, VEGFR = vascular endothelial growth factor receptor.

growth factor receptor, beta polypeptide (PDGFRB). Metastases occur in approximately 20% of patients, generally with advanced disease. On the basis of the potential inhibition of PDGFRB, a multicenter phase 2 study of 800 mg of imatinib daily in 56 patients with advanced chordomas expressing PDGFRB was reported.[27] Among 50 evaluable patients, one partial response was observed at 6 months (2%), 35 patients experienced stable disease as the best response (70%), and a 64% clinical benefit rate (Response Evaluation Criteria In Solid Tumors [RECIST] complete response + partial response + stable disease ≥ 6 months) was noted. The low response rate observed here is further tempered by the indolent natural history of this disease.

Two multicenter phase 2 trials evaluating imatinib in multiple tumors have been reported. The first demonstrated an 8.9% response rate for solid tumors expressing KIT (four complete responses, nine partial responses) treated with 800 mg of imatinib daily.[28] However, all of the complete responses and six of the partial responses were observed in patients with DFSP, and the other two partial responses were in patients with desmoid tumors. In the second trial, imatinib at 300 mg given twice daily was evaluated in 10 subtypes of sarcomas.[29] One complete response (uterine leiomyosarcoma) and three partial responses (one each for myxoid/round cell liposarcoma, pleomorphic undifferentiated sarcoma, and fibrosarcoma) were observed in 185 patients treated (2% response rate). Accordingly, imatinib does not seem to be an active agent in non-GIST sarcomas with the exception of DFSP.

Although not true sarcomas, desmoid-type fibromatoses are clonal fibroblastic proliferations that arise in the deep soft tissues and are characterized by infiltrative growth and local recurrence but an inability to metastasize.[9] A phase 2 trial of imatinib at 800 mg daily in 19 patients was reported.[30] Three patients of 19 (15.7%) had a partial response, with four additional patients having stable disease lasting more than 1 year. The median time to treatment failure was 10.7 months. Sixteen patients of 19 (84%) had mutations involving the Wnt pathway (adenomatous polyposis coli [APC] or β-catenin [CTNNB1]); however, there was no correlation between Wnt pathway mutations and response to imatinib. There was no evidence of KIT, PDGFRA, or PDGFRB activation in any of the tumors. Twenty patients with advanced desmoid tumors were included in the aforementioned multitumor study.[29] Two patients had partial response (10%), and eight patients had stable disease (40%); the median TTP was 9.1 months. The molecular basis for the activity of imatinib in this disease remains unknown.

Sunitinib inhibits vascular endothelial growth factor receptors (VEGFRs) 1 to 3, PDGFRA, PDGFRB, KIT, Fms-like tyrosine kinase 3 (FLT3), rearranged during transfection kinase, and colony-stimulating factor 1 kinase (CSF-1). It was approved by the FDA in 2006 for the treatment of GIST after progression on, or intolerance to, imatinib. This approval was based on a ran-

domized, double-blind, placebo-controlled trial in patients who had disease progression during prior imatinib treatment or who were imatinib intolerant.[31] The primary end point was TTP. Two hundred seven patients were randomized to sunitinib and 105 to a placebo. Most patients enrolled (96% in both treatment arms) had tumors that had progressed on or within 6 months of completing prior imatinib therapy. An interim analysis after 149 TTP events had occurred demonstrated a significant advantage for sunitinib (median, 27 weeks versus 6 weeks, hazard ratio = 0.33; $P < 0.0001$), and an advantage in PFS (median, 24 weeks versus 6 weeks, hazard ratio = 0.33; $P < 0.0001$) was observed. In the sunitinib arm, 6.8% of patients experienced a partial response, compared to 0% in the placebo arm ($P = 0.006$). Subset analysis showed that sunitinib treatment yielded higher rates of antitumor response in tumors with KIT exon 9 mutations compared to KIT exon 11 mutations. Overall survival data have not been updated.

Sunitinib was evaluated for activity in non-GIST sarcomas.[32] Fifty-three patients with other sarcomas received 37.5 mg of sunitinib daily. Of 48 patients eligible for response, 1 patient (DSRCT) achieved a confirmed partial response and remained in the study for 56 weeks (2% response rate). Ten patients (20%) achieved stable disease for at least 16 weeks. Metabolic partial response (percentage change in maximum standardized uptake value less than –25%) was seen in 10 of 21 patients (48%) in whom ^{18}F FDG-PET was done. Like imatinib, sunitinib has limited activity in non-GIST sarcomas.

Sorafenib inhibits B-rapidly accelerated fibrosarcoma kinase (B-raf), VEGFRs 1 to 3, PDGFRB, FLT3, and KIT. It was approved by the FDA in 2005 for the treatment of advanced kidney cancer and in 2007 for the treatment of advanced liver cancer. Sorafenib has activity in imatinib-resistant and sunitinib-resistant GISTs.[33] In this population, 13% partial response and 58% stable disease was achieved. The median PFS was 5.3 months.

In two large phase 2 trials of sorafenib in non-GIST sarcomas, activity was disappointing.[34,35] In the first trial, 145 patients were treated with 400 mg twice daily in a multiarm study in multiple sarcoma subtypes.[34] Only one arm met the response rate primary end point (angiosarcoma, partial response 14%). The median PFS time was 3.2 months for the entire cohort. These results were recapitulated in a study with 51 patients, although this study had no confirmed responses even in the angiosarcoma cohort.[35] The median PFS time was also 3 months. These studies confirm the lack of activity of sorafenib in non-GIST sarcomas.

Regorafenib inhibits B-raf, VEGFRs 2 and 3, KIT, PDGFR, and rearranged during transfection (RET) kinases. A phase 3 trial of regorafenib versus placebo in patients with metastatic or unresectable GIST who failed at least previous imatinib and sunitinib demonstrated improvement in median PFS from 0.9 months to 4.8 months (hazard ratio = 0.27; 95% confidence interval 0.19-0.39; $P < 0.0001$).[36]

Masatinib inhibits KIT, PDGFRA, fibroblast growth factor receptor 3 (FGFR3), and focal adhesion kinase. Masatinib is undergoing evaluation in a phase 3 trial in patients with previously untreated metastatic GIST compared to imatinib, after a phase 2 trial in imatinib-naïve patients with locally advanced or metastatic GIST demonstrated 6.7% complete response, 43.3% partial response, 46.7% stable disease, and 3.3% progressive disease as best response at a median follow-up of 23.7 months. The median PFS was 27.2 months.[36,37]

Pazopanib inhibits VEGFRs 1 to 3, PDGFRA, PDG-FRB, and KIT. It was approved by the FDA in 2009 for the treatment of advanced kidney cancer. In 2009, a phase 2 study of pazopanib in patients with relapsed or refractory advanced STSs was reported.[38] One hundred forty-five patients received 800 mg of pazopanib daily. Four different strata were studied: adipocytic STS (liposarcoma), leiomyosarcomas, synovial sarcomas, and other types. The primary end point was the progression-free rate (PFR) at 12 weeks. The adipocytic stratum was closed early because of insufficient activity (26% PFR at 12 weeks); however, the PFRs at 12 weeks in the leiomyosarcoma stratum (44%), the synovial sarcoma stratum (49%), and the other stratum (39%) were intriguing enough to proceed to a randomized phase 3 trial. In this trial, patients with anthracycline-refractory STS (except liposarcoma) were randomized according to a 2:1 ratio to receive pazopanib or placebo.[39] The primary end point was PFS; 369 patients were randomized. Pazopanib significantly prolonged PFS (4.6 months versus 1.6 months; hazard ratio = 0.31; $P < 0.0001$). Overall survival was nonsignificantly improved with pazopanib (11.9 months versus 10.4 months, hazard ratio = 0.83; $P = 0.256$). The primary adverse effects observed were fatigue, hypertension, anorexia, and diarrhea. These results led the FDA to approve the drug in this setting. Pazopanib adds to the limited armamentarium for treating advanced STS.

Crizotinib inhibits ALK and MET, also known as hepatocyte growth factor receptor, was approved in 2011 for treatment of non–small-cell lung cancer in patients who possess rearrangements of the *ALK* locus. Because 50% of IMTs also carry *ALK* rearrangements, crizotinib was tested and shown to be effective in a patient with *ALK*-translocated IMT, and had no activity in another patient without the translocation.[18]

Cediranib inhibits VEGFRs 1 to 3. A phase 2 trial of cediranib for treatment of ASPS was reported in 2013.[40] Forty-six patients received 30 mg of cediranib daily. In 43 evaluable patients, 15 patients with partial response (35%) and 26 patients with stable disease (60%) were observed. Dynamic contrast-enhanced MRI and ^{18}F FDG-PET showed reduction in tumor blood flow and standard uptake values of target lesions, respectively. Cediranib may be an active agent for this rare STS subtype.

Tivantinib (ARQ 197) inhibits MET. Because the MiT transcription factor family can transactivate *MET*, a phase 2 study of tivantinib was conducted in patients with MiT-associated tumors.[41] Of 28 patients enrolled, 1 patient with partial response (clear cell sarcoma) and 15 patients with stable disease (10 with ASPS, 2 with clear cell sarcoma, 3 with translocation-associated renal cell carcinoma) were observed (4% response rate). The authors concluded that tivantinib demonstrated a favorable safety profile and preliminary evidence of antimalignancy activity in MiT-associated tumors.

Vascular Endothelial Growth Factor Inhibitors

Bevacizumab is a recombinant human monoclonal antibody that binds vascular endothelial growth factor. Angiogenesis is necessary for the growth, migration, and dissemination of sarcomas. A phase 2 trial in 17 patients with metastatic STS was conducted combining doxorubicin (75 mg/m^2) with bevacizumab (15 mg/kg) given intravenously every 3 weeks.[42] Two patients with partial response (12%) and 11 patients with stable disease lasting at least four cycles were observed. The response rate was no greater than that observed for single-agent doxorubicin, and six patients (35%) developed cardiac toxicity at or above grade 2, which is a cautionary note for this combination. More promising was a report of single-agent bevacizumab in 26 patients with angiosarcoma.[43] In a preliminary report, 3 patients with partial response (3 to 16 cycles), 13 patients with stable disease (3 to 32 cycles), and 10 patients with progressive disease were observed (12% response rate). Bevacizumab has definite activity in this STS subset. Additionally, the activity of bevacizumab in combination with the oral DNA alkylating agent temozolomide in advanced hemangiopericytoma and malignant solitary fibrous tumor was reported.[44] In a retrospective analysis of 14 patients treated with this novel combination, 11 patients (79%) achieved a Choi partial response as best response. Toxicity did not appear to be greater than would be observed with temozolomide alone. A phase 2 study of neoadjuvant bevacizumab and radiation therapy is ongoing.[45] Here, 5 of the 12 resected tumors were more than 85% necrotic, which was double the historical rate. Bevacizumab may have its broadest and most significant role here.

IGF1R Inhibitors

R1507 is a monoclonal antibody targeting IGF1R. Chromosomal translocations in Ewing sarcoma, DSRCT, and alveolar rhabdomyosarcoma lead to increased expression of IGF1R.[12,13,15] Increased IGF1R signaling promotes proliferation, differentiation, and prevention of apoptosis. A 10% response rate was observed in a phase 2 study of R1507 in 115 patients with Ewing sarcoma or primitive neuroectodermal tumor.[46] The median duration of response was 29 weeks. Despite these results, development of R1507 was halted by its manufacturer in December 2009.

Ganitumab (AMG 479) is also a monoclonal antibody targeting IGF1R. The response rate was 6%, with objective responses in DSRCT and Ewing sarcoma observed in 35 patients.[47] As a single agent, IGF1R antibodies clearly have modest activity, and this approach is likely to best be used in combination with other cytostatic or cytocidal agents.

mTOR Inhibitors

Ridaforolimus (AP23573), formerly known as deforolimus, is an analog of the natural compound sirolimus, an antifungal agent approved as an immunosuppressant for organ transplantation. A phase 2 trial of intravenous ridaforolimus (12.5 mg/day for 5 days every 2 weeks) in 213 patients with previously treated bone sarcoma and STS demonstrated a clinical benefit rate (defined as complete response, partial response, or stable disease for at least 16 weeks) of 28%.[48] There were five partial responses (three patients with osteosarcoma, one patient with spindle cell sarcoma of bone, and one patient with pleomorphic undifferentiated sarcoma) (2% response rate). These promising results led to an international phase 3 trial of ridaforolimus as maintenance therapy in patients with advanced sarcoma following standard cytotoxic chemotherapy.[49] Seven hundred eleven patients were randomly assigned to 40 mg of ridaforolimus orally for 5 days per week or a placebo. The study reached its primary end point PFS (hazard ratio = 0.72, $P = 0.001$). Median PFS improved by 21%; however, this finding translated to an absolute benefit of only 3.1 weeks (17.7 weeks versus 14.6 weeks). Accordingly, the FDA declined to approve the drug in this setting.

Histone Deacetylase Inhibitors

SB939 is a histone deacetylase inhibitor. Histone deacetylase inhibitors target a core epigenetic mechanism in synovial sarcoma caused by the SYT-SSX fusion protein.[16] A phase 2 study of SB939 in patients with translocation-associated recurrent or metastatic sarcomas is being conducted.[50] Results of this trial have not been reported to date.

MDM2 Inhibitors

RG7112 (RO5045337, Nutlin-3) interferes with the interaction between MDM2 and p53. A neoadjuvant study of RG7112 was conducted in chemotherapy-naive patients with primary or relapsed well-differentiated or dedifferentiated liposarcoma who were eligible for tumor resection.[51] Patients received RG7112 orally at 1,440 mg/m[2] daily for 10 days on a 28-day cycle. Three cycles were planned, followed by complete surgical resection. Twelve patients had well-differentiated liposarcoma, and nine patients had dedifferentiated liposarcoma. Thirteen of 14 evaluable patients had *MDM2* amplification, and 2 of 19 patients had *TP53* mutations. Nine of 14 patients had increased TUNEL activity, 9 of 13 patients had decreased Ki67 by immunohistochemistry, and 2 patients progressed.

The results show that RG7112 neoadjuvant treatment induces apoptosis and decreases proliferation in patients with well-differentiated or dedifferentiated liposarcoma.

Cyclin-Dependent Kinase 4 Inhibitors

PD0332991 selectively inhibits cyclin-dependent kinase 4 (CDK4)/cyclin D1 kinase, which inhibits retinoblastoma (Rb) phosphorylation and prevents Rb-positive tumor cells from entering the S phase of the cell cycle A phase 2 study of PD0332991 in patients with advanced or metastatic liposarcoma reported that the median PFS was 18 weeks, and at 12 weeks, 66% of patients were free from progression. 1 partial response was noted in the 30 patients enrolled.[52]

Heat Shock Protein 90 Inhibitors

IPI-504 and AT13387 are heat shock protein 90 (HSP90) inhibitors. HSP90 is a molecular chaperone that participates in stabilizing and activating more than 200 "client" proteins, many of which are oncoproteins. Secondary mutations in the KIT oncoprotein drive resistance to imatinib in GIST. Accordingly, a phase 3 study of IPI-504 versus placebo in patients with GIST following failure of treatment with imatinib and/or sunitinib was conducted.[53] Forty-seven of the projected 195 patients were enrolled; however, the trial was terminated early because four on-treatment deaths occurred in the IPI-504 arm. A phase 2 trial of AT13387 is ongoing in patients with unresectable and/or metastatic GIST who have progressed following treatment with up to three tyrosine kinase inhibitors.[54] Results have not yet been published.

Receptor Activator of Nuclear Factor-κ B Ligand Inhibitors

Denosumab is a fully humanized monoclonal antibody targeting receptor activator of nuclear factor-κ B (RANK) ligand (RANKL) inhibits osteoclast-mediated bone destruction. Giant cell tumor (GCT) of bone is a primary osteolytic bone tumor of low metastatic potential, with a propensity for metastasis to the lung should it occur; however, it is associated with significant skeletal morbidity.[9] GCT of bone is composed of sheets of neoplastic ovoid mononuclear cells interspersed with uniformly distributed large, osteoclastlike giant cells. The osteoclastlike giant cells express RANK, and some of the mononuclear (stromal) cells express RANKL. An open-label, phase 2 study of denosumab was conducted in patients with GCT of bone.[55] Thirty-seven patients were enrolled and received 120 mg of subcutaneous denosumab monthly with loading doses on days 8 and 15 of month 1. The primary end point was tumor response, defined as elimination of 90% or more of giant cells or no radiologic progression of the target lesion up to week 25. Thirty of 35 evaluable patients had a tumor response (20 of 20 patients with histologic evaluation; 10 of 15 patients with radiologic evaluation)

(86% response rate). The results demonstrate that denosumab, by interfering with the interaction between RANK-positive osteoclastlike giant cells and RANKL-positive stromal cells, has activity as a therapeutic agent for GCT of bone.

Hedgehog and γ-Secretase Inhibitors

Vismodegib (GDC-0449) and RO4929097 are oral hedgehog (Hh) and γ-secretase/Notch signaling pathway inhibitors, respectively. The Hh and Notch signaling pathways inhibit mesenchymal stem cell differentiation and maintain stem cells in an undifferentiated state. Hh and Notch signaling pathways play a similar role in undifferentiated sarcomas, maintaining tumor-initiating cells in a less differentiated state.[56] Vismodegib inhibits Smoothened (Smo), a downstream target of Hh when bound to Ptch1.[56] Vismodegib was approved by the FDA in 2012 for treatment of advanced basal cell carcinoma. RO4929097 inhibits γ-secretase-mediated Notch receptor cleavage upon its activation.[57] A phase 1B/2 study of GDC-0449 plus RO4929097 in advanced or metastatic sarcomas is currently under way.[58] No results from this trial are available.

Oncolytic Viruses

Reolysin (Oncolytics Biotech) is a proprietary form of the naturally occurring double-stranded RNA (dsRNA) reovirus that specifically targets malignant cells with activated Ras signaling pathway by inhibiting dsRNA-activated protein kinase.[59] A phase 2 trial of Reolysin given intravenously daily for 5 days every 28 days to 52 patients showed encouraging results in adult patients with resistant bone and STSs with lung metastases.[59] In this study, 43% of patients achieved stable disease for more than 8 weeks, and 14% achieved stable disease for more than 24 weeks. The therapy was well tolerated and without dose-limiting toxicities. This study shows that oncolytic viruses may have future applications in sarcomas.

Adoptive Immunotherapy

Genetically engineered lymphocytes reactive with New York esophageal squamous cell carcinoma-1 cancer/testis antigen (NY-ESO-1) are genetically modified autologous T lymphocytes harvested from patients expressing high levels of NY-ESO-1, a cancer/testis antigen not normally expressed in adult human tissue except for testis, but expressed in approximately 80% of synovial sarcoma.[60] The T lymphocytes are transduced with a retroviral vector containing a T cell receptor (TCR) with an enhanced ability to recognize NY-ESO-1 in the context of HLA-A*0201 class I restriction. The transduced T lymphocytes are expanded and adoptively transferred into patients after treatment with a lymphodepleting chemotherapy regimen consisting of cyclophosphamide and fludarabine. In a pilot trial using genetically engineered T lymphocytes reactive with NY-ESO-1, six patients with synovial sarcoma, refractory to extensive prior treatment,

were enrolled.[60] Four of the six patients exhibited an objective partial response, with one lasting 18 months (67% response rate). Between 2% and 60% of the CD8+ T cells present in peripheral blood mononuclear cells bound NY-ESO-1 tetramer at 1 month. Peptide-specific and tumor-specific interferon-γ ELISPOT responses were detected in peripheral blood mononuclear cells from most patients 1 month after therapy. Tumor regression was not correlated with the persistence of transferred T lymphocytes or ELISPOT responses. This study is the first adoptive immunotherapy trial to treat synovial sarcoma using genetically engineered T lymphocytes to express a cancer/testis antigen-specific TCR, and raises the hope that this approach can be broadened to other sarcoma subtypes with unique malignancy antigens.

Summary

Significant advancement in the treatment of sarcomas has been achieved with the advent of targeted therapy. This achievement is even more remarkable given the rarity and heterogeneity of these malignancies. Certainly, these types of studies could be conducted only with significant collaboration among groups focused on sarcomas both nationwide and worldwide. It was led by the seminal discovery that imatinib inhibits KIT-mediated GIST oncogenesis more than a decade ago. Driven by new insights into sarcoma biology through the development and application of novel techniques in molecular and cell biology, the resulting breadth of therapeutic options currently ranges from small molecule inhibitors to adoptive immunotherapy (**Table 1**). In addition, novel clinical end points, such as the clinical benefit rate, that encompass response and stable disease should be used given the predominant cytostatic mechanism of these targeted therapies. Analogously, the use of novel response criteria such as the Choi criteria, in which response is defined as decrease in tumor size more than 10% (versus 30% for RECIST) or decrease in tumor density more than 15% on CT, will allow investigators to glean early insight into antitumor activity without unnecessarily withdrawing a patient for RECIST-defined progressive disease.[61] This chapter was not intended to be completely inclusive; rather, it offers insights into the molecular and biologic rationale for these new approaches.

Annotated References

1. Borden EC, Baker LH, Bell RS, et al: Soft tissue sarcomas of adults: State of the translational science. *Clin Cancer Res* 2003;9(6):1941-1956.

2. Hirota S, Isozaki K, Moriyama Y, et al: Gain-of-function mutations of c-kit in human gastrointestinal stromal tumors. *Science* 1998;279(5350):577-580.

3. Heinrich MC, Corless CL, Duensing A, et al: PDGFRA activating mutations in gastrointestinal stromal tumors. *Science* 2003;299(5607):708-710.

4. Joensuu H, Roberts PJ, Sarlomo-Rikala M, et al: Effect of the tyrosine kinase inhibitor STI571 in a patient with a metastatic gastrointestinal stromal tumor. *N Engl J Med* 2001;344(14):1052-1056.

5. Demetri GD, von Mehren M, Blanke CD, et al: Efficacy and safety of imatinib mesylate in advanced gastrointestinal stromal tumors. *N Engl J Med* 2002; 347(7):472-480.

6. Verweij J, Casali PG, Zalcberg J, et al: Progression-free survival in gastrointestinal stromal tumours with high-dose imatinib: randomised trial. *Lancet* 2004;364 (9440):1127-1134.

7. Blanke CD, Rankin C, Demetri GD, et al: Phase III randomized, intergroup trial assessing imatinib mesylate at two dose levels in patients with unresectable or metastatic gastrointestinal stromal tumors expressing the kit receptor tyrosine kinase: S0033. *J Clin Oncol* 2008;26(4):626-632.

   This US-led phase 3 trial of imatinib for unresectable or metastatic GIST led to its approval by the FDA. Level of evidence: I.

8. Mitelman F: Recurrent chromosome aberrations in cancer. *Mutat Res* 2000;462(2-3):247-253.

9. Fletcher CD, Unni KK, Mertens F (eds): *Pathology and Genetics of Tumours of Soft Tissue and Bone.* Lyon, France, IARC Press, 2002.

10. Arvand A, Denny CT: Biology of EWS/ETS fusions in Ewing's family tumors. *Oncogene* 2001;20(40):5747-5754.

11. Torchia EC, Jaishankar S, Baker SJ: Ewing tumor fusion proteins block the differentiation of pluripotent marrow stromal cells. *Cancer Res* 2003;63(13):3464-3468.

12. Prieur A, Tirode F, Cohen P, Delattre O: EWS/FLI-1 silencing and gene profiling of Ewing cells reveal downstream oncogenic pathways and a crucial role for repression of insulin-like growth factor binding protein 3. *Mol Cell Biol* 2004;24(16):7275-7283.

13. Karnieli E, Werner H, Rauscher FJ III, Benjamin LE, LeRoith D: The IGF-I receptor gene promoter is a molecular target for the Ewing's sarcoma-Wilms' tumor 1 fusion protein. *J Biol Chem* 1996;271(32):19304-19309.

14. Davis IJ, Fisher DE: MiT transcription factor associated malignancies in man. *Cell Cycle* 2007;6(14): 1724-1729.

   A general review of genetic strategies associated with disregulation of miT transcription factor is presented.

15. Kolb EA, Gorlick R: Development of IGF-1R inhibitors in pediatric sarcomas. *Curr Oncol Rep* 2009; 11(4):307-313.

   The authors reviewed preclinical data and ongoing clinical trials, along with issues related to development of drugs to treat pediatric malignancies.

16. Su L, Sampaio AV, Jones KB, et al: Deconstruction of the SS18-SSX fusion oncoprotein complex: Insights into disease etiology and therapeutics. *Cancer Cell* 2012;21(3):333-347.

   The authors studied the SS18-SSX fustion complex and determined that its activity results in repression of activating transcription factor 2 target genes.

17. Rubin BP, Schuetze SM, Eary JF, et al: Molecular targeting of platelet-derived growth factor B by imatinib mesylate in a patient with metastatic dermatofibrosarcoma protuberans. *J Clin Oncol* 2002;20(17):3586-3591.

   This is the first case report of a patient with refractory, metastatic DFSP treated successfully with imatinib. Level of evidence: II-3.

18. Butrynski JE, D'Adamo DR, Hornick JL, et al: Crizotinib in ALK-rearranged inflammatory myofibroblastic tumor. *N Engl J Med* 2010;363(18):1727-1733.

   This is the first report of a patient with refractory, metastatic IMT treated successfully with crizotinib. Level of evidence: II-3.

19. Grossmann AH, Layfield LJ, Randall RL: Classification, molecular characterization, and the significance of pten alteration in leiomyosarcoma. *Sarcoma* 2012; 2012:380896.

   A general discussion of the mechanism of leiomyosarcomagenesis and the role of *Pten* in genomic stability is presented.

20. Ghadimi MP, Liu P, Peng T, et al: Pleomorphic liposarcoma: Clinical observations and molecular variables. *Cancer* 2011;117(23):5359-5369.

   The authors studied natural history, patient outcomes, and commonly deregulated protein biomarkers associated with pleomorphic liposarcoma. The 5-year disease-specific survival rate was 53%.

21. Heinrich MC, Owzar K, Corless CL, et al: Correlation of kinase genotype and clinical outcome in the North American Intergroup Phase III Trial of imatinib mesylate for treatment of advanced gastrointestinal stromal tumor: CALGB 150105 Study by Cancer and Leukemia Group B and Southwest Oncology Group. *J Clin Oncol* 2008;26(33):5360-5367.

   This retrospective study correlated c-Kit and PDGFR-A genotype to response and survival in the randomized, phase 3 trial of standard versus high-dose imatinib in advanced or metastatic GIST. Level of evidence: II-1.

22. Blay JY, Le Cesne A, Ray-Coquard I, et al: Prospective multicentric randomized phase III study of imatinib in

patients with advanced gastrointestinal stromal tumors comparing interruption versus continuation of treatment beyond 1 year: The French Sarcoma Group. *J Clin Oncol* 2007;25(9):1107-1113.

This phase 3 study demonstrated that discontinuation of imatinib in patients with metastatic GIST with at least stable disease for 1 year led to significantly reduced PFS, but did not affect overall survival. Level of evidence: I.

23. Le Cesne A, Ray-Coquard I, Bui BN, et al; French Sarcoma Group: Discontinuation of imatinib in patients with advanced gastrointestinal stromal tumours after 3 years of treatment: An open-label multicentre randomised phase 3 trial. *Lancet Oncol* 2010;11(10): 942-949.

This study is a long-term follow-up of the previous French Sarcoma Group discontinuation trial of imatinib in patients with metastatic GIST. Level of evidence: I.

24. Dematteo RP, Ballman KV, Antonescu CR, et al; American College of Surgeons Oncology Group (ACOSOG) Intergroup Adjuvant GIST Study Team: Adjuvant imatinib mesylate after resection of localised, primary gastrointestinal stromal tumour: A randomised, double-blind, placebo-controlled trial. *Lancet* 2009;373(9669):1097-1104.

This phase 3 trial demonstrated that adjuvant imatinib at 400 mg daily for 1 year significantly improved RFS compared to placebo in patients with GISTs ≥ 3 cm. Level of evidence: I.

25. Joensuu H, Eriksson M, Sundby Hall K, et al: One vs three years of adjuvant imatinib for operable gastrointestinal stromal tumor: A randomized trial. *JAMA* 2012;307(12):1265-1272.

This phase 3 trial demonstrated that adjuvant imatinib at 400 mg daily for 3 years significantly improved RFS and overall survival compared to 400 mg daily for 1 year in high-risk GIST patients. Level of evidence: I.

26. Rutkowski P, Van Glabbeke M, Rankin CJ, et al; European Organisation for Research and Treatment of Cancer Soft Tissue/Bone Sarcoma Group; Southwest Oncology Group: Imatinib mesylate in advanced dermatofibrosarcoma protuberans: Pooled analysis of two phase II clinical trials. *J Clin Oncol* 2010;28(10):1772-1779.

This pooled analysis of two phase 2 trials of imatinb for advanced dermatofibrosarcoma protuberans demonstrated an overall response rate of 46%. Level of evidence: II-1.

27. Stacchiotti S, Longhi A, Ferraresi V, et al: Phase II study of imatinib in advanced chordoma. *J Clin Oncol* 2012;30(9):914-920.

A multinational, phase 2 trial demonstrated modest activity of imatinib for chordomas. Level of evidence: II-1.

28. Heinrich MC, Joensuu H, Demetri GD, et al; Imatinib Target Exploration Consortium Study B2225: Phase II,

open-label study evaluating the activity of imatinib in treating life-threatening malignancies known to be associated with imatinib-sensitive tyrosine kinases. *Clin Cancer Res* 2008;14(9):2717-2725.

This multicenter, phase 2 study of imatinib in 40 different malignancies demonstrated clinical benefit confined to diseases with known genomic mechanisms of activation of imatinib target kinases. Level of evidence: II-1.

29. Chugh R, Wathen JK, Maki RG, et al: Phase II multicenter trial of imatinib in 10 histologic subtypes of sarcoma using a bayesian hierarchical statistical model. *J Clin Oncol* 2009;27(19):3148-3153.

This multicenter phase 2 study of imatinib in 10 histologic subtypes of sarcoma demonstrated minimal activity. Level of evidence: II-1.

30. Penel N, Le Cesne A, Bui BN, et al: Imatinib for progressive and recurrent aggressive fibromatosis (desmoid tumors): An FNCLCC/French Sarcoma Group phase II trial with a long-term follow-up. *Ann Oncol* 2011;22(2):452-457.

This phase 2 trial demonstrated a 15.7% partial response rate with imatinib at 800 mg daily in patients with desmoid tumors. Level of evidence: II-1.

31. Demetri GD, van Oosterom AT, Garrett CR, et al: Efficacy and safety of sunitinib in patients with advanced gastrointestinal stromal tumour after failure of imatinib: A randomised controlled trial. *Lancet* 2006; 368(9544):1329-1338.

32. George S, Merriam P, Maki RG, et al: Multicenter phase II trial of sunitinib in the treatment of nongastrointestinal stromal tumor sarcomas. *J Clin Oncol* 2009;27(19):3154-3160.

This multicenter phase 2 trial of sunitinib in non-GIST sarcomas demonstrated notable metabolic responses but rare RECIST-defined responses. Level of evidence: II-1.

33. Wiebe L, Kasza KE, Maki RG, et al: Activity of sorafenib (SOR) in patients (pts) with imatinib (IM) and sunitinib (SU)-resistant (RES) gastrointestinal stromal tumors (GIST): A phase II trial of the University of Chicago Phase II Consortium. *J Clin Oncol 2008 ASCO Annual Meeting Proceedings* 2008; 26(suppl 15):10502.

This multicenter phase 2 trial of sorafenib demonstrated a disease control rate of 71% in patients with imatinib and sunitinib-resistant GIST. Level of evidence: II-1.

34. Maki RG, D'Adamo DR, Keohan ML, et al: Phase II study of sorafenib in patients with metastatic or recurrent sarcomas. *J Clin Oncol* 2009;27(19):3133-3140.

This multicenter phase 2 trial of sorafenib in multiple sarcoma subtypes demonstrated modest activity for angiosarcomas. Level of evidence: II-1.

35. von Mehren M, Rankin C, Goldblum JR, et al: Phase 2 Southwest Oncology Group-directed intergroup trial

(S0505) of sorafenib in advanced soft tissue sarcomas. *Cancer* 2012;118(3):770-776.

This multicenter phase 2 trial of sorafenib in advanced vascular sarcomas, high-grade liposarcomas, and leiomyosarcomas demonstrated no confirmed responses. Level of evidence: II-1.

36. Demetri GD, Reichardt P, Kang Y-K, et al; GRID study investigators: Efficacy and safety of regorafenib for advanced gastrointestinal stromal tumours after failure of imatinib and sunitinib (GRID): An international, multicentre, randomised, placebo-controlled, phase 3 trial. *Lancet* 2013;381(9863):295-302.

    This multinational phase 3 trial demonstrated improvement in PFS from 0.9 months in the placebo arm to 4.8 months in the regorafenib arm in patients with imatinib and sunitinib-resistant GIST. Level of evidence: I.

37. Le Cesne A, Blay J, Bui NB, et al: Masatinib mesylate in imatinib-naïve locally advanced or metastatic gastrointestinal stromal tumor (GIST): Results of the French Sarcoma Group phase II trial. *J Clin Oncol* 2009;15s:10507a.

38. Sleijfer S, Ray-Coquard I, Papai Z, et al: Pazopanib, a multikinase angiogenesis inhibitor, in patients with relapsed or refractory advanced soft tissue sarcoma: A phase II study from the European organisation for research and treatment of cancer-soft tissue and bone sarcoma group (EORTC study 62043). *J Clin Oncol* 2009;27(19):3126-3132.

    This multicenter phase 2 trial demonstrated a promising 12-week progression-free rate in patients with leiomyosarcoma, synovial sarcoma, and other soft-tissue sarcomas. Insufficient activity was observed in the adipocytic sarcoma cohort. Level of evidence: l II-1.

39. van der Graaf WT, Blay JY, Chawla SP, et al; EORTC Soft Tissue and Bone Sarcoma Group; PALETTE study group: Pazopanib for metastatic soft-tissue sarcoma (PALETTE): A randomised, double-blind, placebo-controlled phase 3 trial. *Lancet* 2012;379(9829):1879-1886.

    This phase 3 trial of pazopanib in patients with anthracycline-refractory STS demonstrated significant improvement in PFS compared to placebo. Level of evidence: I.

40. Kummar S, Allen D, Monks A, et al: Cediranib for metastatic alveolar soft part sarcoma. *J Clin Oncol* 2013;31(18):2296-2302.

    This phase 2 trial of cediranib reported an overall response rate of 35% for metastatic alveolar soft part sarcoma. Level of evidence: II-1.

41. Goldberg J, Demetri GD, Choy E, et al: Preliminary results from a phase II study of ARQ 197 in patients with microphthalmia transcription factor family (MiT)-associated tumors. *J Clin Oncol 2009 ASCO Annual Meeting Proceedings* 2009;29(suppl 15): 10502.

    This multicenter phase 2 trial reported modest clinical activity for ARQ 197 in patients with clear cell sarcoma, alveolar soft part sarcoma, and translocation-associated renal cell carcinoma. Level of evidence: II-1.

42. D'Adamo DR, Anderson SE, Albritton K, et al: Phase II study of doxorubicin and bevacizumab for patients with metastatic soft-tissue sarcomas. *J Clin Oncol* 2005;23(28):7135-7142.

43. Agulnik M, Oksuno SH, Von Mehren M, et al: An open-label multicenter phase II study of bevacizumab for the treatment of angiosarcoma. *J Clin Oncol 2009 ASCO Annual Meeting Proceedings* 2009;27(suppl 15):10522.

    This multicenter phase 2 trial reported modest clinical activity (3 PRs in 26 evaluable patients) for bevacizumab in angiosarcoma. Level of evidence: II-1.

44. Park MS, Patel SR, Ludwig JA, et al: Activity of temozolomide and bevacizumab in the treatment of locally advanced, recurrent, and metastatic hemangiopericytoma and malignant solitary fibrous tumor. *Cancer* 2011;117(21):4939-4947.

    The authors present a single-center, retrospective review that revealed significant activity for temozolomide and bevacizumab in hemangiopericytoma and solitary fibrous tumor. Level of evidence: II-3.

45. Yoon SS, Karl D, Rothrock C, et al: Abstract: Interim analysis of a phase II study of neoadjuvant bevacizumab and radiation therapy for resectable soft tissue sarcomas. *Proc CTOS* 2009;15:39179.

    An interim analysis of an ongoing phase 2 trial of neoadjuvant bevacizumab and radiation therapy for soft-tissue sarcomas is presented. Level of evidence: II-2.

46. Pappo AS, Patel SR, Crowley J, et al: R1507, a monoclonal antibody to the insulin-like growth factor 1 receptor, in patients with recurrent or refractory Ewing sarcoma family of tumors: Results of a phase II Sarcoma Alliance for Research through Collaboration study. *J Clin Oncol* 2011;29(34):4541-4547.

    This multicenter phase 2 trial demonstrated a modest 10% response rate for R1507, a monoclonal antibody to the insulin-like growth factor 1 receptor, in patients with Ewing sarcoma family of tumors. Level of evidence: l II-1.

47. Tap WD, Demetri GD, Barnette P, et al: AMG 479 in relapsed or refractory Ewing's family tumors (EFT) or desmoplastic small round cell tumors (DSRCT): Phase II results. *J Clin Oncol 2010 ASCO Annual Meeting Proceedings* 2010;28(suppl 15):10001.

    This multicenter phase 2 trial demonstrated a modest 6% response rate for AMG 479, a monoclonal antibody to the insulin-like growth factor 1 receptor, in patients with Ewing sarcoma family of tumors or desmoplastic small round cell tumors. Level of evidence: II-1.

48. Chawla SP, Tolcher AW, Staddon AP, et al: Updated results of a phase II trial of AP23573, a novel mTOR inhibitor, in patients (pts) with advanced soft tissue or bone sarcomas. *J Clin Oncol 2006 ASCO Annual Meeting Proceedings* 2006;24(suppl 18):9505.

49. Demetri GD, Chawla SP, Ray-Coquard I, et al: Results of an international randomized phase III trial of the mammalian target of rapamycin inhibitor ridaforolimus versus placebo to control metastatic sarcomas in patients after benefit from prior chemotherapy. *J Clin Oncol* 2013;31(19):2485-2492.

This phase 3 study of maintenance therapy with ridaforolimus following standard cytotoxic chemotherapy demonstrated a 3.1-week PFS advantage compared to placebo (*P* = 0.001). Level of evidence: I.

50. National Institutes of Health: A study of SB939 in patients with translocation-associated recurrent/metastatic sarcomas (IND200). http://clinicaltrials.gov/ct2/show/NCT01112384. Accessed September 25, 2013.

51. Ray-Coquard IL, Blay JY, Italiano A, et al: Effect of the MDM2 antagonist RG7112 on the P53 pathway in patients with MDM2-amplified, well-differentiated or dedifferentiated liposarcoma: An exploratory proof-of-mechanism study. *Lancet Oncol* 2012;13(11):1133-1140.

This multicenter phase 2 trial showed molecular changes consistent with MDM2 inhibition and P53 activation in patients with liposarcoma receiving RG7112 in the neoadjuvant setting. Level of evidence: II-1.

52. Dickson MA, Tap WD, Keohan ML, et al: Phase II trial of the CDK4 inhibitor PD0332991 in patients with advanced CDK4-amplified well-differentiated or dedifferentiated liposarcoma. *J Clin Oncol* 2013;31(16):2024-2028.

This phase 2 trial demonstrated promising 66% 12-week PFS in patients with advanced CDK4-amplified well-differentiated or dedifferentiated liposarcoma. Level of evidence: II-1.

53. Demetri GD, Le Cense A, Von Mehren M, et al: Abstract: Final results from a phase II study of IPI-504 (retaspimycin hydrochloride) versus placebo in patients (pts) with gastrointestinal stromal tumors (GIST) following failure of kinase inhibitor therapies. *Proc GI Cancers Symposium* 2010;64.

54. National Institutes of Health: A study to investigate the safety and efficacy of AT13387, alone or in combination with imatinib, in patients with GIST. http://clinicaltrials.gov/ct2/show/NCT01294202. Accessed September 24, 2013.

55. Thomas D, Henshaw R, Skubitz K, et al: Denosumab in patients with giant-cell tumour of bone: An open-label, phase 2 study. *Lancet Oncol* 2010;11(3):275-280.

This open-label, phase 2 trial of denosumab demonstrated efficacy in patients with unresectable GCT. Level of evidence: II-1.

56. Wang CY, Wei Q, Han I, et al: Hedgehog and Notch signaling regulate self-renewal of undifferentiated pleomorphic sarcomas. *Cancer Res* 2012;72(4):1013-1022.

The results of this study indicated that Hedgehog and Notch signaling induce tumor self-renewal. Novel treatment strategies are required for deadly, recurrent unresectabe forms of pleomorphic sarcomas.

57. Takebe N, Harris PJ, Warren RQ, Ivy SP: Targeting cancer stem cells by inhibiting Wnt, Notch, and Hedgehog pathways. *Nat Rev Clin Oncol* 2011;8(2):97-106.

The authors reviewed the role of embryonic signaling pathways in the function of cancer stem cells (CSC), along with new anti-CSC therapeutic agents and potential CSC signaling cross-talk.

58. National Institutes of Health: Vismodegib and gamma-secretase/Notch signalling pathway inhibitor RO4929097 in treating patients with advanced or metastatic sarcoma. http://clinicaltrials.gov/ct2/show/NCT01154452. Accessed September 24, 2013.

59. Mita M, Sankhala K, Sarantopoulos J, et al: Abstract: Phase II study of intravenous reolysin (wild type reovirus) in patients with bone and soft tissue sarcoma metastatic to lung. *Proc CTOS* 2009;15:39323.

60. Robbins PF, Morgan RA, Feldman SA, et al: Tumor regression in patients with metastatic synovial cell sarcoma and melanoma using genetically engineered lymphocytes reactive with NY-ESO-1. *J Clin Oncol* 2011;29(7):917-924.

This study was the first adoptive immunotherapy trial to successfully treat synovial sarcoma using genetically engineered T lymphocytes to express a cancer/testis antigen-specific TCR. Level of evidence: Level II-1.

61. Choi H, Charnsangavej C, Faria SC, et al: Correlation of computed tomography and positron emission tomography in patients with metastatic gastrointestinal stromal tumor treated at a single institution with imatinib mesylate: Proposal of new computed tomography response criteria. *J Clin Oncol* 2007;25(13):1753-1759.

In a retrospective single-center analysis, the authors demonstrated a decrease in tumor size > 10% or decrease in tumor density > 15% had high sensitivity and specificity in identifying PET response in patients with advanced GIST. Level of evidence: II-2.

Chapter 8

Radiation Therapy

Elizabeth H. Baldini, MD, MPH

Introduction

Radiation therapy is an integral component of the treatment of many musculoskeletal malignancies. The roles of radiation therapy are very different for soft-tissue sarcomas compared to bone sarcomas. As described in this chapter, radiation therapy plays a role in the management of most intermediate-grade and high-grade soft-tissue sarcomas, whereas it is used much less frequently for low-grade soft-tissue sarcoma or for bone sarcomas. Accordingly, this chapter primarily focuses on aspects of radiation therapy as they pertain to soft-tissue sarcomas of the extremities.

Radiation Therapy: Indications and Efficacy

Soft-Tissue Sarcoma
High-Grade Soft-Tissue Sarcoma
Three landmark randomized trials have established limb-sparing surgery and radiation therapy as the standard of care for the treatment of intermediate-grade and high-grade soft-tissue sarcoma of the extremity. The first trial was conducted at the National Cancer Institute (NCI) and randomized patients to treatment with amputation or to limb-sparing surgery and postoperative external beam radiation therapy.[1] No difference in survival was seen between the two groups, and the local recurrence rate was 0% for patients who underwent amputation compared to 15% for those treated with limb-sparing surgery and radiation therapy ($P = 0.06$). Prior to this report, amputation had been the standard of care. These results established limb-sparing surgery as a rational alternative. Notably, this study enrolled patients from 1975 to 1981 and predates the era of MRI. The second randomized trial, also at the NCI, compared treatment with limb-sparing surgery alone to treatment with limb-sparing surgery and postoperative external beam radiation therapy.[2] No difference in survival was seen between groups, but the addition of radiation therapy demonstrated a significant improvement in local control. Specifically, for the

high-grade tumors, the local recurrence rate was 20% for limb-sparing surgery alone compared to 0% for limb-sparing surgery and radiation therapy ($P = 0.003$). The third trial was performed at Memorial Sloan-Kettering Cancer Center and randomized participants to limb-sparing surgery alone or to limb-sparing surgery and postoperative brachytherapy.[3] Brachytherapy catheters were sewn into the tumor bed and loaded postoperatively with iridium-192 to deliver a dose of 42 to 45 Gy over 4 to 6 days. Similar to the aforementioned trials, no significant differences in survival rates were seen. For the high-grade tumors, the local recurrence rate was 30% for limb-sparing surgery alone versus 9% for limb-sparing surgery and radiation therapy ($P = 0.0025$), once again establishing the role of radiation therapy in addition to limb-sparing surgery for the treatment of high-grade soft-tissue sarcoma. As a result of these three robust trials, limb-sparing surgery and radiation therapy represent the standard of care for local management of intermediate-grade and high-grade soft-tissue sarcoma of the extremity and trunk. Several retrospective and one prospective report have shown that select high-grade tumors may be adequately treated with surgery alone.[4-7] Typically eligible cases have small, subcutaneous, and readily resectable tumors with wide negative margins. However, other reports have shown high local recurrence rates following surgery alone, so this approach should be used with caution.[8,9]

Low-Grade Soft-Tissue Sarcoma
Conversely, low-grade soft-tissue sarcoma of the extremity is typically managed with limb-sparing surgery alone. For patients who undergo wide excision with negative margins, the local recurrence rate is typically less than 20%.[10] Radiation therapy is indicated in the treatment of low-grade sarcoma in certain situations, such as locally recurrent tumors, those resected with positive margins, and/or those for which a local recurrence would not be amenable to salvage surgery.

Sarcomas of Bone
Osteosarcoma
A detailed description of the management of osteosarcoma is provided in chapter 15. The mainstays of treatment are systemic chemotherapy and surgery. With these treatments, the survival rate for localized disease

---

Dr. Baldini or an immediate family member serves as a board member, owner, officer, or committee member of the Connective Tissue Oncology Society.

Table 1

Relative Advantages and Disadvantages of Preoperative Versus Postoperative Radiation Therapy

	Preoperative RT	Postoperative RT
Advantages	Smaller RT treatment volume Lower RT dose (50 Gy) Lower risk of (irreversible) late toxicities[a] Potential to render unresectable or marginally resectable tumors resectable Potential to prevent tumor seeding of surgical bed and/or systemic circulation Potential for better oxygenation of tissues due to uninterrupted vasculature Relative simplicity of RT target definition for a tumor in situ	Lower risk of wound complications Entire untreated specimen available for pathologic review, which allows for individualized postoperative treatment
Disadvantages	Higher risk of wound complications Potential for less informative pathologic analysis due to treatment	Larger RT treatment volume Higher RT dose (60–66 Gy) Higher risk of (irreversible) late toxicities[a] Potential inability to deliver RT at all if major wound complication occurs Potential increased hypoxic environment due to surgical disruption of vasculature Relative complexity of RT target definition to include prior site of tumor and the surgical bed

RT = radiation therapy.
[a]Late toxicities include subcutaneous fibrosis, joint stiffness, edema, pain, and bone fractures.

is greater than 65%.[11] Typically, adjuvant radiation therapy is not used, given that it does not improve survival and it increases the risk of second tumors.[12] However, radiation therapy is considered in situations of incomplete resection or unresectable disease.[13,14]

Chondrosarcoma

For the most part, localized chondrosarcoma is managed with surgery alone. The appropriate surgical management varies by grade, location, and histology and is described in chapter 17. The relative indications for radiation therapy include cases of incomplete resection of high-grade tumors or cases not amenable to resection without undue morbidity.[15] Proton radiation therapy has been associated with excellent local control rates for unresectable chondrosarcoma of the skull base or spine.[16,17]

Ewing Sarcoma

Subclinical systemic disease is present for the preponderance of patients in whom localized Ewing sarcoma has been diagnosed. Both multiagent chemotherapy and local therapy are necessary components of curative treatment. Appropriate treatment of the primary tumor can include surgery, radiation therapy, or both. Surgery and radiation therapy are considered to be equally effective, but the toxicity profiles vary.[18] Importantly, radiation therapy is associated with an increased risk of second tumors (especially for children).[12,19] For this reason, surgery is the preferred local treatment modality if it can achieve negative resection margins and an accept-

able functional result. The indications for radiation therapy include situations in which resection would result in significant morbidity (such as bulky sacral tumors) or as adjuvant treatment in situations of positive resection margins or residual gross disease. Chapter 16 describes the management of Ewing sarcoma in more detail.

Radiation Timing: Preoperative Versus Postoperative

Limb-sparing surgery and radiation therapy are the standard of care for the treatment of high-grade large soft-tissue sarcomas of the extremity and trunk. It is acceptable to administer radiation therapy preoperatively or postoperatively. In general, preoperative radiation therapy is delivered at a dose of 50 Gy using 2-Gy increments on a daily basis (Monday through Friday) for 5 weeks; postoperative radiation therapy is delivered at a dose of 60 to 66 Gy using 1.8- or 2.0-Gy fractions on a daily basis (Monday through Friday) for 6.5 to 7.5 weeks. Local control and survival rates with the two approaches are similar, but the side-effect profiles are different.[20,21] The relative advantages of preoperative versus postoperative radiation therapy are shown in **Table 1**. Compared with postoperative radiation therapy, preoperative radiation therapy uses a lower dose (50 Gy versus 60 to 66 Gy) and encompasses a smaller treatment volume (gross tumor plus a margin versus the entire surgical bed plus a margin). As a result of the

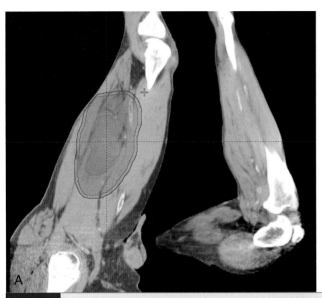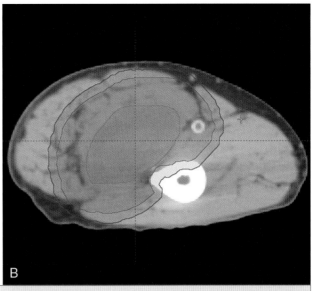

| Figure 1 | Sagittal (**A**) and axial (**B**) CT scans for radiation planning for a 74-year-old man show a high-grade pleomorphic spindle cell sarcoma of the right posterior thigh. The gross tumor volume is depicted in orange; the clinical target volume, in blue; and the planning target volume, in pink. Note the patient's position in **A**: he is on his right side with his left leg flexed forward so that it will not be in the entrance or exit paths of the treatment beams. |

higher dose and larger treatment fields, postoperative radiation therapy is associated with higher permanent rates of limb edema, joint stiffness, and fibrosis.[22] However, preoperative radiation therapy is associated with a higher rate of acute wound complications.[20,23] The NCI Canada sentinel randomized trial comparing preoperative to postoperative radiation therapy reported wound complications following surgery for 35% of patients in the preoperative radiation therapy group compared with 17% of patients in the postoperative radiation therapy group.[20] Other advantages of preoperative radiation therapy include the potential to render unresectable or marginally resectable tumors resectable and the relative simplicity of radiation target definition for a tumor in situ. Additional theoretical advantages for preoperative radiation include the potential to prevent tumor seeding of the surgical bed and/or systemic circulation and the potential for better oxygenation of tissues (and therefore radiation efficacy) due to uninterrupted vasculature. Another advantage of postoperative radiation is the availability of the entire untreated specimen for pathologic review, which allows for individualized postoperative treatment.

Radiation Treatment Techniques

Conventional Radiation Therapy Techniques

The design and implementation of radiation treatment of the extremities can be challenging, especially for tumors that are proximal and for those that encompass most of the limb circumference. To start, patients are positioned on the table in such a way as to allow treatment with optimal beam angles. For example, a tumor of the posterior thigh is often treated with the patient in the decubitus position and with the legs "scissor kicked" so that opposing beams can access the tumor without passing through the anterior aspect of the involved leg or through any aspect of the contralateral leg (note the position of the patient's legs in **Figure 1, A**). For tumors of the proximal medial thigh, patients are usually placed supine with the contralateral leg flexed and abducted out of the way. For males, the genitalia are displaced to the contralateral side using mesh or other devices so that they are out of the path of the treatment beams. Once the treatment position has been established, it is critical to immobilize the patient so that the position is reproducible with high accuracy. Typically, custom casts are made to accomplish this goal. A planning CT scan is obtained with the patient immobilized in the treatment position.

Next, three radiation treatment volumes are contoured on the planning CT scan by the radiation oncologist. If the tumor is not readily visible on the CT, the diagnostic MRI can be fused with the planning CT to help with contouring. For preoperative radiation therapy, the gross tumor volume (GTV) represents the gross tumor and is defined by the T1 gadolinium-enhanced MRI. The clinical target volume (CTV) represents the gross tumor plus potential areas of microscopic disease. The CTV is typically defined as the GTV with expansions of 4 cm in the superior and inferior directions and 1.5 cm in the radial direction.[24] These volumes are edited so as not to extend outside a compartment, through an intact fascial plane, or into bone or skin. The planning target volume (PTV) accounts for potential setup error resulting from inaccurate patient positioning or patient movement, and is usually represented

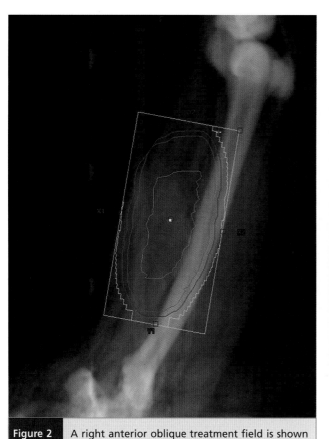

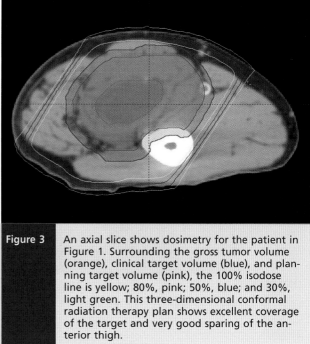

Figure 3 | An axial slice shows dosimetry for the patient in Figure 1. Surrounding the gross tumor volume (orange), clinical target volume (blue), and planning target volume (pink), the 100% isodose line is yellow; 80%, pink; 50%, blue; and 30%, light green. This three-dimensional conformal radiation therapy plan shows excellent coverage of the target and very good sparing of the anterior thigh.

Figure 2 | A right anterior oblique treatment field is shown for the patient in Figure 1. The gross tumor volume (orange), clinical target volume (blue), and planning target volume (pink) are shown, as are the custom blocks (yellow) that shield uninvolved normal tissues.

as a 5- to 7-mm expansion of the CTV. **Figure 1** shows a soft-tissue sarcoma of the posterior thigh with GTV, CTV, and PTV contours in both the sagittal and axial planes. In postoperative radiation therapy, the GTV is usually contoured to correspond to the location of the gross tumor before resection. The CTV includes the entire surgical bed, including the incision and drainage sites plus expansions of approximately 4 cm in the longitudinal direction and 1.5 cm in the radial direction.[24]

The goal of radiation treatment planning is to design a plan that delivers a homogeneous dose that conforms as closely as possible to the PTV with minimal dose delivery to adjacent normal tissues. Some of the normal tissues to be cognizant of in the planning process include the soft tissues of the limb, bone, joints, male genitalia, and skin. Specifically, it is important to spare as much of the uninvolved limb circumference as possible to minimize long-term edema, fibrosis, and pain.[25] The mean and maximum dose to bone as well as the volume of bone receiving more than 40 Gy should be minimized to decrease the risk of fracture.[26] The dose to the whole joint should be less than 45 Gy to minimize joint stiffness, and the dose to the testicles should be as low as possible to avoid infertility.[25] Sperm banking should be discussed in situations when it may not be possible to avoid infertility. Finally, a high dose to the skin should be minimized if possible to avoid moist desquamation requiring a break from treatment and potentially to decrease the risk of postoperative wound complications. **Figure 2** shows a treatment field for a patient with a high-grade pleomorphic spindle cell sarcoma of the posterior thigh, and **Figure 3** shows the corresponding dosimetry for the same case.

The two most common radiation therapy treatment techniques are three-dimensional conformal radiation therapy (3D-CRT) and intensity-modulated radiation therapy (IMRT). In 3D-CRT, several fixed beams irradiate the tumor from chosen angles. Custom blocks are designed to shape the beams (and block normal structures from the path of the beam), and the treatment angles and custom blocks are designed based on the shape and location of the PTV. Each beam delivers a uniform dose. In contrast, IMRT uses beams with variable, computer-controlled intensities. The result is that with IMRT, dose conformality is improved, particularly for complex targets such as those with concave shapes. IMRT can be especially helpful when critical normal structures are adjacent to the treatment target. **Figure 4** shows radiation therapy PTVs and dosimetry for a patient with a high-grade myxofibrosarcoma of the left inguinal region that was treated with IMRT. Although it offers improved dose conformality compared to 3D-CRT, IMRT is more expensive, has a prolonged treatment time, and treats a larger volume of normal tissue with low doses. A theoretical concern exists that IMRT may be associated with an increased risk of radiation-associated second malignancies.[27] Although they have not been compared in a randomized trial, excellent local control rates have been reported for both

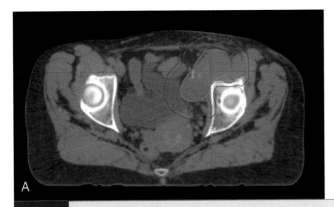
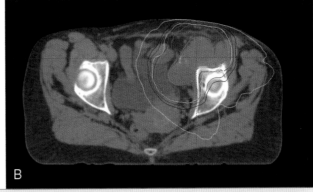

Figure 4   Gross tumor volume (orange), clinical target volume (blue), and planning target volume (pink) (**A, B**) and dosimetry (**B**) are shown for a 62-year-old woman with a high-grade myxofibrosarcoma of the left inguinal region that was treated with intensity-modulated radiation therapy (IMRT). **B**, The 100% isodose line is yellow; 90%, pink; 80%, blue; and 30%, light green. Note how the intensity-modulated radiation therapy (IMRT) dosimetry conforms tightly to the concave target volume abutting the acetabulum.

3D-CRT and IMRT.[21,23,28] Currently, both are acceptable approaches. Some radiation oncologists use 3D-CRT as a starting point and use IMRT only when it yields a superior plan; others use IMRT almost exclusively.

Novel Radiation Therapy Techniques

Several innovative radiation therapy techniques are worthy of mention. First, with IMRT, it is possible to vary the dose within each beam to simultaneously treat different areas within the tumor using different doses. This technique is described as dose painting and has been proposed as a means of delivering a boost dose of radiation therapy to areas of the tumor deemed to be at higher risk of resulting in positive resection margins. It has been used for the treatment of retroperitoneal sarcoma but has not yet been reported for the treatment of extremity sarcoma.[29] Second, the increased availability of kilovoltage portal imaging on linear accelerators has resulted in more frequent use of image-guided radiation therapy (IGRT). IGRT refers to serial (often daily) imaging of patient setup before treatment so that the patient can be repositioned, if appropriate. The result is increased treatment accuracy, and the setup error added to create the PTV can be reduced so that the overall treatment volume is decreased. In addition, many new-generation linear accelerators have CT imaging capabilities. If such images show a substantial change in the contour of the patient or the tumor during the radiation therapy treatment course, a new radiation therapy plan can be generated to adapt to the new geometry. This technique is called adaptive radiation therapy.

All of the preceding techniques refer to radiation therapy treatment using photons. Radiation therapy can also be delivered using particle beams such as protons and carbon ions. These beams have favorable physical characteristics in which most of the energy is deposited at the end of a linear track, called a Bragg peak. The dose deposited beyond this peak is negligi-

ble. The result is the ability to deliver high doses to treatment targets and markedly reduced doses to adjacent normal structures. The availability of these modalities is limited, and no randomized studies have compared particle beams to photons for the treatment of sarcoma. Nonetheless, single-institution reports for the treatment of chondrosarcoma and soft-tissue sarcoma of the skull base of the spine with both protons and carbon ions demonstrate excellent results.[16,17,30,31] These modalities will likely find a permanent place in the armamentarium to treat sarcoma.

Stereotactic body radiation therapy (SBRT) is a novel technique that involves the delivery of focused doses of photons to extracranial tumors. Typical treatment schedules involve large ablative doses of 6 to 30 Gy delivered in a hypofractionated course of one to five treatments. Several studies have documented the use of SBRT for the treatment of medically inoperable non–small cell lung cancer as well as for metastatic sites from various primary tumors.[32,33] A role for this modality may exist for the treatment of sarcomas with oligometastatic disease such as solitary pulmonary or spine metastases.

Radiation Therapy Toxicities

Acute Toxicities

Acute toxicities of radiation therapy are typically related to the tissues within the radiation therapy treatment fields and therefore vary with the part of the body that is irradiated. For treatment of an extremity, acute toxicities include fatigue, skin erythema (sometimes progressing to desquamation), localized pruritus or alopecia, mild muscle aches, and acute wound complications. Except for wound complications, these toxicities usually occur gradually during the treatment course and resolve quickly over a period of about 3 to 6 weeks following completion of radiation therapy. Impaired wound healing is the most significant acute toxicity. As mentioned previously, the rate is higher in preoperative radiation therapy than in postoperative radiation therapy (35% versus 17%).[20] Two studies reported on detailed analyses of risk factors for wound complications.[20,23] On multivariate analyses, in addition to preoperative radiation therapy, independent significant predictors were reported for wound complications that included lower extremity site, tumor size greater than 10 cm, tumor located less than 3 mm from the skin surface, vascularized flap closure, and diabetes mellitus.

Chronic Toxicities

Chronic toxicities following radiation therapy to the extremities are usually permanent and include edema, fibrosis, joint stiffness, and less commonly, pain, bone fracture, peripheral nerve damage, and radiation-associated second tumors. Reported rates vary, but one study reported the following rates for a cohort of 145 patients treated with surgery and radiation therapy: moderate edema, 19%; fibrosis, 57%; moderately or severely decreased range of motion, 32%; pain requiring narcotics, 7%; and bone fracture, 6%.[25] Rates of edema, fibrosis, and decreased range of motion are increased with large treatment volumes and high radiation therapy dose.[20,22,25] The risk of bone fracture is increased with periosteal stripping and high radiation therapy dose.[26,34,35] Furthermore, when fractures do occur, they can be associated with delayed bone union and/or the need for complex surgical intervention as a result of adverse effects of radiation on the local vasculature and osteoblasts.[36,37] For these reasons, consideration of prophylactic intramedullary rod placement is recommended at the time of soft-tissue sarcoma resection for cases deemed to be at high risk of fracture such as the setting of periosteal resection.[34,36,37] Radiation-associated second tumors are a significant concern when treating children but are much less common following radiation therapy for adults.[12,27]

Summary

Limb-sparing surgery and radiation therapy, with or without chemotherapy, is the standard of care for most high-grade soft-tissue sarcomas of the extremities and trunk. Low-grade soft-tissue sarcoma is typically treated with wide excision alone as long as negative margins are achieved. For low-grade soft-tissue sarcoma, radiation therapy may play a role in the presence of locally recurrent disease, positive resection margins, and situations in which a recurrence would not be amenable to function-sparing salvage surgery. Indications for radiation therapy for sarcomas of bone are less common. Radiation therapy is indicated for osteosarcoma in situations of incomplete resection or unresectable disease. In chondrosarcoma, radiation therapy may play a role in situations with incompletely resected high-grade tumors or unresectable tumors. In Ewing

sarcoma, radiation therapy is used for cases in which resection would be associated with significant morbidity and for cases with positive resection margins or gross residual disease.

For soft-tissue sarcoma, radiation therapy may be administered preoperatively or postoperatively with equivalent local control and survival outcomes. However, toxicities vary in that preoperative radiation therapy is associated with a higher risk of wound complications, and postoperative radiation therapy is associated with a higher risk of long-term fibrosis, edema, and joint stiffness. Standard radiation therapy approaches include 3D-CRT and IMRT. New techniques such as dose painting, IGRT, adaptive radiation therapy, SBRT, and proton and carbon ion treatment are being used and tested with increasing frequency and are likely to have an established role in the treatment of sarcoma in the future.

Annotated References

1. Rosenberg SA, Tepper J, Glatstein E, et al: The treatment of soft-tissue sarcomas of the extremities: Prospective randomized evaluations of (1) limb-sparing surgery plus radiation therapy compared with amputation and (2) the role of adjuvant chemotherapy. *Ann Surg* 1982;196(3):305-315.

2. Yang JC, Chang AE, Baker AR, et al: Randomized prospective study of the benefit of adjuvant radiation therapy in the treatment of soft tissue sarcomas of the extremity. *J Clin Oncol* 1998;16(1):197-203.

3. Pisters PW, Harrison LB, Leung DH, Woodruff JM, Casper ES, Brennan MF: Long-term results of a prospective randomized trial of adjuvant brachytherapy in soft tissue sarcoma. *J Clin Oncol* 1996;14(3):859-868.

4. Baldini EH, Goldberg J, Jenner C, et al: Long-term outcomes after function-sparing surgery without radiotherapy for soft tissue sarcoma of the extremities and trunk. *J Clin Oncol* 1999;17(10):3252-3259.

5. Rydholm A, Gustafson P, Rööser B, Willén H, Berg NO: Subcutaneous sarcoma: A population-based study of 129 patients. *J Bone Joint Surg Br* 1991;73(4):662-667.

6. Gibbs CP, Peabody TD, Mundt AJ, Montag AG, Simon MA: Oncological outcomes of operative treatment of subcutaneous soft-tissue sarcomas of the extremities. *J Bone Joint Surg Am* 1997;79(6):888-897.

7. Pisters PW, Pollock RE, Lewis VO, et al: Long-term results of prospective trial of surgery alone with selective use of radiation for patients with T1 extremity and trunk soft tissue sarcomas. *Ann Surg* 2007;246(4):675-681, discussion 681-682.

8. Fabrizio PL, Stafford SL, Pritchard DJ: Extremity soft-

1: General Evaluation and Treatment of Musculoskeletal Tumors

tissue sarcomas selectively treated with surgery alone. *Int J Radiat Oncol Biol Phys* 2000;48(1):227-232.

9. Khanfir K, Alzieu L, Terrier P, et al: Does adjuvant radiation therapy increase loco-regional control after optimal resection of soft-tissue sarcoma of the extremities? *Eur J Cancer* 2003;39(13):1872-1880.

10. Mendenhall WM, Indelicato DJ, Scarborough MT, et al: The management of adult soft tissue sarcomas. *Am J Clin Oncol* 2009;32(4):436-442.

    This is a well done and comprehensive review of the important literature that has defined the management of adult soft tissue sarcoma. Level of evidence: I.

11. Anninga JK, Gelderblom H, Fiocco M, et al: Chemotherapeutic adjuvant treatment for osteosarcoma: Where do we stand? *Eur J Cancer* 2011;47(16): 2431-2445.

    The authors performed a meta-analysis of clinical studies of localized osteosarcoma. Studies from the prechemotherapy era were also included. The meta-analysis showed that three-drug regimens had better outcomes than two-drug regimens, and the latter had a 5-year survival of 70%. Level of evidence: I.

12. Tucker MA, D'Angio GJ, Boice JD Jr, et al: Bone sarcomas linked to radiotherapy and chemotherapy in children. *N Engl J Med* 1987;317(10):588-593.

13. DeLaney TF, Park L, Goldberg SI, et al: Radiotherapy for local control of osteosarcoma. *Int J Radiat Oncol Biol Phys* 2005;61(2):492-498.

14. Ciernik IF, Niemierko A, Harmon DC, et al: Proton-based radiotherapy for unresectable or incompletely resected osteosarcoma. *Cancer* 2011;117(19): 4522-4530.

    Fifty-five patients with unresected or partially resected osteosarcoma were treated with proton or mixed proton-photon therapy. Five-year local control was 72%. The authors concluded that proton therapy allows curative treatment of some patients with unresectable or incompletely resected osteosarcoma. Level of evidence: II-2.

15. Goda JS, Ferguson PC, O'Sullivan B, et al: High-risk extracranial chondrosarcoma: Long-term results of surgery and radiation therapy. *Cancer* 2011;117(11): 2513-2519.

    Sixty patients with extracranial chondrosarcoma were treated with surgery and radiation therapy. Patients with R0, R1, and R2 resections had local control of 100%, 94%, and 42%, respectively. The authors concluded that radiation therapy is a useful treatment of incompletely resected disease. Level of evidence: II-3.

16. Weber DC, Rutz HP, Pedroni ES, et al: Results of spot-scanning proton radiation therapy for chordoma and chondrosarcoma of the skull base: The Paul Scherrer Institute experience. *Int J Radiat Oncol Biol Phys* 2005;63(2):401-409.

17. DeLaney TF, Liebsch NJ, Pedlow FX, et al: Phase II study of high-dose photon/proton radiotherapy in the management of spine sarcomas. *Int J Radiat Oncol Biol Phys* 2009;74(3):732-739.

    Fifty patients with chordoma, chondrosarcoma, or other spine sarcomas were treated with high-dose proton-photon radiation therapy with or without radical resection. Five-year local control was 78%, showing that radiation therapy can be associated with good control rates for spine sarcomas. Level of evidence: II-2.

18. Yock TI, Krailo M, Fryer CJ, et al; Children's Oncology Group: Local control in pelvic Ewing sarcoma: Analysis from INT-0091—a report from the Children's Oncology Group. *J Clin Oncol* 2006;24(24): 3838-3843.

19. McLean TW, Hertel C, Young ML, et al: Late events in pediatric patients with Ewing sarcoma/primitive neuroectodermal tumor of bone: The Dana-Farber Cancer Institute/Children's Hospital experience. *J Pediatr Hematol Oncol* 1999;21(6):486-493.

20. O'Sullivan B, Davis AM, Turcotte R, et al: Preoperative versus postoperative radiotherapy in soft-tissue sarcoma of the limbs: A randomised trial. *Lancet* 2002;359(9325):2235-2241.

21. O'Sullivan B, Davis A, Turcotte R, et al: Abstract: Five-year results of a randomized phase III trial of preoperative vs post-operative radiotherapy in extremity soft tissue sarcoma. *J Clin Oncol 2004 ASCO Annual Meeting Proceedings* 2004;22(14S):9007.

22. Davis AM, O'Sullivan B, Turcotte R, et al; Canadian Sarcoma Group; NCI Canada Clinical Trial Group Randomized Trial: Late radiation morbidity following randomization to preoperative versus postoperative radiotherapy in extremity soft tissue sarcoma. *Radiother Oncol* 2005;75(1):48-53.

23. Baldini EH, Lapidus MR, Wang Q, et al: Predictors for major wound complications following preoperative radiotherapy and surgery for soft-tissue sarcoma of the extremities and trunk: Importance of tumor proximity to skin surface. *Ann Surg Oncol* 2013;20(5):1494-1499.

    This study included 103 patients treated with preoperative radiation therapy and surgery. Major wound complications occurred for 35%. Significant predictors of wound complications included diabetes, tumor size greater than 10 cm, tumor located less than 3 mm from skin, and vascularized flap closure. Four-year freedom from local recurrence was 90%. Level of evidence: II-2.

24. Haas RLM, Delaney TF, O'Sullivan B, et al: Radiotherapy for management of extremity soft tissue sarcomas: Why, when, and where? *Int J Radiat Oncol Biol Phys* 2012;84(3):572-580.

    A critical review of the published literature pertaining to extremity soft-tissue sarcoma regarding the indications and outcomes for radiation therapy is presented. Expert consensus recommendations for radiation therapy target volumes in both the preoperative and post-operative settings are described in detail. Level of evidence: IV.

25. Stinson SF, DeLaney TF, Greenberg J, et al: Acute and long-term effects on limb function of combined modality limb sparing therapy for extremity soft tissue sarcoma. *Int J Radiat Oncol Biol Phys* 1991;21(6): 1493-1499.

26. Dickie CI, Parent AL, Griffin AM, et al: Bone fractures following external beam radiotherapy and limb-preservation surgery for lower extremity soft tissue sarcoma: Relationship to irradiated bone length, volume, tumor location and dose. *Int J Radiat Oncol Biol Phys* 2009;75(4):1119-1124.

   This case-control study analyzed 21 patients who developed fractures following surgery and radiation therapy for soft-tissue sarcoma of the extremity. Risk of fracture was increased for patients who received higher mean and maximum doses to bone. Level of evidence: II-2.

27. Hall EJ, Wuu CS: Radiation-induced second cancers: The impact of 3D-CRT and IMRT. *Int J Radiat Oncol Biol Phys* 2003;56(1):83-88.

28. Alektiar KM, Brennan MF, Healey JH, Singer S: Impact of intensity-modulated radiation therapy on local control in primary soft-tissue sarcoma of the extremity. *J Clin Oncol* 2008;26(20):3440-3444.

   This analysis described 41 patients with soft-tissue sarcoma of the lower extremity who were treated with IMRT. Three-year local control was 94%, and toxicity was comparable to that seen for patients treated with 3D-CRT. Level of evidence: II-2.

29. Tzeng CW, Fiveash JB, Popple RA, et al: Preoperative radiation therapy with selective dose escalation to the margin at risk for retroperitoneal sarcoma. *Cancer* 2006;107(2):371-379.

30. Schulz-Ertner D, Nikoghosyan A, Hof H, et al: Carbon ion radiotherapy of skull base chondrosarcomas. *Int J Radiat Oncol Biol Phys* 2007;67(1):171-177.

   Fifty-four patients with low-grade and intermediate-grade chondrosarcoma of the skull base and gross residual disease following surgery were treated with carbon ions. Three-year local control was 96%. The authors concluded that carbon ions are effective with high local control and low toxicity. Level of evidence: II-2.

31. Kamada T, Tsujii H, Tsuji H, et al; Working Group for the Bone and Soft Tissue Sarcomas: Efficacy and safety of carbon ion radiotherapy in bone and soft tissue sarcomas. *J Clin Oncol* 2002;20(22):4466-4471.

32. Heinzerling JH, Kavanagh B, Timmerman RD: Stereotactic ablative radiation therapy for primary lung tumors. *Cancer J* 2011;17(1):28-32.

   Several multi-institutional trials have established SBRT as a standard treatment of early-stage medically inoperable non–small cell lung cancer. This review article describes the results and toxicities for SBRT in this group of patients. Level of evidence: II-2.

33. Milano MT, Katz AW, Schell MC, Philip A, Okunieff P: Descriptive analysis of oligometastatic lesions treated with curative-intent stereotactic body radiotherapy. *Int J Radiat Oncol Biol Phys* 2008;72(5): 1516-1522.

   This report describes two prospective pilot studies treating 293 oligometastases in 121 patients with hypofractionated SBRT and stereotactic radiosurgery for brain metastases. Good local control was achieved (2-year local control was 77%). Level of evidence: II-2.

34. Lin PP, Schupak KD, Boland PJ, Brennan MF, Healey JH: Pathologic femoral fracture after periosteal excision and radiation for the treatment of soft tissue sarcoma. *Cancer* 1998;82(12):2356-2365.

35. Holt GE, Griffin AM, Pintilie M, et al: Fractures following radiotherapy and limb-salvage surgery for lower extremity soft-tissue sarcomas: A comparison of high-dose and low-dose radiotherapy. *J Bone Joint Surg Am* 2005;87(2):315-319.

36. Lin PP, Boland PJ, Healey JH: Treatment of femoral fractures after irradiation. *Clin Orthop Relat Res* 1998;352:168-178.

37. Pak D, Vineberg KA, Griffith KA, et al: Dose-effect relationships for femoral fractures after multimodality limb-sparing therapy of soft-tissue sarcomas of the proximal lower extremity. *Int J Radiat Oncol Biol Phys* 2012;83(4):1257-1263.

Benign Bone Tumors

SECTION EDITOR:

Albert J. Aboulafia, MD, FACS, MBA

Chapter 9

Cystic and Radiolucent Bone Lesions

John A. Abraham, MD

Introduction

The diagnosis of a cystic bone lesion relates to the anatomic structure of the lesion, namely the presence of a predominant fluid-filled area within the lesion. These lesions appear lucent on plain films. This chapter discusses cystic lesions of bone as well as several solid but radiographically lucent lesions. Care should be taken when describing these lesions because, although most cystic lesions of bone are radiolucent, not all lucent lesions are cystic.

Cystic lesions of bone can be divided into benign, malignant, and nontumorous conditions. Benign cystic lesions include simple, also called unicameral, bone cysts (UBCs), aneurysmal bone cysts (ABCs), and cystic fibrous dysplasia. Certain location-specific diagnoses exist as well, specifically calcaneal simple cysts and liposclerosing myxofibrous tumor (LSMFT), a solid benign tumor that has a marked predilection for the proximal femur. Malignant tumors can have cystic regions due to central necrosis, and can be confused for an ABC. Telangiectatic osteosarcoma is an example of a malignant bone lesion that is expected to have fluid-filled areas evident on imaging. For this reason, care must be taken in the diagnosis and management of these lesions. Nontumorous conditions that have a cystic appearance include bone abscesses and intraosseous ganglions, otherwise known as geodes. Humeral pseudocyst is an example of a normal variant that has a radiolucent appearance on plain radiographic imaging and can be confused with a lesion if incorrectly identified.

Diagnosis of any bone lesion, including cystic lesions, relies on an accurate history and physical examination, as well as an accurate and clear understanding of the patient's imaging. For the majority of bone lesions, plain radiographic imaging is the starting point for evaluation. When plain radiographs of a bone lesion are evaluated, several features are considered, including size, location, the zone of transition or borders of the lesion, and, importantly, the matrix identified within the lesion.

Benign Cystic Lesions

Unicameral Bone Cysts

UBC is a cystic lesion most commonly found at the metaphysis of bone. This lesion also referred to as a simple cyst or a solitary cyst. Although the etiology is not completely elucidated, it is thought that increased pressure in the region of the cyst at development leads to necrosis of local bone and then accumulation of fluid.[1] UBC may thus be more of a reactive lesion than a true neoplasm, although this classification is not yet clearly defined. The fluid contained in the cyst is proteinaceous and straw colored, and is not bloody except in patients with pathologic fracture. The cyst has been shown to contain prostaglandins, interleukins, and metalloproteinases.[2] This characteristic distinguishes UBC from ABC, which has grossly bloody fluid. These lesions typ-

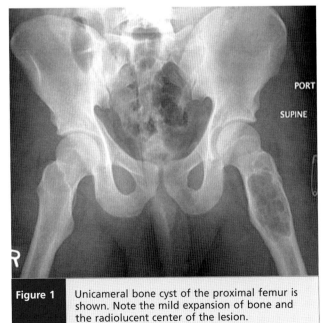

Figure 1 Unicameral bone cyst of the proximal femur is shown. Note the mild expansion of bone and the radiolucent center of the lesion.

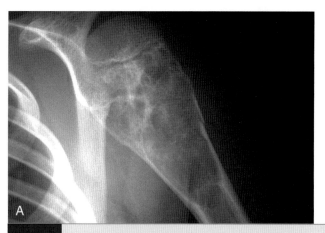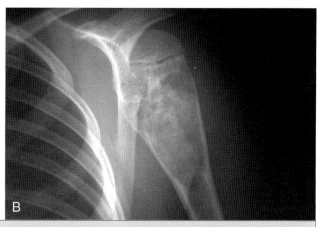

Figure 2 **A,** Unicameral bone cyst of the proximal humerus is shown. Note the small cortical defect in the cortex. **B,** The bone is expanded to the width of the physis but not beyond.

ically occur in the first two decades of life with a 2:1 male predominance. The proximal humerus and proximal femur (**Figure 1**) are the most common sites. The lesions may be painless, but pathologic fracture can occur in up to two thirds of patients and can cause significant pain (**Figure 2**). Lesions large enough to present an impending risk for fracture are also painful. In some instances fracture can precipitate healing, although this is only occasionally the case. Most lesions become evident during childhood, and may grow or be painful, but heal spontaneously with skeletal maturity. The lesions are seen infrequently in adults, in whom they are usually found in less common locations such as the calcaneus or ilium.

Imaging

Plain radiography of UBC is usually diagnostic. The lesion is a lucent cystic lesion at the metaphysis of the bone and has one chamber, but occasionally has a multichamber appearance due to internal septations within the lesion. The lesion is central in the bone and may expand the contour of the bone slightly but not to the extent seen in ABC, and usually not wider than the width of the adjacent physis. The cortex is thinned, but no areas of cortical breakthrough or soft-tissue mass are present. However, pathologic fracture can occur. In some instances a small portion of the cortical wall breaks off and sinks to the floor of the cystic cavity, giving rise radiographically to the classically described "fallen leaf" sign. This finding is considered pathognomonic for a UBC and is a radiographic confirmation that there is no tissue within the cavity, but rather fluid. Periosteal reaction is not seen unless in response to a fracture. UBCs are classified as active or latent on the basis of the relationship to the physis.[3] Historically, lesions within 1 cm of the physis were defined as active, and those farther into the diaphyseal region were called latent. Over time, a lesion may seem to "move" toward the diaphysis. This appearance of movement is due to the new bone growth stemming from the physis, and, in the case of a latent lesion, exceeding the growth of

the cyst, thereby "pushing" it farther into the diaphysis. However, the classification of a lesion as latent or active does not relate to biologic behavior or predictability of progression.

CT imaging will show thinned cortical bone and may better define fallen fragments or pathologic fractures. MRI will show homogenous fluid signal within the cavity. In the absence of fracture, fluid-fluid levels are usually not seen because of the absence of blood in the cavity. If bone scanning is performed, it shows peripheral uptake with central photopenia.

Histology

Histology of the lesion shows a thin, fibrous lining. The lesion has no epithelial or endothelial component. The cells are fibroblastic, and the lining can also contain scattered giant cells, mesenchymal cells, and lymphocytes, all with bland appearance. The lining is not typically bloody unless pathologic fracture has occurred, so the large lakes of red blood cells seen in ABCs are absent. Eosinophilic fibrinous material known as cementum is sometimes seen.

Treatment

Many lesions are painless and found incidentally. If imaging confirms a low level of concern for pathologic fracture, these lesions are generally observed. In the setting of a painful lesion or concern for pathologic fracture, injection or curettage may be considered. In the case of an actual pathologic fracture in the upper extremity, the fracture is generally allowed to heal before surgical intervention for the cyst itself is considered. Following fracture healing, the lesion can then be treated surgically, or can be observed to see if the fracture will precipitate healing. In most cases occurrence of a pathologic fracture is a reasonable indication for treatment of the cyst, because in general the occurrence of fracture does not lead to complete involution of the cyst. In the weight-bearing lower extremity, in particular the proximal femur, depending on the age of the pa-

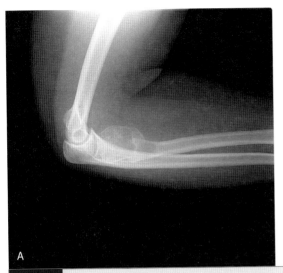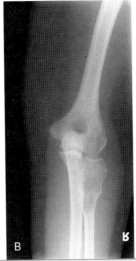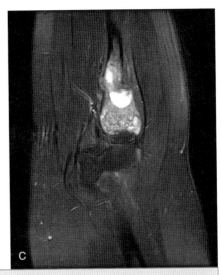

Figure 3 **A,** Lateral radiograph of elbow shows an aneurysmal bone cyst (ABC) in the proximal radius. A thin rim of bone remains as the lesion expands the bone anteriorly. **B,** AP radiograph shows bone expansion beyond the physeal width, typical of ABC but not unicameral bone cyst. **C,** T2-weighted MRI sequence shows characteristic high signal.

tient and the size of the lesion, a more aggressive approach may be taken with curettage, grafting, and internal fixation to avoid hip fracture.

Initial surgical management, particularly in the upper extremity, often consists of cyst aspiration and injection. It is unclear what the best injection material is; various agents have been tested. These agents include methylprednisolone acetate (historically used) as well as autogenous bone marrow, cancellous allograft, demineralized bone matrix, calcium sulfate, high-porosity hydroxyapatite, and fibrosing agents. A recent report described the use of platelet-rich plasma.[4] None of these agents has been shown to demonstrate increased healing rates or lower recurrence rates compared to the others. If a first injection fails, with failure defined as no radiographic signs of healing in a 3-month period, then a second or third injection may precipitate healing. If three injections fail, curettage and bone grafting with or without internal fixation should be considered. In general, the use of bone allograft is associated with adequate healing, so autogenous bone graft harvest is usually not necessary.

Aneurysmal Bone Cysts

ABC is a cystic neoplasm of bone generally affecting patients younger than 20 years, with a slight female predominance. These lesions are usually found in the metaphyses of long bones, most commonly the proximal humerus, distal femur, and proximal tibia. ABCs also occur in locations such as the ilium, sacrum, and spine in 15% to 20% of patients, which may present difficult anatomic challenges for treatment. Spinal lesions are generally located in the posterior elements and may extend into the vertebral body. The clinical presentation is usually one of pain that is mild to moderate and may be associated with swelling. Lesions in

the spine may cause radiculopathy, vertebral collapse, scoliosis, and neurologic deficits. Pathologic fracture can occur as a result of an ABC and can cause exacerbation of pain.

Molecular Biology

ABCs can be seen as a primary lesion or as a secondary component of another bone lesion. Once thought to potentially be a reactive lesion secondary to local circulatory disturbance, ABCs are now known to be a result of the translocation of *USP6* (also known as *TRE17*) leading to its upregulation. The induction of matrix metalloproteinase 9 (MMP-9) in response to the presence of the upregulated ubiquitin-specific protease (USP) fusion protein is thought to be responsible for the pathogenesis of ABCs.[5]

Imaging

Plain radiography of an ABC shows an eccentric lucent bone lesion at the metaphysis of the bone, bounded by a thin cortical rim (**Figure 3, A and B**). Even in the most extensive cases, a thin bony rim, or at least a portion of one, can be seen at the periphery of the cyst. The width of the cyst may be wider than that of the metaphysis; this feature distinguishes ABCs from UBCs, which generally do not expand wider than the adjacent physis. The cyst may have multiple fluid-filled or blood-filled chambers separated by bony septa. Periosteal elevation and new bone formation can be seen at the junction of the cyst with normal host bone. MRI or CT shows multiloculated fluid-filled or blood-filled chambers, and fluid-fluid levels are a characteristic, but not diagnostic, feature (**Figure 3, C**). A soft-tissue mass can arise from the lesion and extend beyond the bone into the adjacent tissues. Bone scan will show uptake in the region of the lesion, and may have an area of decreased uptake centrally.

2: Benign Bone Tumors

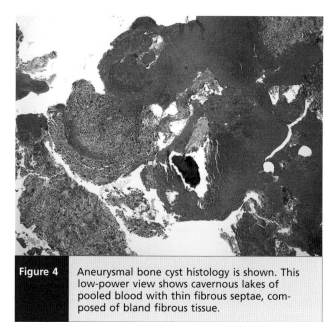

Figure 4 Aneurysmal bone cyst histology is shown. This low-power view shows cavernous lakes of pooled blood with thin fibrous septae, composed of bland fibrous tissue.

Histology

On histologic evaluation, a thin fibrous lining that is usually hemorrhagic is found. A fibrohistiocytic stroma is present, along with chronic inflammatory cells, scattered giant cells, and hemosiderin-laden macrophages. There is no endothelial lining. The cavity itself is usually blood filled, and the microscopic appearance is dominated by large, blood-filled spaces with interspersed lining tissue (**Figure 4**). Reactive osteoid can be seen along the periphery of the lesion. A solid variant exists with identical histology but without the cavernous cystic spaces. A recent study proposed a "healing index" that comprises certain histologic factors that could help predict recurrence risk.[6]

An important differential diagnosis to consider in all patients with ABC is telangiectatic osteosarcoma. This variant of osteosarcoma can have a radiographic appearance similar to ABC and may have a similar clinical presentation.[7] On microscopic examination, however, these malignant tumors demonstrate pleomorphic cells and atypical mitotic figures characteristic of malignancy. Malignant osteoid surrounded by osteoblasts is seen in a lacelike pattern, with malignant-appearing cells infiltrating the entire lesion. Because of the radically different treatment and prognosis of this potentially lethal tumor, the diagnosis must be considered and ruled out in evaluation of ABC. Exposure to ionizing irradiation can also lead to sarcomatous degeneration of ABCs. Additionally, rare instances of metastasis of ABCs have been described, and were confirmed with the presence of *USP6* gene mutation in pulmonary metastases.[8] Genetic testing for ABC and screening for metastases of ABC are not routine at this time.

Treatment

The main treatment of ABC is curettage and bone grafting. As with all bone tumors, surgical management should not proceed until histologic confirmation has been completed. The local recurrence rate is high, with studies of curettage and bone grafting demonstrating up to 31% recurrence.[9] Factors such as young age, periarticular location, incomplete initial curettage, open physes, and high Enneking stage have all been found to be predictors of recurrence.[10,11] Adjuvant therapy with agents such as alcoholic zein,[12] phenol, liquid nitrogen, polymethyl methacrylate, high-speed burring, or argon beam[13] have been described, but none has shown conclusive improvement in the recurrence rate. Historically, radiation therapy has also been described, and although it is effective in treating the lesion, associated risks such as growth arrest, nonunion, arthrofibrosis, organ injury, and malignant transformation prevent it from being a recommended modality of treatment. Alternative treatments include intracyst injection, sclerotherapy with polidocanol,[14] and embolization.[15] In anatomically less accessible locations, such as the spine, parts of the pelvis, or the sacrum, these alternate treatments are promising and may be a better initial treatment to avoid significant surgical morbidity or mortality. En bloc resection can be considered for expendable bones to decrease the recurrence risk.

Intraosseous Ganglions and Degenerative Cysts

Intraosseous ganglions are subchondral lesions that are presumed to be the result of a cartilage defect at a joint surface allowing chronic passage of synovial fluid into the bone. These lesions are often seen in an arthritic joint, and thus tend to affect middle-aged populations more frequently. However, they can also be associated with younger patients who have traumatic or other cartilage defects.

Clinical presentation is often as an incidental finding, or a finding in radiography of a chronically painful arthritic joint. These lesions vary in size and can become quite large. In the case of large lesions, pathologic fractures can occur.

Imaging

Plain radiography demonstrates a lucent subchondral intraosseous lesion with a sclerotic border. There is no associated periosteal reaction or elevation, and no intralesional mineralization. CT scanning may show communication with a joint surface (**Figure 5**). MRI shows a fluid-filled cavity with a dense border and no associated edema in the absence of fracture. The cavity is filled with fluid that appears bright on T2-weighted MRI, and in many cases, with careful evaluation a communication with the joint can be identified.

Treatment

Treatment of these lesions generally consists of observation, and treatment of the underlying joint process. In the cases of large lesions threatening pathologic fracture, curettage and packing of the lesion with bone graft with or without prophylactic stabilization may be considered. In cases where appropriate, these lesions are usually addressed at the time of total joint arthroplasty for the underlying arthritic process.

Calcaneal Bone Cysts

Simple calcaneal bone cysts occur fairly commonly. Although the exact incidence is unknown because the majority are discovered incidentally, several series of simple bone cysts show that the calcaneal variety accounts for anywhere from 2% to 11% of simple cysts. The precise algorithm for management of these lesions remains undefined because their clinical relevance is debated. For asymptomatic lesions under normal loading conditions, it is unclear if there is a risk of pathologic fracture; biomechanical studies have suggested that the strength of the calcaneus remains unchanged even in the presence of a cyst.[16] Other clinical studies present series of pathologic fractures in patients with these lesions, although these fractures usually occur in previously painful lesions, or during sports or impact activities. Pathologic fractures of these cysts can be extremely difficult to manage because of the intraarticular nature of the fractures, which highlights the need for an accurate method of predicting which lesions are at risk of fracture. A subset of patients will have a variable amount of fat within the cyst, leading to the postulation of a corollary diagnosis of calcaneal intraosseous lipoma, but the relationship between these lesions is unknown.[17]

Imaging

Lesions are found in the anterior-central portion of the calcaneus, typically below the sulcus calcanei and the posterior articular facet of the talus. A well-circumscribed lucent area devoid of any trabeculae is seen on plain radiographic imaging (**Figure 6, A**). CT imaging may show some thinning of the cortex in regions where the cyst abuts the endosteal surface. Frequently, extensive sclerosis is evident around the tumor, presumably relating to the remodeling to accommodate

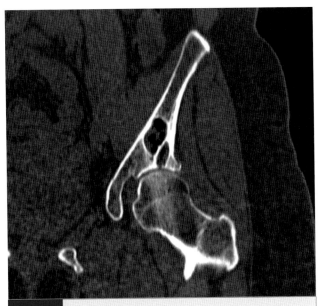

| Figure 5 | An intraosseous ganglion is shown. CT shows communication with joint, and well-circumscribed borders reflecting the benign nature of this lesion. |

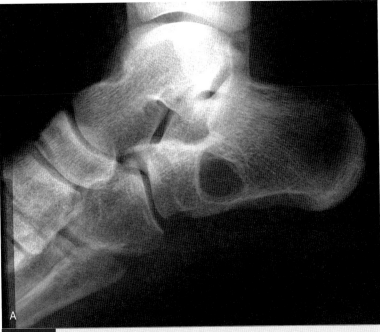
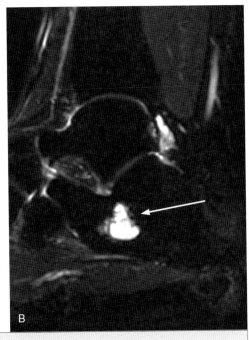

| Figure 6 | **A,** Radiographic appearance of a calcaneal cyst demonstrates its purely lytic nature with no intralesional mineralization. **B,** T2-weighted MRI shows the high water content of the lesion (arrow). |

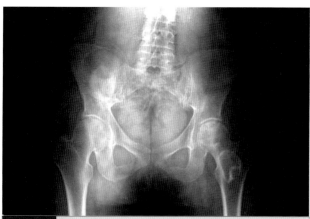

Figure 7 Liposclerosing myxofibrous tumor (LSMFT) of the proximal femur is shown. The intertrochanteric lesion is well circumscribed and has the typical appearance for LSMFT with mixed lytic/sclerotic findings on plain radiograph. This patient had an incidental LSMFT and pain from osteonecrosis of the femoral head, also seen in this image, and underwent total hip arthroplasty. Pathologic analysis at the time of the total hip arthroplasty confirmed LSMFT.

load throughout the calcaneus. MRI shows a fluid signal within the cyst (**Figure 6, B**), although some fat signal may be seen as well.

Histology
Histologically, as with other simple cysts, a thin cyst wall is seen with fibrous lining, scattered giant cells, and thin, scattered trabeculae. Fat seen histologically usually has the appearance of marrow fat.

Treatment
Management of calcaneal bone cysts is controversial. There are no clear parameters that define cysts with pathologic fracture risk. One series of 50 patients suggested the following criteria as determinants of a critical lesion size: completely filling the calcaneus in the coronal plane, and occupying more than 30% of the transverse plane. In that series, 8 of the 17 patients who met the criteria were successfully treated nonsurgically. Below this critical size, however, none of the patients suffered pathologic fracture and none progressed. This finding suggests that these parameters may be used as a reasonable lower-limit threshold of nonsurgical management.[18]

Once the decision for surgical management has been made, several treatment options are available. These options include steroid, demineralized bone matrix or bone marrow aspirate injections, and curettage with or without bone grafting or bone graft substitute. Internal fixation may be necessary in the presence of fracture. Both open and minimally invasive or endoscopic procedures have been described.[19] Most reported procedures have results comparable but not superior to open treat-

ment. Reported success rates for open curettage and bone grafting procedures range from 55% to 65%.

Liposclerosing Myxofibrous Tumor

LSMFT of bone is a benign lesion with a predilection for the proximal femur. The histopathology of the lesion was described in 1986,[20] and recognized as an "almost site specific" proximal femur lesion in 1993.[21] The lesion is usually found incidentally and in more than 80% of patients is located in the intertrochanteric region of the femur.

Imaging
This lesion is well defined with a sclerotic border, and may have some mineralization (**Figure 7**). In most patients the bone contour is normal, but mild to moderate expansion of the cortex has also been described. CT may show lobular irregular mineralization, which can extend to the margins of the lesion. MRI shows a relatively homogenous signal on T1-weighted images, with signal intensity similar to skeletal muscle.[22] Fat signal will not necessarily be seen on these sequences. Nuclear studies can show mild to moderate radioactive tracer uptake. The occurrence of pathologic fracture has been described, so painful lesions warrant investigation to evaluate the risk of fracture. However, careful and thorough clinical evaluation may be necessary to distinguish a truly painful lesion from a lesion that is found incidentally in the setting of another source of hip pain.

Histology
Histologic evaluation of LSMFT demonstrates areas of several differing histologic elements including myxofibrous areas, xanthomatous areas, lipomatous areas and areas of hypertrophic fat, fat necrosis, dystrophic mineralization, ossification, and areas resembling fibrous dysplasia with formation of thin, metaplastic, woven bony trabeculae.[23] The fibrous dysplasia like areas and predilection for the proximal femur have led to the postulation that this lesion is related to fibrous dysplasia and may represent a variant form (**Figure 8**).

Molecular Biology
Molecular studies investigating this possibility have revealed an activating $G_s\alpha$ mutation at the Arg201 codon in some but not all LSMFT samples.[24] This mutation is seen in nearly all patients with fibrous dysplasia, which gives some molecular support to the relationship between these lesions.

Malignant transformation of LSMFT has been described, and in one report was seen in 10% of patients.[22] The most common malignant histology seen was osteosarcoma, but other malignancies such as high-grade and low-grade spindle cell malignancies (for example, unclassified pleomorphic lesions formerly referred to as malignant fibrous histiocytomas) have also been described.

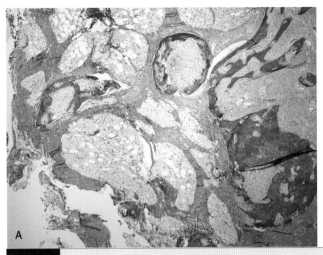
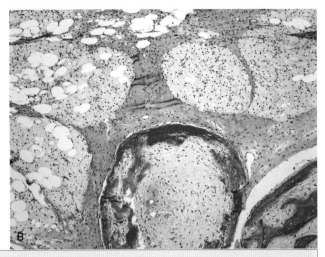

Figure 8 Histology of liposclerosing myxofibrous tumor is shown. **A,** The low-power view shows regions of bone sclerosis and thickened bony trabeculae adjoining myxoid areas with interspersed fibrous bands. **B,** The high-power view confirms low-grade cellular appearance and no significant atypia.

Management of these lesions generally consists of serial radiographic observation, with surgical intervention reserved for pathologic fracture, impending fracture, or lesions that demonstrate aggressive features on imaging or clinical evaluation.

Hemangioma of Bone

Hemangioma of bone is most commonly seen in the calvaria or spine (80% of patients) as an incidental finding. Other areas also have been described, although with far smaller incidence. The lesions are usually asymptomatic and may grow very slowly over time; they do not exhibit rapid growth. In some patients, however, these lesions may have an aggressive appearance and may be called aggressive hemangioma. In symptomatic cases, the patient may notice mild pain or swelling. In the spine, large lesions can cause compression fracture or spinal cord compression.

A recent study of these lesions reviewed 15 patients with the previously described subtypes of intramedullary, subperiosteal, and cortical lesions.[25] Although all of these lesions are rare, the subperiosteal and cortical varieties are extremely rare and may be mistaken for osteoid osteoma or even periosteal osteosarcomas. Imaging findings are usually most suggestive on CT scan.

Imaging

Radiographs may show an area of thickened trabeculae with enlarged vascular channels, sometimes referred to as "Irish lace" or "filigree lace," between them (**Figure 9, A**). Spinal lesions may show similar striations of trabeculae in a vertical direction in response to stress (**Figure 9, B**). On a cross-sectional image such as a CT scan, these vertically oriented, thickened trabeculae can show a polka-dot pattern that is highly suggestive of

hemangioma of bone. MRI can show areas of fat signal intensity on T1-weighted images, which saturate out with fat suppression because of the fat content of these lesions (**Figure 9, C**). T2-weighted images show bright signal, and the lesions enhance avidly with contrast.[25]

Histology

On histologic examination, these lesions show large, cavernous vascular spaces lined by a thin, attenuated endothelial lining. At high magnification, endothelial cells are inconspicuous, with small dark nuclei.

Treatment

Treatment usually consists of observation. For symptomatic lesions, sclerotherapy or alcohol injections have been tried, and recent reports show promising results.[26] Irradiation at a low dose can be used for symptomatic spinal lesions.[27] Curettage and bone grafting is usually reserved for highly symptomatic lesions such as those with associated mechanical compromise, particularly in the spine. These lesions can exhibit significant bleeding with curettage, and adequate preparation with preoperative embolization or other methods of blood loss management should be considered.

Humeral Pseudocyst

Humeral pseudocyst represents a variant of a normal imaging finding that may be confused for a true lesion, and therefore it is important that the practicing orthopaedic surgeon recognize this variant to avoid unnecessary workup or intervention. The variant is described as an area of rarefaction in the humeral head at the junction of the humeral head and greater tuberosity, and the imaging findings can appear to extend into the entire tuberosity. The original reports suggest that this

2: Benign Bone Tumors

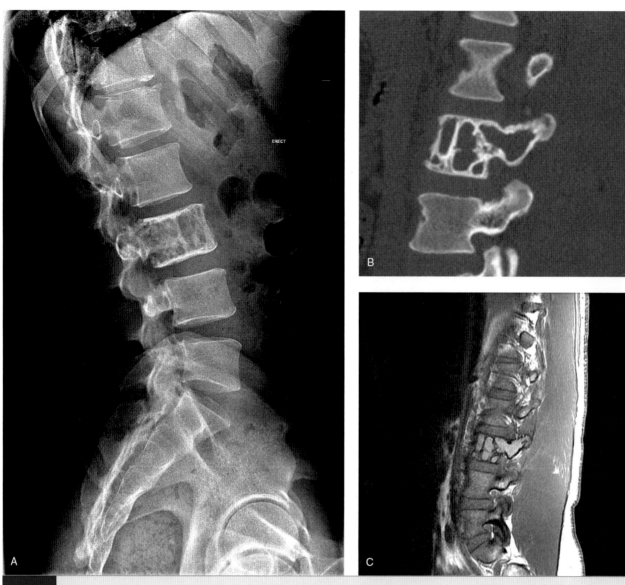

Figure 9 Hemangioma of bone is shown. **A,** Lateral radiograph of the lumbar spine shows a lesion with vertical striations, sometimes called "jailhouse striations" or "corduroy vertebrae," and lytic areas. **B,** CT scan shows striated thickened vertebrae. In cross-section, these striations may appear as "polka dots." **C,** T1-weighted MRI sequence may show areas of signal intensity similar to fat.

pseudotumor is due to a difference in the amount of trabecular bone present in the greater tuberosity and the humeral head.[28] Up to 98% of patients may have some rarefaction of this area compared to the rest of the proximal humerus, so these findings are quite common. In many patients, but not all, the lucent appearance of the pseudotumor region may be similar on the contralateral side, so comparison radiographs can be useful (**Figure 10**). Because most of these lucencies are seen as incidental findings during the workup of a report of shoulder pain, additional pathology such as rotator cuff tear or avulsion can result in positive findings on studies such as bone scan or MRI. Cystic lesions at

the footprint of the rotator cuff can also occur in this setting and may be diagnosed by characteristic MRI findings. True pathology such as giant cell tumor, myeloma, metastatic disease, chondroblastoma, and others can also occur in this region, so more aggressive features such as cortical breakthrough, periosteal reaction or new bone formation, extensive proximal humeral involvement, marrow replacement, or poorly defined margins should be taken seriously and lead to further workup. However, in the absence of these findings, biopsy is not necessary for these imaging variants. If there is a concern for any other benign pathology, serial imaging, usually with plain radiographs, to document stability of the area over time can be considered.

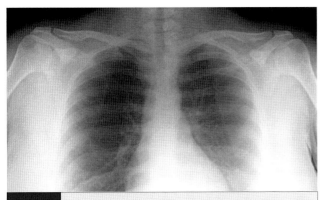

Figure 10 Chest radiograph shows bilateral humeral pseudocysts. These are not true lesions but areas of rarefaction in the proximal humerus, and for this reason the finding is present bilaterally.

Summary

Most cystic lesions of bone are benign, but malignancies can also have a radiographically lucent appearance and be confused for cystic disease. The common cystic lesions of bone generally have relatively classic appearances on imaging and can be readily distinguished. The understanding of the molecular basis of these lesions has progressed in the past several years, and future studies will continue to further delineate the etiologies of these lesions.

Annotated References

1. Harnet JC, Lombardi T, Klewansky P, Rieger J, Tempe MH, Clavert JM: Solitary bone cyst of the jaws: A review of the etiopathogenic hypotheses. *J Oral Maxillofac Surg* 2008;66(11):2345-2348.

   This review article elucidated the suspected etiologies of solitary bone cysts and presented supporting data from prior studies.

2. Komiya S, Kawabata R, Zenmyo M, Hashimoto S, Inoue A: Increased concentrations of nitrate and nitrite in the cyst fluid suggesting increased nitric oxide synthesis in solitary bone cysts. *J Orthop Res* 2000;18(2): 281-288.

3. Capanna R, Campanacci DA, Manfrini M: Unicameral and aneurysmal bone cysts. *Orthop Clin North Am* 1996;27(3):605-614.

4. Pedzisz P, Zgoda M, Kocon H, Benke G, Górecki A: Treatment of solitary bone cysts with allogenic bone graft and platelet-rich plasma: A preliminary report. *Acta Orthop Belg* 2010;76(3):374-379.

   This study reported on nine symptomatic patients without controls who underwent curettage and bone grafting with cancellous graft mixed with platelet-rich

plasma. All nine patients showed complete healing of cysts and became asymptomatic. Although promising, this study has the limitations of no control and a very small sample size. Level of evidence: II.

5. Ye Y, Pringle LM, Lau AW, et al: TRE17/USP6 oncogene translocated in aneurysmal bone cyst induces matrix metalloproteinase production via activation of NF-kappaB. *Oncogene* 2010;29(25):3619-3629.

   This series of molecular experiments delineated that TRE17 is sufficient to initiate tumorigenesis, and identified MMPs as novel TRE17 effectors that likely contribute to ABC pathogenesis and define the underlying signaling mechanism of their induction.

6. Docquier PL, Delloye C, Galant C: Histology can be predictive of the clinical course of a primary aneurysmal bone cyst. *Arch Orthop Trauma Surg* 2010; 130(4):481-487.

   This study examined histology from 21 aneurysmal bone cysts. Healing was seen in 16 cysts and recurrence in 5, with a mean follow-up of 4.43 years. The two groups differed significantly in their proportion of cellular content and their healing index. The ratio of CD68-negative to CD68-positive cells was also significantly different between the groups, suggesting that these tests may help determine prognosis. Level of evidence: III.

7. Murphey MD, wan Jaovisidha S, Temple HT, Gannon FH, Jelinek JS, Malawer MM: Telangiectatic osteosarcoma: Radiologic-pathologic comparison. *Radiology* 2003;229(2):545-553.

8. van de Luijtgaarden AC, Veth RP, Slootweg PJ, et al: Metastatic potential of an aneurysmal bone cyst. *Virchows Arch* 2009;455(5):455-459.

   A case of metastasis of ABC is described. Level of evidence: V.

9. Cottalorda J, Bourelle S: Modern concepts of primary aneurysmal bone cyst. *Arch Orthop Trauma Surg* 2007;127(2):105-114.

   Current concepts regarding aneurysmal bone cyst, including imaging, diagnosis, and treatment, were reviewed.

10. Gibbs CP Jr, Hefele MC, Peabody TD, Montag AG, Aithal V, Simon MA: Aneurysmal bone cyst of the extremities: Factors related to local recurrence after curettage with a high-speed burr. *J Bone Joint Surg Am* 1999;81(12):1671-1678.

11. Başarir K, Pişkin A, Güçlü B, Yildiz Y, Sağlik Y: Aneurysmal bone cyst recurrence in children: A review of 56 patients. *J Pediatr Orthop* 2007;27(8):938-943.

    In this retrospective review of 56 patients with ABC, recurrence rates were higher in younger children, and did not vary based on physeal contact or size of the lesion. Level of evidence: III.

12. George HL, Unnikrishnan PN, Garg NK, Sampath JS, Bass A, Bruce CE: Long-term follow-up of Ethibloc in-

2: Benign Bone Tumors

jection in aneurysmal bone cysts. *J Pediatr Orthop B* 2009;18(6):375-380.

This study included 33 patients treated with injection of alcoholic zein, or Ethibloc. Eleven treatments were for recurrences. Fifty-eight percent showed complete healing, and 36% showed partial healing. There were no controls, but these rates are comparable to repeat injection or curettage rates. Level of evidence: III.

13. Steffner RJ, Liao C, Stacy G, et al: Factors associated with recurrence of primary aneurysmal bone cysts: Is argon beam coagulation an effective adjuvant treatment? *J Bone Joint Surg Am* 2011;93(21):e1221-e1229.

This study provided a retrospective review of 96 patients with primary ABCs. The rate of recurrence was 20.6% after curettage and high-speed-burr treatment alone and 7.5% after curettage and high-speed-burr treatment plus argon beam coagulation, but postoperative fracture was a common complication. Level of evidence: III.

14. Varshney MK, Rastogi S, Khan SA, Trikha V: Is sclerotherapy better than intralesional excision for treating aneurysmal bone cysts? *Clin Orthop Relat Res* 2010; 468(6):1649-1659.

In this study, 94 patients were randomized into sclerotherapy and curettage groups. Healing rates were similar. Higher complication rates were seen in the surgically treated group. Level of evidence: II.

15. Rossi G, Rimondi E, Bartalena T, et al: Selective arterial embolization of 36 aneurysmal bone cysts of the skeleton with N-2-butyl cyanoacrylate. *Skeletal Radiol* 2010;39(2):161-167.

In this study, 36 patients were treated with embolization. Ninety-four percent had healing with one to three injections, including one patient who had prior surgery. There was no control group. Level of evidence: III.

16. Symeonides PP, Economou CJ, Papadimitriou J: Solitary bone cyst of the calcaneus. *Int Surg* 1977;62(1): 24-26.

17. Narang S, Gangopadhyay M: Calcaneal intraosseous lipoma: A case report and review of the literature. *J Foot Ankle Surg* 2011;50(2):216-220.

This case report of a calcaneal intraosseous lipoma suggests that this lesion is distinct from calcaneal cysts, which is a debated topic. Level of evidence: V.

18. Pogoda P, Priemel M, Linhart W, et al: Clinical relevance of calcaneal bone cysts: A study of 50 cysts in 47 patients. *Clin Orthop Relat Res* 2004;424:202-210.

19. Yildirim C, Akmaz I, Sahin O, Keklikci K: Simple calcaneal bone cysts: A pilot study comparing open versus endoscopic curettage and grafting. *J Bone Joint Surg Br* 2011;93(12):1626-1631.

In this study, 26 patients were randomized into open and endoscopic curettage groups. No statistically significant differences regarding radiologic healing were found. Surgical time and mean length of stay were shorter in the endoscopic group. Level of evidence: II.

20. Ragsdale BD, Sweet DE: *The Pathology of Incipient Neoplasia*. Philadelphia, PA, Saunders, 1986, pp 381-423.

21. Ragsdale BD: Polymorphic fibro-osseous lesions of bone: An almost site-specific diagnostic problem of the proximal femur. *Hum Pathol* 1993;24(5):505-512.

22. Kransdorf MJ, Murphey MD, Sweet DE: Liposclerosing myxofibrous tumor: A radiologic-pathologic-distinct fibro-osseous lesion of bone with a marked predilection for the intertrochanteric region of the femur. *Radiology* 1999;212(3):693-698.

23. Gilkey FW: Liposclerosing myxofibrous tumor of bone. *Hum Pathol* 1993;24(11):1264.

24. Matsuba A, Ogose A, Tokunaga K, et al: Activating Gs alpha mutation at the Arg201 codon in liposclerosing myxofibrous tumor. *Hum Pathol* 2003;34(11):1204-1209.

25. Rigopoulou A, Saifuddin A: Intraosseous hemangioma of the appendicular skeleton: Imaging features of 15 cases, and a review of the literature. *Skeletal Radiol* 2012;41(12):1525-1536.

This study is a retrospective review of 15 patients with intraosseous hemangioma; imaging features are detailed. Level of evidence: III.

26. Crawford EA, Slotcavage RL, King JJ, Lackman RD, Ogilvie CM: Ethanol sclerotherapy reduces pain in symptomatic musculoskeletal hemangiomas. *Clin Orthop Relat Res* 2009;467(11):2955-2961.

This study is a retrospective review of 19 patients. Four patients reported full pain relief, 11 had partial relief, and 4 had no relief. The study had a short mean follow-up of 24 months. Level of evidence: III.

27. Miszczyk L, Tukiendorf A: Radiotherapy of painful vertebral hemangiomas: The single center retrospective analysis of 137 cases. *Int J Radiat Oncol Biol Phys* 2012;82(2):e173-e180.

This study describes 137 painful vertebral hemangioma irradiations in 101 patients, with no control group. Mean pain relief percentages (defined as a decrease of primary pain level expressed as a percentage) at 1, 6, 12, and 18 months after radiation therapy were 60.5%, 65.4%, 68.3%, and 78.4%. There was no effect on the ossification of lesions. Level of evidence: III.

28. Helms CA: Pseudocysts of the humerus. *AJR Am J Roentgenol* 1978;131(2):287-288.

Chapter 10

Benign Cartilage Tumors

Adam J. Schwartz, MD

Introduction

Benign cartilage tumors are the most common biopsy-proven benign lesions of bone.[1] The clinical behavior of these tumors ranges from completely benign to having the potential to differentiate into malignancy. Both chromosomal translocations and specific gene mutations are likely to play a significant role in the genesis of these lesions.[2,3] Most benign cartilage tumors are found incidentally during the evaluation of an unrelated disorder and do not require treatment. Rarely, a known lesion can grow, change in radiographic appearance, or cause new symptoms, prompting further investigation. Biopsy of cartilage tumors is notoriously difficult, because the heterogeneity typical of these lesions contributes to a high likelihood of sample error. Furthermore, the pathologic discrimination between benign and malignant cartilage tumors is challenging, often necessitating the input of a multidisciplinary team. The purpose of this chapter is to review the clinical and pathologic features of the more common benign cartilage tumors of bone.

Osteochondroma

Osteochondroma is the most common biopsy-proven benign lesion of bone. The true incidence of this lesion is likely underestimated because most are asymptomatic and may never undergo radiographic evaluation.[4] Approximately 15% of patients in whom an osteochondroma is diagnosed have multiple lesions, referred to as multiple osteochondromatosis. Because of the resemblance of the cartilage cap to the normal physis, the etiology of osteochondroma is believed to be pathologic herniation of the portion of the growth plate through the metaphyseal bone, although this has yet to be firmly established. The ability to produce an osteochondroma in a rabbit model by transplantation of physeal cartilage to the metaphysis has been demonstrated.[5] Molecular pathologic studies suggest an underlying biochemical origin of both solitary and multi-

ple lesions. Grossly, an osteochondroma is a variably sized stalk that is confluent with the normal medullary canal and attached to a cartilage cap that typically is directed away from the normal physis as the bone elongates. A cartilage cap larger than 2 cm in adults has been identified as an indicator of potential malignancy.[6]

Clinical Features and Radiographic Findings

Most osteochondromas are asymptomatic and found as a palpable osseous mass or incidentally during the evaluation of an unrelated complaint. The most common location is the metaphysis of the knee (distal femur, proximal tibia, proximal fibula), followed by the proximal humerus, and less commonly the scapula, pelvis, and spine. Lesions can present with irritation of an overlying bursa, impingement on an adjacent neurovascular structure, or fracture of the stalk (**Figure 1**). In a skeletally mature patient, growth of a lesion or pain that was not previously present in an existing lesion may be an indication of malignant degeneration. Fewer than 1% of solitary osteochondromas and up to 20% of multiple osteochondromas will undergo malignant transformation.[4]

Plain radiographs most commonly reveal a bony growth attached to the bone either with a broad base or stalk that appears to grow away from the adjacent elongating physis. In flat bones or ribs, plain radiographs also show the characteristic continuity of the marrow cavity of the bone with the central portion of the lesion. An osteochondroma may be either sessile or pedunculated, based on the size of the stalk connecting the lesion to the host bone, although the utility of this distinction is debatable. Subtle intralesional calcification is commonly seen on plain radiographs in the cartilage cap, although a disproportionate amount of calcification could indicate malignant transformation. Plain radiographs are particularly useful to document changes in the lesion on serial images.

Although tendon or other soft-tissue irritation is a common clinical finding, ultrasound can be used for dynamic visualization of adjacent tendons or soft tissues that may be mechanically involved with the lesion. Additionally, ultrasound can help to distinguish bursal fluid from the cartilage cap overlying the lesion. Nuclear medicine studies poorly differentiate benign osteochondroma from low-grade chondrosarcoma and are of limited utility.

Axial imaging with either CT (for clearer definition

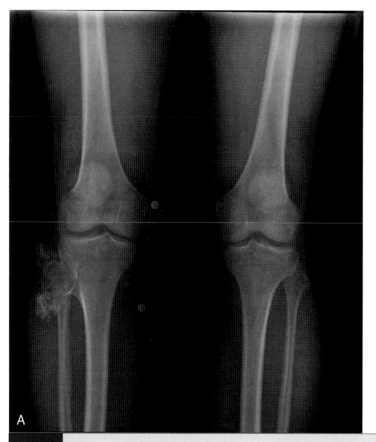
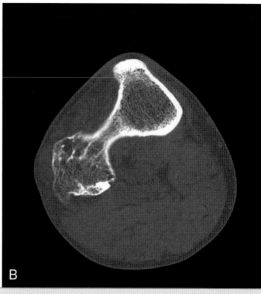

| Figure 1 | Benign osteochondroma is shown in a 42-year-old man. **A**, Plain radiograph shows a benign osteochondroma involving the proximal fibula. **B**, Axial CT scan demonstrates underlying cancellous bone confluent with the lesion that is distorting and flattening the peroneal nerve. The patient reported a mass involving the proximal fibula that had been present for more than 30 years. He developed numbness and weakness in the right lower extremity. Electromyography revealed evidence of chronic peroneal nerve compression. Removal of the lesion resulted in complete resolution of the patient's symptoms. |

of bony anatomy) or MRI (to demonstrate surrounding soft tissue) is helpful in symptomatic cases. Noncontrast CT is superior for bone anatomy, whereas MRI is useful for identifying the size and thickness of the cartilage cap. A recent study compared the MRI and CT findings of 67 benign osteochondromas to 34 biopsy-proven secondary chondrosarcomas.[7] The authors describe the use of a novel method to measure cap thickness. Using this method, the sensitivity and specificity of MRI and CT were 100% and 98%, and 100% and 95%, respectively, when a cartilage cap of 2 cm was used to distinguish benign osteochondroma from secondary chondrosarcoma. The authors cautioned that formation of bursae, particularly adjacent to lesions involving the ventral surface of the scapula or the hip, may confound accurate measurement of the cartilage cap. The use of fluid-sensitive sequences (particularly a cartilage-sensitive, fat-suppressed, spoiled gradient-echo sequence) can reduce the incidence of false-positive measurements of cap thickness due to adjacent bursal fluid collections. A recommended approach to the patient included an initial measurement of cap thickness on CT, followed by selective MRI or ultra-sound to distinguish lesions with cap thickness greater than 2 cm from bursal fluid.

Pathology and Genetics

The gross appearance of an osteochondroma is that of a sessile or pedunculated bony mass with a cartilage cap of variable thickness. A thick (larger than 2 cm), irregular cap is worrisome but is not diagnostic of malignant degeneration. The cortex of the lesion's base on gross inspection is confluent with the underlying bone, or alternatively and more frequently stated, the medullary bone from the host and the lesion are in continuity. This feature is essential in distinguishing osteochondroma from other surface lesions such as periosteal chondroma, periosteal or parosteal osteosarcoma, or juxtacortical heterotopic ossification.

Histology classically reveals three layers, including the perichondrium, cartilage, and bone. The fibrous perichondrium is confluent with the surrounding periosteum of the normal host bone. Between the underlying bone and the perichondrium lies a variably sized cartilage cap. In the regions closest to bone, the cartilage cap resembles the cords seen in the normal growth plate. This site of enchondral ossification results in lesion growth and expansion. Toward the periphery of the lesion, the cartilage cells are less organized. Features that signal malignant transformation include myxoid change, increased cellularity or nuclear atypia, and mitotic activity. Growth or enlargement of an osteochondroma following skeletal maturity is indicative of malignant transformation.

The preponderance of genetic evidence points to the cartilage cap as the only neoplastic component of a benign osteochondroma, because homozygous deletion of the *EXT-1* gene is found only in this location.[8] Mutations involving the *EXT-1* gene are neither present in the perichondrial ring nor the bony stalk. Single mutations in the *EXT-1* gene, resulting in loss of function of the normal product exostosin-1, have been demonstrated in numerous studies to occur in solitary lesions.

Treatment

Asymptomatic osteochondromas do not require treatment, and the use of routine surveillance films for a solitary lesion is debatable. A reasonable approach would be to inform the patient of the rare (less than 1%) incidence of malignant degeneration, and to return for evaluation if symptoms develop, or if the patient notices growth of the lesion.

Surgical excision should be considered for symptomatic lesions. The goal of resection is to remove the entire cartilage cap, the stalk at its base, and in skeletally immature patients, the perichondral ring while minimizing associated morbidity. Osteochondromas infrequently encroach upon neurovascular structures that make removal difficult. Although recurrence is rare with complete excision, one series cited osteochondroma as the most common precursor of chondrosarcoma (127 of 151 cases; 81%).[1] This would suggest that in locations in which it is difficult to achieve complete excision, adequate clinical follow-up and radiographic surveillance are important. At the time of removal, the perichondral ring should be included in the resection so as to reduce the incidence of local recurrence. The decision to remove an osteochondroma prior to skeletal maturity should be individualized based on the location of the lesion and the amount of growth remaining. In the forearm, removal of a lesion may necessitate ulnar lengthening or radial hemiepiphysiodesis, corrective osteotomy, or radial head excision. In recurrent cases, a one-bone forearm is a possible solution as a salvage procedure. In the lower extremity, periarticular deformity can result in early degenerative joint disease, varus or valgus deformity or limb length inequality. It is not uncommon to perform multiple corrective procedures in such cases.

Multiple Osteochondromas

Multiple osteochondromatosis, or multiple hereditary exostosis (MHE), is an autosomal dominant condition that results in multiple skeletal deformities. The incidence is approximately 1:50,000, with males more commonly affected possibly because of incomplete penetrance in females. More than one half of patients with MHE have a positive family history.[4] Remodeling defects are common as growth is inhibited from osteochondroma enlargement. Common deformities include ulnar shortening with secondary radial bowing, limb-length inequality, and short stature. A diagnosis of MHE can be made with either plain radiographs demonstrating two separate osteochondromas, or through genetic testing. MHE is caused by mutation in either the exostosis (multiple) – 1 EXT1, or exostosis (multiple) – 2 EXT2 gene, located on chromosomes 8q24.11-q24.13 and 11p11-12 (OMIM Nos. 133700 and 133701), respectively.[9] Most mutations result in a loss of protein function encoded by the gene, and are heterozygous. Both EXT1 and EXT2 proteins function in heparan sulfate proteoglycan biosynthesis, which is critical to signaling pathways in normal physis, including the Indian hedgehog (IHH), parathyroid hormone related peptide, and fibroblast growth factor pathways. A recent molecular analysis demonstrated that biallelic inactivation of the *EXT1* gene is present only in the cartilage cap of nonhereditary osteochondromas.[8]

In the presence of multiple osteochondromas, histology alone is insufficient to diagnose malignant transformation. Lesions can frequently exhibit nodularity, irregular calcification, mucoid changes, and necrosis, and binucleate cells can be present. Measurement of thickness of the cartilage cap, along with careful review of the history and radiographic appearance in these cases, is important in differentiating benign from malignant lesions. Growth of a lesion following skeletal maturity suggests malignant transformation. In one recent study, interobserver variability was determined between 12 experienced musculoskeletal pathologists who interpreted 38 surgical specimens.[10] Although there was substantial agreement among pathologists (correlation coefficient, 0.78), the authors noted that interpretation should take into account the entire clinical picture, including the thickness of the cartilage cap and radiographic appearance.

Enchondroma

An enchondroma is a benign growth of hyaline cartilage, typically located in the medullary bone. Enchondromas are thought to be a portion of enchondral ossification that has become trapped in the medullary space.

Clinical Features and Radiographic Findings

Enchondromas are most frequently found incidentally (**Figure 2**). The true incidence of this lesion is unknown because many are asymptomatic and likely do not come to the attention of the patient or the clinician. Lesions can be identified at any age, although they are

2: Benign Bone Tumors

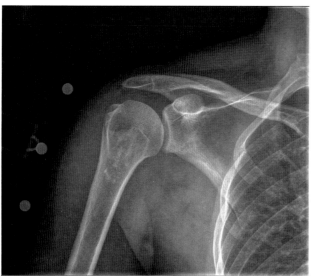

Figure 2 Benign enchondroma is shown. This lesion was noted incidentally on a chest radiograph obtained in a routine preoperative evaluation. The lesion is characterized by areas of rounded calcification (so-called popcorn calcification). Note the lack of endosteal scalloping, cortical thickening or erosion, or associated soft-tissue mass.

radiographic features demonstrate worrisome findings such as expansion of the bone, cortical thinning, or large intralesional lucencies, then referral to an orthopaedic oncologist is appropriate. CT and MRI are both useful in the evaluation of a symptomatic benign enchondroma. The bone windows of an axial CT image are most useful for determining the presence or absence of endosteal scalloping and cortical thickening or breakthrough. MRI can demonstrate surrounding T2 enhancement and edema in the case of impending fracture. An associated soft-tissue lesion on MRI is indicative of a more aggressive lesion that should be investigated further.

Pathology and Genetics

Enchondromas are composed of nodules of cartilage separated by cancellous bone. Lesions typically demonstrate hypocellular areas of chondrocytes sitting within clearly defined lacunae, surrounded by copious amounts of hyaline cartilage.[11]

Distinguishing a benign from a malignant cartilaginous tumor is perhaps one of the more challenging tasks facing the musculoskeletal pathologist. It is extremely important to correlate the clinical presentation, radiographic appearance, and histologic analysis to arrive at an overall understanding of the expected behavior of the lesion. Therefore, the pathologist, radiologist, and surgeon must arrive at a collaborative consensus in the evaluation and management of a particular lesion. In a study similar to the one discussed previously, an analysis of interobserver variability was performed among 18 specialized pathologists charged with distinguishing benign enchondroma from low-grade chondrosarcoma.[12] Considerable discord was noted, with a kappa coefficient of 0.54. Five factors were most likely to differentiate between enchondroma and low-grade chondrosarcoma: high cellularity, presence of host bone entrapment, open chromatin, mucoid matrix, and age older than 45 years. Lamellar trapping refers to the permeation of a more aggressive lesion through host bone that surrounds and entraps preexisting bony trabeculae, and is suggestive of a low-grade chondrosarcoma.

Although it is always true that the best care is delivered in musculoskeletal oncology with the close multidisciplinary cooperation of radiologist, pathologist, and surgeon, this reality is never more salient than in the diagnosis of cartilage lesions of bone. For example, high cellularity in a cartilage lesion of the digit may be radiographically and clinically characteristic of an enchondroma, whereas the exact same histologic finding likely would be considered malignant if it were obtained from the pelvis of a middle-aged person.

Parathyroid hormone-like hormone (PTHLH) and IHH work in concert to regulate and inhibit differentiation of proliferating growth plate chondrocytes. Approximately 8% of patients with multiple enchondromatosis demonstrate a mutation in the gene encoding the PTHLH receptor, PTHR1. Studies of tumor cultures have revealed that IHH may be sensitive to the extracellular environment, explaining the difference

most commonly identified in the second through fourth decades of life.

Approximately one half of all enchondromas occur in the hands and feet, with the proximal humerus and metaphyseal regions of the femur next in frequency. Solitary enchondromas are only very rarely seen in the axial skeleton. Radiographically, a benign enchondroma is typically metaphyseal in location, characterized by a well-marginated border and central area filled with variable amounts of mineralization.

A variety of radiographic features exist that distinguish a simple benign enchondroma from a more aggressive cartilaginous tumor. Central location, lack of endosteal scalloping or cortical breakthrough, and uniform prominent mineralization are typical characteristics of benign lesions. Although an asymptomatic lesion does not require further workup, more aggressive features, including the appearance of radiolucencies within the lesion, changes in cortical thickness, and expansion of the bone, should prompt further investigation with axial imaging and referral.

A common clinical scenario is a middle-aged patient with an enchondroma of the proximal humerus and coexisting shoulder pathology (for example, subacromial bursitis, rotator cuff tear, biceps tendinitis, or degenerative joint disease of the acromioclavicular joint). If the patient's history and physical examination findings are consistent with the shoulder pathology, and radiographic features of the lesion are suggestive of a benign enchondroma, then treatment should proceed independently of the lesion. Localized injections may be useful both diagnostically and therapeutically in this situation. If plain seen among the various blocking agents. In one recent study, c-propeptides of procollagens Ia1 and II (PC1CP and PC3CP) were shown to have a variable effect on chondrocyte proliferation and viability depending on the extracellular environment. Although PC1CP increased angiogenesis and tumor progression, PC2CP acted to induce apoptosis in the immobilized state. Interestingly, while in the soluble state, PC2CP also induced tumor progression and metastasis. Animal studies have demonstrated that loss of p53 in the presence of Gli2 overexpression leads to the development of chondrosarcoma.

Treatment

As with other benign cartilaginous tumors, asymptomatic enchondromas are typically treated with observation. In younger patients with open physes, treatment is generally delayed until the distance between the lesion and the physis is sufficient to avoid premature growth arrest at the time of treatment. Enchondromas rarely are diagnosed in children, and when they do are sometimes confused with benign cystic tumors because mineralization has not yet developed.

For symptomatic lesions that have not caused a fracture, the mainstay of treatment is simple curettage, bone grafting, and supplemental fixation as necessary. The recurrence rate for benign enchondromas treated in this manner is low, typically less than 5%.

When fracture occurs through a benign enchondroma, the decision to proceed with surgery should be based on the stability of the fracture. Particularly in young patients with healthy periosteum, fractures heal reliably even in the presence of a large lesion. When the lesion is close to the physis, treatment should be delayed until the fracture heals and the lesion is far enough away to prevent injury to the growth plate at the time of curettage. If the fracture warrants fixation (for example, fracture of the proximal femur), extended curettage is performed at the time of surgery. Care should be taken to avoid spreading the lesion to other parts of the bone with intramedullary devices, and if such implants are to be used, the lesion should be completely removed before placement of the device through the pathologic area. Although good results have been reported with curettage alone, grafting of the lesion can be performed with either allograft or autograft. A thorough review of grafting materials is provided elsewhere in this book.

Cryosurgery is a useful adjunct to curettage, particularly in cases where extended margins may be difficult to achieve. In a recent review of 75 lesions treated with extended curettage and cryosurgery, only two recurrences were identified.[13] An additional 55 grade 1 chondrosarcomas were treated in a similar fashion with no reported recurrences. A major concern with this method of treatment is the integrity of the surrounding normal bone that may be compromised by temperature-induced necrosis. The authors of this particular study cited a 14% incidence of postoperative

fracture, many of which occurred even with prophylactic stabilization. The authors also cited one case of nitrogen gas emboli, which caused transient hemodynamic changes. In children, mineralization may not have developed in the enchondroma, and the radiographically apparent lytic lesion can be confused with benign cystic tumors of bone. Once enchondroma has been identified, treatment can usually be delayed until the distance between the lesion and the physis is sufficient to avoid premature growth arrest at the time of treatment.

Periosteal (Juxtacortical) Chondroma

Periosteal chondroma is a benign lesion that arises juxtacortically from the host-bone periosteum. Lesions are typically painful, palpable masses that can occur in any age group, most commonly involving the long bones. The classic radiographic appearance is a radiolucent lesion that abuts and erodes the cortical bone into a saucer-shaped contour (saucerization). Axial imaging reveals saucerization but no evidence of frank cortical penetration, which is confirmed by histologic analysis at the time of removal. Treatment is symptomatic and removal is uniformly curative. Infrequently, juxtacortical chondromas left untreated can gradually extend to the medullary cavity, although they remain benign.

Enchondromatosis

The rarer forms of multiple enchondromatosis have been classified numerous times, although sporadic case reports tend to undermine any comprehensive system. Perhaps the most widely cited classification system was described in 1978, but this system omits some of the more recently described entities.[14] More recently, a concise diagnostic algorithm was proposed based on spinal involvement and genetic transmission.[15] Ollier disease (Spranger type I), a nonhereditary disorder that lacks spinal involvement, is the most common clinical presentation of multiple enchondromatosis[16,17] (**Figure 3**). The original description of this disease cited unilateral involvement, suggesting a postzygotic mutation. Maffucci syndrome (Spranger type II) is similar to Ollier disease but with the added finding of multiple soft-tissue hemangiomas.[18] Both Maffucci syndrome and Ollier disease are considered sporadic and nonhereditary, but genetic mutations in PTH1R have been documented. Both disorders carry a significant risk of malignant transformation of benign osseous lesions. The risk of developing malignant bone tumors, particularly chondrosarcoma, is approximately 15% to 30% in patients with Ollier disease.[4]

Similar to Ollier disease and Maffucci syndrome, metachromatosis (Spranger type III) and genochromatosis typically lack spinal involvement, but are distinguished by their autosomal dominant mode of inheri-

2: Benign Bone Tumors

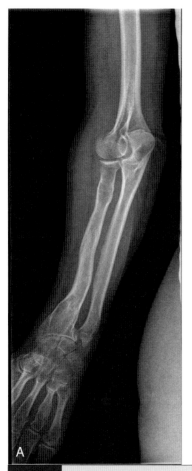
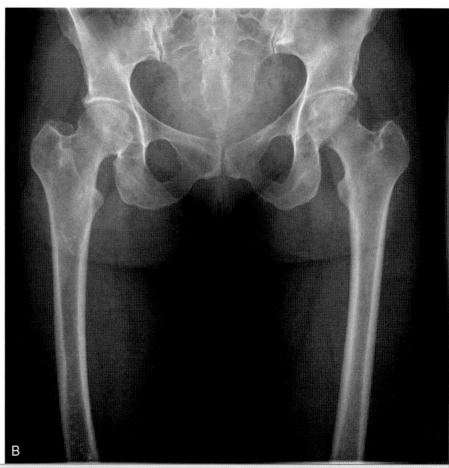

Figure 3   **A** and **B**, Multiple enchondromatosis is shown on plain radiographs from a 62-year-old woman who had a chief report of wrist pain. The patient had a known history of multiple lesions in the long bones of the lower and upper extremity. A rapidly enlarging mass over the wrist was biopsied and found to be consistent with a low-grade chondrosarcoma involving the hamate bone.

tance. The hallmark of metachondromatosis is the presence of exostoses, whereas type I genochrondromatosis exhibits marked thickening of the clavicles and symmetric lesions.

Spinal involvement is seen in both inherited and sporadic enchondromatosis syndromes. Spondyloenchondrodysplasia (Spranger type IV) is thought to be an autosomal recessive disorder; patients have short stature, platyspondyly, and increased lumbar lordosis. Classic type I spondyloenchondrodysplasia does not demonstrate the central nervous system involvement typical of type II.[19] Cheirospondyloenchondromatosis (Spranger type VI) demonstrates marked hand and foot involvement, and frequent mental retardation. Dysspondyloenchondromatosis is distinguished from other multiple enchondromatosis syndromes by the variety of vertebral anomalies, including severe segmentation and progressive kyphoscoliosis. Sporadic case reports continue to refine and add to the spectrum of multiple enchondromatosis syndromes. The true incidence of malignant degeneration for many of these syndromes is unknown.[20]

Chondroblastoma

Chondroblastoma is a benign neoplasm of cartilage that typically arises in the epiphyses of young patients.[21-23] Most lesions involve the long bones and are typically unifocal. Although chondroblastoma is considered to be a benign condition, pulmonary metastasis is rare.

Clinical Features and Radiographic Findings

Most patients with chondroblastomas present with a chief report of pain that is frequently of long duration. Because lesions are typically epiphyseal in location, concomitant joint swelling, stiffness, and associated limitation in motion can be present.

Chondroblastomas most frequently affect the epiphyses of long bones; however, involvement of flat bones and sesamoid bones has also been reported. Lesions are typically radiolucent and sharply demarcated, occasionally with a thin sclerotic border. Calcification of the matrix can help to differentiate this lesion from giant cell tumor, which tends to occur in older patients.

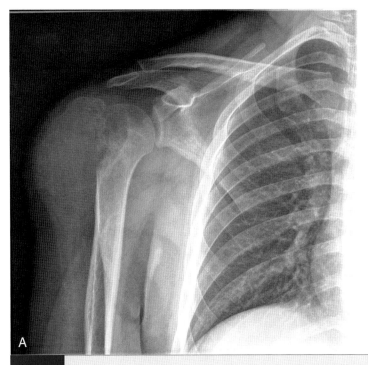
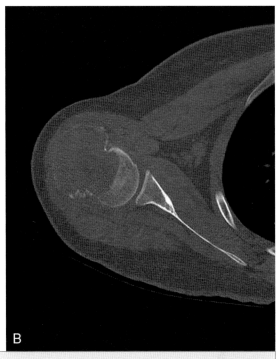

Figure 4 Chondroblastoma is shown. **A,** Plain radiograph of the right shoulder of a 20-year-old man reveals a radiolucent lesion arising from the apophysis of the proximal humerus with significant cortical expansion from a secondary aneurysmal bone cyst. **B,** CT scan reveals complete obliteration of the lateral cortex by the tumor with a large soft-tissue extension. Biopsy was consistent with benign chondroblastoma. Three years after extended intralesional curettage, argon beam cautery, and cementation, the patient remained pain free without evidence of local recurrence or pulmonary metastasis.

Lesions can infrequently penetrate the cortical bone and appear quite aggressive with soft-tissue extension and large areas of secondary aneurysmal bone cyst formation (Figure 4).

Pathology and Genetics
Histologically, chondroblastoma consists of nodules of chondroid surrounding sheets of variably shaped chondroblasts. The cells are typically bordered by weaving calcification (chicken-wire calcification). Giant cells are frequently present, as are secondary aneurysmal bone cysts. Primary giant cell tumor can be differentiated from chondroblastoma by patient age, lesion location, and presence of chondroid matrix.

Limited differentiation of chondrocytes is typical of chondroblasts, and as a result, type II cartilage is not expressed by tumor cells. Immunostains are positive for S100 protein, vimentin, and neuron-specific enolase. No recurrent chromosomal abnormalities have been identified in chondroblastoma. Multiple chromosomes have been implicated in the development of chondroblastoma, including chromosomes 5, 17, and 8.

Treatment
Because of the aggressive nature of chondroblastoma, local treatment typically consists of extended intralesional curettage and grafting. (See chapter 14 for a discussion on surgical management of benign bone tumors.) Local recurrence is more common following treatment than with other benign cartilage tumors, particularly in larger lesions and those with a secondary aneurysmal bone cyst component.

An alternative treatment method for smaller lesions is radiofrequency ablation. In a recent review of 17 patients with relatively small lesions (mean volume, 2.4 mL), percutaneous radiofrequency ablation proved effective in 12 (mean follow-up, 41.3 months), all of whom reported immediate relief of symptoms following the procedure.[24] The authors cautioned against the use of radiofrequency ablation in larger lesions, particularly those beneath weight-bearing surfaces. One patient with a relatively large lesion (volume, 10.5 mL) suffered collapse of the lateral tibial plateau overlying a previously treated lesion. During subsequent surgery, residual viable tumor was found. Similar results are documented in other recent reports involving limited numbers of patients.

Patients should be counseled regarding the possible incidence of pulmonary metastasis. Annual plain chest radiographs for surveillance, at the time of routine follow-up for the local site, is likely sufficient. When pulmonary metastasis does occur, it can be adequately treated with surgical excision.

2: Benign Bone Tumors

Chondromyxoid Fibroma

Chondromyxoid fibroma (CMF) was first described as an entity distinct from chondrosarcoma.[25] It was theorized that this lesion represented a fibroma with chondroid metaplasia. It was later thought that this lesion may represent a chondroma with fibroid characteristics, or perhaps an intermediate lesion between chondroblastoma and enchondroma. More recently, there is evidence to support the notion that this lesion most likely originates from fetal cartilage in the epiphysis.[26]

Clinical Features and Radiographic Findings

CMF represents fewer than 1% of all biopsy-proven bone lesions. It is more common in males than females, and most frequently occurs in the second and third decades of life. Most cases involve the long bones, although axial lesions and lesions of the flat bones have also been reported.

Pain, frequently of long duration, is the most common presenting symptom, along with soft-tissue swelling and rarely an associated mass. Some lesions, particularly those in axial locations, are found incidentally.

Lesions are typically metaphyseal, eccentric, and well defined with sharp sclerotic borders. MRI is useful to demonstrate the demarcation between fibrous (low signal intensity on fluid-weighted images, with postcontrast enhancement) and myxoid (high signal intensity, no enhancement) portions of the lesion.

Pathology and Genetics

Macroscopically, CMF is a firm, bluish lesion that does not demonstrate any evidence of central necrosis or liquefaction.[27] The lesion occasionally shows areas of cortical erosion and expansion into the surrounding soft tissues, particularly in cases involving the feet. Histology reveals chondroid lobules with stellate or spindle-shaped mesenchymal cells within a myxoid matrix. Densely cellular areas may demonstrate nuclear atypia, and can be difficult to distinguish from more aggressive lesions.

A recent study cited characteristic histologic similarities between pathological findings in CMF and fetal cartilage as evidence that this lesion represents a neoplasm originating from immature cartilage.[26] The authors found that among 10 cases of CMF and 4 fetal femora, common findings included immature fibrous tissue of vascularized stroma with accumulation of macrophages in areas of superficial sinusoidal proliferation and variable amounts of lobulated chondroid tissue. Although S100 protein positivity has been reported in CMF, the large amount of matrix compared to the positive chondroid areas makes this test of limited value. Smooth muscle actin and CD34 are also useful markers, particularly in peripheral regions of the tumor.

Rearrangements of the long arm of chromosome 6 at bands q13 and q25 are common in CMF. In a recent study, 16 chondromyxoid fibromas arising in 14 patients underwent cytogenetic analysis to elucidate the 6q13 breakpoint.[28] The authors found the breakpoint to reside within the *COL12A1* gene, implicating this as the most likely oncogene involved in development of this lesion. The *COL12A1* gene encodes the α chain of type XII collagen, although its exact function remains poorly understood. The authors encouraged the use of a fluorescent in situ hybridization probe aimed at identifying this particular 6q13 aberration as a useful piece of evidence to distinguish CMF from chondrosarcoma in difficult cases.

Treatment

As with other benign cartilage lesions, curettage and grafting is the mainstay of treatment. A recurrence rate of up to 15% is expected with this method, although even in the presence of recurrence, prognosis is uniformly good. No evidence currently exists that CMF is a precursor to chondrosarcoma or other malignancy.

Summary

Benign cartilage lesions are common, typically slowly growing or indolent tumors, many of which are found incidentally. When symptomatic, treatment usually consists of excision with a low likelihood of local recurrence. Asymptomatic lesions without radiographically or clinically concerning features may be observed. A significant diagnostic challenge is identifying the source of symptoms, as common musculoskeletal complaints can occur in juxtaposition to incidentally identified asymptomatic benign lesions. Evaluation of cartilage tumors usually requires multidisciplinary collaboration between surgeon, pathologist, and radiologist. Cross-sectional MRI and CT can help in diagnostic accuracy and surgical planning. There is a low risk of malignant degeneration in some benign cartilage tumors, and distinguishing benign from malignant cartilage tumors may be difficult.

Annotated References

1. Unni K, Inwards C: *Dahlin's Bone Tumors: General Aspects and Data on 10,165 Cases*, ed 6. Baltimore, MD, Lippincott Williams & Wilkins, 2009.

   This book presents the Mayo Clinic's experience with bone tumors and is a succinct summary of well-diagnosed bone tumors.

2. Romeo S, Hogendoorn PC, Dei Tos AP: Benign cartilaginous tumors of bone: From morphology to somatic and germ-line genetics. *Adv Anat Pathol* 2009;16(5): 307-315.

   The authors provide a concise review of recent advances in somatic and germ-line mutations as applicable to benign cartilage tumors of bone. Level of evidence: IV.

3. Bovée JV, Hogendoorn PC, Wunder JS, Alman BA: Cartilage tumours and bone development: Molecular pathology and possible therapeutic targets. *Nat Rev Cancer* 2010;10(7):481-488.

    A review of the signaling pathways and genetic mutations involved in the genesis of cartilage tumors is provided. Level of evidence: IV.

4. Fletcher CD Unni KK, Mertens F (eds): *Pathology and Genetics of Tumours of Soft Tissue and Bone.* Lyon, France, IARC Press, 2002.

5. D'Ambrosia R, Ferguson AB Jr: The formation of osteochondroma by epiphyseal cartilage transplantation. *Clin Orthop Relat Res* 1968;61:103-115.

6. Garrison RC, Unni KK, McLeod RA, Pritchard DJ, Dahlin DC: Chondrosarcoma arising in osteochondroma. *Cancer* 1982;49(9):1890-1897.

7. Bernard SA, Murphey MD, Flemming DJ, Kransdorf MJ: Improved differentiation of benign osteochondromas from secondary chondrosarcomas with standardized measurement of cartilage cap at CT and MR imaging. *Radiology* 2010;255(3):857-865.

    The authors describe and validate a technique for reproducible measurement of the osteochondroma cartilage cap with CT and MRI. With 2 cm used as a cutoff for distinguishing benign versus malignant lesions, respective sensitivities and specificities were 100% and 98% for MRI and 100% and 95% for CT. Level of evidence: III.

8. Hameetman L, Szuhai K, Yavas A, et al: The role of EXT1 in nonhereditary osteochondroma: Identification of homozygous deletions. *J Natl Cancer Inst* 2007;99(5):396-406.

    Eight nonhereditary osteochondroma samples underwent resolution, array-based, comparative genomic hybridization. All eight had a large deletion of 8q, and five had additional deletions of the other 8q allele containing the gene *EXT1*. Fluorescence in situ hybridization was used to isolate the location of clonal origin to the cartilage cap only. Level of evidence: IV.

9. Kitsoulis P, Galani V, Stefanaki K, et al: Osteochondromas: Review of the clinical, radiological and pathological features. *In Vivo* 2008;22(5):633-646.

    The authors provided a well-organized review of the current literature regarding solitary and multiple osteochondromas. A review of the current understanding of the molecular pathogenesis is provided. Level of evidence: V.

10. de Andrea CE, Kroon HM, Wolterbeek R, et al: Interobserver reliability in the histopathological diagnosis of cartilaginous tumors in patients with multiple osteochondromas. *Mod Pathol* 2012;25(9):1275-1283.

    Thirty-eight lesions in patients with multiple enchondromas were reviewed by 12 experienced musculoskeletal pathologists. Interobserver reliability was high (interclass correlation coefficient = 0.78). The most important factors to indicate malignancy included nodularity, the presence of binucleated cells, irregular calcification, cystic/mucoid changes, and necrosis. Histology alone was insufficient to distinguish benign from malignant lesions in patients with multiple enchondromas; cartilage cap size and radiographic appearance were cited as additional important distinguishing indicators. Level of evidence: III.

11. Mirra JM, Gold R, Downs J, Eckardt JJ: A new histologic approach to the differentiation of enchondroma and chondrosarcoma of the bones: A clinicopathologic analysis of 51 cases. *Clin Orthop Relat Res* 1985;201:214-237.

12. Eefting D, Schrage YM, Geirnaerdt MJ, et al; EuroBoNeT consortium: Assessment of interobserver variability and histologic parameters to improve reliability in classification and grading of central cartilaginous tumors. *Am J Surg Pathol* 2009;33(1):50-57.

    Twenty enchondromas and 37 central grade 1 chondrosarcomas were reviewed by 18 musculoskeletal pathologists. A classification scheme based upon two features (mucoid degeneration more than 20% and/or host bone entrapment) resulted in 94.7% accuracy in diagnosis (95% sensitivity, 95% specificity). Level of evidence: IV.

13. van der Geest IC, de Valk MH, de Rooy JW, Pruszczynski M, Veth RP, Schreuder HW: Oncological and functional results of cryosurgical therapy of enchondromas and chondrosarcomas grade 1. *J Surg Oncol* 2008;98(6):421-426.

    The authors performed extended curettage and cryosurgery on 123 patients (130 lesions). Lesions were identified as active enchondromas (*n* = 18), aggressive enchondroma (*n* = 57), and grade 1 chondrosarcoma (*n* = 55). Follow-up ranged from 2 to 12 years for the entire cohort. Two recurrences were identified, one involving an active enchondroma and one an aggressive enchondroma. No recurrences among patients treated for grade 1 chondrosarcoma were identified using this method. Both recurrences were treated with repeat curettage and cryosurgery, with no evidence of re-recurrence at 3 and 5 years, respectively. The authors reported a relatively high (14%) fracture rate, and one case of nitrogen gas emboli caused transient hemodynamic changes. Level of evidence: III.

14. Spranger J, Kemperdieck H, Bakowski H, Opitz JM: Two peculiar types of enchondromatosis. *Pediatr Radiol* 1978;7(4):215-219.

15. Pansuriya TC, Kroon HM, Bovée JV: Enchondromatosis: Insights on the different subtypes. *Int J Clin Exp Pathol* 2010;3(6):557-569.

    The authors provide a concise review of the different subtypes of multiple enchondromatosis along with a review of pertinent clinical and pathological features of each. Level of evidence: IV.

16. Ollier L: Exostoses osteogeniques multiples. *Lyon Med* 1898;88:484-486.

17. Ollier L: Dyschondroplasie. *Lyon Med* 1900;93:23-25.

2: Benign Bone Tumors

18. Maffucci A: Di un caso di enchondroma ed angioma multiplo: Contribuzione ell genesi embrionale dei tumor. *Mov Med Chir Napoli.* 1881;3:399-412.

19. Ghatan A, Scharschmidt T, Conrad E: Extreme enchondromatosis: A report of two cases and review of the literature. *J Bone Joint Surg Am* 2010;92(13):2336-2343.

    The authors reported a case of extreme enchondromatosis with a review of the literature. A concise review of the classification systems commonly used for enchondromatosis is provided. Level of evidence: IV.

20. Schwartz HS, Zimmerman NB, Simon MA, Wroble RR, Millar EA, Bonfiglio M: The malignant potential of enchondromatosis. *J Bone Joint Surg Am* 1987;69(2):269-274.

21. Jaffe HL, Lichtenstein L: Benign chondroblastoma of bone: A reinterpretation of the so-called calcifying or chondromatous giant cell tumor. *Am J Pathol* 1942;18(6):969-991.

22. Ramappa AJ, Lee FY, Tang P, Carlson JR, Gebhardt MC, Mankin HJ: Chondroblastoma of bone. *J Bone Joint Surg Am* 2000;82-A(8):1140-1145.

23. Springfield DS, Capanna R, Gherlinzoni F, Picci P, Campanacci M: Chondroblastoma: A review of seventy cases. *J Bone Joint Surg Am* 1985;67(5):748-755.

24. Rybak LD, Rosenthal DI, Wittig JC: Chondroblastoma: Radiofrequency ablation—alternative to surgical resection in selected cases. *Radiology* 2009;251(2):599-604.

    The authors reported results for 13 male and 4 female patients treated for symptomatic chondroblastoma with radiofrequency ablation. Lesions were located in the proximal humerus ($n = 7$), proximal tibia ($n = 4$), proximal femur ($n = 3$), and distal femur ($n = 3$). The mean size of the lesion was 2.46 mL, and the mean follow-up was 41.3 months (range, 4 to 134 months). Probe sizes ranged from 5 mm to 2 cm, and the number of treatments required ranged from 1 to 10. Total time for the procedure ranged from 6 to 71 minutes (mean, 17.6 minutes). All patients in this series reported complete relief of their preprocedure pain on day one. Three patients were lost to follow-up. Twelve patients reported continued pain relief with no evidence of recurrence at the time of most recent follow-up. One patient developed collapse of the lateral tibial plateau overlying a previously treated lesion. Viable tumor was found at the time of revision surgery. Another patient developed hip pain following treatment of a proximal femoral lesion, and was successfully treated with hip arthroscopy. Level of evidence: IV.

25. Jaffe HL, Lichtenstein L: Chondromyxoid fibroma of bone; a distinctive benign tumor likely to be mistaken especially for chondrosarcoma. *Arch Pathol (Chic)* 1948;45(4):541-551.

26. Zustin J, Akpalo H, Gambarotti M, et al: Phenotypic diversity in chondromyxoid fibroma reveals differentiation pattern of tumor mimicking fetal cartilage canals development: An immunohistochemical study. *Am J Pathol* 2010;177(3):1072-1078.

    The authors analyzed 4 fetal femora and 10 CMF samples through the use of histochemistry and immunohistochemical markers. Two characteristic components were demonstrated in each CMF sample: immature fibrous tissue of vascularized stroma with accumulation of macrophages in areas of superficial sinusoidal proliferation, and variable amounts of lobulated chondroid tissue. The authors suggested, on the basis of the morphological similarity between fetal cartilage and CMF, that this lesion represented a neoplasm originating from or mimicking fetal cartilage canals. Level of evidence: IV.

27. Dahlin DC, Wells AH, Henderson ED: Chondromyxoid fibroma of bone; report of two cases. *J Bone Joint Surg Am* 1953;35-A(4):831-834.

28. Yasuda T, Nishio J, Sumegi J, et al: Aberrations of 6q13 mapped to the COL12A1 locus in chondromyxoid fibroma. *Mod Pathol* 2009;22(11):1499-1506.

    Cytogenetic analysis of 16 CMF samples from 14 patients revealed rearrangements of chromosome 6 in 10 of 11 clonally abnormal specimens. Fluorescence in situ hybridization based positional cloning localized the breakpoint on 6q13 within the *COL12A1* gene. The authors suggested that this gene is likely involved in recurrent 6q13 mutation and may help with diagnosis in more challenging cases. Level of evidence: IV.

2: Benign Bone Tumors

Chapter 11

Benign Bone-Forming Tumors

Robert Mikael Henshaw, MD   Emily E. Carmody Soni, MD

Introduction

Benign bone-forming tumors are neoplasms characterized by the presence of bone (osteoid) formation within the lesion, leading to distinctive radiographic and histologic features. Tumors in this group have variable clinical and biologic behavior and presentation, and can occur as painless or painful lesions, and can be biologically latent or extremely aggressive. These tumors were first recognized as a distinct group in 1932; many lesions within this group were further classified over the following two decades. Treatment options, determined by the biologic potential of each lesion, range from simple observation to percutaneous ablation to complete resection.

Osteoid Osteoma

Definition and Clinical Features

An osteoid osteoma is characterized by the radiographic presence of a small (usually less than 1.5 cm), lucent central region of fibro-osseous tumor (referred to as a nidus), surrounded by a zone of reactive bone sclerosis (**Figure 1**).[1] This fascinating primary lesion of bone classically occurs with a characteristic pain pattern, often compared to a severe toothache by patients, which is rapidly alleviated temporarily by the administration of NSAIDs and aspirin. Patients frequently have months of pain, with some patients experiencing symptoms for years before diagnosis. This pain, which can be distinguished from mechanical symptoms on the basis of the presence of pain at rest and at night, may be so severe that some patients self-medicate with toxic doses of over-the-counter NSAIDs. The ability of NSAIDs to alleviate pain from osteoid osteomas is explained by the well-documented production of prosta-

glandin E_2 and prostacyclin by the tumor; NSAIDs block the production of prostaglandins through inhibition of cyclo-oxygenase enzymes (COX-1 and COX-2). The characteristic symptoms of osteoid osteoma—dull, aching pain that is nonmechanical and occurs at night, and the typical relief seen with administration of NSAIDs or aspirin—are extremely useful to the clinician in establishing the diagnosis. The production of prostaglandins results in an inflammatory cascade that can affect surrounding structures.[2] Osteoid osteomas that occur adjacent to or within joints frequently occur with symptoms mimicking a monoarticular inflammatory arthritis, with joint effusion and stiffness (**Figure 2**). When lesions occur along the spine, a reactive scoliosis may be present. Patients can often precisely localize the source of their pain; however, when the lesion occurs adjacent to a major nerve, referred pain due to the generalized inflammation from the lesion can make localization difficult.[3] Referred pain can occur in the form of hip pain or knee pain with pelvic lesions, and knee pain with hip lesions, particularly in children and young adults.

Demographics

Osteoid osteomas represent 10% to 12% of all benign bone tumors analyzed by biopsy, with a peak incidence in the second decade of life. Although more than 80% of lesions occur in patients between the ages of 5 and 25 years, rare lesions have been observed in patients as young as 2.5 years of age. Males are more commonly affected, with a male-female ratio of 3:1. At least 50% of these tumors occur in the long bones of the lower extremities. Upper extremity and posterior elements of the spine are other common locations. Lesions can occur along the endosteal or periosteal surfaces of the bone, with some lesions entirely contained within the cortex. Although most of these lesions are solitary, the presence of a second nidus, sometimes after treatment of the original lesion, is occasionally noted.

Radiographic Appearance

The appearance of a nidus on plain radiographs, consisting of a central lucency surrounded by a sclerotic rim of bone, is highly suggestive of an osteoid osteoma. Because of the small size of these lesions, high-resolution CT imaging usually is necessary to visualize the actual nidus and its relationship to the surrounding bone (**Figure 3, A**). MRI imaging often demonstrates

Dr. Henshaw or an immediate family member serves as a paid consultant to or is an employee of Amgen; has received research or institutional support from Amgen; and serves as a board member, owner, officer, or committee member of the Mattie Miracle Cancer Foundation. Neither Dr. Carmody Soni nor any immediate family member has received anything of value from or has stock or stock options held in a commercial company or institution related directly or indirectly to the subject of this chapter.

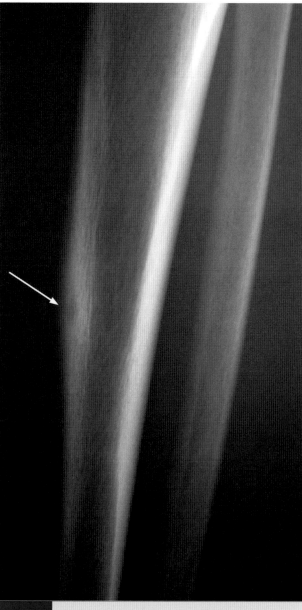

Figure 1 Lateral radiograph of the leg demonstrates a small (<1 cm) lytic nidus located within the anterior tibial diaphyseal cortex (arrow), consisting of a small radiolucent area that is surrounded by thickened reactive cortical bone formation. The presence of osteoid matrix within the nidus can often be difficult to visualize on plain radiographs because of the small size of the nidus.

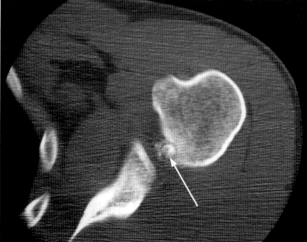

Figure 2 Axial CT image of an intra-articular osteoid osteoma (arrow) of the glenohumeral joint in a patient with shoulder pain at rest and with motion. The patient was found to have joint irritability on physical examination that persisted even after the referring physician had done an aspiration and steroid injection of the joint.

ticularly in patients where referred pain may obscure the anatomic location.[6] Positron emission tomography (PET) of osteoid osteomas is characterized by intense focal hypermetabolic activity that has been shown to resolve rapidly following radiofrequency ablation (RFA).[7] Currently, PET is not clinically indicated for the evaluation of suspected osteoid osteoma.

Pathology

The central radiolucent portion of the nidus, which rarely measures more than 1.0 to 1.5 mm in diameter, is filled with a red, relatively soft and friable tissue that is easily separated from the surrounding sclerotic bone (**Figure 6**). Microscopically, the nidus is characterized by an interlacing network of osteoblast-lined trabeculae (**Figure 7, A**). Calcification of the osteoid may be prominent, particularly in the center, and cement lines are common. Scattered multinucleated giant cells are commonly noted. The intertrabecular stroma consists of a richly vascular connective tissue, devoid of hematopoietic elements (**Figure 7, B**). Electron microscopy with axonal silver stain has been used to demonstrate the presence of nerve endings within the nidus. The bone surrounding the nidus usually reveals nonspecific sclerotic changes.

Differential Diagnosis

Radiographically, osteoid osteoma must be distinguished from a stress fracture, Brodie abscess, and osteoblastoma, which occur in this age group and can appear as a radiolucent lesion with a surrounding sclerotic border. High-resolution CT, particularly with coronal and sagittal reconstructions, can be very helpful in identifying stress fractures, which do not

substantial amounts of bone and soft-tissue edema, which occurs in response to the inflammatory action of prostaglandin production (**Figure 3, B**). Frequently, significant amounts of reactive cortical bone can be seen surrounding the nidus (**Figure 4**).[4] Evaluation with MRI alone in the absence of radiographs or CT imaging can result in misdiagnosis of this condition because of the extensive bone marrow inflammation. Bone scanning is extremely sensitive for detection of osteoid osteoma[5] and can help localize a nidus (**Figure 5**), par-

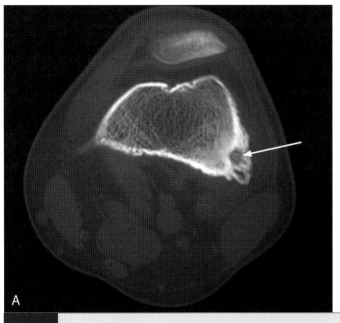

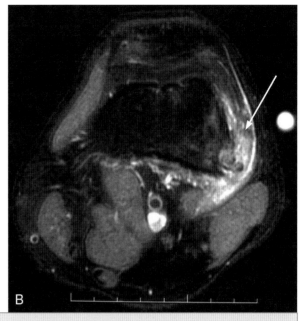

Figure 3 **A,** Axial CT image of the distal femur demonstrates an osteoid osteoma, with classic nidus containing osteoid within the radiolucent zone of the lesion (arrow). Because of the small size of the nidus, CT often is needed to visualize the nidus, especially when significant reactive bone formation has occurred. **B,** Axial T2-weighted MRI of the same nidus demonstrates the reactive bone and soft-tissue edema frequently seen in patients with osteoid osteoma.

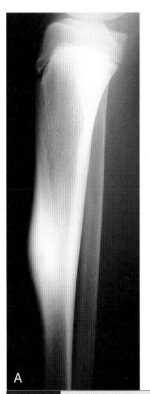

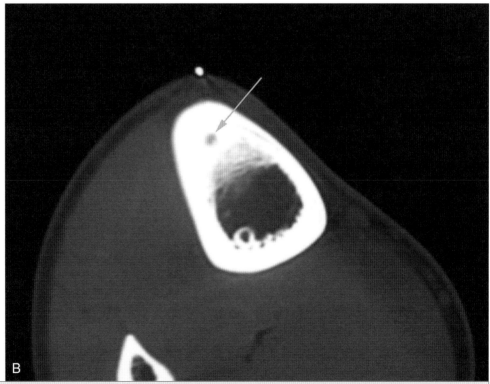

Figure 4 **A,** Lateral radiograph of the leg demonstrates substantial reactive hyperplasia of the anterior tibial cortex completely obscuring the nidus of this patient's osteoid osteoma. **B,** Corresponding axial CT image reveals a small intracortical nidus (arrow) that was obscured by the cortical reaction on plain radiographs.

2: Benign Bone Tumors

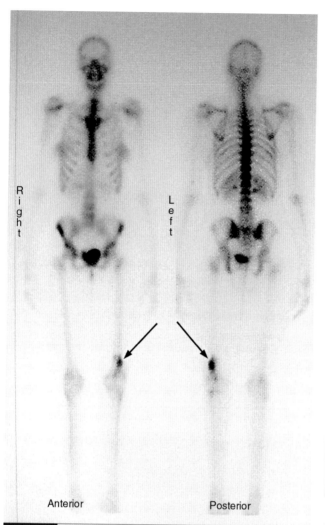

Figure 5   Static technetium Tc-99m total-body bone scan demonstrates intense focal uptake associated with a osteoid osteoma located in the posterior lateral portion of the left distal femur (arrows). Note that the lesion is more visible on the posterior view, corresponding to the anatomic location of the lesion.

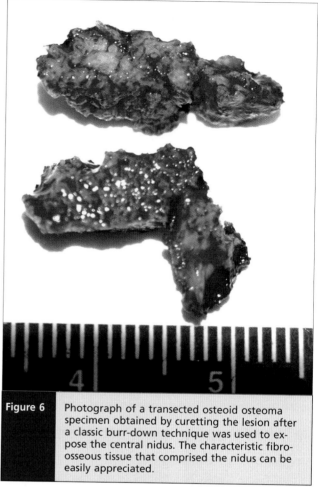

Figure 6   Photograph of a transected osteoid osteoma specimen obtained by curetting the lesion after a classic burr-down technique was used to expose the central nidus. The characteristic fibro-osseous tissue that comprised the nidus can be easily appreciated.

contain a nidus. Occasionally, it may be difficult to distinguish a large osteoid osteoma from a small osteoblastoma.[8,9] The presence or absence of the typical pain pattern seen with osteoid osteoma, as well as the response of pain to aspirin or other NSAIDs, helps to differentiate these entities. Other conditions to consider in the radiographic differential diagnosis include osteomyelitis, bone island of the medullary canal, intracortical hemangioma, and intracortical osteosarcoma for cortically based lesions.

Treatment

Osteoid osteomas have limited growth potential and no malignant potential. Removal or complete destruction of the central nidus is necessary to eliminate the source of pain. Some patients have mild symptoms that can be managed with chronic NSAID administration; some of these lesions have been reported to resolve, or burn out, over time.[10] Historically, wide resection was performed to ensure complete removal; subsequently, the burr-down technique was used. Better imaging led to the introduction of less aggressive contemporary methods of intralesional removal, including CT-guided thermal RFA (**Figures 8** and **9**).[11] Because of the significant pain associated with placing a needle or probe into a nidus, such ablations must be performed with regional or general anesthesia.

Complications associated with RFA include incomplete ablation of the lesion, recurrence of the lesion, fracture of the treated bone (particularly around the hip), and damage to surrounding structures including overlying skin and adjacent nerves.[12] Such complications are rare in high-volume centers, attesting to the learning curve associated with this form of treatment. Lesions in difficult-to-access or challenging anatomic locations, including intra-articular and spinal locations, although typically treated with minimally invasive surgical excision, may also respond to RFA.[13] Intraoperative C-arm or O-arm fluoroscopy, CT-guided wire localization, and, more recently, navigation systems using preoperative CT overlay have been used to facilitate

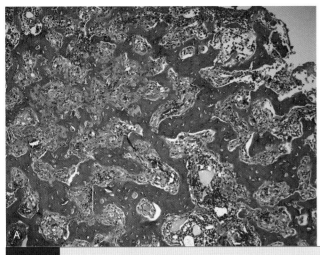
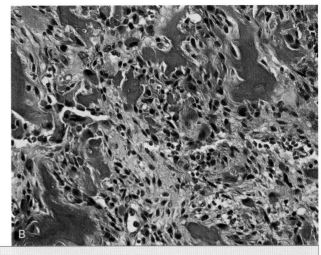

Figure 7 Low-power (**A**) and high-power (**B**) photomicrographs of an osteoid osteoma nidus demonstrate the classic findings of interlacing trabeculae of immature bone lined with osteoblasts surrounding a vascular fibrous stroma. Note the absence of marrow elements.

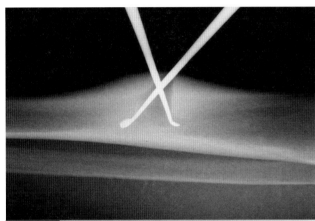

Figure 8 Intraoperative radiograph demonstrates complete removal of the involved cortex of the intracortical osteoid osteoma shown in **Figure 4**. Following CT-guided wire localization of the lesion, a high-speed burr inserted through a minimal skin incision was used to burr down and through the lesion.

localization of the nidus during open surgical approaches.[14] Arthroscopically assisted curettage of intraarticular osteoid osteomas involving joints such as the hip, wrist, knee, and ankle has been reported in a limited number of patients.[15]

Osteoblastoma

Definition and Clinical Features

Osteoblastoma, a rare fibro-osseous tumor arising from bone, was first described in 1956 as a lesion related to osteoid osteoma, but characterized by its greater growth potential.[16,17] A more aggressive form, termed aggressive osteoblastoma, was described in 1973 on the

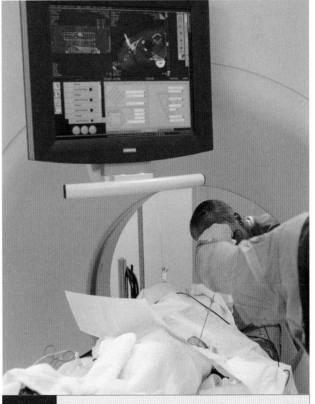

Figure 9 Percutaneous radiofrequency ablation of a scapular osteoid osteoma in an anesthetized pediatric patient being done under CT image guidance. Complete resolution of the patient's classic symptoms of persistent pain requiring NSAIDs was achieved in less than 12 hours.

basis of histologic and radiographic features overlapping osteosarcoma of bone. Osteoblastoma is differentiated from osteoid osteoma by size greater than 1.5 cm, frequently without the classic nocturnal pain re-

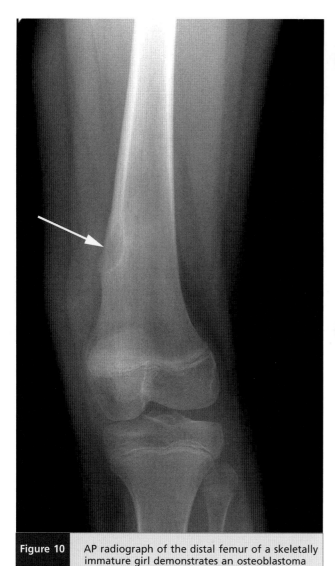

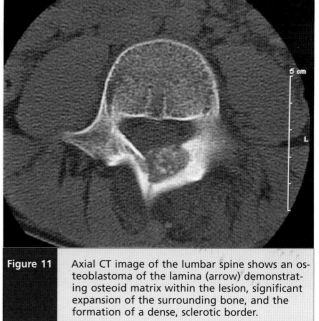

Figure 11 Axial CT image of the lumbar spine shows an osteoblastoma of the lamina (arrow) demonstrating osteoid matrix within the lesion, significant expansion of the surrounding bone, and the formation of a dense, sclerotic border.

Figure 10 AP radiograph of the distal femur of a skeletally immature girl demonstrates an osteoblastoma of the medial metadiaphyseal junction (arrow) characterized by a well-defined, relatively large, central lucent zone surrounded by a sclerotic zone of bone formation.

Demographics

Osteoblastoma accounts for fewer than 1% of bone tumors analyzed by biopsy, with a peak incidence in the second decade of life. Most patients are between the ages of 5 and 45 years, a slightly older population than that seen with osteoid osteoma, whereas a similar male-female ratio of 3:1 is seen. Osteoblastoma has a predilection for the axial skeleton, with more than 50% of lesions involving the posterior elements of the vertebral column, sacrum, and skull.[21] Lesions that occur in the appendicular skeleton mirror the distribution seen with osteoid osteoma. Unlike osteoid osteomas, which frequently involve the cortex, osteoblastomas typically involve cancellous bone.

Radiographic Appearance

The classic radiographic appearance of osteoblastoma is similar to that of osteoid osteoma, with a central, well-defined lytic region surrounded by a sclerotic, reactive border of bone (**Figure 10**). Unlike osteoid osteomas, the lytic area exceeds 1.5 cm in size, which is often used as a distinguishing feature between the two lesions. Lesions involving the spine predominantly involve the posterior elements of the neural arch (**Figure 11**), resulting in thinning and occasional destructive expansion of the bone, particularly when secondary ABC formation occurs (**Figure 12**). Aggressive osteoblastomas have a similar radiographic appearance, but typically exceed 4 cm in diameter, with some documented lesions reaching 10 cm in size. Depending on the location of the lesion, cortical destruction and resultant periosteal reaction may be present even with relatively small lesions, and can easily mimic the radiographic features seen with osteosarcoma. Plain radiographs and axial CT imaging that can demonstrate the presence of

lieved by NSAIDs that is associated with osteoid osteoma.[18] Unlike osteoid osteomas, osteoblastomas can exceed 4 cm in diameter, leading to pain. Frequently, however, the classic nocturnal pain pattern (dull, aching nonmechanical pain) seen with osteoid osteomas is absent. When osteoblastoma is present in the jaw along the roots of teeth, it is referred to as a cementoblastoma. Secondary aneurysmal bone cyst (ABC) formation may occur in an area of osteoblastoma, leading to rapid enlargement and bone destruction. Osteoblastoma must be differentiated from osteosarcoma and osteoid osteoma.[19] Clinical correlation of age, site, and histologic finding often indicates the correct diagnosis. A recently described subtype, epithelioid multinodular osteoblastoma, features multiple nidi within a single lesion and appears to have a benign prognosis.[20]

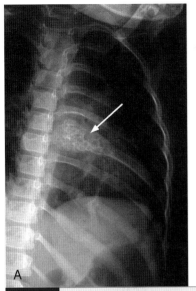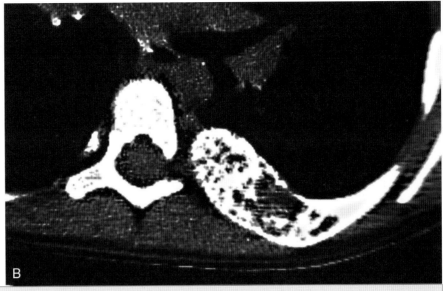

| **Figure 12** | Chest radiograph (**A**) and axial CT image (**B**) of an osteoblastoma involving the posterior rib (**A**, arrow) demonstrating significant bone expansion and cystic changes associated with secondary aneurysmal bone cyst formation. |

osteoid matrix and the relationship of the lesion to the surrounding bone are best suited for the diagnostic workup of a suspected osteoblastoma (**Figure 13**). MRI may be misleading because of the inflammatory response often seen with osteoblastoma, potentially simulating a more aggressive or malignant lesion.[22]

Pathology
Benign osteoblastoma has an appearance similar to that of osteoid osteoma. Grossly, the lesion is a highly vascular tumor with areas of gritty osteoid formation (**Figure 14**). The basic architecture of this lesion consists of a complex network of osteoid trabeculae that are lined by large but uniform osteoblasts. A variable number of multinucleated giant cells are usually present, occasionally causing confusion with giant cell tumor of bone. The extent of ossification varies from a few small foci to prominent confluent areas. The mitotic rate can be high in focal areas, but atypical cells should not be present. Aggressive osteoblastomas are characterized by the presence of epithelioid osteoblasts rimming the bony trabeculae and filling the intertrabecular spaces. Secondary aneurysmal cystic changes are frequently present. Limited cytogenetic data suggest that aggressive osteoblastoma may be a distinct entity.[23,24]

Differential Diagnosis
Osteoblastoma must be differentiated radiographically from osteosarcoma, ABC, infection, and osteoid osteoma.[25] Size is typically used to distinguish osteoid osteoma from osteoblastoma. Secondary ABC formation can make the differential diagnosis challenging, particularly when cortical destruction and periosteal reaction are present. The distinguishing characteristics of osteosarcoma include a high mitotic rate and the presence of

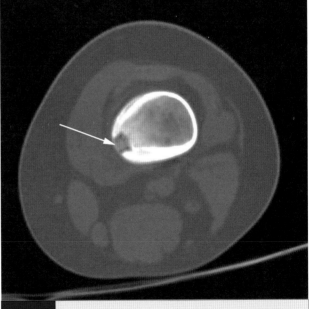

| **Figure 13** | Axial CT image of an osteoblastoma of the distal femur demonstrating the presence of osteoid matrix (arrow) that could not be appreciated on plain radiographs (Figure 10). Note the substantial reactive bone formation surrounding the central lesion. |

atypical cells and atypical mitotic figures, along with a permeative growth pattern and poor margination.

Treatment
Accurate diagnosis is necessary to ensure proper treatment of these bone-forming lesions. Complete surgical removal is needed to minimize the risk of recurrence,

2: Benign Bone Tumors

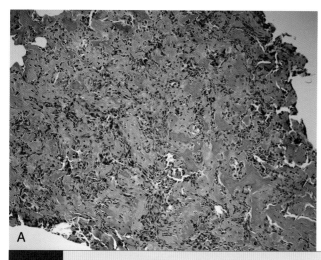
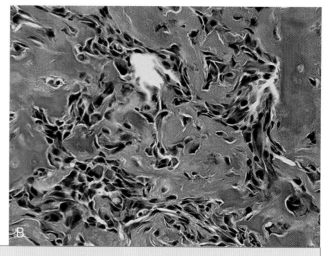

Figure 14 Low-power (**A**) and high-power (**B**) photomicrographs of an osteoblastoma demonstrating a network of osteoid trabeculae rimmed with large uniform osteoblasts along with a cellular stroma. Although these findings are similar to those seen in osteoid osteoma (Figure 7), the size of the lesion distinguishes the two clinical entities, whereas the lack of cellular atypia excludes osteosarcoma.

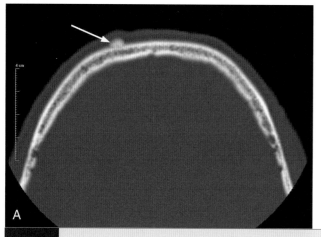
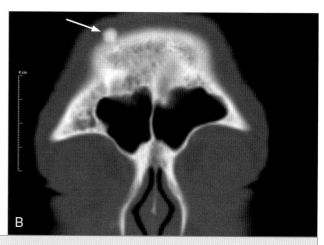

Figure 15 Axial (**A**) and coronal (**B**) CT images of a frontal osteoma (arrow) that occurred as a visible mass on the forehead demonstrating a very dense, mature-appearing bony lesion arising from the external cortex of the skull.

which can approach 25% following simple curettage.[26] Use of a high-speed burr to remove the surrounding reactive zone after curettage of the central lytic lesion (curettage and resection) can reduce the risk of recurrence. Chemical intraoperative adjuvants, including cryotherapy and phenol, are frequently used to improve the chances of local control. Aggressive osteoblastomas are thought to have a much greater risk of recurrence, making wide resection the treatment of choice when clinically feasible. Although surgical treatment of osteoblastoma is preferred when possible, the use of external beam irradiation, particularly for lesions involving the anterior portion of the vertebral body where en bloc resection is not feasible, can be effective.[27] Outcomes following RFA of osteoblastoma remain undefined.

Osteoma

Definition and Clinical Features
An osteoma is a benign bone-forming tumor involving a membranous bone, classically demonstrating a mature bony structure with a well-demarcated smooth border. Lesions are typically classified as either an ivory (compact) or a spongy (trabecular) osteoma on the basis of their dominant radiographic features. Lesions involving the skull frequently occur as slow-growing bony prominences that may be visually obvious (**Figure 15**). When these lesions are present within sinus cavities, headaches and recurrent sinusitis and visual alterations can occur. Orbital involvement can occur with exophthalmos and even blindness. Similar osteomas

can occasionally be found on the surface of long bones,[28] but whether they represent a true neoplasm or a hamartomatous lesion remains unclear.

Demographics

Osteomas are most commonly encountered in patients in their 50s, although they have been described in teenage patients. Several studies have demonstrated a 3:1 female-male ratio. The presence of multiple ivory osteomas has been associated with Gardner syndrome (intestinal polyposis, osteomas, desmoid tumors, and sebaceous cysts, arising from mutation of the *APC* gene on chromosome band 5q21), although they can occur in the absence of this syndrome.[29]

Radiographic Appearance

Because of the dense bone formation seen with osteomas, radiographs and CT imaging are ideal for visualizing these lesions. The characteristic appearance is of a well-defined, dense lesion with smooth, noninvasive borders arising in the skull. Because these lesions are similar in density and structure to cortical bone, osteomas can be easily overlooked on MRI. Because of the complex geometry of the skull, axial CT imaging with sagittal and coronal reconstruction is frequently required to fully characterize these lesions (**Figure 15**).

Pathology

Ivory osteomas are composed of mature lamellar bone, typically contiguous with the cortex from which they originate (**Figure 16**). Osteons with haversian canals are present, demonstrating the presence of focal osteoclastic resorption. Spongy osteoma also features central regions of cancellous-appearing bone, with active remodeling demonstrating osteoblastic activity and osteoclastic resorption. Osteomas involving the ethmoid and frontal sinuses can have regions that are histologically indistinguishable from osteoblastomas; these lesions are more clincally aggressive.

Differential Diagnosis

The primary differential diagnosis of osteoma includes osteochondroma, exostosis due to trauma or inflammation, and fibrous dysplasia. Care must be taken not to overlook the much more likely diagnosis of a parosteal osteosarcoma when a dense bone-forming lesion is found on the surface of a long bone. CT imaging is usually sufficient for diagnosis.[30]

Treatment

Osteomas of the skull rarely require treatment once a radiographic diagnosis has been made.[31] Lesions causing pain or disfiguring asymmetry, or lesions involving the sinus or orbits, are best treated with simple excision. Occasional recurrences have been noted. Several series of endoscopic excision of frontal sinus osteomas have been published, demonstrating excellent symptomatic relief and no evidence of recurrence with short-term follow-up.[32,33]

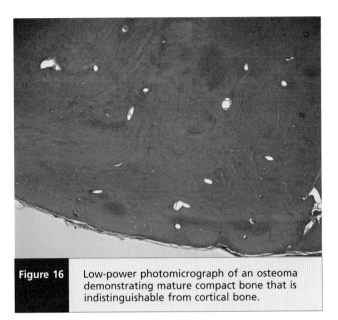

Figure 16 Low-power photomicrograph of an osteoma demonstrating mature compact bone that is indistinguishable from cortical bone.

Enostosis (Bone Island)

Definition and Clinical Features

Enostoses, commonly referred to as bone islands, are common, asymptomatic sclerotic lesions composed of oval or round regions of dense compact bone within the medullary cavity.[34] Classically, enostoses are found as asymptomatic, incidental findings on plain radiographs. Thus, their primary clinical significance lies in proper recognition and diagnosis to avoid unnecessary diagnostic studies and procedures.

Demographics

Bone islands are found in all age groups and have no specific gender predilection. They are frequently seen in the pelvis, spine, and ribs as well as in the metaphysis and epiphysis of long bones.

Radiographic Appearance

The characteristic features of an enostosis on plain radiographs is a homogeneous, dense sclerotic lesion within the cancellous bone, usually less than 2 cm in diameter (**Figure 17**). CT shows a diffusely sclerotic lesion with normal surrounding trabecular bone.[35] MRI typically shows low signal intensity on both T1-weighted and T2-weighted imaging because of the dense mineralization. Bone scanning shows little to modest uptake.

Pathology

Histologically, an enostosis is composed of compact lamellar bone with normal architecture. The lesion typically has radiating streaks that blend in to the surrounding trabeculae of the host bone ("thorny radiation"). A prominent haversian canal network with osteoblasts and osteoclasts is present, with larger lesions often showing evidence of bone deposition and remodeling.

2: Benign Bone Tumors

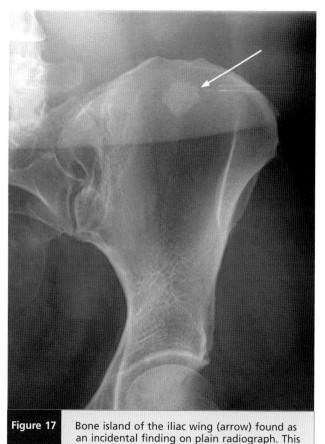

Figure 17 Bone island of the iliac wing (arrow) found as an incidental finding on plain radiograph. This very dense bone lesion is characterized by a geographic, smooth border, intramedullary location, and homogeneous density throughout the lesion.

Differential Diagnosis

It is important to differentiate large or "giant" bone islands from intramedullary sclerosing osteosarcoma or blastic metastatic disease.[36,37] Most sclerosing osteosarcomas have some areas that show lytic, cortical destruction and/or a soft-tissue component. In addition, osteosarcoma and blastic metastases typically demonstrate intense uptake on a bone scan. Concerning radiographic features, progression of the lesion, or a clinical history of otherwise unexplained pain should warrant a biopsy.

Treatment

Enostoses are stable lesions and are rarely, if ever, symptomatic; therefore, treatment of these lesions is seldom warranted. Their chief importance lies in distinguishing them from other lesions.

Osteopoikilosis (Spotted Bone Disease)

Definition and Clinical Features

Osteopoikilosis is characterized by multiple sclerotic lesions within the carpal, tarsal, and long bones.[38] These lesions are closely related to enostoses, which may represent a unifocal variant of this condition.[39] Because the lesions are asymptomatic, the condition is usually discovered incidentally. Osteopoikilosis can be an autosomal dominant disorder, particularly when it occurs with multiple cutaneous elastic nevi, a condition known as Buschke-Ollendorff syndrome.[40]

Demographics

Lesions generally develop in childhood but do not regress, and are therefore seen in all age groups.

Radiographic Appearance

Radiographs illustrate numerous round or oval sclerotic foci, generally 2 to 10 mm in size and symmetrically located throughout the skeleton. Lesions are usually located in the metaphysis and the epiphysis of long bones. The ribs, clavicle, spine, and skull are usually spared. Because of the small size of some of these lesions, CT imaging often reveals the multiple nature of this condition (**Figure 18**). On MRI, lesions appear dark on both T1-weighted and T2-weighted images. Bone scanning should show minimal uptake, which is an important distinction when differentiating this condition from diffuse osteoblastic metastases.[41]

Pathology

Histologically, these lesions are composed of dense, mature lamellar bone with normal architecture. Recently, osteopoikilosis has been associated with a deletion mutation in the *LEMD3* gene.[42] This mutation has also been identified in patients with both osteopoikilosis and melorheostosis in combination, but not in patients with melorheostosis alone.

Differential Diagnosis

The primary differential diagnosis is diffuse osteoblastic bone metastases, such as metastatic prostate cancer in males. A key differentiating feature is that metastases show diffuse uptake on a technetium Tc-99m bone scan, whereas osteopoikilosis shows little to no uptake.[43]

Treatment

Because the lesions associated with osteopoikilosis are asymptomatic, no treatment is warranted beyond the initial diagnosis.

Melorheostosis

Definition and Clinical Features

Melorheostosis, also known as Leri disease, is a rare, nonheritable sclerosing bone dysplasia, with abnormalities in both enchondral and intramembranous ossification.[44] Unlike most sclerosing bone disorders, melorheostosis is usually progressive and symptomatic, interspersed with periods of disease arrest.[45] In addition

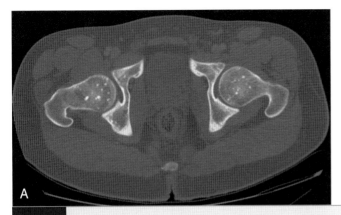
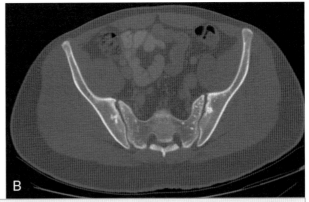

Figure 18   Axial CT imaging of the hips (**A**) and pelvis (**B**) demonstrating classic osteopoikilosis (spotted bone disease) involving multiple bones, which was found incidentally in a 20-year-old man.

to pain and limb deformity, patients often also have soft-tissue involvement that can lead to disabling joint contractures. Joint ankylosis can also be seen. Melorheostosis has been associated with osteopoikilosis and osteopathia striata.[46] This manifestation is commonly referred to as overlap syndrome. There have been case reports of osteosarcoma occurring in the setting of melorheostosis.

Demographics
Melorheostosis typically manifests in adolescence or early adulthood.

Radiographic Appearance
Radiographs illustrate characteristic cortical or medullary hyperostosis along one side of a long bone or multiple adjacent bones in a sclerotomal distribution (**Figure 19**). This periosteal hyperostosis has been described as "dripping candle wax" and gave the condition its name, which is derived from Greek (*melos*, limb; *rhein*, to flow; *ostos*, bone). CT reveals cortical hyperostosis and demonstrates the amount of endosteal involvement, whereas MRI can help determine the amount of soft-tissue fibrosis.[47] Lesions show uptake on bone scan.[48]

Pathology
Microscopically, these lesions show diffuse cortical sclerosis with small haversian systems, similar to that seen in osteomas and enostoses. Soft-tissue masses can be composed of a mixture of bone, cartilage, fibrous, and adipose tissue.

Differential Diagnosis
Polyostotic disease is readily distinguishable from other conditions on the basis of its characteristic radiographic appearance. However, monostotic disease can be confused with mature myositis ossificans, osteoid osteoma (with no visible nidus), and parosteal osteosarcoma.

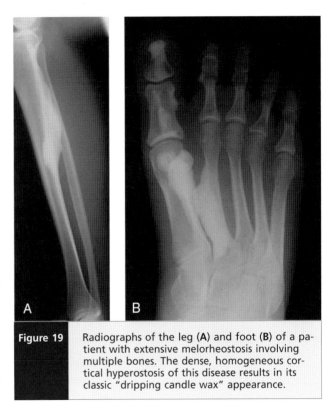

Figure 19   Radiographs of the leg (**A**) and foot (**B**) of a patient with extensive melorheostosis involving multiple bones. The dense, homogeneous cortical hyperostosis of this disease results in its classic "dripping candle wax" appearance.

Treatment
No treatment exists for melorheostosis; however, surgery is often used to manage limb deformity and for contracture release. Recurrent contractures often occur, complicating management. Recently, a case report described a patient successfully treated with bisphosphonates for pain management.[49]

Osteopathia Striata

Definition and Clinical Features
Osteopathia striata, also known as Voorhoeve disease, is rare, genetic sclerosing bone dysplasia characterized

2: Benign Bone Tumors

by fine linear streaks of dense bone within the ends of tubular bones.[50] The inheritance pattern was initially thought to be autosomal dominant, but more recently, an X-linked dominant inheritance pattern has been suggested.[51] The specific genetic mutation is not known. The condition is usually discovered incidentally, and the lesions are asymptomatic. Subsets of patients with this condition also have associated cranial sclerosis, a condition known as osteopathia striata with cranial sclerosis (OSCS), characterized by an X-linked dominant inheritance pattern.[52] Patients often have symptoms related to cranial nerve palsies. Many female patients have associated cleft lip and palate, as well as hearing loss. Male patients are more severely affected and exhibit multiple malformations involving the brain, heart, and skeleton, as well as the respiratory, intestinal, and urogenital tracts. This more severe form often results in neonatal lethality. OSCS is associated with mutations in the Wilms tumor gene on the X chromosome (*WTX*), although these patients do not appear to have an associated risk of malignancy.[53,54]

Demographics

Osteopathia striata can be diagnosed at any age and, because the lesions do not regress, it persists throughout life. Lesions are typically bilateral.

Radiographic Appearance

Radiographs characteristically show dense linear striations in the metaphysis and epiphysis. In the long bones, these striations run parallel to the long axis of the bone, giving rise to the descriptive term celery stalk metaphysis. In the ilium, this pattern is often described as fan-like.

Differential Diagnosis

The presence of bilateral prominent vertical striations is essentially pathognomonic for this condition. Other considerations include osteopetrosis, enchondromatosis, and osteopoikilosis.

Treatment

The classic appearance on radiographs is generally all that is needed for diagnosis. Biopsy is not warranted.

Summary

Benign bone-forming tumors, characterized by the presence of benign osteoid on histologic evaluation, exhibit a variety of clinical and radiographic features ranging from latent to aggressive. Recognition and proper diagnosis of these lesions is necessary to avoid overtreatment in many cases. Proper radiographic assessment is key to the correct diagnosis of these tumors, which then determines the optimal course of treatment for each patient.

Annotated References

1. Jaffe H: Osteoid osteoma: A benign osteoblastic tumor composed of osteoid and atypical bone. *Arch Surg* 1935;31:709-728.

2. Ciabattoni G, Tamburrelli F, Greco F: Increased prostacyclin biosynthesis in patients with osteoid osteoma. *Eicosanoids* 1991;4(3):165-167.

3. Schulman L, Dorfman HD: Nerve fibers in osteoid osteoma. *J Bone Joint Surg Am* 1970;52(7):1351-1356.

4. Norman A, Dorfman HD: Osteoid-osteoma inducing pronounced overgrowth and deformity of bone. *Clin Orthop Relat Res* 1975;110:233-238.

5. Bilchik T, Heyman S, Siegel A, Alavi A: Osteoid osteoma: The role of radionuclide bone imaging, conventional radiography and computed tomography in its management. *J Nucl Med* 1992;33(2):269-271.

6. Beck SE, Schwab JH, Rosenthal DI, Rosenberg AE, Grottkau BE: Metachronous osteoid osteoma of the tibia and the T7 vertebral body: A case report. *J Bone Joint Surg Am* 2011;93(13):e73.

   This case report of vertebral osteoid osteoma observed 9 years after initial workup and RFA treatment of a tibial osteoid osteoma is presented as the first reported multicentric metachronous osteoid osteoma. Level of evidence: IV.

7. Purandare NC, Rangarajan V, Shah SA, et al: Therapeutic response to radiofrequency ablation of neoplastic lesions: FDG PET/CT findings. *Radiographics* 2011;31(1):201-213.

   Focal hypermetabolic uptake of osteoid osteoma on fluorodeoxyglucose PET-CT imaging resolves within 4 hours following RFA, suggesting that PET-CT may be a useful tool to monitor the response of bone tumors to RFA. Level of evidence: IV.

8. Atesok KI, Alman BA, Schemitsch EH, Peyser A, Mankin H: Osteoid osteoma and osteoblastoma. *J Am Acad Orthop Surg* 2011;19(11):678-689.

   The authors discuss histology, frequency, and treatment of osteoid osteoma and osteoblastoma.

9. Bettelli G, Capanna R, van Horn JR, Ruggieri P, Biagini R, Campanacci M: Osteoid osteoma and osteoblastoma of the pelvis. *Clin Orthop Relat Res* 1989;247:261-271.

10. Kneisl JS, Simon MA: Medical management compared with operative treatment for osteoid-osteoma. *J Bone Joint Surg Am* 1992;74(2):179-185.

11. Campanacci M, Ruggieri P, Gasbarrini A, Ferraro A, Campanacci L: Osteoid osteoma: Direct visual identification and intralesional excision of the nidus with minimal removal of bone. *J Bone Joint Surg Br* 1999; 81(5):814-820.

12. Rosenthal DI, Alexander A, Rosenberg AE, Springfield D: Ablation of osteoid osteomas with a percutaneously placed electrode: A new procedure. *Radiology* 1992; 183(1):29-33.

13. Akhlaghpoor S, Aziz Ahari A, Arjmand Shabestari A, Alinaghizadeh MR: Radiofrequency ablation of osteoid osteoma in atypical locations: A case series. *Clin Orthop Relat Res* 2010;468(7):1963-1970.

    Twenty-one patients with osteoid osteoma in unusual locations such as the hip, radioulnar joint, and proximal phalanx reliably achieved pain relief within 1 to 7 days following RFA. No recurrences or major complications were noted. Level of evidence: IV.

14. Nagashima H, Nishi T, Yamane K, Tanida A: Case report: Osteoid osteoma of the C2 pedicle: Surgical technique using a navigation system. *Clin Orthop Relat Res* 2010;468(1):283-288.

    Curettage of an osteoid osteoma that was deemed unsuitable for RFA because of its anatomic location was successfully performed using an intraoperative navigation system to facilitate a minimally invasive surgical approach. Level of evidence: IV.

15. Lee DH, Jeong WK, Lee SH: Arthroscopic excision of osteoid osteomas of the hip in children. *J Pediatr Orthop* 2009;29(6):547-551.

    Intra-articular osteoid osteomas involving the hip joint in two children were successfully excised arthroscopically, with excellent postoperative outcomes. This small series, in conjunction with several case reports, suggests that arthroscopic excision is a viable surgical technique for intra-articular tumors. Level of evidence: IV.

16. Jaffe HL: Benign osteoblastoma. *Bull Hosp Joint Dis* 1956;17(2):141-151.

17. Lichtenstein L, Sawyer WR: Benign osteoblastoma: Further observations and report of twenty additional cases. *J Bone Joint Surg Am* 1964;46:755-765.

18. Gitelis S, Schajowicz F: Osteoid osteoma and osteoblastoma. *Orthop Clin North Am* 1989;20(3): 313-325.

19. Healey JH, Ghelman B: Osteoid osteoma and osteoblastoma: Current concepts and recent advances. *Clin Orthop Relat Res* 1986;204:76-85.

20. Zon Filippi R, Swee RG, Krishnan Unni K: Epithelioid multinodular osteoblastoma: A clinicopathologic analysis of 26 cases. *Am J Surg Pathol* 2007;31(8):1265-1268.

    A series of 26 osteoblastomas that demonstrated a multinodular growth pattern of multiple nidi within a single tumor were reviewed. The characteristic finding was multiple nodules of epithelioid cells with a lacy blue-bone matrix. Although these lesions mimic osteosarcoma, of 14 patients with long-term follow-up, no deaths occurred due to disease. Level of evidence: IV.

21. Nemoto O, Moser RP Jr , Van Dam BE, Aoki J, Gilkey FW: Osteoblastoma of the spine: A review of 75 cases. *Spine (Phila Pa 1976)* 1990;15(12):1272-1280.

22. Chakrapani SD, Grim K, Kaimaktchiev V, Anderson JC: Osteoblastoma of the spine with discordant magnetic resonance imaging and computed tomography imaging features in a child. *Spine (Phila Pa 1976)* 2008;33(25):E968-E970.

    The inflammatory features associated with osteoblastoma as seen on MRI may result in misdiagnosis unless the images are compared to similar CT images, which may more accurately reflect the benign nature of this lesion. Level of evidence: IV.

23. Baker AC, Rezeanu L, Klein MJ, et al: Aggressive osteoblastoma: A case report involving a unique chromosomal aberration. *Int J Surg Pathol* 2010;18(3):219-224.

    Cytogenetic analysis of an aggressive osteoblastoma demonstrated a pseudodiploid clone with a balanced translocation involving chromosomes 4, 7, and 14. Level of evidence: IV.

24. Giannico G, Holt GE, Homlar KC, Johnson J, Pinnt J, Bridge JA: Osteoblastoma characterized by a three-way translocation: Report of a case and review of the literature. *Cancer Genet Cytogenet* 2009;195(2):168-171.

    Cytogenetic analysis of an osteoblastoma reviewed a novel three-way translocation involving chromosomes 1, 2, and 14, t(1;2;14)(q42;q13;q24). Rearrangement of 1q42 was identified in a previously reported case. Level of evidence: IV.

25. Dorfman HD, Weiss SW: Borderline osteoblastic tumors: Problems in the differential diagnosis of aggressive osteoblastoma and low-grade osteosarcoma. *Semin Diagn Pathol* 1984;1(3):215-234.

26. Berry M, Mankin H, Gebhardt M, Rosenberg A, Hornicek F: Osteoblastoma: A 30-year study of 99 cases. *J Surg Oncol* 2008;98(3):179-183.

    The recurrence rate of osteoblastoma in this large series was 24%, mostly occurring after curettage and packing. Although this finding supports the role of primary resection in selected patients, the data increase support for the use of physical adjuvants following curettage. Level of evidence: IV.

27. Boriani S, Amendola L, Bandiera S, et al: Staging and treatment of osteoblastoma in the mobile spine: A review of 51 cases. *Eur Spine J* 2012;21(10):2003-2010.

    This retrospective study of 51 patients stratified according to the Enneking staging system showed that irradiation was effective for adjuvant treatment when en bloc resection was not feasible or would result in unacceptable functional loss. Patients with recurrent disease fared worse than patients treated primarily. Level of evidence: IV.

28. Geschickter CF, Copeland MM: Parosteal osteoma of bone: A new entity. *Ann Surg* 1951;133(6):790-807.

2: Benign Bone Tumors

29. Gardner EJ, Plenk HP: Hereditary pattern for multiple osteomas in a family group. *Am J Hum Genet* 1952; 4(1):31-36.

30. Efune G, Perez CL, Tong L, Rihani J, Batra PS: Paranasal sinus and skull base fibro-osseous lesions: When is biopsy indicated for diagnosis? *Int Forum Allergy Rhinol* 2012;2(2):160-165.

    In patients with fibro-osseous lesions of the skull, the positive predictive value of preoperative imaging was 100% for 10 osteomas, suggesting that classic radiologic features of osteoma are sufficient for diagnosis and subsequent observation; surgical resection is warranted only for those with clinical symptoms. Level of evidence: IV.

31. Gil-Carcedo LM, Gil-Carcedo ES, Vallejo LA, de Campos JM, Herrero D: Frontal osteomas: Standardising therapeutic indications. *J Laryngol Otol* 2011; 125(10):1020-1027.

    A staging system for frontal osteomas based on the relationship of the tumor mass to sinus size, tumor proximity to the infundibulum, destruction of sinus walls, and complications helped determine which lesions could be observed safely without surgery. Level of evidence: IV.

32. Lai CH, Sun IF, Huang SH, Lai CS, Lin SD: Forehead osteoma excision by endoscopic approach. *Ann Plast Surg* 2008;61(5):533-536.

    Complete endoscopically assisted excision of frontal osteoma was performed safely and effectively in six patients with small lesions. Level of evidence: IV.

33. Seiberling K, Floreani S, Robinson S, Wormald PJ: Endoscopic management of frontal sinus osteomas revisited. *Am J Rhinol Allergy* 2009;23(3):331-336.

    Endoscopically assisted excision of large frontal osteoma can be performed by removing the inferior portion of the interfrontal septum, the superior portion of the nasal septum, and the frontal sinus floor to the orbit laterally (modified Lothrop procedure). Level of evidence: IV.

34. Greenspan A, Stadalnik RC: Bone island: Scintigraphic findings and their clinical application. *Can Assoc Radiol J* 1995;46(5):368-379.

35. Hall FM, Goldberg RP, Davies JA, Fainsinger MH: Scintigraphic assessment of bone islands. *Radiology* 1980;135(3):737-742.

36. Ehara S, Kattapuram SV, Rosenberg AE: Giant bone island: Computed tomography findings. *Clin Imaging* 1989;13(3):231-233.

37. Smith J: Giant bone islands. *Radiology* 1973;107(1): 35-36.

38. Benli IT, Akalin S, Boysan E, Mumcu EF, Kiş M, Türkolğu D: Epidemiological, clinical and radiological aspects of osteopoikilosis. *J Bone Joint Surg Br* 1992; 74(4):504-506.

39. Lagier R, Mbakop A, Bigler A: Osteopoikilosis: A radiological and pathological study. *Skeletal Radiol* 1984;11(3):161-168.

40. Burger B, Hershkovitz D, Indelman M, et al: Buschke-Ollendorff syndrome in a three-generation family: Influence of a novel LEMD3 mutation to tropoelastin expression. *Eur J Dermatol* 2010;20(6):693-697.

    DNA sequencing of three generations of a Swiss family with osteopoikilosis and associated Buschke-Ollendorff syndrome revealed a frameshift mutation in the coding sequence of *LEMD3*, located on chromosome band 12q14. Level of evidence: IV.

41. Tuncel M, Caner B: Osteopoikilosis: A major diagnostic problem solved by bone scintigraphy. *Rev Esp Med Nucl Imagen Mol* 2012;31(2):93-96.

    Bone scanning played a key role in distinguishing between osteopoikilosis and osteoblastic metastases in two patients. Level of evidence: IV.

42. Baasanjav S, Jamsheer A, Kolanczyk M, et al: Osteopoikilosis and multiple exostoses caused by novel mutations in LEMD3 and EXT1 genes respectively—coincidence within one family. *BMC Med Genet* 2010;11: 110.

    DNA sequencing of five patients from three generations of a Polish family affected with osteopoikilosis revealed a novel mutation in *LEMD3* that was not found in 200 ethnically matched controls. Level of evidence: IV.

43. Whyte MP, Murphy WA, Siegel BA: 99mTc-pyrophosphate bone imaging in osteopoikilosis, osteopathia striata, and melorheostosis. *Radiology* 1978; 127(2):439-443.

44. Brown RR, Steiner GC, Lehman WB: Melorheostosis: Case report with radiologic-pathologic correlation. *Skeletal Radiol* 2000;29(9):548-552.

45. Younge D, Drummond D, Herring J, Cruess RL: Melorheostosis in children: Clinical features and natural history. *J Bone Joint Surg Br* 1979;61-B(4): 415-418.

46. Greenspan A: Sclerosing bone dysplasias—a target-site approach. *Skeletal Radiol* 1991;20(8):561-583.

47. Suresh S, Muthukumar T, Saifuddin A: Classical and unusual imaging appearances of melorheostosis. *Clin Radiol* 2010;65(8):593-600.

    A current review of melorheostosis illustrates the associations and rare complications of this disorder. MRI and CT help differentiate this condition from other disease entities. Level of evidence: IV.

48. Sonoda LI, Halim MY, Balan KK: Detection of extensive melorheostosis on bone scintigram performed for suspected metastases. *Clin Nucl Med* 2011; 36(3):240-241.

    Melorheostosis involving the bilateral upper and lower

extremities of a patient with breast cancer was discovered following a bone scan for suspected metastases, demonstrating the utility of this modality to help detect this condition. Level of evidence: IV.

49. Hollick RJ, Black A, Reid D: Melorheostosis and its treatment with intravenous zoledronic acid. *BMJ Case Rep* 2010;2010.

    A patient's painful melorheostosis was successfully managed with bisphosphonate therapy. Level of evidence: IV.

50. Gehweiler JA, Bland WR, Carden TS Jr , Daffner RH: Osteopathia striata: Voorhoeve's disease. Review of the roentgen manifestations. *Am J Roentgenol Radium Ther Nucl Med* 1973;118(2):450-455.

51. Viot G, Lacombe D, David A, et al: Osteopathia striata cranial sclerosis: Non-random X-inactivation suggestive of X-linked dominant inheritance. *Am J Med Genet* 2002;107(1):1-4.

52. Holman SK, Daniel P, Jenkins ZA, et al: The male phenotype in osteopathia striata congenita with cranial sclerosis. *Am J Med Genet A* 2011;155A(10):2397-2408.

Osteopathia striata with cranial sclerosis is an X-linked disease caused by mutations in *WTX* leading to different phenotypic expressions in males and females. Level of evidence: IV.

53. Jenkins ZA, van Kogelenberg M, Morgan T, et al: Germline mutations in WTX cause a sclerosing skeletal dysplasia but do not predispose to tumorigenesis. *Nat Genet* 2009;41(1):95-100.

    Abnormal Wnt signaling is implicated in a broad range of developmental anomalies and tumorigenesis, but despite having germline mutations, individuals with osteopathia striata and cranial sclerosis showed no predisposition to tumor development. Level of evidence: IV.

54. Perdu B, Lakeman P, Mortier G, Koenig R, Lachmeijer AM, Van Hul W: Two novel WTX mutations underscore the unpredictability of male survival in osteopathia striata with cranial sclerosis. *Clin Genet* 2011; 80(4):383-388.

    Two novel mutations in the *WTX* gene were found in members of two families affected by OSCS; despite the X-linked nature of these mutations, an affected boy remains alive in his teens. Level of evidence: IV.

2: Benign Bone Tumors

Chapter 12

Benign Fibrous and Histiocytic Lesions of Bone

William M. Parrish, MD

Introduction

Benign fibrous and histiocytic lesions of bone occur most commonly in children. These lesions are often diagnosed as incidental findings on plain radiographs obtained for other reasons. Plain radiographs can be diagnostic and preclude the need for biopsy for confirmation. Treatment is often observation but when surgical intervention is required, the goal should be to stabilize the affected bone and maximize function.[1,2]

Fibrous Dysplasia

Fibrous dysplasia is a developmental anomaly of bone in which the normal bone marrow and cancellous bone are replaced with abnormal fibrous and fibro-osseous tissue. Fibrous dysplasia can be isolated to one bone or may be diffuse, causing substantial deformity and disability. Fibrous dysplasia can be classified clinically into four categories: monostotic, polyostotic, McCune-Albright syndrome, and Mazabraud syndrome.[3]

The incidence of fibrous dysplasia is equal between males and females. Monostotic fibrous dysplasia is usually diagnosed before age 30 years and most commonly during childhood or adolescence as an incidental finding. Monostotic disease accounts for approximately 70% of patients with fibrous dysplasia. Polyostotic fibrous dysplasia is more often diagnosed at a younger age, with a mean age at diagnosis of 8 years, and often presents with pain or pathologic fracture.

The etiology of fibrous dysplasia is not fully understood but thought to be a postzygotic mutation affecting the cell membrane-bound protein G. Both monostotic and polyostotic forms of fibrous dysplasia exhibit an abnormal proliferation of mesenchymal osteoblastic precursor cells with this mutation. Chromosome 12 has been postulated as the location of this mutation. Patients with McCune-Albright syndrome exhibit an increased level of interleukin-6 that may be responsible

for increased bone resorption secondary to increased activity of osteoclasts.[3]

The diagnosis of fibrous dysplasia may be made as an incidental radiographic finding.[1,2,4] Patients can present with vague symptoms, including swelling or tenderness, or a stress fracture. Seventy percent of patients with fibrous dysplasia report bone pain. Deformity can develop as a result of repetitive stress that causes fractures to heal and then remodel. Bones most commonly affected by fibrous dysplasia include the femur (91%), the tibia (81%), the pelvis (78%), bones in the foot (73%), and craniofacial bones (50%).[3] Chronic fracture and remodeling of the proximal femur in this condition can lead to the classic shepherd's crook deformity. Craniofacial involvement can lead to

Table 1

Extraosseous Findings in Fibrous Dysplasia

± Café-au-lait areas with "coast of Maine" irregular contour. 50% occurrence in polyostotic disease and proportional to skeletal involvement. Most commonly located on the dorsal neck, lower lumbar region, face, lips, and oral mucosa.

Solitary and multiple myxomas (predilection for the right side) especially with polyostotic form (Mazabraud syndrome). The myxomas may originate from primitive mesenchymal cells that differentiate to fibroblasts that lose the ability to produce collagen, but instead produce hyaluronic acid.

Precocious puberty (females > males) (McCune-Albright syndrome) may present as vaginal bleeding within the first few months of life.

Albright's triad: multiple bone lesions (predominantly unilateral), precocious puberty, café-au-lait spots (tend to be unilateral and may be overlying involved bone).

Myriad endocrine abnormalities are possible.

Most common single entity causing oncogenic osteomalacia, from renal phosphate wasting caused by fibroblast growth factor-23.

(Reproduced from Pitcher JD Jr, Weber KL: Benign fibrous and histiocytic lesions, in Schwartz HS: *Orthopaedic Knowledge Update Musculoskeletal Tumors*, ed 2. American Academy of Orthopaedic Surgeons, Rosemont, IL, 2007, pp 121-132.)

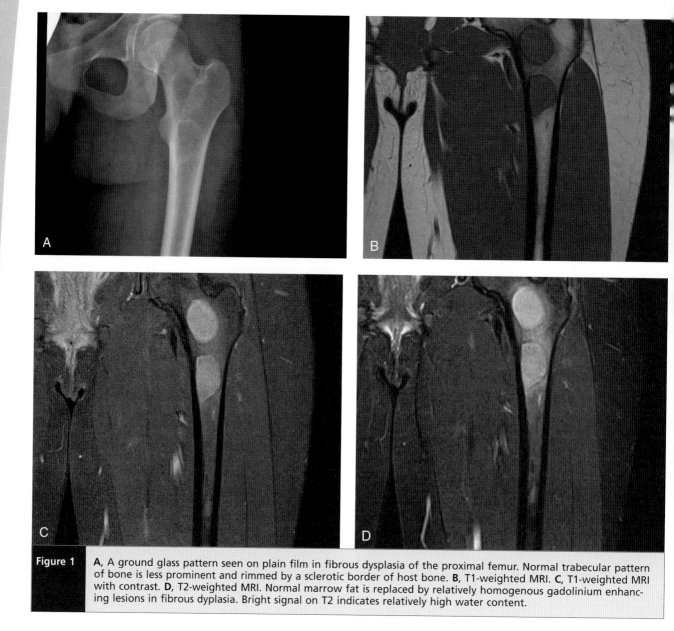

Figure 1 **A,** A ground glass pattern seen on plain film in fibrous dysplasia of the proximal femur. Normal trabecular pattern of bone is less prominent and rimmed by a sclerotic border of host bone. **B,** T1-weighted MRI. **C,** T1-weighted MRI with contrast. **D,** T2-weighted MRI. Normal marrow fat is replaced by relatively homogenous gadolinium enhancing lesions in fibrous dyplasia. Bright signal on T2 indicates relatively high water content.

proptosis and blindness in rare cases. Extraskeletal manifestations associated with fibrous dysplasia can be substantial (**Table 1**).

Most cases of fibrous dysplasia can be diagnosed with plain radiographs.[1,2,4] The diaphysis or metaphysis of long bones are the most common location (**Figure 1**). The normal trabecular pattern of bone is replaced by woven bone and fibrous tissue producing the classic ground glass appearance. The radiographic changes in the bone exhibit a sharp geographic border in keeping with a benign process. Periosteal elevation can be seen in the case of healing stress fractures. Shepherd's crook deformity or bowing of the tibia can be evident on plain films.[3] Other changes, such as islands of cartilage forming popcorn calcifications or a secondary aneurysmal bone cyst, may also be seen. Technetium bone scans demonstrate mild to moderate uptake. MRI

shows decreased signal intensity on T1-weighted images and increased signal intensity on T2-weighted images[1] (**Figure 1**).

The gross appearance of fibrous dysplasia is a firm tan to gray/white tissue with a gritty texture from the spicules of bone that are present in the tissue. Histologically, the tissue has a fibrous stroma with bone spicules scattered throughout that form curvilinear structures commonly referred to as alphabet soup or Chinese letters. The tissue is of low cellularity and mitotic figures are rare.[1,2,5]

A clinical triad of polyostotic fibrous dysplasia, café-au-lait spots, and precocious puberty characterizes McCune-Albright syndrome (**Figure 2**). This syndrome is characterized by increased rates of growth and development of premature secondary sexual characteristics. The causes of these symptoms can be multifactorial.

Only 3% to 4% of patients with McCune-Albright syndrome will exhibit all three characteristics of the triad.[1,3]

Mazabraud syndrome is a rare form of polyostotic fibrous dysplasia in association with multiple soft-tissue myxomas. The myxomas are often found overlying bone with fibrous dysplastic changes. These patients can present with enlarging soft-tissue myxomas.[1]

Malignant transformation of fibrous dysplasia is rare but has been reported. The incidence is between 0.5% and 1.0% for monostotic disease. Patients with McCune-Albright syndrome or polyostotic disease have a malignant transformation rate of 4%. Radiation to the affected bone increases the risk of malignant change.[1,6]

The treatment of fibrous dysplasia is generally conservative. The main goal of treatment should be to prevent deformity. Surgical indications include persistent pain, deformity, nonunion, and femoral fractures. Bone grafting is often unsuccessful because new ingrowth of bone is affected by the same processes, so treatment should focus on structural restoration and maintenance rather than attempts at extirpation of the disease.[7] Cortical struts can be helpful in selected cases. When bone grafting is required, some think that the use of cortical bone graft is preferable to cancellous bone graft. Pharmacologic therapy can be used in patients with polyostotic disease, or those with monostotic disease unsuitable for or refractory to surgery, using bisphosphonates to inhibit osteoclast activity. Fracture rates are decreased and pain can be improved for patients with polyostotic disease who are treated with bisphosphonates.[1,3,6,8-14] Denosumab, a receptor activator of nuclear factor-κ B (RANK) ligand (RANKL) inhibitor of bone, also has recently been reported effective in controlling pain and progression of disease in fibrous dysplasia.[12]

Nonossifying Fibroma

Nonossifying fibroma is a benign fibrous lesion most commonly found in the metaphysis of skeletally immature patients and occasionally in young adults. These lesions are usually eccentrically located and are most commonly seen in the distal femur, proximal tibia, distal tibia, and proximal fibula.

There has been great confusion regarding this lesion due to the plethora of diagnostic terms applied, including fibrous cortical defect (for smaller lesions predominantly involving the cortex), fibroxanthoma, nonosteogenic fibromas of bone, and metaphyseal fibrous defect.

These lesions are thought to develop as a result of the failure of normal subperiosteal membrane to ossify during development and instead fill in with fibrous tissue.[15] Eighty percent of nonossifying fibromas occur in individuals younger than 20 years. Lesions found in older patients are often regressing. These lesions occur more commonly in males with a ratio of 1.6 to 1.[3]

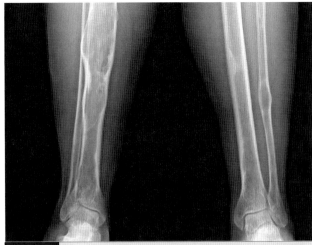

Figure 2 Polyostotic fibrous dysplasia seen in bilateral tibiae and fibulae. Weakening of the bone can lead to bowing of the tibia, or, in the femur (not pictured), development of a varus deformity in the femoral neck referred to as a shepherd's crook deformity.

Nonossifying fibromas are most commonly discovered as an incidental finding. They are generally asymptomatic unless associated with a pathologic fracture. Physical examination is generally unremarkable.[3,16,17] Pain in the area of a suspected nonossifying fibroma in the absence of a fracture or acute injury should raise the suspicion of a more aggressive process. Secondary aneurysmal bone cysts can develop with the nonossifying fibroma.[18]

Nonossifying fibromas are seen in 30% to 40% of children and may occur bilaterally. Multiple lesions, café-au-lait spots, multiple nevi, mental retardation, hypogonadism, ocular disorders, and cardiovascular abnormalities characterize the rare Jaffe-Campanacci syndrome.

Plain radiographs demonstrate eccentric metaphyseal lesions (**Figure 3**). Fibrous cortical defects are generally between 1 and 3 cm in diameter. These may be intracortical and do not involve the medullary canal. Nonossifying fibromas are larger and are longer than they are wide. The outer edges are lobulated, and internal septation creates a bubbly appearance. A rind of sclerotic bone provides the margin, and the sclerosis progresses as the lesion matures. Bone scans may demonstrate faint uptake and do not contribute to the diagnosis. Cross-sectional imaging is usually unnecessary to confirm the diagnosis, but CT scans demonstrate thinning of the cortex. MRI studies are consistent with fibrous lesions on T2-weighted images, and T1 images may show areas of hemosiderin deposits. Secondary aneurysmal bone cysts can develop within a nonossifying fibroma.[3,6,16,17,19]

Gross examination of a nonossifying fibroma demonstrates soft, fibrous tissue with brownish-tan tissue and foci of hemorrhage. Histologically, the nonossifying

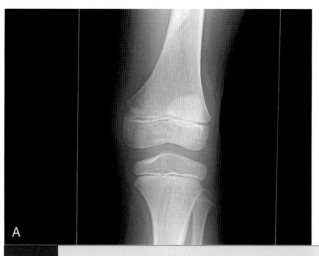
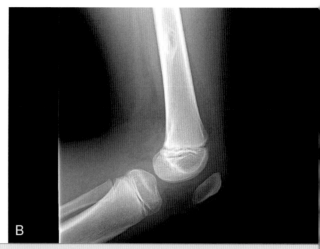

Figure 3 **A,** Nonossifying fibroma (fibroxanthoma) discovered as an incidental finding in an 8-year-old boy. **B,** Nonossifying fibroma is seen more characteristically on the lateral view. Biplanar radiography is helpful in establishing the diagnosis.

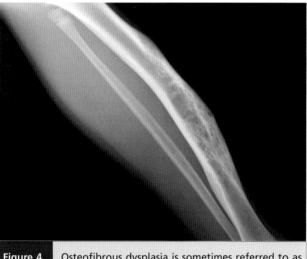

Figure 4 Osteofibrous dysplasia is sometimes referred to as Campanacci disease. The bubbly appearance involving the mid tibia is a classic radiographic finding.

fibroma demonstrates monotonous fibroblastic cells with little atypia and few mitoses.[3,16,17]

In most cases, management of fibrous cortical defects and nonossifying fibroma is with serial radiographs as needed to monitor the progression and ultimate regression of the lesion, which typically coincides with skeletal maturity, often 5 to 10 years after diagnosis. Although most of these lesions are treated nonsurgically, those that become quite large can cause pain due to mechanical insufficiency and place the patient at risk for fracture. Curettage and bone grafting are indicated in these situations with prophylactic fixation if needed. Recurrence of these lesions is rare after surgical intervention.[3,19]

Osteofibrous Dysplasia

Osteofibrous dysplasia (OFD), also known as Campanacci disease, is a rare congenital dysplasia made up of fibrous and osseous tissue. This condition occurs most commonly in the tibia but occasionally in the fibula. Males are more often affected, and the condition is almost always observed in patients younger than 10 years and in those younger than 5 years in 66% of the cases.[3,20,21]

The clinical presentation is classic expansion of the anterior cortex of the mid diaphysis of the tibia in a child that may lead to anterior bowing. The condition is generally painless unless pathologic fracture occurs. OFD rarely can occur bilaterally.

OFD presents on radiographs as an eccentric intracortical area with the appearance of multiloculated lucencies[22] (**Figure 4**). The subperiosteal cortical surface is generally expanded and thinned (**Figure 5**). Pathologic fractures may be seen and are generally incomplete and involve the anterior cortex. OFD can appear identical to an adamantinoma, a low-grade malignant lesion that also is most commonly seen in the tibia,[15,23] although typically adamantinoma occurs in a much older age group.

Histologically, OFD is characterized by fibrous tissue surrounded by osteoblast-bordered bony trabeculae. The fibrous component is spindle shaped and may be arranged in a swirling, storiform pattern or a loose myxomatous pattern. If a biopsy is performed, experienced histologic review precludes misdiagnosis of adamantinoma, an error that can lead to inappropriate treatment.[3,24,25]

Treatment of OFD should be as conservative as possible until the patient reaches skeletal maturity. Excision should not be performed in young children because the dysplasia could recur even more aggressively. If fractures occur in children, casting should be used as

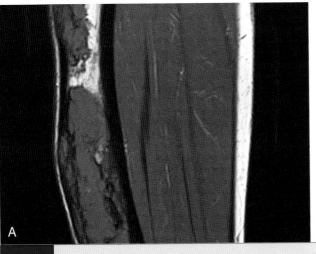
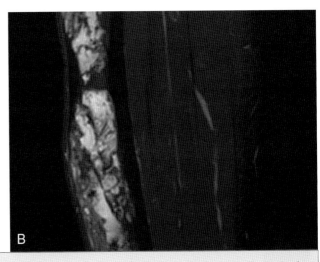

Figure 5 A, Sagittal T1-weighted image of osteofibrous dysplasia. Low signal change and lobular appearance are seen in the lesion. B, Sagittal T2-weighted image of osteofibrous dysplasia. Note the increased signal intensity seen within the lesion.

the treatment of choice. If bowing becomes excessive or fractures recur, osteotomy may be required but should be delayed until after age 15 years if possible.[3,26]

The prognosis for OFD is variable, but the disease is most active before age 10 years. The lesions generally begin to improve as the patient reaches skeletal maturity. If the lesion has not resolved by adulthood and is clinically symptomatic, resection and bone grafting can be performed.

Desmoplastic Fibroma

Desmoplastic fibroma (DF) is an exceptionally rare benign but aggressive lesion of bone that behaves much like a soft-tissue fibromatosis. The lesion is composed of dense fibrous tissue that infiltrates the local bone but does not have the ability to metastasize. DF occurs most commonly between the ages of 15 and 40 years and is more common in women than men. More than 50% of these lesions occur in the femur, tibia, and pelvis. The mandible is also a common site.[3,15,27]

Pain lasting several months is the most common presenting symptom. Fifteen percent to 20% of these patients may have an initial presentation with a pathologic fracture. Physically, findings are nonspecific without a fracture, but there can be some subtle swelling about the affected bone.

Radiographically, desmoplastic fibroma is characterized by osteolytic defects with slight to moderate expansion of the bone and lobulated margins (**Figure 6**). The tumor can break through the cortex and appear loculated. Periosteal reaction is rare unless a fracture has occurred. Bone scans demonstrate increased central uptake. CT scan can be valuable to assess the extent of bony involvement.[3,15,28]

Desmoplastic fibroma is grossly a firm intramedullary tissue and histologically is similar to an aggressive

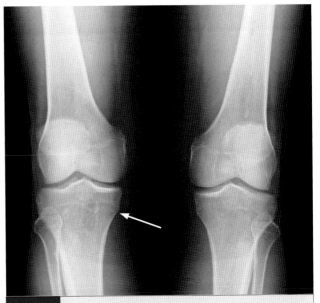

Figure 6 Desmoplastic fibroma of the tibia (arrow). Radiographic findings of desmoplastic fibroma are nonspecific, but usually show a lucent lesion with some surrounding sclerosis.

soft-tissue fibromatosis. It is relatively hypocellular with spindled fibroblasts seen in a mature collagen matrix. Genetic abnormalities have been observed. Loss of 5q21-22 gene location has been reported. That is also the gene location for familial adenomatous polyposis and Gardner syndrome.[3,15]

Treatment can vary, from aggressive intralesional curettage to wide en bloc resection and reconstruction, in cases involving extensive bone loss. Local recurrence rates of up to 40% have been reported.[3,20]

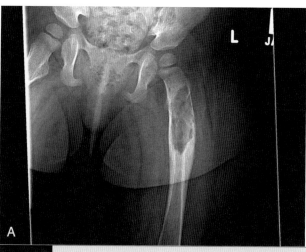
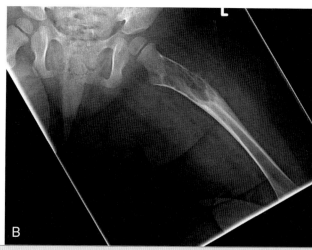

Figure 7 Radiographs showing eosinophilic granuloma of the femur in an 18-month-old patient. **A**, A significant periosteal reaction is shown. **B**, Eosinophilic granuloma of the femur seen on a frog-lateral view of the hip. Patients in this age group with confirmed eosinophilic granuloma of bone should be referred for evaluation of other sites of disease and consideration of systemic therapy.

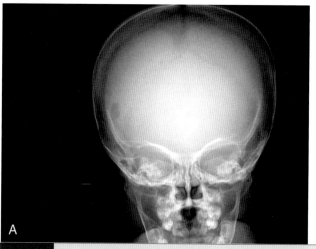
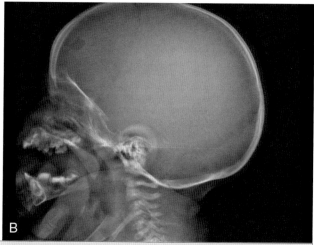

Figure 8 **A**, Eosinophilic granuloma of the skull. The atypical punched-out lesion demonstrates sharp geographic boundaries. **B**, Lateral view of calvarial eosinophilic granuloma.

Langerhans Cell Histiocytosis (Histiocytosis X, Eosinophilic Granuloma)

Langerhans cell histiocytosis (LCH) is a disease with a protean presentation characterized by an abnormal proliferation of macrophages (histiocytes). The disease has been divided into four forms: eosinophilic granuloma, Hand-Schuller-Christian syndrome, Letterer-Siwe disease, and congenital self-healing reticulohistiocytosis, also termed Hashimoto-Pritzker disease. Eosinophilic granuloma disease is the most commonly encountered form for orthopaedic surgeons, in which the lesions are limited to bone. Hans-Christian syndrome is multifocal and widely disseminated, often with a characteristic triad of diabetes insipidus, exopthalmos, and lytic bone lesions, usually diagnosed in patients age 2 to 10 years. Letterer-Siwe disease is a fulminant, multi-organ form that presents in infancy with hepatosplenomegaly, and is usually fatal.[3,29-31] Congenital self-healing reticulohistiocytosis is a spontaneously resolving form characterized by skin eruptions within the first months of life.[3,27,29,30,32]

The skull, spine, pelvis, or ribs are involved in 70% of cases (**Figures 7** and **8**). Children exhibit spine changes in approximately 10% of cases and adults in 3% of cases. The thoracic spine and the lumbar spine are the most common spine locations. Rib lesions occur in 25% of adults and 8% of children. LCH occurs most commonly in patients younger than 21 years. Sixty-one percent of cases occur in this age group and of those, 55% are males and 45% are females. LCH in patients older than 21 years is even more common in males, with an incidence of 75% males and 25% females.[3,29,30]

Clinically, patients with eosinophilic granuloma have

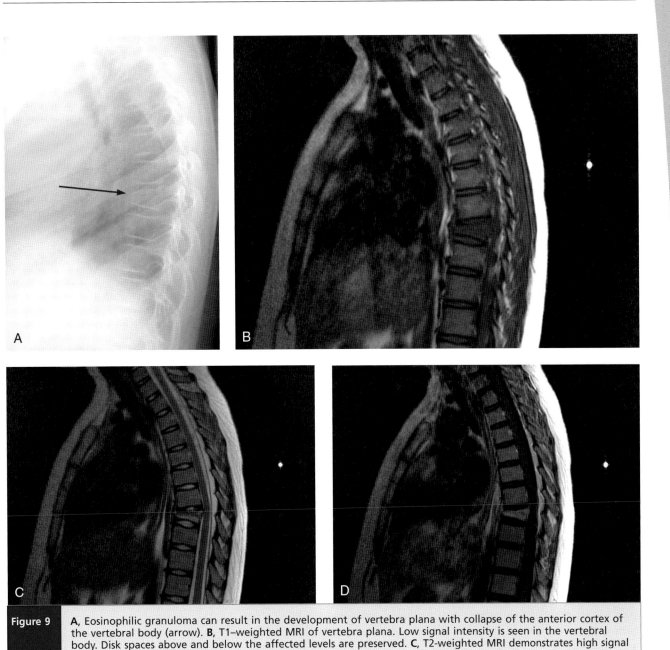

Figure 9   **A,** Eosinophilic granuloma can result in the development of vertebra plana with collapse of the anterior cortex of the vertebral body (arrow). **B,** T1–weighted MRI of vertebra plana. Low signal intensity is seen in the vertebral body. Disk spaces above and below the affected levels are preserved. **C,** T2-weighted MRI demonstrates high signal intensity. **D,** T1-weighted MRI with contrast. The lesion demonstrates diffuse enhancement.

a solitary bone lesion and sometimes a visible or palpable mass. Localized pain, sometimes worse at night, is common. Back pain could be present if the spine is involved, and low-grade fevers are sometimes seen. These patients may present with a limp if the lower extremity is involved.

Radiographically, vertebra plana is a classic finding with LCH (**Figure 9**). When LCH occurs in the spine, vertebra plana is seen in 15% of cases.[33] The lesion only affects the body of the vertebrae. The pedicles, posterior elements, and disk spaces are spared. Flat bones are commonly affected and radiographically present as punched-out lesions. In long bones, the metaphysis is involved in 42% of children and 23% of adults. Diaphyseal lesions occur in 54% of children

and 75% of adults. The epiphysis is rarely involved. Eosinophilic granuloma has been called "the great mimicker" because plain radiographs can demonstrate periosteal reaction (onion skin), which can be seen in more aggressive tumors such as Ewing sarcoma or osteomyelitis (**Figure 10**). Because a single scan demonstrates only 35% of lesions, a skeletal survey is more reliable for identifying multifocal bone disease.

Pathologically, LCH is seen as a soft red-brown tissue or as firm white tissue. Microscopically, Langerhans-type histiocytes with eosinophils are seen. The histiocytes are large, with granular pink-blue cytoplasm. Nuclei are oval and multilobulated and have a kidney bean shape. Immunohistochemical examination is positive for S-100, OKT6, and intracellular lysozyme

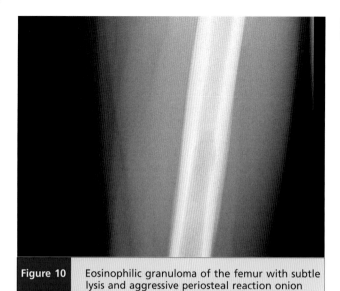

Figure 10 Eosinophilic granuloma of the femur with subtle lysis and aggressive periosteal reaction onion skin is seen. The radiographic differential diagnosis for this lesion proved histologically to be eosinophilic granuloma, and includes Ewing sarcoma and osteomyelitis.

staining.[3,29,30] Electron microscopy demonstrates Birbeck bodies, although this finding is seldom clinically relevant.

Biopsy is recommended for lesions with an aggressive appearance unless the disease is disseminated or the diagnosis established. Solitary bone lesions are often self-limiting and heal reliably with curettage or steroid injection. Multiple steroid injections may be required. Spine lesions rarely require surgical intervention. Disseminated forms of disease require systemic treatment, and young children in whom LCH of bone has been diagnosed should be referred for screening for visceral disease and possible medical management. Methotrexate and vinblastine have been used, along with external beam radiation, especially in patients with spinal compression.[31,34,35]

Summary

Benign fibrous lesions of bone can generally be diagnosed based on clinical history and imaging studies. Classic radiographic findings are seen for patients with fibrous dysplasia, nonossifying fibroma and osteofibrous dysplasia. Treatment of these lesions should be observation, unless clinical symptoms develop or the patient is at risk for pathologic fracture. Desmoplastic fibromas require aggressive surgical management. LCH of bone with solitary bone lesions responds to intralesional steroid injection or curettage, or can even be self-limited. Disseminated forms of LCH carry a worse prognosis and should be referred for medical management.

Annotated References

1. Pitcher JD, Weber KL: Benign fibrous and histiocytic lesions, in Schwartz HS (ed): *Orthopaedic Knowledge Update Musculoskeletal Tumors*, ed 2. American Academy of Orthopaedic Surgeons, Rosemont, IL, 2007, pp 121-132.

   An excellent overview of commonly occurring benign and fibrohistiocytic lesions of bone is presented. Lesions covered include nonossifying fibroma, fibrous cortical defects, fibrous dysplasia, osteofibrous dysplasia, desmoplastic fibroma, and histiocytosis X.

2. Fibrous dysplasia, in Campanacci M, Bertoni F, Bacchini P, Enneking W, Notini S (eds): *Bone and Soft Tissue Tumors.* New York, Springer-Verlag, 1990, pp 391-418.

3. Hillock R, Zuppan C: Fibrous dysplasia. *Orthopaedic Knowledge Online* 2007;5(4).

4. Osseous tumors of intramedullary origin, in Mirra JM, Picci P, Gold RH (eds): *Bone Tumors: Clinical, Radiologic and Pathologic Correlations.* Philadelphia/London, Lea and Febiger, 1989, pp 143-438.

5. de Sanctis C, Lala R, Matarazzo P, et al: McCune-Albright syndrome: A longitudinal clinical study of 32 patients. *J Pediatr Endocrinol Metab* 1999;12(6):817-826.

6. Ruggieri P, Sim FH, Bond JR, Unni KK: Malignancies in fibrous dysplasia. *Cancer* 1994;73(5):1411-1424.

7. Moretti VM, Slotcavage RL, Crawford EA, Lackman RD, Ogilvie CM: Curettage and graft alleviates athletic-limiting pain in benign lytic bone lesions. *Clin Orthop Relat Res* 2011;469(1):283-288.

   The study involved a series of athletes with disabling benign bone lesions that were treated with curettage and bone grafting. This treatment resulted in pain relief and allowed the patients to return to full athletic activity. Level of evidence: IV.

8. Chapurlat RD, Hugueny P, Delmas PD, Meunier PJ: Treatment of fibrous dysplasia of bone with intravenous pamidronate: Long-term effectiveness and evaluation of predictors of response to treatment. *Bone* 2004;35(1):235-242.

9. Guille JT, Kumar SJ, MacEwen GD: Fibrous dysplasia of the proximal part of the femur: Long-term results of curettage and bone-grafting and mechanical realignment. *J Bone Joint Surg Am* 1998;80(5):648-658.

10. Lane JM, Khan SN, O'Connor WJ, et al: Bisphosphonate therapy in fibrous dysplasia. *Clin Orthop Relat Res* 2001;382:6-12.

11. Ozaki T, Hamada M, Sugihara S, Kunisada T, Mitani S, Inoue H: Treatment outcome of osteofibrous dysplasia. *J Pediatr Orthop B* 1998;7(3):199-202.

12. Boyce AM, Chong WH, Yao J, et al: Denosumab treatment for fibrous dysplasia. *J Bone Miner Res* 2012; 27(7):1462-1470.

    Denosumab is a humanized monoclonal antibody RANKL approved for treatment of osteoporosis and bone metastasis. This article describes the use of denosumab in the treatment of a 9-year-old patient with severe fibrous dysplasia. The patient demonstrated decreased bone turnover and decrease in pain and tumor growth over a 7-month period while being treated. Level of evidence: IV.

13. DiMeglio LA: Bisphosphonate therapy for fibrous dysplasia. *Pediatr Endocrinol Rev* 2007;4(suppl 4):440-445.

    The author of this study reviewed and acknowledged the many observational reports of pain relief associated with the use of bisphosphonates in the treatment of fibrous dysplasia, bringing into question the true effectiveness of this therapy in the overall course of the disease; in particular, the incidence of fracture or deformity. A case in which a patient developed hypophosphatemia and secondary hyperparathyroidism requiring medical management is presented. It was concluded that although the patient responded well, the side effects warrant further study. Level of evidence: IV.

14. Mansoori LS, Catel CP, Rothman MS: Bisphosphonate treatment in polyostotic fibrous dysplasia of the cranium: Case report and literature review. *Endocr Pract* 2010;16(5):851-854.

    This article provides a literature review of bisphosphonate treatment of fibrous dysplasia. The experience of a patient with extensive fibrous dysplasia of the skull is presented. This patient demonstrated a significant decrease in bone-specific alkaline phosphate levels and dramatic radiographic improvement with treatment. Clinically, the patient's headaches improved rapidly with treatment. Level of evidence: IV.

15. Most MJ, Sim FH, Inwards CY: Osteofibrous dysplasia and adamantinoma. *J Am Acad Orthop Surg* 2010; 18(6):358-366.

    This study examined the potential relationship between osteofibrous dysplasia and adamantinoma. Differences in behavior and treatment of each of these are reviewed. Recent information describing the possibility of an intermediate form called osteofibrous dysplasia-like adamantinoma is also reviewed. Level of evidence: III.

16. Histiocytic fibroma, in Campanacci M, Bertoni F, Bacchini P, Enneking W, Notini S (eds): *Bone and Soft Tissue Tumors*. New York, Springer-Verlag, 1990, pp 93-110.

17. Fibrous cortical defect and nonossifying fibroma, in Mirra JM, Picci P, Gold RH (eds): *Bone Tumors: Clinical, Radiologic and Pathologic Correlations*. Philadelphia/London, Lea and Febiger, 1989, pp 691-800.

18. Tabrizi R, Nejhad ST, Özkan BT: Nonossifying fibroma secondary to aneurysmal bone cyst in the man-

dibular condyle. *J Craniofac Surg* 2011;22(3):1157-1158.

    Nonossifying fibroma associated with aneurysmal bone cyst is rare. The authors describe a case in which a nonossifying fibroma of the mandible was diagnosed with an aneurysmal component. This combination is more aggressive than a simple nonossifying fibroma and requires more aggressive treatment. Level of evidence: IV.

19. Moser RP Jr, Sweet DE, Haseman DB, Madewell JE: Multiple skeletal fibroxanthomas: Radiologic-pathologic correlation of 72 cases. *Skeletal Radiol* 1987;16(5):353-359.

20. Domson G, Scarbourough M, Gibbs C: Fibrous bony lesions. *Orthopaedic Knowledge Online* 2007;5(8).

    This article provides an overview of several fibrous bony lesions including osteofibrous dysplasia, nonossifying fibroma, and desmoplastic fibroma.

21. Karol LA, Brown DS, Wise CA, Waldron M: Familial osteofibrous dysplasia: A case series. *J Bone Joint Surg Am* 2005;87(10):2297-2307.

22. Taconis WK, Schütte HE, van der Heul RO: Desmoplastic fibroma of bone: A report of 18 cases. *Skeletal Radiol* 1994;23(4):283-288.

23. Ramanoudjame M, Guinebretière JM, Mascard E, Seringe R, Dimeglio A, Wicart P: Is there a link between osteofibrous dysplasia and adamantinoma? *Orthop Traumatol Surg Res* 2011;97(8):877-880.

    This article reports a case of osteofibrous dysplasia-like adamantinoma that developed in a child with a previous diagnosis of osteofibrous dysplasia. The authors recommend surveillance because of the possible progression from osteofibrous dysplasia to adamantinoma. Level of evidence: IV.

24. Osteofibrous dysplasia of long bones, in Campanacci M, Bertoni F, Bacchini P, Enneking W, Notini S (eds): *Bone and Soft Tissue Tumors*. New York, Springer-Verlag, 1990, pp 419-432.

25. Adamantinoma and osteofibrous dysplasia, in Mirra JM, Picci P, Gold RH (eds): *Bone Tumors: Clinical, Radiologic and Pathologic Correlations*. Philadelphia/London, Lea and Febiger, 1989, pp 1203-1232.

26. Kosuge DD, Pugh H, Ramachandran M, Barry M, Timms A: Marginal excision and Ilizarov hemicallotasis for osteofibrous dysplasia of the tibia: A case report. *J Pediatr Orthop B* 2011;20(2):89-93.

    A technique using distraction osteogenesis combined with excision of only the anterior cortex of the tibia rather than a complete segment for the treatment of tibial deformity in osteofibrous dysplasia is described. Level of evidence: IV.

27. Abla O, Egeler RM, Weitzman S: Langerhans cell histiocytosis: Current concepts and treatments. *Cancer Treat Rev* 2010;36(4):354-359.

2: Benign Bone Tumors

A review of three studies sponsored by the Histiocyte Society since 1991 is presented. The results of these studies suggest that patients with involvement of so-called risk organs have a higher incidence of mortality. Risk organs include blood-forming organs, the liver, and/or the spleen. Patients without involvement of risk organs have a lower mortality but may need treatment of disease control. Treatment protocols and results are presented. Level of evidence: III.

28. Zhang F, Ni B, Zhao L, et al: Desmoplastic fibroma of the cervical spine: Case report and review of the literature. *Spine (Phila Pa 1976)* 2010;35(14):E667-E671.

An excellent review of desmoplastic fibroma is presented, along with an unusual case of desmoplastic fibroma involving the cervical spine. The patient demonstrated symptoms similar to those seen with disk disease. An aggressive wide resection/reconstruction is described, with immediate pain relief and no recurrence at 36 months after surgery. Level of evidence: IV.

29. Histiocytosis X, in Campanacci M, Bertoni F, Bacchini P, Enneking W, Notini S (eds): *Bone and Soft Tissue Tumors*. New York, Springer-Verlag, 1990, pp 769-791.

30. Histiocytosis, in Mirra JM, Picci P, Gold RH (eds): *Bone Tumors: Clinical, Radiologic and Pathologic Correlations*. Philadelphia/London, Lea and Febiger, 1989, pp 1021-1086.

31. Yasko AW, Fanning CV, Ayala AG, Carrasco CH, Murray JA: Percutaneous techniques for the diagnosis and treatment of localized Langerhans-cell histiocyto-sis (eosinophilic granuloma of bone). *J Bone Joint Surg Am* 1998;80(2):219-228.

32. Kilpatrick SE, Wenger DE, Gilchrist GS, Shives TC, Wollan PC, Unni KK: Langerhans' cell histiocytosis (histiocytosis X) of bone: A clinicopathologic analysis of 263 pediatric and adult cases. *Cancer* 1995;76(12):2471-2484.

33. Raab P, Hohmann F, Kühl J, Krauspe R: Vertebral remodeling in eosinophilic granuloma of the spine: A long-term follow-up. *Spine (Phila Pa 1976)* 1998;23(12):1351-1354.

34. Moralis A, Kunkel M, Kleinsasser N, Müller-Richter U, Reichert TE, Driemel O: Intralesional corticosteroid therapy for mandibular Langerhans cell histiocytosis preserving the intralesional tooth germ. *Oral Maxillofac Surg* 2008;12(2):105-111.

Solitary eosinophilic granuloma of the mandible was treated with intralesional injection of methylprednisolone. Pain and associated swelling receded quickly. These results are similar to those seen in long bone treatment with steroid injection. Level of evidence: IV.

35. Minkov M: Multisystem Langerhans cell histiocytosis in children: Current treatment and future directions. *Paediatr Drugs* 2011;13(2):75-86.

This article discusses a current treatment protocol and possible future treatments for multisystem Langerhans cell histiocytosis.

Chapter 13

Giant Cell Tumor of Bone

David Cheong, MD   G. Douglas Letson, MD

Introduction

Giant cell tumor of bone (GCTB) was first described in 1818. Previously this tumor was referred to as myeloid sarcoma, osteoclastoma, and osteoblastoclastoma. GCTB is considered benign, although it is locally aggressive and has the potential to metastasize in its benign form, paradoxically referred to as "benign metastasizing" giant cell tumor. Adding to the confusion, there is a rare malignant variant of giant cell tumor, which is clinically and histologically distinctive, as well as cases of malignancy arising in benign giant cell tumor. Cases of malignant transformation are most commonly reported following radiation.

Historically, the diagnosis and treatment of GCTB involved assessment with plain radiographs and surgical intervention. With advances in diagnostic imaging and recently available medical management, the evaluation and treatment of GCTB has evolved. Much has been learned about the behavior of GCTB via cellular pathways, leading to targeted medical therapy and new and more effective management strategies.

Epidemiology

GCTB accounts for 4% to 5% of biopsy-analyzed primary bone tumors in North America. In Asia, where the reported incidence of GCTB is higher, it accounts for 20% of all primary bone tumors.[1] GCTB has a slightly higher female-to-male preponderance. The peak incidence of occurrence is between the third and fourth decades of life. GCTB has been identified and reported in nearly every bone of the appendicular and axial skeleton, with a predilection for the metaphyseal-epiphyseal region of long bones. The most common location of GCTB is around the knee, with most frequent incidence in the distal femur, followed by the proximal tibia and the distal radius as the third most common sites[2] (Figure 1). Benign GCTB has been observed to metastasize to the lungs in 4% of cases. Speculation has

occurred regarding the relationship of growth or appearance of GCTB and the use of hormone replacement therapy and pregnancy; however, this has not been definitively confirmed. GCTB in skeletally immature patients is uncommon, and other diagnostic considerations in this patient population should include solid variant of aneurysmal bone cyst or giant cell rich osteosarcoma.

Presentation

The chief complaint of patients with GCTB is pain that often begins insidiously, with reports of a dull ache that gradually increases over time. As pain increases, the patient may notice swelling of the adjacent joint, soft-tissue fullness, and even a soft-tissue mass overlying the area of concern. A painful limp associated with weight-bearing activities may accompany these progressively worsening symptoms. The patient may relate symptom onset to a trauma. Approximately 10% of patients will present with pathologic fracture, usually preceded by prodromal symptoms of pain and decreased motion (Figure 2). Giant cell tumor of the spine can present with radicular symptoms.[3]

Imaging

After a detailed history and physical examination, plain radiographs should be obtained. Frequently, the patient presents with radiographs that have been taken at the request of the primary physician or emergency room when the patient is first seen. GCTB is typically described as metaphyseal-epiphyseal lesions. Orthogonal views of the extremity demonstrate an eccentric geographic border most commonly without sclerosis (80% to 85%). It should be noted that there can be areas of sclerosis opposite the side of the fading border. The lesion can be quite large and encompass the metaphysis and epiphysis up to the subchondral bone (Figure 3). Cortical erosion and periosteal elevation with expansion of the cortex can also be seen. Only 5% of GCTBs show complete sclerotic rimming, usually on CT scan or a mineralization pattern.[4] When presenting with pathologic fracture and subsequent fracture changes of periosteal elevation, it can be difficult to distinguish the GCTB from a malignant tumor of bone.

2: Benign Bone Tumors

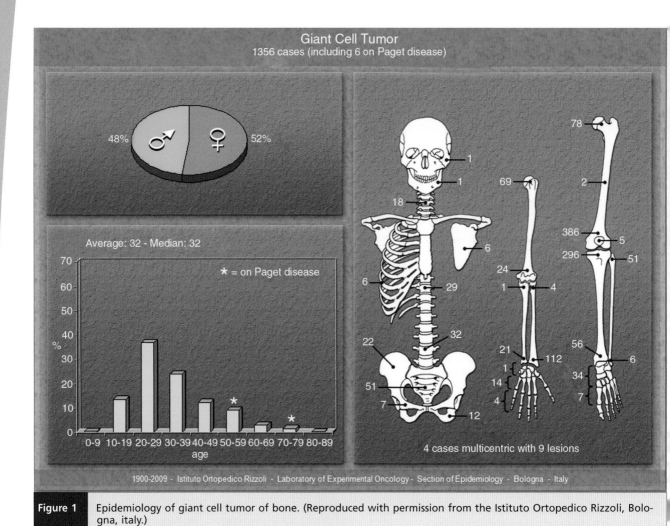

1900-2009 - Istituto Ortopedico Rizzoli - Laboratory of Experimental Oncology - Section of Epidemiology - Bologna - Italy

Figure 1 Epidemiology of giant cell tumor of bone. (Reproduced with permission from the Istituto Ortopedico Rizzoli, Bologna, Italy.)

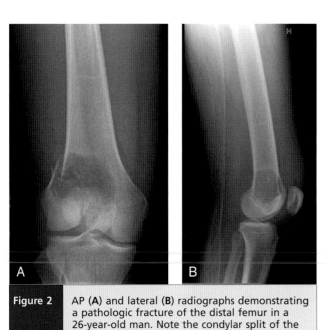

Figure 2 AP (**A**) and lateral (**B**) radiographs demonstrating a pathologic fracture of the distal femur in a 26-year-old man. Note the condylar split of the intra-articular fracture. Biopsy revealed giant cell tumor of bone.

After plain films, MRI is the diagnostic modality of choice because it will demonstrate the extraosseous soft-tissue component as well as the marrow extent of disease for surgical planning and/or treatment response assessment. T1-weighted MRI demonstrates a low to intermediate signal, homogenous in most lesions. T2 sequences show heterogeneity, as the hemosiderin produces a lower signal and the high water content a high signal. Gadolinium-enhanced images confirm a solid lesion with enhancement throughout. MRI details the marrow replacement by the lesion, particularly in regard to the involvement of the metaphysis and epiphysis extending to the articular surface of the adjacent joint (**Figure 4**). MRI can also reveal a soft-tissue component representing a potentially more aggressive process, although there is no correlation between this finding and the development of metastatic disease.

CT can also be used to evaluate for cortical erosions or sclerosis around the tumor-bone interface and assess for intralesional mineralization or fracture. A thin sclerotic border is often seen on CT, which helps distinguish GCTB from malignancies. The absence of a thick sclerotic border helps to differentiate this lesion from more indolent lesions. Cartilage tumors can be ruled

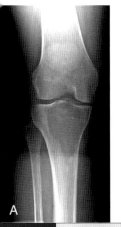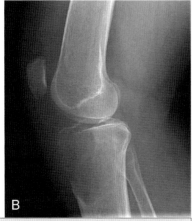

Figure 3 AP (**A**) and lateral (**B**) radiographs of a 38-year-old man with a giant cell tumor of bone involving the proximal tibia. Note the metaphyseal-epiphyseal eccentric location with extension to the subchondral surface of the bone.

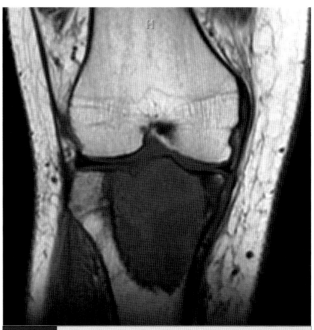

Figure 4 T1-weighted MRI of a giant cell tumor of bone of the proximal tibia. Note the low signal characteristics and narrow geographic margin.

out by the absence of any significant matrix or mineralization pattern within the tumor; however, many cartilage tumors do not show significant matrix or mineralization. Occasionally, GCTB will appear multiloculated on CT or MRI, usually because of osseous ridges and trabecular remnants left behind from areas of bone that have been removed because of osteoclast resorption.[4] The observation of these multiloculated cavities may also suggest the presence of an aneurysmal bone cyst component of GCTB, which occurs in 14% of cases. Bone scintigraphy is uninformative in characterizing the lesion. Technetium bone scans can screen for multifocal disease, which may arise with hyperparathyroidism, which produces multiple brown tumors radiologically and histologically indistinguishable from solitary GCTB. Although not contributing substantially to the diagnosis, most GCTBs will have increased radiotracer uptake, and at times exhibit a peripheral rim of enhancement with a central void or photopenia. Described as a donut sign, the appearance of this rim of enhancement is not from increased blood flow as some have presumed, but rather this finding is believed to be from increased reactive bone formation caused by both endosteal and periosteal reaction. Most cases studied with bone scintigraphy will also demonstrate increased radiotracer uptake across adjacent joints. It has been reported that 62% of cases with this phenomenon are the result of the increased blood flow and disuse osteoporosis rather than tumor extension.[4]

Positron emission tomography (PET) scan has no role in the evaluation of GCTB. Radiolabeled glucose in fluorodeoxyglucose-PET imaging studies of GCTB will reveal increased fluorodeoxyglucose avidity, but this is nonspecific and does not change diagnosis or management.

Histopathology

Biopsy and resected specimens of GCTB demonstrate the classic multinucleated giant cells, from which the neoplasm derives its name. These osteoclasts are often distributed evenly throughout a vascular stroma of mononuclear cells that resemble histiocytes (**Figure 5**). The nuclei of the giant cells, when compared to the stromal cells, are very similar in size and appearance; both the stromal cells and the nuclei of the giant cells take on round, ovoid, and even polygonal forms (**Figures 6 and 7**). Mitotic activity can be plentiful, and it is not uncommon to see scarce osteoid production. The presence of giant cells alone does not singularly make the diagnosis. The differential diagnosis based on pathology alone for a giant cell-rich lesion is extensive, and would include tumors such as giant cell-rich osteosarcoma, chondroblastoma, aneurysmal bone cyst, and chondroblastoma. For this reason, correlation of radiographic and clinical data are required.

Recent literature has highlighted the role of osteoclast-like macrophages with a high receptor activator of nuclear factor kappa–B ligand (RANKL) expression. The true neoplastic cells of GCTB are the ovoid mononuclear cells of the stroma, which display markers of mesenchymal origin, and partial differentiation along an osteoblastic lineage. This differentiation is altered by inflammatory cytokines to subsequently favor an environment of multinucleated osteoclastic cells.[5] This is the molecular basis of the use of RANKL inhibition for medical management, in which targeted medications interfere with osteoclastic stimulation.

2: Benign Bone Tumors

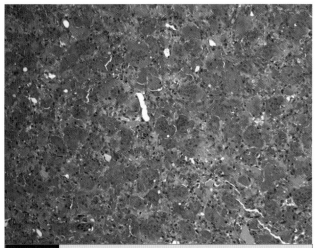

Figure 5   A giant cell tumor is shown (hematoxylin and eosin, magnification 10X). Histologic section demonstrates a uniform distribution of large, osteoclast-like giant cells with interspersed oval to elongated mononuclear cells. The nuclei of the mononuclear cells are similar to those of the osteoclast-like giant cells, with an open chromatin pattern with one or two small nucleoli.

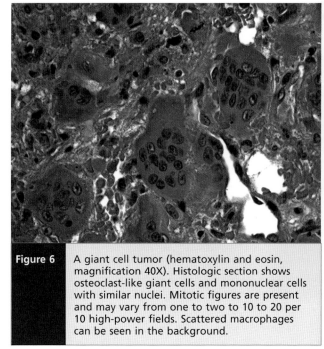

Figure 6   A giant cell tumor (hematoxylin and eosin, magnification 40X). Histologic section shows osteoclast-like giant cells and mononuclear cells with similar nuclei. Mitotic figures are present and may vary from one to two to 10 to 20 per 10 high-power fields. Scattered macrophages can be seen in the background.

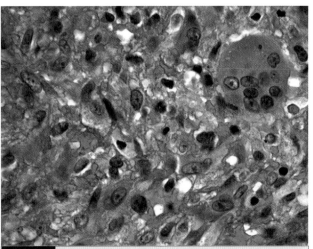

Figure 7   Giant cell tumor (hematoxylin and eosin, magnification 60X). Histologic section shows the open chromatin pattern and nucleoli present in the osteoclast-like giant cells and adjacent mononuclear cells. Fibroblasts are also present in the background.

Multicentric Giant Cell Tumor

Multicentric giant cell tumor, also known as synchronous giant cell tumor, is an extremely rare subset of the disease process. Comprising less than 1% of all giant cell tumors, case reports of multicentric giant cell tumor involve the discovery of synchronous disease or multiple lesions believed to have developed in close temporal association with one another. Reports suggest that as opposed to the more common solitary presentation of GCTB, which demonstrates higher female-to-male ratio as well as the more common presentation in location such as the knee and distal radius, cases of multicentric giant cell tumor commonly involve the short bones of the hands and feet and have a higher incidence in males.[6] Treatment of this diagnosis is similar to that of a solitary GCTB, using surgery and adjuvant therapies to address the symptomatic lesions. Serum calcium, phosphate, and parathyroid hormone evaluation should be obtained to rule out brown tumors of hyperparathyroidism.[7]

Surgical Treatment

The management of GCTB has evolved considerably over the past three decades. Treatment initially was simple curettage of the cavitary lesion with filling of the defect. This method provided suboptimal results with high local recurrence rates; therefore, the intensity of local treatment was increased. Historically, wide en bloc resections, a seemingly aggressive surgical approach for benign disease, were common and maintained published local recurrence rates as low as 5%.[8] Currently, en bloc wide resection of giant cell tumor is generally reserved for recurrent disease or in the setting of intra-articular pathologic fracture.

Subsequently, extended intralesional curettage was performed, which involves the use of a high-speed burr to remove tumor beyond the area of curettage. Visualization of the entire defect through a cortical fenestration optimizes the opportunity for complete removal (**Figure 8**). See chapter 14 for a more detailed description of this technique. With this added mechanical ad-

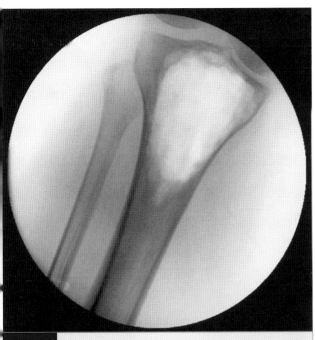

Figure 8 Intraoperative fluoroscopic image after aggressive curretting. Note the extent of affected area is larger than seen in preoperative images (**Figure 3**), as the margins of the tumor are extended to an area beyond grossly involved bone; hence, the description extended intralesional curettage.

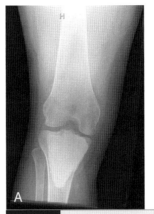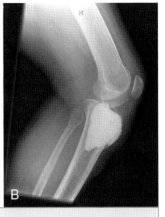

Figure 9 Postoperative AP (**A**) and lateral (**B**) radiographs of the knee demonstrating fill of bone void with polymethyl methacrylate, providing mechanical support to articular surface and thermal (heat) adjuvant therapy to surrounding bone.

junct, there appeared to be improvement in local recurrence; however, an unacceptably high rate of local recurrence remained. Although en bloc resections could be performed in these recalcitrant cases,[8] patients would then be subject to the subsequent series of complications, revisions, and activity restrictions inherent in megaprosthetic or allograft limb reconstructions.

The challenge of adequate local disease control and distaste for large resections in this patient population ushered in the era of adjuvant treatments, which broadly fall under the categories of thermal and chemical adjuvants. The idea behind the cavitary adjuvants, whether thermal or chemical, is that the zone of tumor kill is extended beyond what has been structurally removed, thereby providing a few extra millimeters of bone that are now tumor free without removal of the trabeculae or cortex (the structural elements), but rendering the tumor cells nonviable. Extended intralesional curettage with adjuvants is now the most common treatment of GCTB, with a local recurrence rate of 6% to 25%.[9-11]

Thermal adjuvants are often used on the tumor cavity following removal of all gross tumor. Initially, freezing with liquid nitrogen poured directly into tumor cavities was performed. Although this method led to a substantial reduction of the rate of local recurrence, it also created secondary complications of osteonecrosis and fracture, which necessitated additional stabilization of the construct. The relatively uncontrolled extension

of the freeze zone with the pour technique was improved with the more recent utilization of thermal probes with considerably more control of the cooling mechanism and intraoperative ease of use.

Heat as an adjuvant has been evaluated primarily with two mechanisms: the heat resulting from polymerization of polymethyl methacrylate (PMMA) or heat from cauterization from argon beam coagulation. PMMA is advantageous because it provides not only a thermal adjuvant, but also a structural fill to the cavity that ideally allows for earlier weight bearing (**Figures 9** and **10**). An additional benefit of PMMA compared with bone grafting is the improved identification of recurrences. The remodeling associated with bone graft integration can lead to difficulties in image interpretation when looking for local recurrences (**Figures 11** and **12**).

Argon beam coagulation is a temperature-variable modality that uses high-frequency energy to produce tissue desiccation and subsequent protein coagulation. The energy is delivered via an applicator, and the depth of tissue treatment is both wattage and time dependent. Argon beam coagulation has been reported in the surgical management of GCTB utilized in conjunction with PMMA.[12]

Chemical adjuvants such as phenol (carbolic acid) historically have been readily available and determined to be an appropriate locally cytotoxic agent. However, concerns regarding potential systemic and host toxicity of phenol led to the exploration of other chemical adjuvants such as ethanol and hydrogen peroxide.[10,11]

No randomized controlled studies exist that discuss the utilization of any of the adjuvants in comparison with extended curettage, and study results reporting on the efficacy of adjuvants have been inconsistent, with some studies suggesting an improvement in local control[9,13] and others suggesting no difference.[14-16]

Despite a relatively acceptable local control rate[1,9,17] in the extremities with current mechanical and adju-

2: Benign Bone Tumors

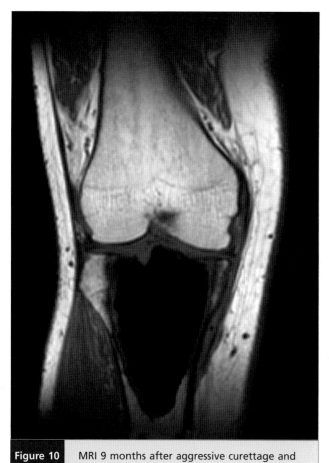

Figure 10   MRI 9 months after aggressive curettage and cementation. The patient presented with new reports of pain. Note the apparent recurrence of disease at the subchondral border of the proximal tibia.

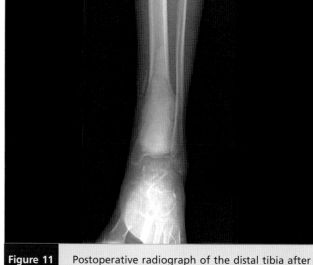

Figure 11   Postoperative radiograph of the distal tibia after aggressive curetting, adjuvant intraoperative phenol, and particulate bone allograft.

vant treatment, several problems remain in the management of giant cell tumor. Difficult anatomic locations where harsh adjuvants would be in proximity with critical structures, such as the spine and sacrum, made utilization of adjuvants difficult.[16] Reports on the use of serial embolization showed reasonable control rates in these areas.[18-20] Radiotherapy has been used and is efficacious,[21,22] but early reports of malignant transformation of radiated giant cell tumors have caused radiotherapy to be a last-resort treatment. Although contemporary radiotherapeutic techniques for the treatment of giant cell tumor can reduce or remove the concern about malignancy of radiated giant cell tumors, the advent of effective medical therapy has decreased the indications for radiotherapy.

Systemic Treatment

Adjuvant medical management of giant cell tumors has been attempted on a variety of levels and expands with the advent of new medications and the understanding of signaling pathways. Early recognition of inhibitors of angiogenesis, such as interferon alfa-2b, have led to

a small series of successful treatments with the medication being reported,[23-25] primarily in areas difficult to access surgically.

Bisphosphonates, used either systemically or as a local adjuvant (when placed in local media such as PMMA) have been reported in the treatment of GCTB in the adjuvant or recurrent setting. These drugs, including pamidronate and zoledronate, induce apoptosis and inhibit osteoclast function. Local recurrences as low as 4% are reported both in systemic and local adjuvant applications; this modality has been applied primarily when further local control techniques are challenging or impossible in locations such as the pelvis or spine.[13,26-29]

Denosumab, a fully human monoclonal antibody and a RANKL inhibitor, has enjoyed great success in the management of bone metastatic disease and in a short time radically changed the options for unresectable GCTB, or disease where resection would leave significant functional deficit. A recent phase II clinical trial evaluating the efficacy and toxicity of denosumab resulted in a significant reduction of tumor size and near-complete disappearance of giant cells from pathologic specimens, replacing them with increasing amounts of densely woven new bone.[30,31]

In a recently published phase II study of 282 patients with GCTB, denosumab was studied in three groups of patients: unresectable GCTB, resectable GCTB but with severe mobidity, or those previously treated with denosumab from a prior study. Ninety-six percent of patients with unresectable disease had no further progression, with a median follow-up of 13 months. Of the patients with resectable disease but with severe morbidity likely from potential resection, 74% were able to defer surgery and 62% were able to undergo surgery of a lesser magnitude at a median 9 months follow-up.[32] Results from this study with longer follow-up are eagerly anticipated, but based on the available data from this and other preliminary reports, FDA clearance for denosumab in the treatment of GCTB was given in June 2013. Denosumab is administered as a monthly injection. It is well tolerated and has few toxicities. As with bisphosphonates, denosumab has been associated with osteonecrosis of the jaw, and patients who are considered for this treatment should have dental examinations and any necessary dental remedial treatment before therapy begins.[33] The optimal duration of therapy and the timing of surgery with neoadjuvant denosumab have yet to be determined.

The plethora of treatment options now available for GCTB can lead to some confusion in decision making. The National Comprehensive Cancer Network recently published evidence-based and consensus-based guidelines for the evaluation, treatment, and surveillance of GCTB.[34] Initial imaging should include the local site as well as the chest (**Figure 13**). Treatment is generally surgical if possible, using a chemical or thermal adjuvant. Denosumab therapy or other management strategies as needed should be considered if the lesion is unresectable, or if anticipated surgical resection results in excessive morbidity that includes joint sacrifice (**Figure 14**).

Local Recurrence

Recurrence following treatment for giant cell tumor can be anticipated at a rate from 4% to 30%, given

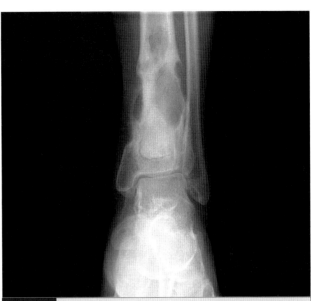

Figure 12 Radiograph of the distal tibia after recurrence of giant cell tumor, managed initially with intracavitary treatment and bone graft. After diagnosis of recurrence, the patient was treated medically with systemic denosumab. The patient was ambulating without an assistive device and with minimal pain.

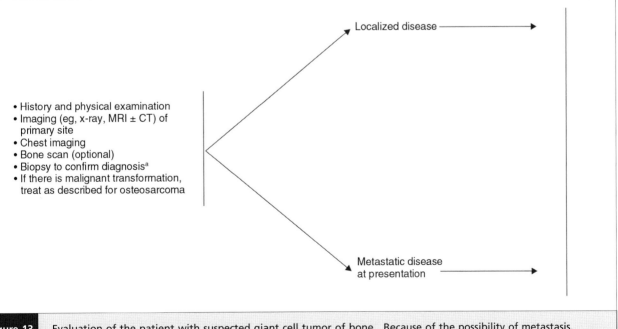

Localized disease ──────────►

- History and physical examination
- Imaging (eg, x-ray, MRI ± CT) of primary site
- Chest imaging
- Bone scan (optional)
- Biopsy to confirm diagnosis[a]
- If there is malignant transformation, treat as described for osteosarcoma

Metastatic disease at presentation ──────────►

Figure 13 Evaluation of the patient with suspected giant cell tumor of bone. Because of the possibility of metastasis, imaging of both local site and chest should be performed. Bone scan is relatively uninformative. [a]Brown tumor of hyperparathyrodism should be considered as a differential diagnosis. (Adapted with permission from Biermann JS, Adkins DR, Agulnik M, et al: Bone cancer. *J Natl Compr Canc Netw* 2013;11:688-723.)

2: Benign Bone Tumors

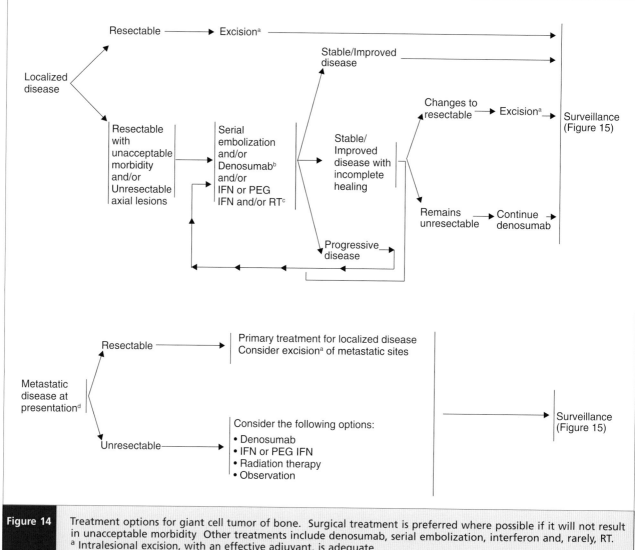

Figure 14	Treatment options for giant cell tumor of bone. Surgical treatment is preferred where possible if it will not result in unacceptable morbidity Other treatments include denosumab, serial embolization, interferon and, rarely, RT. [a] Intralesional excision, with an effective adjuvant, is adequate. [b] Denosumab should be continued until disease progression in responding patients. [c] Radiation therapy has been associated with increased risk of malignant transformation. [d] Treatment of primary tumor is as described for local disease. IFN = interferon; PEG = pegylated; RT = radiation therapy. (Adapted with permission from Biermann JS, Adkins DR, Agulnik M, et al: Bone Cancer. *J Natl Compr Canc Netw* 2013;11:688-723.)

modern treatment modalities of surgery and the use of local adjuvants.[35] The risk of recurrence is highest in the first 24 months after treatment, and often is detected because of changes in the radiographic evaluation of the surgical site. Locally recurrent disease can be visualized in both the bone and soft tissues around the primary site of disease. Surveillance using plain radiographs, CT, and MRI, similar to screening for the local recurrence of malignant tumors, should be conducted, as well as interval chest imaging[33] (**Figure 15**). Surveillance visits should include physical examination of the surgical site. Interpretation of plain films should include the evaluation of consolidation of bone graft if present, stability of polymethyl methacrylate, and/or fixation, presence of fracture, and assessment of any increased lucency. If MRI is obtained, areas of new soft tissue mass or or increased contrast enhancement are suspicious for recurrent disease. Many local recurrences in the setting of an initial intralesional surgery with adjuvants can be treated successfully with repeat intralesional surgery.[36] Failure of local control could result from inability to sufficiently treat the entire tumor cavity. Additionally, the risk of local recurrence seems to be higher with specific locations within the skeleton. GCTB in the proximal femur, distal radius, and small bones of the wrist and feet all have a reported higher risk of local recurrence compared to sites about the knee.[37] This is often attributed to the difficulty with adequate exposure and access to these sites with intralesional approaches. The recurrent disease often will be discovered as a smaller portion of its initial presentation, thereby lending itself to potentially more focused

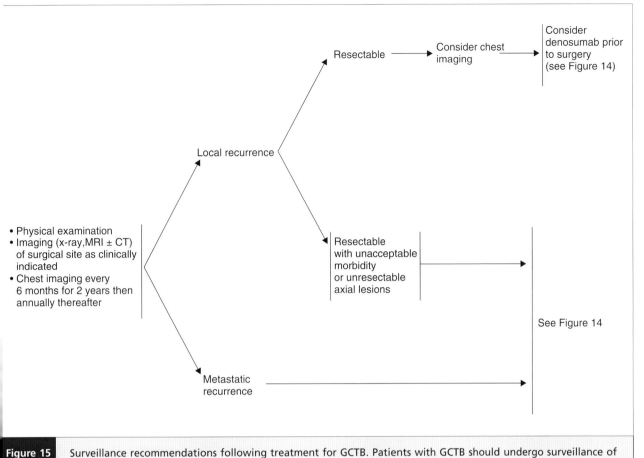

Figure 15 Surveillance recommendations following treatment for GCTB. Patients with GCTB should undergo surveillance of both the local site and chest following treatment, because local relapse is not uncommon and chest metastases can occur. (Adapted with permission from Biermann JS, Adkins DR, Agulnik M, et al: Bone Cancer. *J Natl Compr Canc Netw* 2013;11:688-723.)

intralesional surgery and adjuvant therapy. En bloc resection following local recurrence is becoming less common because of the possibility that denosumab or other systemic treatment will facilitate less aggressive surgery[31,38] (**Figures 11, 12,** and **16**). Poor prognostic indicators for functional preservation include recurrent subchondral disease, pathologic fracture, and malignant degeneration.

Metastasis From GCTB

GCTB, although a benign neoplasm, has a known ability for the development of pulmonary metastases (**Figure 17**). The term benign metastasizing tumor may at first appear contradictory; however, several series indicate a rate of metastases of approximately 2% to 4%. The appearance of chest metastasis is often associated with recurrent disease.[1,35] Some have speculated a correlation between p53 expression and the development of pulmonary disease. The pulmonary metastases are histologically identical to the primary bone lesion,[39-42] classically displaying numerous large multinucleated osteoclast-like giant cells with interspersed mononuclear cells demonstrating similar nuclear features in

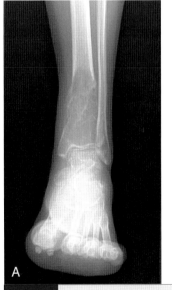
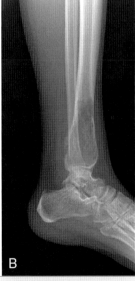

Figure 16 AP (**A**) and lateral (**B**) radiographs of giant cell tumor of bone diagnosed during pregnancy of a 28-year-old woman. Note the pseudotrabeculation of the bone.

2: Benign Bone Tumors

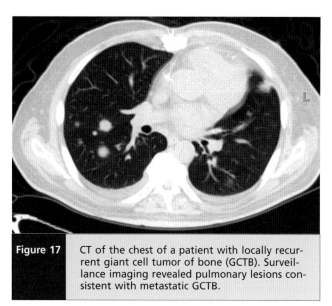

Figure 17 CT of the chest of a patient with locally recurrent giant cell tumor of bone (GCTB). Surveillance imaging revealed pulmonary lesions consistent with metastatic GCTB.

both cell types. There have been reports of other benign tumors that demonstrate histologically "benign" metastases such as leiomyoma, pleomorphic adenoma, solitary fibrous tumor, and meningioma.[43-46]

Clinically, the behavior of a pulmonary metastasis from a benign GCTB can be unpredictable; some metastatic GCTB lesions grow with a slow, indolent course and are successfully treated with surgical resection; in others, the lesion can stop growing spontaneously, and in still others there is aggressive growth with subsequent pulmonary compromise.[47] Metastasis is almost always exclusively to the lungs. Treatment of metastatic disease is often dictated by several factors such as the number of metastatic foci, resectability of the lesions, and patient performance status. Limited metastasis can readily be treated with pulmonary metastasectomy, whereas numerous lesions may rule out surgery and thus favor systemic therapies. Researchers have previously used interferon for the treatment of unresectable disease on the basis that embolization of pelvic lesions has been curative. This finding implies that limiting the blood supply to these lesions can be an effective treatment option. Interferon is capable of inhibiting both basic fibroblast growth factor receptor and vascular endothelial growth factor receptors. Unfortunately, tolerance to interferon can be difficult because of the many associated side effects. Denosumab is likely to play a significant role in the management of pulmonary metastases from GCTB;[48] however, more data will be needed to identify optimal management of these patients.

Malignancy in GCTB

Giant cell tumors can, on rare occasions, be malignant, either degenerating from a previously benign tumor or arising de novo as a malignant tumor.[49,50] On occasion primary malignancy in GCTB is seen where an area of

highly pleomorphic cells are present in an otherwise conventional giant cell tumor of bone, or secondary malignant transformation to an undifferentiated sarcoma is identified in a pre-existing giant cell tumor. Diagnosis of malignant transformation relies on overt malignant cytological features and presence of atypical mitotic figures, because necrosis and mitoses are seen in the usual benign GCTB[51] as well as lymph-vascular invasion. Reportedly, in a case of recurrent giant cell tumor of bone with malignant transformation, pulmonary metastases were present but the metastases were histologically benign, nontransformed.[51] Given these findings, histologically benign-appearing giant cell tumor metastases may arise from a primary lesion of either histologically benign or malignant appearance.

Treatment of malignant GCTB generally follows that of osteosarcomas (Figure 13), although the rarity of this entity precludes definitive recommendations regarding its management.

Summary

GCTB is a benign but relatively aggressive bone tumor, with a rare potential to metastasize. Thermal or chemical adjuvants are often used in conjunction with intralesional removal. Although surgery is the mainstay of treatment of localized GCTB, it is no longer the sole treatment option. The use of systemic adjuvant therapies has allowed for less morbid procedures in areas difficult to resect and nonsurgical treatment strategies in selected patients. The availability of medical therapy has created new therapeutic options, either as standalone treatment or in concert with procedural modalities.

Acknowledgment

The authors of this article would like to acknowledge the contributions of Evita Henderson-Jackson, MD (Pathology) and Tony Conley, MD (Medical Oncology).

Annotated References

1. Niu X, Zhang Q, Hao L, et al: Giant cell tumor of the extremity: Retrospective analysis of 621 Chinese patients from one institution. *J Bone Joint Surg Am* 2012;94(5):461-467.

   Metastatic disease developed from benign giant cell tumor has been documented at a rate ranging from 2% to 9%. Most metastases are to the lungs, but metastases to the endobronchium, lymph nodes, bone, skin, scalp, calf muscles, brain, liver, adrenal glands, kidneys, and breast have been reported.

2. Errani C, Ruggieri P, Asenzio MA, et al: Giant cell tumor of the extremity: A review of 349 cases from a single institution. *Cancer Treat Rev* 2010;36(1):1-7.

   The results of this study suggest that an aggressive curettage reduces the recurrence rate. Special attention must be given to giant cell tumors not only in the distal radius, but also in the proximal femur, where the treatment is associated with a higher rate of local recurrence.

3. Boriani S, Bandiera S, Casadei R, et al: Giant cell tumor of the mobile spine: A review of 49 cases. *Spine (Phila Pa 1976)* 2012;37(1):E37-E45.

 A retrospective analysis of giant cell tumors of the mobile spine was performed. Age younger than 25 years was associated with a worse relapse-free survival (*P* = 0.03). En bloc resection was associated with better local control with Enneking stage III tumors (*P* = 0.01)

4. Murphey MD, Nomikos GC, Flemming DJ, Gannon FH, Temple HT, Kransdorf MJ: From the archives of AFIP: Imaging of giant cell tumor and giant cell reparative granuloma of bone. Radiologic-pathologic correlation. *Radiographics* 2001;21(5):1283-1309.

5. Kim Y, Nizami S, Goto H, Lee FY: Modern interpretation of giant cell tumor of bone: Predominantly osteoclastogenic stromal tumor. *Clin Orthop Surg* 2012; 4(2):107-116.

 The modern interpretation of giant cell tumor is predominantly osteoclastogenic stromal cell tumors of mesenchymal origin. An array of inflammatory cytokines and chemokines disrupts osteoblastic differentiation and promotes excessive osteoclastic cells. Recombinant RANK-Fc protein and bisphosphonates are currently being tried for giant cell tumor treatment in addition to surgical excision and conventional topical adjuvant therapies.

6. Novais EN, Shin AY, Bishop AT, Shives TC: Multicentric giant cell tumor of the upper extremities: 16 years of ongoing disease. *J Hand Surg Am* 2011; 36(10):1610-1613.

 A case report of a 13-year-old patient with multicentric giant cell tumor is presented. Over 16 years, giant cell tumors occurred in eight separate sites, including the distal radius, lunate, middle metacarpal, ring finger, proximal phalanx, radial head, distal humerus, and proximal humerus.

7. Werner M: Giant cell tumour of bone: Morphological, biological and histogenetical aspects. *Int Orthop* 2006; 30(6):484-489.

8. Yu XC, Xu M, Song RX, Fu ZH, Liu XP: Long-term outcome of giant cell tumors of bone around the knee treated by en bloc resection of tumor and reconstruction with prosthesis. *Orthop Surg* 2010;2(3):211-217.

 Nineteen patients (11 men, 8 women, average age 35.4 years) were treated with en bloc resection and reconstruction. En bloc resection and reconstruction with prosthesis is a feasible method for treating giant cell tumor of bone around the knee. Complications related to the prosthesis, mainly prosthesis loosening and limb shortening, increased gradually with longer survival time.

9. Becker WT, Dohle J, Bernd L, et al; Arbeitsgemeinschaft Knochentumoren: Local recurrence of giant cell tumor of bone after intralesional treatment with and without adjuvant therapy. *J Bone Joint Surg Am* 2008; 90(5):1060-1067.

 The overall recurrence rate after the intralesional procedures was 49% when no adjuvants had been used, 22% when polymethyl methacrylate only had been used as an adjuvant, 27% when polymethyl methacrylate had been used after phenolization, and 15% when phenol or other local toxins had been used.

10. Lin WH, Lan TY, Chen CY, Wu K, Yang RS: Similar local control between phenol- and ethanol-treated giant cell tumors of bone. *Clin Orthop Relat Res* 2011; 469(11):3200-3208.

 Local recurrence rates were similar in two groups of patients treated with intralesional surgery and a chemical adjuvant: 11% in the ethanol group and 12% in the phenol group. The survival curves (using local recurrence as an end point) of the two groups were similar.

11. Algawahmed H, Turcotte R, Farrokhyar F, Ghert M: High-speed burring with and without the use of surgical adjuvants in the intralesional management of giant cell tumor of bone: A systematic review and meta-analysis. *Sarcoma* 2010;2010.

 In a meta-analysis of six studies and 387 patients, improved local control with the use of surgical adjuvants was not observed. Given the available data, this study suggests that surgical adjuvants are not required when meticulous tumor removal is performed.

12. Lewis VO, Wei A, Mendoza T, Primus F, Peabody T, Simon MA: Argon beam coagulation as an adjuvant for local control of giant cell tumor. *Clin Orthop Relat Res* 2007;454(454):192-197.

13. Balke M, Campanacci L, Gebert C, et al: Bisphosphonate treatment of aggressive primary, recurrent and metastatic giant cell tumour of bone. *BMC Cancer* 2010;10:462.

 Bisphosphonates are antiresorptive drugs that act mainly on osteoclasts. Findings suggest that bisphosphonates could be useful in controlling disease progression in GCTB and that these agents directly inhibit GCTB-derived osteoclast resorption.

14. Trieb K, Bitzan P, Lang S, Dominkus M, Kotz R: Recurrence of curetted and bone-grafted giant-cell tumours with and without adjuvant phenol therapy. *Eur J Surg Oncol* 2001;27(2):200-202.

15. Turcotte RE, Wunder JS, Isler MH, et al; Canadian Sarcoma Group: Giant cell tumor of long bone: A Canadian Sarcoma Group study. *Clin Orthop Relat Res* 2002;397:248-258.

16. Ruggieri P, Mavrogenis AF, Ussia G, Angelini A, Papagelopoulos PJ, Mercuri M: Recurrence after and complications associated with adjuvant treatments for sacral giant cell tumor. *Clin Orthop Relat Res* 2010; 468(11):2954-2961.

2: Benign Bone Tumors

Thirty-one patients with giant cell tumor of the sacrum underwent intralesional management. Forty-eight percent had one or more complications, including wound healing, intraoperative hemodynamic instability due to massive intraoperative hemorrhage, sacral nerve root deficits, and death. The use of intraoperative adjuvants did not change the local recurrence rate (10%) in this small sample. Level of evidence: IV.

17. Klenke FM, Wenger DE, Inwards CY, Rose PS, Sim FH: Giant cell tumor of bone: Risk factors for recurrence. *Clin Orthop Relat Res* 2011;469(2):591-599.

Wide resection had a lower recurrence rate than intralesional surgery (5% versus 25%). Pulmonary metastases occurred in 4%. Multidisciplinary treatment including wedge resection, chemotherapy, and radiotherapy achieved disease-free survival or stable disease in all of these patients.

18. Emori M, Kaya M, Sasaki M, Wada T, Yamaguchi T, Yamashita T: Pre-operative selective arterial embolization as a neoadjuvant therapy for proximal humerus giant cell tumor of bone: Radiological and histological evaluation. *Jpn J Clin Oncol* 2012;42(9):851-855.

Selective arterial embolization was used as precursor to intralesional management of a periarticular proximal humeral GCTB. Histologic examination of the specimen revealed massive fibrosis and remodeling of destroyed bone. The authors advocated a role for preoperative arterial embolization in selected cases of GCTB. Level of evidence: V.

19. Onishi H, Kaya M, Wada T, Nagoya S, Sasaki M, Yamashita T: Giant cell tumor of the sacrum treated with selective arterial embolization. *Int J Clin Oncol* 2010; 15(4):416-419.

The authors reported successful treatment of giant cell tumor of the sacrum in a 58-year-old woman with a series of five arterial embolizations at 5-week intervals. At 28 months follow-up she had returned to normal activity with radiographic improvement noted. Level of evidence: V.

20. Hosalkar HS, Jones KJ, King JJ, Lackman RD: Serial arterial embolization for large sacral giant-cell tumors: Mid- to long-term results. *Spine (Phila Pa 1976)* 2007; 32(10):1107-1115.

Nine patients with sacral giant cell tumor of bone were treated with serial embolizations at 6-week intervals with a median followup of 7.8 years. Seven of nine patients had successful local control. Level of evidence: IV.

21. Ruka W, Rutkowski P, Morysiński T, et al: The megavoltage radiation therapy in treatment of patients with advanced or difficult giant cell tumors of bone. *Int J Radiat Oncol Biol Phys* 2010;78(2):494-498.

Seventy-seven patients with giant cell tumor of bone deemed to be inappropriate candidates for surgery were treated with megavoltage radiation (range, 26 to 89 Gy) in a single center. Local control was achieved with 84%. Three patients developed lung metastases and malignant transformation of the tumor occurred in two patients. Level of evidence: IV.

22. Bhatia S, Miszczyk L, Roelandts M, et al: Radiotherapy for marginally resected, unresectable or recurrent giant cell tumor of the bone: A rare cancer network study. *Rare Tumors* 2011;3(4):e48.

In this multicenter study, 58 patients were treated with a median 50-Gy radiation dose for unresectable or marginally resected giant cell tumor of bone. Five-year local control was 85% with a median follow-up of 8 years. There were no reported cases of malignant transformation, although one patient developed a uterine carcinoma in the radiation field. No patient experience grade 3 or higher toxicity. The authors conclude radiotherapy for GCTB can provide excellent local control of incompletely resected, unresectable or recurrent GCTB with acceptable morbidity.

23. Kaban LB, Troulis MJ, Ebb D, August M, Hornicek FJ, Dodson TB: Antiangiogenic therapy with interferon alpha for giant cell lesions of the jaws. *J Oral Maxillofac Surg* 2002;60(10):1103-1111, discussion 1111-1113.

24. Wei F, Liu X, Liu Z, et al: Interferon alfa-2b for recurrent and metastatic giant cell tumor of the spine: Report of two cases. *Spine (Phila Pa 1976)* 2010;35(24): E1418-E1422.

Two patients with giant cell tumor arising in bone but with multiple sites of disease were treated with interferon alfa-2B for 3 years each. There were no complications related to interferon use, and the lesions disappeared or regressed significantly. Level of evidence: V.

25. Kaiser U, Neumann K, Havemann K: Generalised giant-cell tumour of bone: Successful treatment of pulmonary metastases with interferon alpha, a case report. *J Cancer Res Clin Oncol* 1993;119(5):301-303.

26. Tse LF, Wong KC, Kumta SM, Huang L, Chow TC, Griffith JF: Bisphosphonates reduce local recurrence in extremity giant cell tumor of bone: A case-control study. *Bone* 2008;42(1):68-73.

A retrospective case-control study was performed in which intravenous and oral bisphosphonates were given perioperatively along with surgical intervention. Clinical use of bisphosphonates as an adjuvant therapy for giant cell tumor of bone demonstrated a lower local recurrence rate.

27. Zwolak P, Manivel JC, Jasinski P, et al: Cytotoxic effect of zoledronic acid-loaded bone cement on giant cell tumor, multiple myeloma, and renal cell carcinoma cell lines. *J Bone Joint Surg Am* 2010;92(1):162-168.

Zoledronic acid is released from bone cement, remains biologically active despite the polymerization of cement, and inhibits the in vitro growth of cell lines from giant cell tumor of bone, myeloma, and renal cell carcinoma.

28. Nishisho T, Hanaoka N, Endo K, Takahashi M, Yasui N: Locally administered zoledronic acid therapy for giant cell tumor of bone. *Orthopedics* 2011;34(7):e312-e315.

The first report of local administration of bisphosphonates for the treatment of giant cell tumor of bone is presented. Eighteen months after curettage, the patient had regained full range of motion and good function of the knee, and radiographs at 18 months after curettage revealed no recurrence of GCTB.

29. Lau CP, Huang L, Tsui SK, Ng PK, Leung PY, Kumta SM: Pamidronate, farnesyl transferase, and geranylgeranyl transferase-I inhibitors affects cell proliferation, apoptosis, and OPG/RANKL mRNA expression in stromal cells of giant cell tumor of bone. *J Orthop Res* 2011;29(3):403-413.

30. Branstetter DG, Nelson SD, Manivel JC, et al: Denosumab induces tumor reduction and bone formation in patients with giant-cell tumor of bone. *Clin Cancer Res* 2012;18(16):4415-4424.

     Denosumab treatment in patients with GCTB significantly reduced or eliminated RANK-positive tumor giant cells. In on-study samples from 20 of 20 patients (100%), a decrease of 90% or more in tumor giant cells and a reduction in tumor stromal cells were observed.

31. Thomas D, Henshaw R, Skubitz K, et al: Denosumab in patients with giant-cell tumour of bone: An open-label, phase 2 study. *Lancet Oncol* 2010;11(3):275-280.

     Thirty-seven patients with recurrent or unresectable giant cell tumor were enrolled and received subcutaneous denosumab 120 mg monthly. Thirty of 35 evaluable patients had a tumor response. Adverse events were reported in 33 of 37 patients; the most common were pain in an extremity, back pain, and headache.

32. Chawla S, Henshaw R, Seeger L, et al: Safety and efficacy of denosumab for adults and skeletally mature adolescents with giant cell tumour of bone: Interim analysis of an open-label, parallel-group, phase 2 study. *Lancet Oncol* 2013;14(9):901-908.

     In this phase 2 study of 282 patients with GCTB, authors reported 96% (163 of 169) patients with unresectable GCT had no disease progression, and 74% of patients (74/100) whose tumor had been identified as requiring severely morbid surgery to control were able to defer surgery; 62 of these were later able to undergo surgeries of a lesser magnitude. This was an interim report with relatively short follow-up.

33. Kyrgidis A, Tzellos TG, Toulis K, Arora A, Kouvelas D, Triaridis S: An evidence-based review of risk-reductive strategies for osteonecrosis of the jaws among cancer patients. *Curr Clin Pharmacol* 2013; 8(2):124-134.

34. Biermann JS, Adkins DR, Agulnik M, et al: Bone cancer. *J Natl Compr Canc Netw* 2013;11(6):688-723.

35. Kremen TJ Jr, Bernthal NM, Eckardt MA, Eckardt JJ: Giant cell tumor of bone: Are we stratifying results appropriately? *Clin Orthop Relat Res* 2012;470(3):677-683.

     A retrospective review of 230 patients is presented. The incidence of local recurrence among patients undergoing intralesional curettage (12%) was greater than in those undergoing resection (2%). The incidence of local recurrence among primary tumors was 9%, whereas the incidence of local recurrence after treatment of recurrent lesions was 16%.

36. Klenke FM, Wenger DE, Inwards CY, Rose PS, Sim FH: Recurrent giant cell tumor of long bones: Analysis of surgical management. *Clin Orthop Relat Res* 2011; 469(4):1181-1187.

     The rate of rerecurrence after wide resection was 6%. Intralesional curettage showed an overall rerecurrence rate of 32%. Implantation of PMMA instead of bone grafting was associated with a lower risk of subsequent recurrence in intralesional procedures (14% versus 50%). Extracompartmental disease did not increase the risk of rerecurrence. Pulmonary metastases occurred in seven patients and appeared independent of the surgical treatment.

37. Cho HS, Park IH, Han I, Kang SC, Kim HS: Giant cell tumor of the femoral head and neck: Result of intralesional curettage. *Arch Orthop Trauma Surg* 2010; 130(11):1329-1333.

     Although the recurrence rate of the current study was rather high (41.7%, in 5 of 12 hips), 9 of 12 native hips (75%) were preserved at last follow-up, including 2 hips that underwent repeat curettage. Functional outcomes of the preserved hips were satisfactory.

38. Thomas DM, Skubitz KM: Giant cell tumour of bone. *Curr Opin Oncol* 2009;21(4):338-344.

     Recent discoveries have identified a key role for the osteoclast differentiation factor (RANKL), in the genesis of giant cell tumor. Denosumab presents a new treatment option for patients with previously untreatable giant cell tumor.

39. Rock MG, Pritchard DJ, Unni KK: Metastases from histologically benign giant-cell tumor of bone. *J Bone Joint Surg Am* 1984;66(2):269-274.

     The authors present a review of eight cases of benign GCTB and the histologic review of known metastatic lesions. They report that the lungs are the principle site of metastasis, and appear to be pathologically indistinguishable from the primary tumor.

40. Bertoni F, Present D, Sudanese A, Baldini N, Bacchini P, Campanacci M: Giant-cell tumor of bone with pulmonary metastases: Six case reports and a review of the literature. *Clin Orthop Relat Res* 1988;237:275-285.

     The authors report on 6 cases of giant cell tumor of bone with pulmonary metastasis. After review of the histopathology, 3 of the six metastatic cases were identified with histologically benign lesions.

41. Kay RM, Eckardt JJ, Seeger LL, Mirra JM, Hak DJ: Pulmonary metastasis of benign giant cell tumor of bone: Six histologically confirmed cases, including one of spontaneous regression. *Clin Orthop Relat Res* 1994;302:219-230.

     The authors reported a metastatic rate of 9.1% in a series encompassing 14 years, of benign GCTB.

42. Tubbs WS, Brown LR, Beabout JW, Rock MG, Unni KK: Benign giant-cell tumor of bone with pulmonary metastases: Clinical findings and radiologic appearance of metastases in 13 cases. *AJR Am J Roentgenol* 1992;158(2):331-334.

    The authors emphasized the potential for histologically benign pulmonary metastasis in GCTB. In this series of 13 cases, pulmonary disease was discovered from 3.8 to 10.7 years after diagnosis of the GCTB.

43. Rodríguez-Fernández J, Mateos-Micas M, Martínez-Tello FJ, et al: Metastatic benign pleomorphic adenoma: Report of a case and review of the literature. *Med Oral Patol Oral Cir Bucal* 2008;13(3):E193-E196.

    This is an illustrative case of a histologically benign neoplasm of the salivary glands that has given rise to a metastatic lesion, showing histopathology similar to the primary lesion.

44. Sasaki H, Kurihara T, Katsuoka Y, et al: Distant metastasis from benign solitary fibrous tumor of the kidney. *Case Rep Nephrol Urol* 2013;3(1):1-8.

    An illustrative case of a histologically benign neoplasm giving rise to a similarly histologically benign metastatic lesion.

45. Pramesh CS, Saklani AP, Pantvaidya GH, et al: Benign metastasizing meningioma. *Jpn J Clin Oncol* 2003;33(2):86-88.

46. Abramson S, Gilkeson RC, Goldstein JD, Woodard PK, Eisenberg R, Abramson N: Benign metastasizing leiomyoma: Clinical, imaging, and pathologic correlation. *AJR Am J Roentgenol* 2001;176(6):1409-1413.

    An illustrative case of a histologically benign neoplasm giving rise to a recurrent extrapleural location, successfully managed with wide resection.

47. Viswanathan S, Jambhekar NA: Metastatic giant cell tumor of bone: Are there associated factors and best treatment modalities? *Clin Orthop Relat Res* 2010;468(3):827-833.

    Distant metastases were identified in 24 of 470 patients with giant cell tumors during a 20-year period. Thirteen of the 24 patients had local recurrence before or at the time of metastasis. None of the patients died of their metastatic disease. Although the overall outcome was favorable, metastasectomy is recommended where feasible. Level of evidence: Level IV.

48. Karras NA, Polgreen LE, Ogilvie C, Manivel JC, Skubitz KM, Lipsitz E: Denosumab treatment of metastatic giant-cell tumor of bone in a 10-year-old girl. *J Clin Oncol* 2013;31(12):e200-e202.

49. Boriani S, Sudanese A, Baldini N, Picci P: Sarcomatous degeneration of giant cell tumours. *Ital J Orthop Traumatol* 1986;12(2):191-199.

50. Anract P, De Pinieux G, Cottias P, Pouillart P, Forest M, Tomeno B: Malignant giant-cell tumours of bone: Clinico-pathological types and prognosis. A review of 29 cases. *Int Orthop* 1998;22(1):19-26.

51. Miller IJ, Blank A, Yin SM, McNickle A, Gray R, Gitelis S: A case of recurrent giant cell tumor of bone with malignant transformation and benign pulmonary metastases. *Diagn Pathol* 2010;5:62.

    The authors emphasize the finding that histologically benign-appearing metastases arise from similar histologically benign primary GCTB.

Chapter 14

Surgical Treatment of Benign Bone Tumors

Bruce Rougraff, MD

Introduction

Although the diagnosis and radiographic evaluation of benign bone tumors has not changed significantly in the past 15 years, the surgical management of these lesions has evolved. Open curettage with autogenous bone graft was the most frequent surgical option for benign bone tumors for many years. Subsequently, open curettage and defect filling with polymethyl methacrylate (PMMA) bone cement became commonly used for the treatment of giant cell tumors of bone. Unicameral bone cyst (UBC) treatment has evolved from open curettage and grafting to injection techniques using steroids. More recently, injection with bone marrow and bone grafting materials has become increasingly used for cystic skeletal lesions. Radiofrequency ablation (RFA) was used initially for osteoid osteomas of bone, and its use has been expanded to include other lesions in skeletal sites where curettage is difficult, including eosinophilic granuloma, recurrent giant cell tumors, and chondroblastoma. Embolization of aneurysmal bone cysts (ABCs) is also an effective technique for lesions in difficult surgical locations such as the spine and pelvis. Increased availability of allograft bone and bone graft substitutes and recognition of their effectiveness in the treatment of contained benign skeletal defects has largely obviated the need for large autogenous grafts.

This chapter discusses the most recent findings and recommendations in the surgical treatment of benign bone tumors using open curettage, embolization, bone graft or bone marrow injection, RFA, and bone cement.

Observation

Many benign bone lesions are inactive, asymptomatic, and found only as an incidental radiographic finding.[1] These lesions include one third of UBCs that will resolve without treatment, nonossifying fibromas, en-

chondromas, and fibrous dysplasia. Clinical and radiographic follow-up is all that is typically needed. Reassurance based on a sound radiographic diagnosis can allow the patient to avoid unnecessary surgery and its complications.

Open Curettage

Open curettage of bone lesions is typically reserved for benign skeletal tumors. Malignant bone lesions and, occasionally, highly aggressive benign tumors can be treated with wide resection and allograft or endoprosthetic reconstruction.[2,3] Giant cell tumors with soft-tissue invasion can be treated successfully with extended curettage with high-speed burring and the addition of phenol and bone cement; local recurrence rates have been reported from 14% to 30%.[4] Intralesional curettage is performed in patients with giant cell tumor of bone, large nonossifying fibroma of bone, chondroblastoma, chondromyxoid fibroma, eosinophilic granuloma, ABC, painful enchondromas, osteoblastoma, desmoplastic fibroma of bone, reparative granuloma of bone, and other lesions. Intralesional curettage is a surgical procedure in which a longitudinal incision is made directly over the skeletal lesion. An oval window is created in the cortex, usually in the weakest portion of the bone directly over the lesion. Curets are used to remove the gross majority of the tumor, and then adjuvant treatment is typically used as well. Adjuvant treatment after curettage of the lesion is a high-speed mechanical burr, electrocautery, argon beam coagulation, phenol and alcohol irrigation, liquid nitrogen, and PMMA. Liquid nitrogen also can be used as an adjuvant but has a high postoperative fracture rate. Prophylactic fixation at the time of curettage has diminished this risk.

High-speed mechanical burring, sometimes referred to as extended curettage, has been shown to lower the risk of recurrence of ABCs and giant cell tumors of bone. The authors of a 1999 study showed that 90% of ABCs were successfully treated with open curettage and high-speed burring.[5] They did not add phenol, liquid nitrogen, PMMA, or argon beam coagulation. They also showed that younger patients with open growth

Dr. Rougraff or an immediate family member serves as a board member, owner, officer, or committee member of the American Academy of Orthopaedic Surgeons.

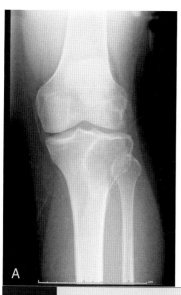
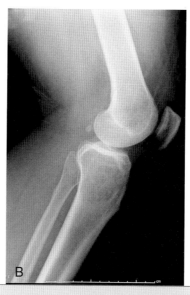
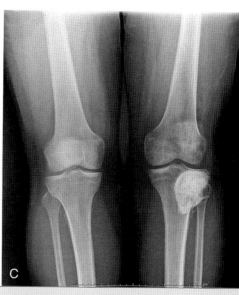

Figure 1 **A** and **B,** Plain radiographs of the knee of a 24-year-old man with severe left lateral knee pain that worsened with weight bearing. A lytic, destructive lesion of the lateral tibial epiphysis is highly suggestive of a benign giant cell tumor. Biopsy was diagnostic of giant cell tumor, and the lesion was treated with extended curettage and cementation. **C,** Three years postoperatively, the patient has no pain and no evidence of tumor recurrence.

plates had a higher recurrence rate. In a similar study in 2007, the authors found a correlation between risk of recurrence of ABCs and younger age (5 years or younger) as well as open growth plates.[6] They did not use high-speed burring but used PMMA in most patients and reported a higher recurrence rate (17%) than the authors of the previously mentioned study (10%).[5] This higher recurrence rate may be the result of not using high-speed burring, but no direct comparison has been made in a randomized fashion to determine whether burring is a better adjuvant than PMMA. In 2012, researchers studied a large cohort of 621 patients with giant cell tumor of bone and found that high-speed burring and curettage lowered the recurrence rate to 9% from the rate of 56% that was found when no burring was performed.[7] They also found no correlation with the type of bone grafting used, and they did not use other adjuvant treatments, including PMMA. It is generally recommended that all curettage procedures include the use of high-speed burring.

Methyl methacrylate polymerizes as an exothermic reaction, and this heat during surgery has been considered by many surgeons to be an adjuvant treatment, particularly in giant cell tumors of bone. However, this thermal effect on tumor control has been controversial. The authors of a 2011 study reported on series of 330 patients with giant cell tumor of bone in which 84 patients received PMMA and 246 patients did not.[8] The study consisted of retrospective and nonrandomized data. The authors reported a much lower risk of recurrence when cement was used (14% versus 30%; $P = 0.001$) and concluded that PMMA was an effective adjuvant in the treatment of giant cell tumors of bone. In contrast, the authors of a 2012 study published a meta-analysis of PMMA versus no PMMA in patients with giant cell tumors of the distal radius.[3] Patients with giant cell tumors of the distal radius are at highest risk for recurrence compared with patients with giant cell tumors of other skeletal sites. In the six studies (80 patients) that were evaluated, the use of cement versus no cement did not lower the recurrence rate of giant cell tumors in the distal radius (32% versus 30%, respectively). Whether the use of cement lowers the recurrence rate as a result of the exothermic reaction or whether a more extensive curettage is performed with the anticipation of an essentially limitless source of filling material has not been determined. Further studies are needed to answer this question. Despite some controversy, bone cement is commonly used to fill defects after curettage of giant cell tumors, recurrent chondroblastoma, and some ABCs.[4,9-11]

Recent studies have evaluated secondary arthritis as a late complication after the use of bone cement (Figure 1) for giant cell tumors of bone.[4,9-11] Although these studies varied in methodology, they concluded that degenerative changes are rare after bone cement filling for giant cell tumors and that the closer to the subchondral bone the cement is, or if irregularity of the subchondral bone is present postoperatively, the higher the risk of secondary arthritis.[12] This risk of secondary arthritis is similar to those for bone grafting of the defect without cement.

Argon beam coagulation is sometimes used as an adjuvant after extended curettage and burring are performed.[13] In 2010, researchers reported a retrospective, comparative study of 29 patients with ABCs and found no recurrences in the 17 patients who were treated with argon beam coagulation and 4 recurrences in the 12 patients who were treated with curettage only.[14] In

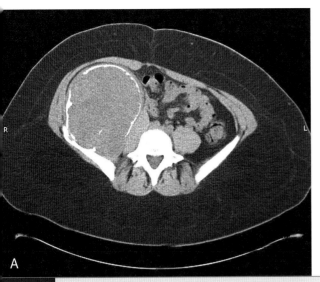
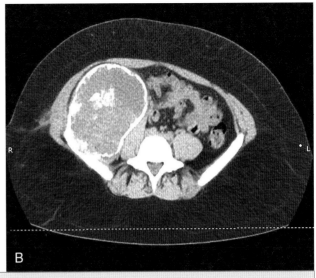

Figure 2   **A,** Pelvis CT scan shows an 18-year-old woman in whom hip pain developed 4 months after the delivery of her second child. The CT shows a large lesion of the inner table of the right iliac crest. Biopsy was consistent with a benign aneurysmal bone cyst. Because the lesion was highly vascular on biopsy, and because of the risk of significant blood loss, embolization of the lesion was performed. **B,** Four-month postembolization CT scan shows increased ossification of the outer shell of the cyst. Resection was performed. The patient remains pain free and disease free 2 years postoperatively.

2012, researchers reported a retrospective study of 93 benign bone tumors that were treated either with phenol or argon beam coagulation.[15] They found a comparable recurrence rate between the two techniques (17% versus 15%). Because argon beam coagulation has lower morbidity, they recommended it over phenol with alcohol extraction. The authors of a 2007 study[16] reported on 37 patients with giant cell tumors treated with argon beam coagulation, curettage, and cementation and found good functional results, a low recurrence rate (4 patients; 11%), and no cases of secondary arthritis at 6-year average follow-up. Their local recurrence rate is very similar to that of patients treated with curettage and cement without argon beam coagulation.[1,4,5,10] More prospective randomized studies need to be done to address the efficacy of argon beam coagulation in benign bone tumors, but these data support its use.

Phenol applied to the bone after extended curettage with burring and then cleansed with 96% ethanol has been used with benign bone tumors and low-grade chondrosarcoma.[15,17] Researchers in 2011 reported on a retrospective study of giant cell tumor comparing curettage and cement with phenol and ethanol to the same regimen without phenol, and found no difference when phenol was not used.[18] It appears that extended curettage and some other adjuvant, such as argon beam coagulation, phenol, or cement, help prevent recurrence in giant cell tumor of bone. It does not appear that multiple adjuvants improve recurrence rates further (that is, using two adjuvant treatments instead of only one would not be expected to lower the recurrence rate further).

Embolization

Embolization of bone lesions has most commonly been used for ABCs and metastatic bone lesions. Embolization of bone tumors can be used either to decrease hemorrhagic risks during surgery or to primarily treat lesions[19] (**Figure 2**). Particularly when the bone lesion is in a difficult anatomic area such as the cervical spine,[20] preoperative embolization and intralesional surgery can be highly successful. Agents used for embolization include particulate emboli, stainless steel or platinum coils, polyvinyl alcohol particles, microspheres, absolute alcohol, gelatin sponge, or liquid anabolic agents.[21] Selective embolization of ABCs is based on the premise that ABCs represent a vascular malformation that can be ablated by injection and that the bone lesion can then heal secondarily without surgical intervention. Embolization has been reported by several authors as a combined treatment with surgical curettage of lesions in the pelvis, thoracic cage, cervical spine, lumbar spine, and sacrum.[20-27] Researchers in a 2010 study[27] reported serial embolization without surgical excision in 36 patients with ABCs; 61% (22 patients) were successfully treated with a single embolization, and the authors reported 94% success with up to three injections. The authors emphasized the need for accurate diagnosis before treatment and found that embolization does not compromise surgical treatment in patients with failed embolization. Sclerotherapy of ABCs using polidocanol also has been studied. In another 2010 study,[28] the authors randomized 94 patients with ABCs to either intralesional curettage or repetitive sclerotherapy. They found comparable local control rates (93% for sclerotherapy versus 85% for surgery) but a much

2: Benign Bone Tumors

lower complication rate with sclerotherapy than with surgery.

Injection for Unicameral Bone Cyst

The treatment of UBCs has varied over the years and has included open curettage, serial steroid injections, placement of a cannulated screw for drainage,[29] and bone graft or marrow injections. The approach to the treatment of UBCs probably incites more divergent and dogmatic opinions from musculoskeletal tumor surgeons than any other bone tumor. The multiplicity of opinions is confounded by several factors that make comparison of studies difficult and thus fuel the debate. These factors include the definition of "active cysts" that require treatment (65% of cysts) and "inactive cysts" (35%) that will never require intervention.[29] Inclusion of inactive lesions, which have a better prognosis, may skew the results of clinical series. The next confounding factor is the definition of a recurrence after initial treatment. Different studies have included radiographic progression, recrudescence of symptoms, and reinjection of the lesion as failure end points, making comparison between studies difficult. Failure defined as reinjection is particularly problematic, because clinicians may decide on reinjection on the basis of different factors. True success in the management of these lesions is not clearly defined. Incomplete ossification of the original cystic void observed in radiographic studies when the patient is asymptomatic can be deemed a clinical success or a radiographic failure. This lack of a consistent definition of success makes success rates between studies difficult to compare.

The authors of a 2002 study reported their initial experience with 23 consecutive patients who had active UBCs, which were irrigated and injected with demineralized bone matrix (DBM) and autogenous bone marrow[30] (Figure 3). In this study, 78% of patients were successfully treated with one injection, and all patients were successfully treated with additional injections.

Several other authors have reported success (defined as no further fractures or need for surgical intervention during the study time frame) with the injection of DBM with and without autogenous marrow.[31,32] Researchers in 2011 reported a comparison study using either DBM or injectable calcium sulfate in 56 patients.[33] They found success rates of 86% and 89%, respectively, with no significant difference in time to healing of the cyst, but lower cost with calcium sulfate. In one of the only randomized prospective studies of the treatment of UBCs,[34] researchers in 2008 looked at injections with bone marrow without DBM versus repeat steroid injections for any patient who had cysts that were considered by the authors to be at risk for repetitive fractures without further surgical intervention, based on the radiographic appearance. The authors found a 42% success rate with steroids and 23% with bone marrow, suggesting that bone marrow alone is not a good op-

tion. A 2010 study[35] reported on a retrospective group of 184 patients treated with either steroid injection or DBM with autogenous bone marrow and found a significantly better initial success rate with DBM (38% versus 71%). A 2008 study provided another valuable comparison of steroids versus steroids with DBM with bone marrow.[36] The authors had a 16% success rate with steroids, a 36% success rate with open curettage, and a 50% success rate with single injection with DBM, steroids, and bone marrow. Their lower success rate (50%) compared with four other studies that did not add steroids to DBM may suggest that the steroids negatively affect bone healing with DBM. More studies are needed to see if adding steroids to DBM has any indication, but at this point, it does not appear to be helpful. The authors of a 2012 study reported on 56 patients with benign tumors treated with injectable calcium sulfate–calcium phosphate bone graft substitute and found a high rate of functional recovery.[37] One of 13 patients with UBCs had recurrence when treated with a two-needle injection technique. Although this is a small series, it points to a promising option for bone graft substitute that is injectable for cavitary skeletal defects for non–weight-bearing bones.

Radiofrequency Ablation

RFA uses low-voltage, high-frequency electrical energy to produce directed heat to destroy neoplastic tissue. RFA creates necrotic tissue with this target heat zone that induces tissue coagulation. The heat is greatest in the tissue in direct contact with the probe and decreases in proportion to the fourth power of the distance away from the probe. Cellular death occurs at 50°C. Typically, the RFA probe is heated to between 90° and 95°C, and that temperature is maintained by the probe for 4 minutes. The procedure is done under general anesthesia, and local anesthesia can be injected into the periosteum for additional pain management after the procedure. Biopsy and culture of every lesion is recommended, when feasible. After RFA, most patients are allowed to bear weight as tolerated and are told to avoid aggressive sporting activities for 6 weeks.

The initial use of RFA in bone tumors was for the percutaneous management of osteoid osteoma. Because these tumors are very painful when viable and asymptomatic when necrotic, early pain relief is strongly associated with clinical success. Likewise, because these lesions are typically small and have cortical hypertrophy, fracture after RFA for osteoid osteoma is rare.[38] Most series find primary success rates of 90% to 97% for the treatment of osteoid osteomas with RFA.[38-51] Typically the RFA probe is placed into the lesion with CT guidance;[52,53] however, fluoroscopy also has been used for placement. Chondroblastoma is another benign bone tumor that has been treated with RFA.[54-58] A 2009 study[57] found that 11 of 13 patients were successfully treated with RFA, whereas 2 patients required second-

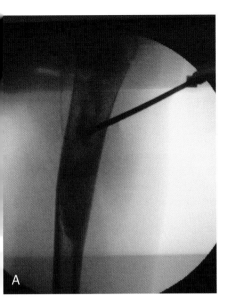
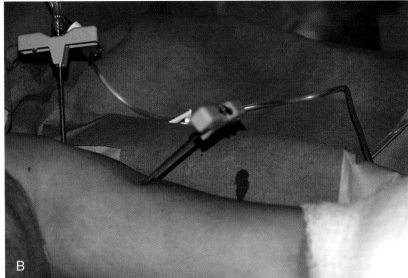
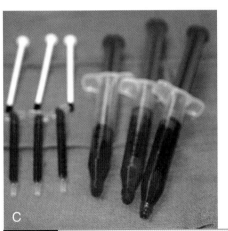
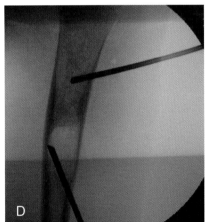
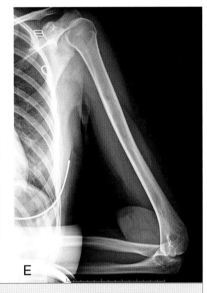

Figure 3 **A,** Intraoperative cystogram of a 12-year-old girl with persistent pain and a UBC of the humerus. **B,** The intraoperative placement of two 11-gauge needles at each end of the cyst as a percutaneous access procedure is shown. **C,** DBM and autogenous bone marrow are mixed in 1-mL syringes. **D,** The contrast material is displaced as the bone graft is injected into the inferior needle. The entire cyst is filled with bone graft from both needle sites until no further material can be injected. The patient returned to full activities 6 weeks postoperatively. **E,** AP radiograph 6 years postoperatively shows no recurrence.

ary surgical curettage. One surgery was for recurrence and subchondral collapse, whereas the other was for structural collapse without recurrence. Those results were similar to previously published reports using open curettage, but with less overall morbidity. Because chondroblastomas frequently occur in areas that are difficult to approach surgically, RFA appears to be a very attractive percutaneous option with a low complication rate. Skin necrosis around the probe, articular damage (with or without subchondral collapse), and fracture have been reported.[38,56]

Summary

The treatment of benign tumors of bone has progressed rapidly in the last two decades to include less open surgery and fewer en bloc resections. Percutaneous injection techniques, arterial embolizations, and percutaneous ablations can be used to address many cysts and smaller benign bone tumors that were previously treated with open curettage and autogenous bone grafting. In patients who require open curettage, adjuvants, such as high-speed burring, phenol, ethanol, argon beam coagulation, and PMMA, enhance the curettage and lead to lower recurrence rates. In the few patients

2: Benign Bone Tumors

with benign bone tumors that require en bloc resection, reconstructive procedures that are typically used in patients with bone sarcomas have improved the functional outcome of these patients as well.

These advances, however, do not change the need for careful radiographic and pathologic confirmation of the diagnosis before intervening. With less invasive approaches, obtaining adequate biopsy material must not be compromised.

Annotated References

1. Rougraff BT: Incidental bone lesions. *Instr Course Lect* 2002;51:451-456.

2. Guo W, Sun X, Zang J, Qu H: Intralesional excision versus wide resection for giant cell tumor involving the acetabulum: Which is better? *Clin Orthop Relat Res* 2012;470(4):1213-1220.

   This article describes a retrospective study of 27 patients with periacetabular giant cell tumor of bone. None of the patients with wide surgical resection had local recurrence, and 4 of 13 patients with intralesional surgery had recurrence. Level of evidence: IV.

3. Liu YP, Li KH, Sun BH: Which treatment is the best for giant cell tumors of the distal radius? A meta-analysis. *Clin Orthop Relat Res* 2012;470(10):2886-2894.

   The authors performed a meta-analysis of six relevant articles and found that the local recurrence rate of giant cell tumors of the distal radius was lowest with wide resection and higher with intralesional surgery. The use of bone cement did not lower the recurrence rate, and curettage was associated with the lowest major complication rate. Level of evidence: IV.

4. Lackman RD, Hosalkar HS, Ogilvie CM, Torbert JT, Fox EJ: Intralesional curettage for grades II and III giant cell tumors of bone. *Clin Orthop Relat Res* 2005; 438:123-127.

5. Gibbs CP Jr, Hefele MC, Peabody TD, Montag AG, Aithal V, Simon MA: Aneurysmal bone cyst of the extremities: Factors related to local recurrence after curettage with a high-speed burr. *J Bone Joint Surg Am* 1999;81(12):1671-1678.

6. Başarir K, Pişkin A, Güçlü B, Yildiz Y, Sağlik Y: Aneurysmal bone cyst recurrence in children: A review of 56 patients. *J Pediatr Orthop* 2007;27(8):938-943.

   A retrospective study of 56 children with ABCs found that the recurrence rate was associated with younger age (5 years and younger) and intralesional curettage. Level of evidence: III.

7. Niu X, Zhang Q, Hao L, et al: Giant cell tumor of the extremity: Retrospective analysis of 621 Chinese patients from one institution. *J Bone Joint Surg Am* 2012;94(5):461-467.

   A retrospective review of 621 patients with giant cell tumor of bone showed that intralesional curettage had a 56% local recurrence rate, whereas extended curettage with or without bone graft was associated with a 9% to 11% recurrence rate. Curettage was associated with a higher functional score than resection. Three patients with multifocal giant cell tumors of bone were reported. Level of evidence: III.

8. Gaston CL, Bhumbra R, Watanuki M, et al: Does the addition of cement improve the rate of local recurrence after curettage of giant cell tumours in bone? *J Bone Joint Surg Br* 2011;93(12):1665-1669.

   This large retrospective study compared 340 patients with giant cell tumor of bone treated with intralesional curettage with and without bone cement. The local recurrence rate without cement was 30%, and with cement the rate was 14%. With multivariate analysis, the stage of the disease and the use of cement were independent variables associated with local recurrence. The data suggest that the use of cement decreases the risk of local recurrence. Level of evidence: II.

9. Balke M, Ahrens H, Streitbuerger A, et al: Treatment options for recurrent giant cell tumors of bone. *J Cancer Res Clin Oncol* 2009;135(1):149-158.

   In this nonrandomized study, 214 patients with giant cell tumor of bone were studied. No tumors recurred after wide resection, 59% recurred after intralesional curettage, and 22% recurred after power burring and cementation of the lesion. Level of evidence: III.

10. Kafchitsas K, Habermann B, Proschek D, Kurth A, Eberhardt C: Functional results after giant cell tumor operation near knee joint and the cement radiolucent zone as indicator of recurrence. *Anticancer Res* 2010; 30(9):3795-3799.

    This retrospective study of 38 patients with giant cell tumor of bone near the knee joint found a 53% recurrence rate with curettage and 22% recurrence after curettage and bone cement filling. The authors found that cement filling was not associated with osteoarthritis and that cement enhanced the ability to find local recurrence at follow-up. Level of evidence: IV.

11. Suzuki Y, Nishida Y, Yamada Y, et al: Re-operation results in osteoarthritic change of knee joints in patients with giant cell tumor of bone. *Knee* 2007;14(5):369-374.

    This retrospective study of 30 patients with giant cell tumor of the bone near the knee found that 33% of tumors locally recurred after curettage and addition of either bone cement or bone graft. The rate of osteoarthritis progression was higher in patients who had recurrence of tumor than in those with residual subchondral bone after curettage. Level of evidence:IV.

12. Aboulafia AJ, Rosenbaum DH, Sicard-Rosenbaum L, Jelinek JS, Malawer MM: Treatment of large subchondral tumors of the knee with cryosurgery and composite reconstruction. *Clin Orthop Relat Res* 1994;307: 189-199.

13. Steffner RJ, Liao C, Stacy G, et al: Factors associated

with recurrence of primary aneurysmal bone cysts: Is argon beam coagulation an effective adjuvant treatment? *J Bone Joint Surg Am* 2011;93(21):e1221-e1229.

This retrospective review of 96 patients with ABCs treated with curettage, high-speed burring, and argon beam coagulation or with curettage, high-speed burring, and no argon beam coagulation found an 11% recurrence rate with argon beam coagulation and a 21% recurrence rate without it. Level of evidence: III.

14. Cummings JE, Smith RA, Heck RK Jr: Argon beam coagulation as adjuvant treatment after curettage of aneurysmal bone cysts: A preliminary study. *Clin Orthop Relat Res* 2010;468(1):231-237.

This retrospective review of 40 consecutive patients with ABCs showed that those treated with argon beam coagulation had a lower recurrence rate (zero versus 33%) than those treated without argon beam coagulation. Level of evidence: IV.

15. Benevenia J, Patterson FR, Beebe KS, Abdelshahed MM, Uglialoro AD: Comparison of phenol and argon beam coagulation as adjuvant therapies in the treatment of stage 2 and 3 benign-aggressive bone tumors. *Orthopedics* 2012;35(3):e371-e378.

This was a retrospective review of 93 consecutive patients with benign bone tumors and a minimum of 10 months of follow-up. Patients were treated with either curettage and phenol or curettage and argon beam coagulation. Recurrence developed in 17 patients, and there was no difference in the recurrence rate between the phenol group and the argon beam coagulation group. Level of evidence: II.

16. Lewis VO, Wei A, Mendoza T, Primus F, Peabody T, Simon MA: Argon beam coagulation as an adjuvant for local control of giant cell tumor. *Clin Orthop Relat Res* 2007;454:192-197.

This article reports a series of 37 patients treated with curettage of giant cell tumors with argon beam coagulation. Recurrences developed in four patients (11%), three of which were in bone and one of which was in soft tissue. Level of evidence: III.

17. Wan R, Zhang W, Xu J, et al: The outcome of surgical treatment for recurrent giant cell tumor in the appendicular skeleton. *J Orthop Sci* 2012;17(4):464-469.

This small retrospective study of 27 patients with recurrent giant cell tumor of bone found that local recurrence was lowest when patients were treated with wide resection and endoprosthetic reconstruction. Functional outcomes were better in patients treated with intralesional surgery. Metastatic cell tumor in both lungs developed in one patient. Level of evidence: IV.

18. Lin WH, Lan TY, Chen CY, Wu K, Yang RS: Similar local control between phenol- and ethanol-treated giant cell tumors of bone. *Clin Orthop Relat Res* 2011; 469(11):3200-3208.

This study was a retrospective review of 26 patients with giant cell tumor of the long bones treated with curettage, high-speed burring, and cementation, with either alcohol or phenol used as an additional adjuvant. The authors noted an 11% recurrence rate, which was similar between the two groups, suggesting that ethanol and phenol have similar adjuvant therapeutic value. Level of evidence: III.

19. Rossi G, Mavrogenis AF, Papagelopoulos PJ, Rimondi E, Ruggieri P: Successful treatment of aggressive aneurysmal bone cyst of the pelvis with serial embolization. *Orthopedics* 2012;35(6):e963-e968.

This case report of a 3-year-old boy with a pelvic ABC treated with serial embolizations is well illustrated and discusses the technical aspects of the procedure. Level of evidence: IV.

20. Novais EN, Rose PS, Yaszemski MJ, Sim FH: Aneurysmal bone cyst of the cervical spine in children. *J Bone Joint Surg Am* 2011;93(16):1534-1543.

This review of seven children treated for ABCs of the cervical spine using curettage after arterial embolization followed by a spinal fusion found satisfactory results with a low recurrence rate. Level of evidence: IV.

21. Owen RJ: Embolization of musculoskeletal bone tumors. *Semin Intervent Radiol* 2010;27(2):111-123.

This discussion of transarterial embolization of bone tumors provides a technical review of the procedure. Level of evidence: IV.

22. Boriani S, De Iure F, Campanacci L, et al: Aneurysmal bone cyst of the mobile spine: Report on 41 cases. *Spine (Phila Pa 1976)* 2001;26(1):27-35.

23. de Kleuver M, van der Heul RO, Veraart BE: Aneurysmal bone cyst of the spine: 31 cases and the importance of the surgical approach. *J Pediatr Orthop B* 1998;7(4):286-292.

24. Geffroy L, Hamel O, Odri GA, et al: Treatment of an aneurysmal bone cyst of the lumbar spine in children and teenagers, about five cases. *J Pediatr Orthop B* 2012;21(3):269-275.

This article provides case reports of five patients with ABCs of the lumbar spine treated with intralesional surgery. None of the patients experienced recurrence and two had a mild skeletal deformity after surgical intervention. Level of evidence: IV.

25. Lambot-Juhan K, Pannier S, Grévent D, et al: Primary aneurysmal bone cysts in children: Percutaneous sclerotherapy with absolute alcohol and proposal of a vascular classification. *Pediatr Radiol* 2012;42(5):599-605.

This retrospective review of 29 children with ABCs treated with alcohol sclerotherapy found a good response in 59% of patients. Level of evidence: IV.

26. Rapp TB, Ward JP, Alaia MJ: Aneurysmal bone cyst. *J Am Acad Orthop Surg* 2012;20(4):233-241.

This article discusses the physiology, presentation, classification, imaging characteristics, histology, and management of ABCs. Level of evidence: IV.

2: Benign Bone Tumors

27. Rossi G, Rimondi E, Bartalena T, et al: Selective arterial embolization of 36 aneurysmal bone cysts of the skeleton with N-2-butyl cyanoacrylate. *Skeletal Radiol* 2010;39(2):161-167.

    In this retrospective series of 36 patients with ABCs treated with selective arterial embolization, 61% of patients were adequately treated with one embolization procedure, 25% required two embolizations, and 14% required three embolizations. Level of evidence: IV.

28. Varshney MK, Rastogi S, Khan SA, Trikha V: Is sclerotherapy better than intralesional excision for treating aneurysmal bone cysts? *Clin Orthop Relat Res* 2010; 468(6):1649-1659.

    This randomized study of 94 patients with ABCs treated with either repetitive sclerotherapy or intralesional curettage with high-speed burring found that repetitive sclerotherapy was a safer treatment option and had a similar tumor recurrence rate. Level of evidence: II.

29. Hou HY, Wu K, Wang CT, Chang SM, Lin WH, Yang RS: Treatment of unicameral bone cyst: A comparative study of selected techniques. *J Bone Joint Surg Am* 2010;92(4):855-862.

    This article reports a retrospective review of 40 patients with UBCs treated with four different surgical techniques, including a new technique that involves curettage, ethanol injection, synthetic calcium sulfate bone graft substitute, and a cannulated screw for drainage. Level of evidence: III.

30. Rougraff BT, Kling TJ: Treatment of active unicameral bone cysts with percutaneous injection of demineralized bone matrix and autogenous bone marrow. *J Bone Joint Surg Am* 2002;84(6):921-929.

31. Kanellopoulos AD, Yiannakopoulos CK, Soucacos PN: Percutaneous reaming of simple bone cysts in children followed by injection of demineralized bone matrix and autologous bone marrow. *J Pediatr Orthop* 2005;25(5):671-675.

32. Killian JT, Wilkinson L, White S, Brassard M: Treatment of unicameral bone cyst with demineralized bone matrix. *J Pediatr Orthop* 1998;18(5):621-624.

33. Kim JH, Oh JH, Han I, Kim HS, Chung SW: Grafting using injectable calcium sulfate in bone tumor surgery: Comparison with demineralized bone matrix-based grafting. *Clin Orthop Surg* 2011;3(3):191-201.

    This article describes a clinical series of 56 patients with various benign bone tumors in which 28 patients were treated with injectable calcium sulfate and 28 patients were treated with DBM grafting. The authors found no significant difference in healing rates or recurrence rates. Level of evidence: II.

34. Wright JG, Yandow S, Donaldson S, Marley L; Simple Bone Cyst Trial Group: A randomized clinical trial comparing intralesional bone marrow and steroid injections for simple bone cysts. *J Bone Joint Surg Am* 2008;90(4):722-730.

    This randomized study of 90 patients with UBCs, separated into treatment groups of bone marrow injection and cortisone injection, found a better healing rate with cortisone than with bone marrow injection. DBM was not used in this study. Level of evidence: I.

35. Di Bella C, Dozza B, Frisoni T, Cevolani L, Donati D: Injection of demineralized bone matrix with bone marrow concentrate improves healing in unicameral bone cyst. *Clin Orthop Relat Res* 2010;468(11):3047-3055.

    This retrospective study of 184 patients with UBCs treated with either steroid injection or DBM with bone marrow concentrate found that the DBM with bone marrow concentrate was more successful than steroid injection. Level of evidence: III.

36. Sung AD, Anderson ME, Zurakowski D, Hornicek FJ, Gebhardt MC: Unicameral bone cyst: A retrospective study of three surgical treatments. *Clin Orthop Relat Res* 2008;466(10):2519-2526.

    This retrospective study comparing 167 patients with UBCs treated with either steroid injection, curettage with bone grafting, or DBM with bone marrow aspirate found that bone injection and curettage with bone grafting had a lower failure rate than steroid injection. Level of evidence: IV.

37. Fillingham YA, Lenart BA, Gitelis S: Function after injection of benign bone lesions with a bioceramic. *Clin Orthop Relat Res* 2012;470(7):2014-2020.

    This retrospective review of 56 patients with benign bone lesions treated with bioceramic grafting found two postoperative fractures, two healing complications, and good overall functional results 24 months after surgery. Level of evidence: IV.

38. Dierselhuis EF, Jutte PC, van der Eerden PJ, Suurmeijer AJ, Bulstra SK: Hip fracture after radiofrequency ablation therapy for bone tumors: Two case reports. *Skeletal Radiol* 2010;39(11):1139-1143.

    This article presents case reports of two patients in whom a hip fracture developed after RFA of chondrosarcoma in one patient and metastatic thyroid carcinoma in the other. Level of evidence: IV.

39. Welch BT, Welch TJ: Percutaneous ablation of benign bone tumors. *Tech Vasc Interv Radiol* 2011;14(3):118-123.

    This review article discusses percutaneous ablation of benign bone tumors using RFA. Level of evidence: IV.

40. Ahrar K: The role and limitations of radiofrequency ablation in treatment of bone and soft tissue tumors. *Curr Oncol Rep* 2004;6(4):315-320.

41. Atesok KI, Alman BA, Schemitsch EH, Peyser A, Mankin H: Osteoid osteoma and osteoblastoma. *J Am Acad Orthop Surg* 2011;19(11):678-689.

    This review article discusses differences between osteoid osteoma and osteoblastoma, including the histology, radiographic presentation, and treatment. Level of evidence: IV.

42. Bosschaert PP, Deprez FC: Acetabular osteoid osteoma treated by percutaneous radiofrequency ablation: Delayed articular cartilage damage. *JBR-BTR* 2010; 93(4):204-206.

This case report describes a patient with osteoid osteoma of the acetabulum treated with percutaneous RFA, which was complicated by delayed articular cartilage damage. Level of evidence: IV.

43. Gangi A, Buy X: Percutaneous bone tumor management. *Semin Intervent Radiol* 2010;27(2):124-136.

The authors reviewed image-guided techniques of primary and secondary bone tumors, which included vertebroplasty, ethanol injection, RFA, laser photocoagulation, cryoablation, and radiofrequency ionization (coblation). The principles, the indications, and the results were presented for each modality. Level of evidence: IV.

44. Liberman B, Gerniak A, Eshed I, Chechick A, Weiss I, Shabshin N: Percutaneous CT guided radio-frequency ablation of osteoid osteoma and osteoblastoma [in Hebrew]. *Harefuah* 2010;149(8):494-497, 552.

Thirty-three of 34 patients (97%) followed retrospectively after CT-guided RFA for osteoid osteoma and osteoblastoma had good results. Level of evidence: IV.

45. Neumann D, Berka H, Dorn U, Neureiter D, Thaler C: Follow-up of thirty-three computed-tomography-guided percutaneous radiofrequency thermoablations of osteoid osteoma. *Int Orthop* 2012;36(4):811-815.

This study is a clinical series of 33 patients with osteoid osteoma treated with CT-guided RFA, with 5-year follow-up. The authors reported a 97% success rate for the initial procedure. One failure occurred 28 months after the initial treatment, and the patient was successfully treated with a second RFA. Level of evidence: IV.

46. Omlor G, Merle C, Lehner B, et al: CT-guided percutaneous radiofrequency ablation in osteoid osteoma: Re-assessments of results with optimized technique and possible pain patterns in mid-term follow-up. *Rofo* 2012;184(4):333-339.

This study reported on a clinical series of 40 patients with CT-directed RFA for osteoid osteoma of bone. The authors had a 98% success rate with the first intervention, and 100% success after the second procedure. Level of evidence: IV.

47. Papagelopoulos PJ, Mavrogenis AF, Galanis EC, et al: Minimally invasive techniques in orthopedic oncology: Radiofrequency and laser thermal ablation. *Orthopedics* 2005;28(6):563-568.

48. Papathanassiou ZG, Petsas T, Papachristou D, Megas P: Radiofrequency ablation of osteoid osteomas: Five years experience. *Acta Orthop Belg* 2011;77(6):827-833.

In this clinical series, 29 patients with osteoid osteoma were treated with CT-directed RFA. The authors had a primary success rate of 90% with the initial treatment and a secondary success rate of 93%. The median

follow-up was 27 months, and the authors found that follow-up CT scans did not predict treatment success well. Level of evidence: IV.

49. Sabharwal T, Katsanos K, Buy X, Gangi A: Image-guided ablation therapy of bone tumors. *Semin Ultrasound CT MR* 2009;30(2):78-90.

This review article discusses image-guided ablation therapy for bone tumors, including RFA, laser photocoagulation, microwave ablation, cryoablation, ablation for metastatic disease, and ablation for benign bone tumors. Level of evidence: IV.

50. Volkmer D, Sichlau M, Rapp TB: The use of radiofrequency ablation in the treatment of musculoskeletal tumors. *J Am Acad Orthop Surg* 2009;17(12):737-743.

This review article discusses the use of RFA in patients with bone tumors, including osteoid osteoma, metastatic disease, and sacral chordoma. Level of evidence: IV.

51. Ward E, Munk PL, Rashid F, Torreggiani WC: Musculoskeletal interventional radiology: Radiofrequency ablation. *Radiol Clin North Am* 2008;46(3):599-610, vi-vii.

52. Martel Villagrán J, Bueno Horcajadas A, Ortiz Cruz EJ: Percutaneous radiofrequency ablation of benign bone tumors: Osteoid osteoma, osteoblastoma, and chondroblastoma [in Spanish]. *Radiologia* 2009;51(6):549-558.

In this retrospective review, 100 patients with osteoid osteoma, osteoblastoma, or chondroblastoma were treated with RFA and had good results. Level of evidence: IV.

53. Mylona S, Patsoura S, Galani P, Karapostolakis G, Pomoni A, Thanos L: Osteoid osteomas in common and in technically challenging locations treated with computed tomography-guided percutaneous radiofrequency ablation. *Skeletal Radiol* 2010;39(5):443-449.

This retrospective study of 23 patients with osteoid osteoma treated with CT-guided percutaneous RFA reported 91% clinical success. Two of 23 patients had a failure of the initial procedure and were treated with a second RFA, with good results. Level of evidence: IV.

54. Christie-Large M, Evans N, Davies AM, James SL: Radiofrequency ablation of chondroblastoma: Procedure technique, clinical and MR imaging follow up of four cases. *Skeletal Radiol* 2008;37(11):1011-1017.

This review of four patients with chondroblastoma treated with RFA reported excellent results in three patients and good results in one patient. Radiographic follow-up with MRI was available for all four patients. Level of evidence: IV.

55. Erickson JK, Rosenthal DI, Zaleske DJ, Gebhardt MC, Cates JM: Primary treatment of chondroblastoma with percutaneous radio-frequency heat ablation: Report of three cases. *Radiology* 2001;221(2):463-468.

2: Benign Bone Tumors

56. Petsas T, Megas P, Papathanassiou Z: Radiofrequency ablation of two femoral head chondroblastomas. *Eur J Radiol* 2007;63(1):63-67.

This article is a report of two cases of chondroblastoma of the femoral head treated with RFA. Both patients had only 1 year of follow-up and did not show any evidence of osteonecrosis at follow-up. One patient did not appear to have radiographic resolution of the tumor. Level of evidence: IV.

57. Rybak LD, Rosenthal DI, Wittig JC: Chondroblastoma: Radiofrequency ablation. Alternative to surgical resection in selected cases. *Radiology* 2009;251(2): 599-604.

This clinical series reported on 17 patients with chondroblastoma who were treated with RFA at two different medical centers. Twelve patients were found to have complete relief of symptoms, and two patients required further surgery, one for recurrent tumor and the other for articular collapse. Level of evidence: IV.

58. Sailhan F, Chotel F, Parot R; SOFOP: Chondroblastoma of bone in a pediatric population. *J Bone Joint Surg Am* 2009;91(9):2159-2168.

This was a retrospective study of 87 children with chondroblastoma treated with intralesional curettage, with or without bone grafting, or en bloc resection, with a minimum of 2 years of follow-up. The authors reported a 32% local recurrence rate. Level of evidence: II.

2: Benign Bone Tumors

Malignant Primary Bone Tumors

SECTION EDITOR:

Carol D. Morris, MD. MS

Chapter 15

Osteosarcoma of Bone

Alexander J. Chou, MD   Farbod Malek, MD

Introduction

Osteosarcoma, or osteogenic sarcoma, is a rare disease but not a new one. With the advent of systemic chemotherapy in the 1960s, osteosarcoma was transformed from an essentially lethal disease to one in which 70% of patients with localized disease can now expect to be cured. In contrast, patients with metastatic disease have, at best, survival in the 20% range. Furthermore, for the estimated 30% who experience relapse after localized disease, survival remains poor.[1-3] This chapter provides an update on the current understanding and clinical management of high-grade osteosarcoma.

Epidemiology of Osteosarcoma

Osteosarcoma is the most common primary bone cancer in adults and children. Classically, the highest incidence occurs during the second decade of life, with a second peak during the seventh and eighth decades of life. In the elderly, osteosarcoma often occurs as a secondary cancer as a result of previous radiation therapy or an underlying bone disease such as Paget disease. In children, osteosarcoma accounts for 5% to 10% of all new pediatric cancer diagnoses in the United States.[4] In the adolescent age range, it is the second most common malignancy, with only lymphoma surpassing it in incidence. Osteosarcoma is diagnosed in 400 children and adolescents each year in the United States. Many studies have linked periods of rapid growth to the development of osteosarcoma, and therefore, not surprisingly, incidence of this disease peaks during the second decade of life, at the time of the adolescent growth spurt. Osteosarcoma has a predilection for the metaphyseal portions of the long bones, with the distal femur and proximal tibia accounting for almost 50% of all osteosarcomas.[5]

Pathogenesis of Osteosarcoma

The World Health Organization classifies osteosarcoma as either primary or secondary osteosarcoma. Primary osteosarcomas are subdivided into intramedullary and surface osteosarcomas.[6]

Conventional osteosarcoma is a primary intramedullary, high-grade malignant tumor in which neoplastic cells of mesenchymal origin produce osteoid (**Figure 1**). Conventional osteosarcoma has historically been classified into osteoblastic, chondroblastic, and fibroblastic histologic subtypes. Several other rare subtypes have been described, including telangiectatic, osteoblastoma-like, small cell, and giant cell rich. Historically, such subtyping of conventional osteosarcoma has had little prognostic significance. However, recent data appear to indicate some predictable survival differences.[7,8]

Telangiectatic osteosarcoma (4% of osteosarcomas) is a subtype of osteosarcoma that radiographically and histologically mimics aneurysmal bone cyst (ABC). Like ABC, telangiectatic osteosarcoma has radiolucent bone destruction and blood-filled spaces with minimal solid tissue. The presence of nuclear pleomorphism and spindle cells producing osteoid distinguish telangiectatic osteosarcoma from ABC.[9,10]

Small cell osteosarcoma (1.5% of osteosarcomas) is

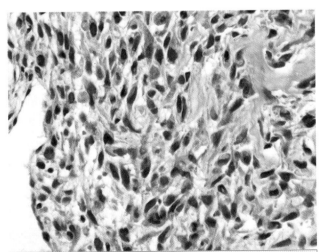

Figure 1 Photomicrograph of a hematoxylin and eosin stain of a conventional high-grade osteosarcoma. (Courtesy of Carol D. Morris, MD, New York, NY.)

Neither of the following authors nor any immediate family member has received anything of value from or has stock or stock options held in a commercial company or institution related directly or indirectly to the subject of this chapter: Dr. Chou and Dr. Malek.

3: Malignant Primary Bone Tumors

composed of small round blue cells with variable osteoid production. The presence of osteoid is necessary to distinguish this entity from Ewing sarcoma. It has a slightly worse prognosis than conventional osteosarcoma.[9,11]

Low-grade central osteosarcoma, or well-differentiated intramedullary osteosarcoma, accounts for 1% to 2% of osteosarcomas. It is composed of a hypocellular to moderately cellular fibroblastic stroma with variable amounts of osteoid production.[9,12] The histologic appearance mimics that of fibrous dysplasia, and therefore radiographic and clinical correlation is often necessary to make an accurate diagnosis.

Surface or juxtacortical osteosarcomas are commonly referred to as parosteal and periosteal. Parosteal osteosarcoma typically refers to a low-grade osteosarcoma that arises on the surface of the bone (4% of osteosarcomas). Approximately 70% of parosteal osteosarcomas involve the surface of the distal posterior femur. The spindle cells in the stroma show minimal atypia. Chromosomal alterations in parosteal osteosarcomas are different from those in conventional osteosarcomas. They are characterized by one or more ring chromosomes. Prognosis is excellent, with 91% overall survival at 5 years.[9,13] Dedifferentiated parosteal osteosarcoma refers to a surface tumor in which a high-grade component is juxtaposed to an underlying low-grade tumor. The prognosis is related to the least differentiated portion of the tumor.

Periosteal osteosarcoma is most often an intermediate-grade chondroblastic osteosarcoma arising on the surface of bone (less than 2% of osteosarcomas). The cartilaginous component can show varied degrees of cytologic atypia.[9,14]

High-grade surface osteosarcoma is a high-grade bone-forming malignancy that arises from the surface of the bone (less than 1% of osteosarcomas). This tumor has the same features seen in conventional osteosarcoma.[9,15]

Secondary osteosarcomas are bone-forming sarcomas occurring in bones that are affected by preexisting conditions, the most common being Paget disease (1% develop osteosarcoma) and bone changes caused by ionizing radiation. Other conditions that have been reported in association with secondary osteosarcoma are bone infarct, chronic osteomyelitis, and fibrous dysplasia.[9,16]

Several genetic syndromes associated with osteosarcoma include Li-Fraumeni syndrome (autosomal dominant disorder with germline mutation of the gene *TP53*), Rothmund-Thomson syndrome (autosomal recessive disorder with a heterogeneous clinical profile and a mutation in the *RECQL4* gene), Werner syndrome (mutation in the *WRN* [*RECQL2*] gene), and Bloom syndrome (mutations in the *BLM* [*RECQL3*] gene).[16] Patients with hereditary retinoblastoma have a high incidence of osteosarcoma. This predisposition is characterized by a germline mutation of the *RB1* gene. The prognosis for patients with *RB1* alterations seems to be poorer than that for patients without *RB1* alterations.[9]

The genetic complexity of osteosarcoma escapes simple characterization. The RB and p53 tumor suppressor pathways are involved in pathogenesis of osteosarcoma. The inactivation of these tumor suppressor genes (*RB1*, *TP53*, *ARF*, *CDKN2B*, *CDKN2A*, *WWOX*, *FGFR2*, *BUB3*, and *RECQL4*) and overexpression of oncogenes (*MYC*, *FOS*, *ERBB2* [formerly *HER2/neu*], *RUNX2*, *CDC5L*, *VEGFA*, *PIM1*, *E2F3*, *TWIST1*, *MET*, *PRIM1*, *CDK4*, *MDM2*, *COPS3*, *PMP22*, and *MAPK7*) are shown to be related to the development of osteosarcoma.[9,16,17]

The Wnt/low density lipoprotein receptor-related protein 5 (LRP5) pathway is one of the pathways involved in cell-to-cell interactions during embryogenesis. A significant correlation between LRP5 expression and worse event-free survival in patients has been identified. Additionally, patients with LRP5 expression have a higher risk of developing metastasis. Blocking Wnt/LRP5 signaling has been reported to halt invasiveness of the tumor.[18]

Clinical Features of Osteosarcoma

Osteosarcoma can occur in any bone of the body. The most common sites of disease are the distal femur, the proximal tibia, and the proximal humerus. Tumors occurring in the appendicular skeleton outnumber those in the axial skeleton. Pain and swelling are the most common complaints; these complaints often are ignored for several months. The initial reports of pain in the growing adolescent are attributed to common benign conditions such as growing pains and trauma.[5] The median time from onset of symptoms to diagnosis is 4 months.

Although only one fourth of all newly diagnosed patients have radiographically detectable metastatic disease, all patients are assumed to have micrometastatic disease. This assumption is based on data from the prechemotherapy era, which showed that metastatic disease developed within 3 to 6 months after resection of the primary tumor in most patients with what was once considered "nonmetastatic" osteosarcoma on the basis of available imaging modalities.[3] The most common site of distant metastasis is the lungs, accounting for 80% of all metastases. Other sites of metastatic spread include bones and soft tissue.[3] Osteosarcoma, like all primary bone tumors, is staged according to the American Joint Committee on Cancer staging system (Table 1).

Few true, robust prognostic factors exist for clinicians to consider in osteosarcoma. The presence of clinically detectable metastatic disease remains the most powerful clinical factor in predicting prognosis in osteosarcoma.[3] As noted previously, whereas survival for patients with nonmetastatic disease is approximately 70% with modern cytotoxic therapy and wide surgical

Table 1		
AJCC Staging System for Malignant Bone Tumors		
Stage	**Tumor Grade**	**Tumor Size**
IA	Low	< 8 cm
IB	Low	> 8 cm
IIA	High	< 8 cm
IIB	High	> 8 cm
III	Any tumor grade, skip metastases[a]	
IV	Any tumor grade, any tumor size, distant metastases	

[a]Skip metastases: discontinuous tumors in the primary bone site
Reprinted from American Joint Committee on Cancer: Bone, in Edge SB, Byrd DR, Compton CC, et al eds: *AJCC Cancer Staging Manual*, ed 7. New York, NY, Springer, 2010, pp 281-290.

resection, long-term survival for patients with metastatic disease at diagnosis is, at best, 20%. Similarly, patients with recurrent or progressive disease have a long-term survival of less than 20%.[1,19] Other prognostic factors that have been used in osteosarcoma include age, tumor size, anatomic site of primary disease, lactate dehydrogenase level, and alkaline phosphatase level.[20,21] Thus far, none of these variables has demonstrated sufficient predictive value to serve as a basis for risk-adapted therapy stratification at diagnosis, such as the schemas used in the treatment of rhabdomyosarcoma. One predictor of outcome that has been used to stratify therapy in some studies is the percentage of tumor necrosis following induction chemotherapy (Huvos grade). The percentage of necrosis is assessed histologically at the time of definitive resection, typically after 10 weeks of preoperative chemotherapy in most studies. Although Huvos grading has been shown to have a strong correlation to disease-free survival, it cannot be evaluated at initial diagnosis and thus cannot serve as a true prognostic factor to help in risk stratification of therapy.[22] Despite this limitation, attempts have been made to modify therapy on the basis of necrosis assessment in an effort to improve survival. Unfortunately, these strategies have not proven to be of significant benefit. One explanation is that tumor necrosis in response to preoperative chemotherapy reflects innate tumor biology rather than chemotherapy effectiveness.

Imaging

According to recent guidelines,[23] plain radiographs, MRI of the entire bone, CT scan of the chest, and whole-body bone scan (with or without positron emission tomography [PET] scan) are recommended for the initial evaluation of patients with suspected osteosarcoma.

Plain radiographs are still the preferred imaging method in the primary workup but are not sensitive in

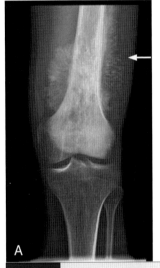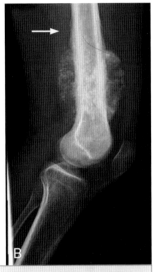

Figure 2	Plain AP (**A**) and lateral (**B**) radiographs of a high-grade classic osteoblastic osteosarcoma of a distal femur show the typical sunburst appearance and Codman triangle (arrows).

identifying the extent of the soft-tissue involvement of the tumor. The radiographic appearance of osteosarcoma is usually a radiodense metaphyseal lesion with ill-defined margins. The normal trabecular pattern of the bone is distorted, and characteristic radiographic features such as the Codman triangle and sunburst appearance are common (**Figure 2**).

MRI demonstrates the extent of soft-tissue involvement, neurovascular proximity, the extent of bone marrow involvement, and the presence of skip lesions (**Figure 3**). The whole length of the bone needs to be visualized in at least one plane. Axial cuts are useful to delineate the relationship of the tumor to the neurovascular structures and hence are most useful in determining limb salvage resectability (**Figure 4**). Dynamic MRI is a method by which vascularity is quantified following contrast administration and has been investigated

3: Malignant Primary Bone Tumors

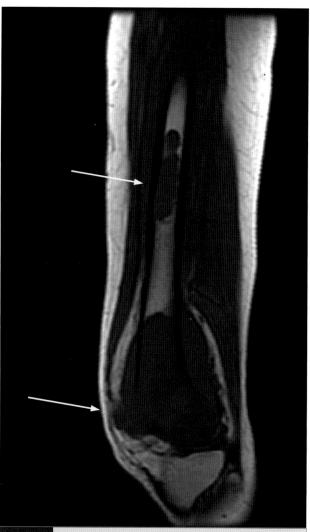

Figure 3 T1-weighted MRI coronal bone view of the femur demonstrating an osteosarcoma of the distal femur with a skip metastasis in the diaphysis (arrows). (Courtesy of Carol D. Morris, MD, New York, NY.)

in osteosarcoma is evolving. Several studies have evaluated the PET-CT scan to predict the histologic response to neoadjuvant chemotherapy in patients with osteosarcoma. In a series of 40 patients with osteosarcoma who had fluorodeoxyglucose (FDG) PET scans before and after induction chemotherapy, favorable FDG PET responses, defined as a standardized uptake value (SUV) of less than 2.5 after induction chemotherapy or a ratio of SUV before chemotherapy to SUV after chemotherapy of less than or equal to 0.5, were associated with improved progression-free survival. The FDG PET responses only partially correlated with histologic response to chemotherapy.[27] In addition, PET has been shown to be useful in differentiating between benign and malignant solitary lung nodules.[28,29]

FDG PET could have several potential uses in orthopaedic oncology. By identifying patients who are more likely to have an unfavorable histologic response to chemotherapy, response-adapted therapy could have a role in the future treatment of patients with poor response.

Current Therapy for Osteosarcoma

Multiagent chemotherapy and surgery are the standard approach to the treatment of patients with osteosarcoma. Historical series demonstrated that most patients who undergo only surgery for treatment of osteosarcoma experience pulmonary metastases within 6 months. Multiagent chemotherapy regimens pioneered in the 1970s markedly improved survival in osteosarcoma. Currently all modalities used in the treatment of malignancy are being brought to bear in the treatment of this disease, including surgery, chemotherapy, radiation therapy, immunotherapy, gene therapy, and therapies aimed at the tumor microenvironment.

Systemic Chemotherapy

Cytotoxic agents with the highest single-agent activity in osteosarcoma include high-dose methotrexate (30% to 40% response rate), cisplatin (approximately 30% response rate), doxorubicin (30% to 40% response rate), and ifosfamide (approximately 30% response rate).[28] Oncologists quickly learned that single-agent regimens did not achieve significant long-term survival in osteosarcoma. Optimal therapy relies on combinations of these effective agents. Early combination chemotherapy studies using methotrexate and doxorubicin in combination or as the mainstay for other combinations demonstrated relapse-free survival as high as 60%.[30] Additionally, trials with combination methotrexate and cisplatin consistently demonstrated a high percentage of tumor necrosis, and response rates of 60% were reported.[30]

Randomized controlled trials in the 1980s firmly established the crucial role of systemic therapy in curing osteosarcoma.[21,31] Most treatment regimens typically administer 10 weeks (two cycles) of induction (or pre-

to predict the tumor response to preoperative chemotherapy.[24]

Chest CT is more sensitive than chest radiographs in detecting lung metastasis smaller than 1 cm. Studies have demonstrated that nodules that are small (less than 5 mm), solitary, or unchanged on serial radiologic studies are typically benign. Peripheral lesions larger than 5 mm are likely to be metastatic (**Figure 5**). Lesions that do not fit into these criteria should still be followed with serial CT examinations, and any increase in size should prompt a biopsy to clarify the diagnosis.[25] Although the CT scan is the most sensitive tool available, CT scanning of the chest has been shown to underestimate the number of histologically proven osteosarcoma nodules.[26]

Technetium Tc-99 whole-body bone scanning is still the standard of care for the evaluation of distant bone metastasis in osteosarcoma (**Figure 6**). The role of PET

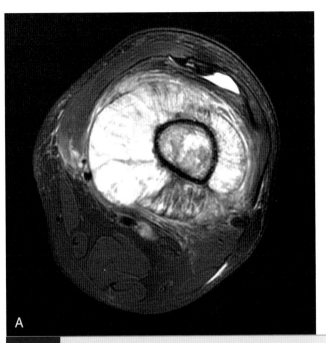
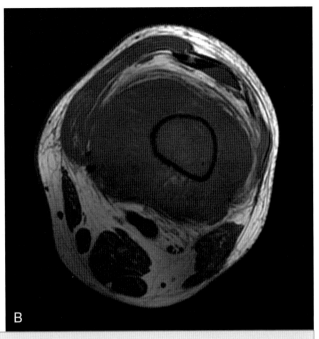

Figure 4   Axial, fat-suppressed T2-weighted (**A**) and T1-weighted (**B**) MRIs of the distal femur show osteosarcoma with extensive soft-tissue extension.

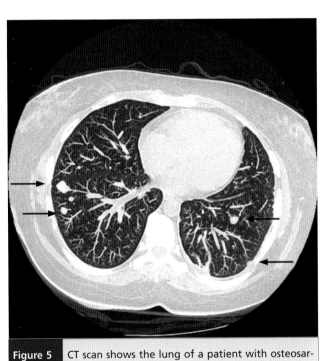

Figure 5   CT scan shows the lung of a patient with osteosarcoma with multiple metastatic lung nodules (arrows).

was a way to bridge the time between diagnosis and surgery. In the modern era, modular prostheses allow definitive surgery to take place at the time of diagnosis; however, this clinically is not the preferred time line.

In the United States and Europe, the most commonly used chemotherapeutic regimen consists of cisplatin, doxorubicin, and high-dose methotrexate preoperatively. After recovery from definitive surgery, patients then receive "maintenance" therapy with the same three cytotoxic agents. Recent clinical trials focused on the addition of other agents (such as ifosfamide/etoposide and interferon-α) during this maintenance phase to improve survival (see discussion on additional EURAMOS-1 trial later in this section).

Current studies suggest that 70% of patients with localized osteosarcoma treated with combination three-drug chemotherapy and wide surgical resection can expect long-term relapse-free survival.[3,32,33] Patients with metastatic disease at presentation will receive the same general treatment schema (preoperative chemotherapy, resection of all sites of disease, and postoperative chemotherapy); unfortunately, the chances of long-term relapse-free survival are vastly different (less than 20%) despite aggressive therapy.

Ifosfamide in combination with etoposide can produce response rates of 30% to 40% in patients with recurrent and/or metastatic disease.[1,34] It stands to reason that the use of this combination in the upfront therapy setting should significantly improve outcomes. However, the data supporting its use at initial diagnosis have been confusing. The largest North American osteosarcoma study conducted in the 1990s (the Children's Oncology Group Intergroup 0133 study) was unable to

operative) chemotherapy. After resection of the primary tumor, patients then receive an additional 20 weeks of systemic therapy. The concept of preoperative chemotherapy for this disease evolved during the 1970s, when custom prostheses for limb salvage procedures took 6 to 8 weeks for fabrication;[28] therefore, systemic therapy

3: Malignant Primary Bone Tumors

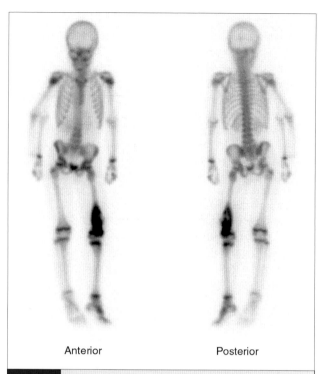

Anterior   Posterior

Figure 6 Whole-body bone scan with intense uptake in a left distal femur osteosarcoma. (Courtesy of Carol D. Morris, MD, New York, NY.)

show a clear benefit to adding ifosfamide to the standard regimen of cisplatin, doxorubicin, and methotrexate.[35] Starting with a mainstay consisting of cisplatin, doxorubicin, and methotrexate, three pilot studies evaluated the feasibility of doxorubicin intensification and ifosfamide intensification. The first pilot study focused on dose intensification of doxorubicin with the support of dexrazoxane (an iron chelate that serves as a cardioprotectant), the second added ifosfamide to doxorubicin dose intensification with dexrazoxane support, and the third evaluated the feasibility of dose intensification of ifosfamide and etoposide. These studies showed that although dose intensification was feasible for both doxorubicin and ifosfamide in patients with osteosarcoma,[36] additional studies were needed to demonstrate any improvement over existing regimens. In contrast to North American studies, concurrent data from several European cooperative groups did suggest improved disease-free survival with the addition of ifosfamide to standard three-drug chemotherapy regimens.[37,38]

In 2005, in part because of these conflicting studies, the largest coordinated international effort in osteosarcoma, the EURAMOS-1 study, was launched; the study was closed in June 2011 when its accrual target was met. This randomized, prospective clinical trial aimed to provide definitive answers to the following questions: (1) whether the addition of ifosfamide and etoposide to postoperative chemotherapy with cisplatin, doxorubicin, and methotrexate improved event-free survival and overall survival for patients with resect-

able osteosarcoma and a poor histologic response (90% necrosis or less) to 10 weeks of preoperative chemotherapy; and (2) whether the addition of pegylated interferon alfa-2b as maintenance therapy after postoperative chemotherapy with cisplatin, doxorubicin, and methotrexate improves the event-free survival and overall survival for patients with resectable osteosarcoma and a good histologic response (more than 90% necrosis) to 10 weeks of preoperative chemotherapy. Preliminary analysis from the EURAMOS group suggested that the addition of interferon-α as a maintenance regimen did not confer a survival advantage in the group of patients who had a good response to chemotherapy.[39] The question regarding the addition of ifosfamide and etoposide to poor responders is still being analyzed.

Surgery

Complete en bloc resection of the tumor for local control of osteosarcoma is the standard of care. There is no agreement as to how wide the margin of resection should be, but tumor-free margins are pivotal for local control. No randomized studies have been performed to compare the outcomes of limb salvage surgery to the outcomes of amputation. However, multiple retrospective studies have shown no statistically significant difference in overall survival of patients with osteosarcoma treated with amputation versus limb salvage.[40] One area of controversy is pathologic fracture of bone in osteosarcoma. It is generally accepted that not all pathologic fractures require amputation. Limb salvage surgery is advocated when local control can be reasonably expected.[41]

Amputation is still performed for local control of osteosarcoma under several circumstances. The only absolute indication for amputation to achieve local control in osteosarcoma is when a functional and disease-free extremity cannot be achieved with limb salvage surgery. The choice of amputation versus limb salvage is often complex and always requires the involvement of the patient and the family in making the decision. Of the factors that are important in this decision, the first priority is local control. Other important factors to consider before finalizing the surgical plan include the use of effective adjuvant therapy, involvement of the major neurovascular structures, presence of a pathologic fracture, potential remaining skeletal growth, and the patient's expectations and goals after the procedure. With the advent of modern prostheses, functional results after lower extremity amputations are quite good. For patients with high physical demands or those desiring advanced athletic activities, amputations are associated with fewer complications, including prosthetic failure or allograft fracture, in comparison with limb salvage.[42]

Limb salvage surgery is possible for more than 85% of patients with extremity osteosarcoma.[40] Although limb salvage is associated with greater psychosocial satisfaction, less oxygen consumption, and a faster rate of ambulation, it is also associated with higher complication and revision surgery rates. No long-term difference has been revealed between limb salvage and amputation when comparing patients' overall satisfaction on the basis of SF-36 and Toronto Extremity Salvage Scores.[42,43]

Recent and adequate imaging is essential to preoperative planning. Plain radiographs and MRI are the most common imaging modalities used. A full-length view of the entire involved bone is essential. Axial imaging provides important details regarding the proximity of key neurovascular structures.

Once the affected bone has been removed, several reconstruction options are available for limb salvage, which are discussed in great detail in chapter 20, Surgical Management of Malignant Primary Bone Tumors. Briefly, the primary options include metallic endoprostheses and allografts alone or in combination (allograft-prosthetic composites). Modular megaprostheses have the advantage of immediate stability, intraoperative flexibility, and extensibility for children at growing age, but have limited longevity.[44,45] Allograft reconstructions allow reconstruction of articular surfaces and, most important, provide reliable soft-tissue attachments, but they require a long period of postoperative limited weight bearing. Allograft-prosthetic composites exploit the strengths of each option.

Radiation Therapy

Although standard therapy for osteosarcoma includes only multiagent chemotherapy and surgery, radiation therapy has been used in select patients. With improvements in technology, limitations that prevented its widespread use in osteosarcoma are dwindling. Historically, radiation therapy has not been used in the upfront treatment of osteosarcoma because studies in the prechemotherapy era did not show a benefit to its use when compared to surgery alone. In addition, osteosarcoma is not sensitive to radiation therapy at doses that would allow safe administration of systemic combination chemotherapy. Dosages in excess of 50 Gy are needed for tumor sterilization.[46] At these doses, complications are common, and the risks of radiation therapy typically outweighed any potential benefits. However, with advances in techniques such as intensity-modulated radiation therapy and other image-guided technologies, several small series reported excellent symptom and even tumor control in patients with large unresectable tumors.[46-49] Furthermore, recent studies have shown that radiation therapy can be incredibly useful in palliation of symptoms in patients with terminal disease.[50] As technologies improve, it is expected that radiation therapy will play a larger role in the treatment of osteosarcoma in the future.

Radiopharmaceuticals can also be used in treating osteosarcoma. Samarium Sm-153 ethylene diamine tetramethylene phosphonate ([153]Sm EDTMP) has been shown to have high bone specificity and could be effective in the palliative setting.[51]

Emerging Therapies for Osteosarcoma

For the past 20 years, survival after osteosarcoma treatment has plateaued in the face of a dizzying pace of continual advances in supportive care, surgical techniques, and development of novel therapeutics. It appears that conventional cytotoxic agents have been maximally used in osteosarcoma. New drug development has shifted from nondiscriminant agents such as ifosfamide and methotrexate to more "targeted" therapies, such as small molecule inhibitors of protein kinases and monoclonal antibodies. Continuing to better understand the biology of osteosarcoma remains critical to the identification of new effective treatment modalities. Efforts to elucidate tumor suppressor pathways, cell signaling pathways, and aberrantly expressed proteins are important to the development of more effective therapy in osteosarcoma. The conventional cytotoxic agents currently used in the treatment of osteosarcoma were discovered more than 20 years ago, without the benefit of understanding of tumor biology. Therefore, these agents are characterized by their narrow therapeutic index, and their use is limited by their high toxicity profiles.

Currently, several new agents are being evaluated for their potential role in the treatment of osteosarcoma. Some agents that held early promise, including long-acting octreotide pamoate[52,53] (an agent capable of reducing serum levels of insulinlike growth factor 1), and trabectedin[54] (a marine-derived alkaloid that interferes with DNA function by several different mechanisms), ultimately failed to demonstrate benefit. Targeting human epidermal growth factor receptor 2 (HER2) with trastuzumab, a monoclonal antibody directed against HER2, was supported by studies showing HER2 overexpression correlated with poor outcome in a sizable number of patients with metastatic disease. Although patients were able to safely receive this agent in combination with conventional cytotoxic chemotherapy, trastuzumab did not improve survival in patients with metastatic disease.[55] Although the scientific rationale for these agents was sound and preclinical data supported their use in osteosarcoma, these agents did not demonstrate efficacy in the initial phases of testing and therefore are no longer pursued.

Liposomal muramyl tripeptide phosphatidylethanolamine (L-MTP-PE), an immune modulator that activates monocytes and macrophages to become tumoricidal, was found to be highly active in animal models, and a phase 3 clinical trial incorporating L-MTP-PE into upfront therapy (INT-0133) demonstrated a statistically significant improvement (an almost one third reduction in the risk of death) in overall survival for patients with localized disease.[35] These data led to its licensure for use in localized osteosarcoma in Europe as well as Mexico. The Food and Drug Administration has not yet approved its use in the United States. The data from INT-0133 demonstrated a trend toward improved survival in metastatic patients who received

L-MTP-PE.[56] The data do not yet strongly support its use in patients with metastatic disease; additional studies are required in this patient population.

The early data for other novel agents, including mammalian target of rapamycin inhibitors (temsirolimus), insulinlike growth factor 1 receptor antagonists (cixutumumab), and inhibitors of the tumor microenvironment (zoledronate), are encouraging. Their utility in osteosarcoma remains undefined.

Summary of Current Therapy for Newly Diagnosed Osteosarcoma

Patients with newly diagnosed localized osteosarcoma should receive treatment with combination chemotherapy using a regimen that contains at least three drugs (cisplatin, doxorubicin, and high-dose methotrexate are the most common). These regimens can achieve a 5-year event-free survival of at least 70% in patients with localized osteosarcoma. The EURAMOS-1 study built upon this three-drug combination backbone by introducing interferon-α for patients with good response (more than 90% necrosis) to preoperative chemotherapy and combination ifosfamide and etoposide for patients with poor response (90% necrosis or less) to preoperative chemotherapy. The study closed in June 2011. The initial report from the good-responder arm demonstrated that maintenance therapy with interferon-α did not improve survival. Final results of this study are eagerly awaited.

Surgery is the key to local control in patients with osteosarcoma. The decision of limb salvage versus amputation is based on the possibility of performing complete removal of the primary tumor and preserving a functional limb for the patient. The timing of the surgery is usually after two cycles of preoperative chemotherapy, when the patient's cell counts have adequately recovered. Complete up-to-date imaging after induction chemotherapy is essential for preoperative planning. Postoperative chemotherapy ideally resumes within 3 weeks after surgery. A delay in the resumption of chemotherapy is associated with inferior outcomes.[57]

Strategies at Relapse

There is no widely accepted treatment regimen for patients whose tumors do not respond to standard therapy or for those who experience relapse. Because recurrent tumors are more likely to be resistant to the agents already used, several factors inform the treatment options available to these patients; these factors include therapy previously given, site(s) of relapse, and timing of recurrence. The standard approach in the relapse setting includes surgery for all sites of metastasis when feasible; the patient whose disease is not resectable is not curable. Systemic chemotherapy in the relapse setting remains a matter of debate. Investigators in a 2005

study demonstrated that for a select group of patients, chemotherapy can improve outcome, especially for patients who have not yet received ifosfamide.[1] Supporting the use of chemotherapy in relapse, the authors of a 1995 study reported that survival was improved in patients who received salvage chemotherapy in addition to surgery.[58] A 2005 study demonstrated that for a cohort of 576 patients treated for relapse of osteosarcoma, the use of chemotherapy was correlated with overall survival for patients who did not achieve a second complete remission ($n = 229$, $P = 0.0001$). Chemotherapy use was also correlated with event-free survival for patients who were able to achieve a second complete remission ($n = 339$, $P = 0.016$).[59] In contrast, the authors of a 2003 study reported that salvage chemotherapy did not affect overall survival in patients with relapse who were able to achieve a second surgical remission.[2] Further supporting the surgery-only approach at relapse, other researchers reported in 2003 that for patients with solitary pulmonary relapse, surgical resection alone provided a better 4-year survival compared to chemotherapy combined with surgery.[19] The data supporting chemotherapy for the patient with relapse remain conflicting.

A patient with a solitary pulmonary nodule diagnosed more than 24 months after initial diagnosis can be effectively treated by resection of the nodule and close observation.[19] Patients with a shorter relapse-free interval (less than 24 months from initial diagnosis) and a single site of disease recurrence may benefit from systemic chemotherapy and aggressive resection of all known areas of tumor involvement.[1,19] Ifosfamide (in doses of 9 to 14 g/m^2) in combination with etoposide should be considered, especially when ifosfamide has not already been used. High-dose ifosfamide could be justified in the relapse setting because its effectiveness appears to be somewhat dose dependent.[34]

Patients with unresectable disease could benefit from additional chemotherapy, although a cure cannot be expected. One study showed that patients who had unresectable disease treated with chemotherapy alone had an average survival of almost 15 months after the first relapse, although none of these patients ultimately survived.[1] In this situation, the wishes of the patient and family must be paramount in making the decision to administer systemic chemotherapy. Finally, although osteosarcoma has long been thought to be resistant to radiation therapy, several groups have reported improvement in symptoms (pain) by using high-dose radiation therapy in patients with unresectable tumors or patients who refused surgery.[60]

Although the presence of distant metastatic disease remains an overwhelming determinant of prognosis in patients with osteosarcoma, a small percentage of patients (4% to 7%) will experience a local recurrence.[59,61,62] Factors associated with worse outcome in patients with locally recurrent osteosarcoma include concomitant distant metastatic recurrence, positive margins, short local disease-free interval, and surgical inoperability. The strategy for patients with local recurrence is similar to the strategy for patients who have a distant recurrence: resection of all sites of disease and systemic chemotherapy in appropriate patients (especially for those with short local disease-free intervals). Five-year survival after local recurrence ranges from 19% to 30%.[59,61-63]

Summary

Although osteosarcoma is a rare disease, it is the most common primary bone tumor in children and adults. The current multidisciplinary approach with complete surgical resection and multiagent chemotherapy with a minimum of three active agents affords a long-term, disease-free survival of almost 70% in patients with localized disease. The prognosis remains poor for patients with overt metastatic disease at presentation and for those patients with relapsed disease. Emerging therapies focus on agents with novel and more targeted mechanisms of action. The new generation of therapeutic agents for this disease will need to be informed by the emerging knowledge of the basic biology of osteosarcoma.

Annotated References

1. Chou AJ, Merola PR, Wexler LH, et al: Treatment of osteosarcoma at first recurrence after contemporary therapy: The Memorial Sloan-Kettering Cancer Center experience. *Cancer* 2005;104(10):2214-2221.

2. Ferrari S, Briccoli A, Mercuri M, et al: Postrelapse survival in osteosarcoma of the extremities: Prognostic factors for long-term survival. *J Clin Oncol* 2003; 21(4):710-715.

3. Marina N, Gebhardt M, Teot L, Gorlick R: Biology and therapeutic advances for pediatric osteosarcoma. *Oncologist* 2004;9(4):422-441.

4. Arndt CA, Crist WM: Common musculoskeletal tumors of childhood and adolescence. *N Engl J Med* 1999;341(5):342-352.

5. Meyers PA, Gorlick R: Osteosarcoma. *Pediatr Clin North Am* 1997;44(4):973-989.

6. Fletcher CDM, Bridge JA, Hogendoorn P, Mertens F (eds): *WHO Classification of Tumours of Soft Tissue and Bone*, ed 4, volume 5. Geneva, Switzerland, The International Agency for Research on Cancer/World Health Organization, 2013.

7. Bacci G, Bertoni F, Longhi A, et al: Neoadjuvant chemotherapy for high-grade central osteosarcoma of the extremity: Histologic response to preoperative chemotherapy correlates with histologic subtype of the tumor. *Cancer* 2003;97(12):3068-3075.

8. Hauben EI, Weeden S, Pringle J, Van Marck EA, Hogendoorn PC: Does the histological subtype of high-grade central osteosarcoma influence the response to treatment with chemotherapy and does it affect overall survival? A study on 570 patients of two consecutive trials of the European Osteosarcoma Intergroup. *Eur J Cancer* 2002;38(9):1218-1225.

9. Martin JW, Squire JA, Zielenska M: The genetics of osteosarcoma. *Sarcoma* 2012;2012:627254.

   In this article, the authors reviewed studies of the genetics of osteosarcoma to comprehensively describe the considerable heterogeneity and complexity of this disease. Level of evidence: V.

10. Sangle NA, Layfield LJ: Telangiectatic osteosarcoma. *Arch Pathol Lab Med* 2012;136(5):572-576.

11. Nakajima H, Sim FH, Bond JR, Unni KK: Small cell osteosarcoma of bone: Review of 72 cases. *Cancer* 1997;79(11):2095-2106.

12. Malhas AM, Sumathi VP, James SL, et al: Low-grade central osteosarcoma: A difficult condition to diagnose. *Sarcoma* 2012;2012:764796.

13. Schwab JH, Antonescu CR, Athanasian EA, Boland PJ, Healey JH, Morris CD: A comparison of intramedullary and juxtacortical low-grade osteogenic sarcoma. *Clin Orthop Relat Res* 2008;466(6):1318-1322.

14. Grimer RJ, Bielack S, Flege S, et al; European Musculo Skeletal Oncology Society: Periosteal osteosarcoma—a European review of outcome. *Eur J Cancer* 2005; 41(18):2806-2811.

15. Okada K, Unni KK, Swee RG, Sim FH: High grade surface osteosarcoma: A clinicopathologic study of 46 cases. *Cancer* 1999;85(5):1044-1054.

16. PosthumaDeBoer J, Witlox MA, Kaspers GJ, van Royen BJ: Molecular alterations as target for therapy in metastatic osteosarcoma: A review of literature. *Clin Exp Metastasis* 2011;28(5):493-503.

    This review aims to give an overview of the biologic changes in metastatic osteosarcoma cells as well as the preclinical and clinical efforts targeting the different steps in osteosarcoma metastases and how these contribute to designing a metastasis-directed treatment of osteosarcoma. Level of evidence: V.

17. Ottaviani G, Jaffe N: The etiology of osteosarcoma. *Cancer Treat Res* 2009;152:15-32.

    In this article, the authors described the factors related to patient characteristics, genetic abnormalities, and syndromes associated with osteosarcoma. Level of evidence: V.

18. McQueen P, Ghaffar S, Guo Y, Rubin EM, Zi X, Hoang BH: The Wnt signaling pathway: Implications for therapy in osteosarcoma. *Expert Rev Anticancer Ther* 2011;11(8):1223-1232.

This article discusses the use of Wnt pathway inhibitors and the targeting of *MET*, a Wnt-regulated proto-oncogene, as possible mechanisms for treatment of osteosarcoma. Level of evidence: V.

19. Hawkins DS, Arndt CA: Pattern of disease recurrence and prognostic factors in patients with osteosarcoma treated with contemporary chemotherapy. *Cancer* 2003;98(11):2447-2456.

20. Davis AM, Bell RS, Goodwin PJ: Prognostic factors in osteosarcoma: A critical review. *J Clin Oncol* 1994; 12(2):423-431.

21. Eilber FR, Rosen G: Adjuvant chemotherapy for osteosarcoma. *Semin Oncol* 1989;16(4):312-322.

22. Gorlick R, Meyers PA: Osteosarcoma necrosis following chemotherapy: Innate biology versus treatment-specific. *J Pediatr Hematol Oncol* 2003;25(11):840-841.

23. Biermann JS, Adkins DR, Agulnik M, et al: Bone cancer. *J Natl Compr Canc Netw* 2013;11(6):688-723.

This article presents consensus-based and evidence-based guidelines for the management of bone sarcoma. Level of evidence: III.

24. Reddick WE, Wang S, Xiong X, et al: Dynamic magnetic resonance imaging of regional contrast access as an additional prognostic factor in pediatric osteosarcoma. *Cancer* 2001;91(12):2230-2237.

25. Grampp S, Bankier AA, Zoubek A, et al: Spiral CT of the lung in children with malignant extra-thoracic tumors: Distribution of benign vs malignant pulmonary nodules. *Eur Radiol* 2000;10(8):1318-1322.

26. Kayton ML, Huvos AG, Casher J, et al: Computed tomographic scan of the chest underestimates the number of metastatic lesions in osteosarcoma. *J Pediatr Surg* 2006;41(1):200-206, discussion 200-206.

27. Hawkins DS, Conrad EU III, Butrynski JE, Schuetze SM, Eary JF: [F-18]-fluorodeoxy-D-glucose-positron emission tomography response is associated with outcome for extremity osteosarcoma in children and young adults. *Cancer* 2009;115(15):3519-3525.

This study evaluated 40 patients with extremity osteosarcoma. All patients received neoadjuvant and adjuvant chemotherapy. FDG PET SUVs before neoadjuvant chemotherapy and after neoadjuvant chemotherapy were analyzed and correlated with histopathologic response. Level of evidence: I.

28. Rosen G, Marcove RC, Caparros B, Nirenberg A, Kosloff C, Huvos AG: Primary osteogenic sarcoma: The rationale for preoperative chemotherapy and delayed surgery. *Cancer* 1979;43(6):2163-2177.

29. Cistaro A, Lopci E, Gastaldo L, Fania P, Brach Del Prever A, Fagioli F: The role of 18F-FDG PET/CT in the metabolic characterization of lung nodules in pediatric patients with bone sarcoma. *Pediatr Blood Cancer* 2012;59(7):1206-1210.

30. Link MP, Eilber F: Osteosarcoma, in Pizzo PA, Poplack DG (eds): *Principles and Practice of Pediatric Oncology*, ed 1. Philadelphia, PA, Lippincott, 1989, pp 689-711.

31. Link MP, Goorin AM, Miser AW, et al: The effect of adjuvant chemotherapy on relapse-free survival in patients with osteosarcoma of the extremity. *N Engl J Med* 1986;314(25):1600-1606.

32. Meyers PA, Schwartz CL, Krailo M, et al: Osteosarcoma: A randomized, prospective trial of the addition of ifosfamide and/or muramyl tripeptide to cisplatin, doxorubicin, and high-dose methotrexate. *J Clin Oncol* 2005;23(9):2004-2011.

33. Meyers PA, Heller G, Healey J, et al: Chemotherapy for nonmetastatic osteogenic sarcoma: The Memorial Sloan-Kettering experience. *J Clin Oncol* 1992;10(1): 5-15.

34. Carli M, Passone E, Perilongo G, Bisogno G: Ifosfamide in pediatric solid tumors. *Oncology* 2003; 65(suppl 2):99-104.

35. Meyers PA, Schwartz CL, Krailo MD, et al; Children's Oncology Group: Osteosarcoma: The addition of muramyl tripeptide to chemotherapy improves overall survival—a report from the Children's Oncology Group. *J Clin Oncol* 2008;26(4):633-638.

36. Schwartz, CL, Wexler, LH, Devidas, M, et al. P9754 therapeutic intensification in non-metastatic osteosarcoma: a COG trial. *Proc Am Soc Clin Oncol* 2004; 23: 798a.

37. Bacci G, Ferrari S, Bertoni F, et al: Long-term outcome for patients with nonmetastatic osteosarcoma of the extremity treated at the istituto ortopedico rizzoli according to the istituto ortopedico rizzoli/osteosarcoma-2 protocol: An updated report. *J Clin Oncol* 2000;18(24):4016-4027.

38. Fuchs N, Bielack SS, Epler D, et al: Long-term results of the co-operative German-Austrian-Swiss osteosarcoma study group's protocol COSS-86 of intensive multidrug chemotherapy and surgery for osteosarcoma of the limbs. *Ann Oncol* 1998;9(8):893-899.

39. Bielack S, Smeland S, Whelan J, et al: MAP plus maintenance pegylated interferon α-2b (MAPIfn) versus MAP alone in patients with resectable high-grade osteosarcoma and good histologic response to preoperative MAP: First results of the EURAMOS-1 "good response" randomization. 2013 ASCO Annual Meeting Proceedings (Post-Meeting Edition). *J Clin Oncol* 2013;31(suppl 18): LBA10504.

40. Rougraff BT, Simon MA, Kneisl JS, Greenberg DB, Mankin HJ: Limb salvage compared with amputation

for osteosarcoma of the distal end of the femur: A long-term oncological, functional, and quality-of-life study. *J Bone Joint Surg Am* 1994;76(5):649-656.

41. Ferguson PC, McLaughlin CE, Griffin AM, Bell RS, Deheshi BM, Wunder JS: Clinical and functional outcomes of patients with a pathologic fracture in high-grade osteosarcoma. *J Surg Oncol* 2010;102(2):120-124.

    This study retrospectively reviewed and compared oncologic and functional outcomes of 201 patients with high-grade osteosarcoma without pathologic fractures to 31 patients with pathologic fractures. The authors concluded that a pathologic fracture in osteosarcoma did not preclude limb salvage surgery in most patients. Level of evidence: III.

42. Malek F, Somerson JS, Mitchel S, Williams RP: Does limb-salvage surgery offer patients better quality of life and functional capacity than amputation? *Clin Orthop Relat Res* 2012;470(7):2000-2006.

    This study compared functional status and quality of life for patients treated with above-knee amputation versus limb salvage surgery. The data suggested that limb salvage surgery offers better gait efficiency and return to normal living compared with above-knee amputation, but does not improve the patient's perception of quality of life. Level of evidence: III.

43. Ottaviani G, Robert RS, Huh WW, Jaffe N: Functional, psychosocial and professional outcomes in long-term survivors of lower-extremity osteosarcomas: Amputation versus limb salvage. *Cancer Treat Res* 2009;152:421-436.

44. Nystrom LM, Morcuende JA: Expanding endoprosthesis for pediatric musculoskeletal malignancy: Current concepts and results. *Iowa Orthop J* 2010;30:141-149.

    This article reviews different options for reconstruction of the salvaged limb in pediatric patients after wide resection of extremity sarcoma. The authors also described the surgical technique, outcomes, and complications of the expandable prosthesis. Level of evidence: V.

45. Palumbo BT, Henderson ER, Groundland JS, et al: Advances in segmental endoprosthetic reconstruction for extremity tumors: A review of contemporary designs and techniques. *Cancer Control* 2011;18(3):160-170.

46. Hristov B, Shokek O, Frassica DA: The role of radiation treatment in the contemporary management of bone tumors. *J Natl Compr Canc Netw* 2007;5(4):456-466.

    The authors offer a comprehensive review of the data supporting radiation therapy in the contemporary treatment of bone tumors. Level of evidence: V.

47. DeLaney TF, Trofimov AV, Engelsman M, Suit HD: Advanced-technology radiation therapy in the management of bone and soft tissue sarcomas. *Cancer Control* 2005;12(1):27-35.

48. Nagarajan R, Clohisy D, Weigel B: New paradigms for therapy for osteosarcoma. *Curr Oncol Rep* 2005;7(6):410-414.

49. Ozaki T, Flege S, Kevric M, et al: Osteosarcoma of the pelvis: Experience of the Cooperative Osteosarcoma Study Group. *J Clin Oncol* 2003;21(2):334-341.

50. Merimsky O, Kollender Y, Inbar M, Meller I, Bickels J: Palliative treatment for advanced or metastatic osteosarcoma. *Isr Med Assoc J* 2004;6(1):34-38.

51. Anderson PM, Wiseman GA, Dispenzieri A, et al: High-dose samarium-153 ethylene diamine tetramethylene phosphonate: Low toxicity of skeletal irradiation in patients with osteosarcoma and bone metastases. *J Clin Oncol* 2002;20(1):189-196.

52. Khanna C, Prehn J, Hayden D, et al: A randomized controlled trial of octreotide pamoate long-acting release and carboplatin versus carboplatin alone in dogs with naturally occurring osteosarcoma: Evaluation of insulin-like growth factor suppression and chemotherapy. *Clin Cancer Res* 2002;8(7):2406-2412.

53. Mansky PJ, Liewehr DJ, Steinberg SM, et al: Treatment of metastatic osteosarcoma with the somatostatin analog OncoLar: Significant reduction of insulin-like growth factor-1 serum levels. *J Pediatr Hematol Oncol* 2002;24(6):440-446.

54. Laverdiere C, Kolb EA, Supko JG, et al: Phase II study of ecteinascidin 743 in heavily pretreated patients with recurrent osteosarcoma. *Cancer* 2003;98(4):832-840.

55. Ebb D, Meyers P, Grier H, et al: Phase II trial of trastuzumab in combination with cytotoxic chemotherapy for treatment of metastatic osteosarcoma with human epidermal growth factor receptor 2 overexpression: A report from the children's oncology group. *J Clin Oncol* 2012;30(20):2545-2551.

    The authors report the results of a phase 2 trial of trastuzumab in metastatic osteosarcoma. Level of evidence: II.

56. Chou AJ, Kleinerman ES, Krailo MD, et al; Children's Oncology Group: Addition of muramyl tripeptide to chemotherapy for patients with newly diagnosed metastatic osteosarcoma: A report from the Children's Oncology Group. *Cancer* 2009;115(22):5339-5348.

57. Imran H, Enders F, Krailo M, et al: Effect of time to resumption of chemotherapy after definitive surgery on prognosis for non-metastatic osteosarcoma. *J Bone Joint Surg Am* 2009;91(3):604-612.

58. Saeter G, Høie J, Stenwig AE, Johansson AK, Hannisdal E, Solheim OP: Systemic relapse of patients with osteogenic sarcoma: Prognostic factors for long term survival. *Cancer* 1995;75(5):1084-1093.

59. Kempf-Bielack B, Bielack SS, Jürgens H, et al: Osteosarcoma relapse after combined modality therapy: An

3: Malignant Primary Bone Tumors

analysis of unselected patients in the Cooperative Osteosarcoma Study Group (COSS). *J Clin Oncol* 2005; 23(3):559-568.

60. DeLaney TF, Park L, Goldberg SI, et al: Radiotherapy for local control of osteosarcoma. *Int J Radiat Oncol Biol Phys* 2005;61(2):492-498.

61. Nathan SS, Gorlick R, Bukata S, et al: Treatment algorithm for locally recurrent osteosarcoma based on local disease-free interval and the presence of lung metastasis. *Cancer* 2006;107(7):1607-1616.

62. Rodriguez-Galindo C, Shah N, McCarville MB, et al: Outcome after local recurrence of osteosarcoma: The St. Jude Children's Research Hospital experience (1970-2000). *Cancer* 2004;100(9):1928-1935.

63. Brosjö O: Surgical procedure and local recurrence in 223 patients treated 1982-1997 according to two osteosarcoma chemotherapy protocols: The Scandinavian Sarcoma Group experience. *Acta Orthop Scand Suppl* 1999;285:58-61.

Chapter 16

Ewing Sarcoma

Matthew R. Steensma, MD

Introduction

Ewing sarcoma was originally described in 1921[1,2] as a "diffuse endothelioma" or "endothelial myeloma of bone," and was later referred to as a "round cell sarcoma of bone" in an effort to differentiate presentations of Ewing sarcoma from osteosarcoma. The fundamental observations of Ewing sarcoma as a clinical entity, including its histologic appearance, natural history, and favorable initial response to radiation therapy, continue to stand the test of time. The early nomenclature for Ewing sarcoma ("diffuse endothelioma") was based on its resemblance to blood vessels in the bone. At that time, the cell of origin was thought to be an endothelial cell. The cell of origin for Ewing sarcoma is still a matter of intense debate. More than an academic discussion, defining the cell of origin for Ewing sarcoma has significant implications in identifying the molecular pathogenesis and potential therapeutic targets of this malignancy.

Ewing sarcoma refers to a group of tumors with varied degrees of neuroectodermal differentiation that possess common cytogenetics, immunohistochemical profiles, and proto-oncogene expression. The common Ewing sarcomas include bone and extraskeletal Ewing sarcoma and primitive neuroectodermal tumor. Several more rare morphologic variants, including large cell, adamantinoma-like, spindle cell sarcoma-like, and vascular-like Ewing sarcoma, have been described.[3] Askin tumor is defined as a Ewing sarcoma arising from the chest wall or peripheral lung.[4] Historically, the term Ewing sarcoma has been applied to tumors that lack demonstrable features of neuroectodermal differentiation based on light microscopy, immunohistochemistry, and electron microscopy, whereas primitive neuroectodermal tumor demonstrates evidence of neuroectodermal differentiation (for example, S-100 positivity, Homer Wright rosettes, or pseudorosettes). Apart from these few histologic distinctions, the management and natural history of all Ewing sarcomas is the same. The general principles of treatment of Ewing sarcoma include local and systemic control measures that are applied on the basis of the stage at presentation. Local control measures consist of surgical resection, radiation therapy, or a combination of the two in the setting of a positive margin, local contamination, or poor chemotherapy-induced histologic necrosis. Both surgical treatment options, limb salvage and amputation, are effective means of local control and offer a chance at restoring meaningful function. Currently, most affected individuals in the United States undergo limb-sparing surgery for extremity-based lesions. Definitive irradiation is usually reserved for unresectable lesions, often in axial locations. Systemic control is achieved through a combination of durable local control and multiagent chemotherapy. Autologous stem cell transplantation is an additional treatment option, and is currently used in patients at the highest risk of disease progression.[5]

Epidemiology

Ewing sarcoma is the second most common primary malignancy of bone. Surveillance, Epidemiology, and End Results (SEER) data confirm the annual incidence to be two to three cases per million individuals in the United States, with most affected individuals younger than 21 years of age.[6] Infantile Ewing sarcoma is a rare but defined entity with a generally favorable prognosis. A baseline incidence of Ewing sarcoma exists among individuals of all ages, with the oldest patient reported as 81 years of age.[7] SEER data also confirm that US whites are nine times more likely to develop Ewing sarcoma than blacks, indicating a disparate incidence among certain ethnicities. This observation has been confirmed by others, and is the basis of a recent genome-wide association study in which 401 French individuals with Ewing sarcoma and 684 unaffected French individuals were compared with 3,668 unaffected individuals of European descent living in the United States to identify genetic susceptibility markers.[8] Two risk haplotypes were identified and replicated in an independent case-control analysis. Two common variants were located near the genetic loci TARDBP and EGR2, both of which were confirmed to be less prevalent in Africans. The precise mechanism whereby TARDBP and/or EGR2 influence Ewing sarcoma risk is under investigation. This impressive study offers the most detailed look at the genetic susceptibility markers of Ewing sar-

3: Malignant Primary Bone Tumors

coma to date. Although not included in the genomewide association study, individuals of Chinese descent and other Asian ethnicities are also known to develop Ewing sarcoma at a much lower rate than whites.

Notably, the overall incidence in the United States has not changed significantly in the past 30 years. Studies support a slight male predominance (59% male; 41% female). Anatomically, the most common osseous sites of presentation are the lower extremity (41%) and pelvis (26%), followed by the chest wall (16%), upper extremity (9%), spine (6%), and skull (2%). Extraosseous Ewing sarcoma has been reported in truncal regions (32%), extremities (26%), the head and neck (18%), the retroperitoneum (16%), and other sites (9%). Within the long bones, diaphyseal location is not uncommon.

Clinical Presentation

The symptoms of Ewing sarcoma are variable and often nonspecific, and include swelling, pain, fever, weight loss, fatigue, and loss of appetite. Spine-based presentations can be associated with bowel or bladder dysfunction, radiculopathy, or myelopathy. Patients with Ewing sarcoma typically have an enlarging, painful mass; minor trauma frequently draws attention to the mass. Growth can be rapid. The presence of pain may indicate a pathologic fracture in bone-based lesions, whereas radiating pain raises concern for tumor compression or frank invasion of peripheral nerves. In painless presentations of both extremity and axial lesions, the most common complaint is stiffness or fullness. The median time from symptom onset to diagnosis varies, but the latency period is typically between 5 and 9 months. Pelvic or other axial sites are usually subject to the longest delay in presentation.

Physical examination frequently reveals a mass, or asymmetric fullness of the affected extremity or anatomic compartment. Erythema may be present, particularly in patients who have a rapidly growing mass attenuating the overlying skin. Neurovascular deficits can be subtle, so a thorough examination should be performed to rule out any peripheral nerve or vessel involvement. Regional lymphadenopathy can also be present, but rarely indicates spread of tumor in Ewing sarcoma. Metastases almost always occur by hematogenous spread, and the lungs are the primary site of involvement, followed by bone. Primary lymphoma of bone mimics Ewing sarcoma both clinically and radiographically, and often involves regional lymph nodes.

Staging and Workup

Staging studies are performed to define the extent of local and systemic disease spread at the time of diagnosis. Stage assignments have important implications for both prognosis and treatment (**Figures 1** and **2**). The key el-

ements in the staging of Ewing sarcoma are tumor grade, tumor size, extent of local spread, and the presence or absence of metastasis. Several systems for staging bone malignancies are relevant to Ewing sarcoma. The two most frequently used are the American Joint Committee on Cancer (AJCC) staging system and the Enneking surgical staging system.[9] The most common stage of Ewing sarcoma at presentation is Enneking Stage IIB or AJCC Stage IIA or IIB. Ewing sarcoma is a uniformly high-grade malignancy with a strong propensity for metastasis. The National Comprehensive Cancer Network publishes diagnosis, staging, and treatment recommendations for primary bone malignancies, including Ewing sarcoma.[10] These guidelines are updated regularly to reflect advances in diagnostic and treatment strategies.

In addition to a thorough history and physical examination, the initial workup includes plain radiographs. Ewing sarcoma typically occurs as a permeative, lytic lesion within the diaphysis or metadiaphysis of long bones. The shadow from the associated soft-tissue mass can frequently be seen on plain radiographs. Soft-tissue mineralization outside of the bone is less common and can indicate a bone-forming tumor such as osteosarcoma. Reactive bone formation, such as periosteal reaction (onion skinning or Codman triangle) or marginal sclerosis, is present in more than 30% of Ewing sarcomas. Lytic tumor progression can make the identification of subtle pathologic fractures challenging. CT imaging can be useful if pathologic fracture is suspected and cannot be ruled out on the basis of plain radiographs alone.

Laboratory evaluation is useful for determining the health status of the patient at presentation, and has bearing on prognosis. Complete blood count, comprehensive metabolic panel, erythrocyte sedimentation rate, C-reactive protein level, and lactate dehydrogenase (LDH) studies are recommended. The erythrocyte sedimentation rate and C-reactive protein level are nonspecific and are often elevated in Ewing sarcoma, particularly if the patient exhibits fever, malaise, or decreased appetite leading up to diagnosis. Microcytic anemia can be present, indicating a chronic marrow response to tumor cytokine production. If significant marrow infiltration occurs, white blood cell and platelet counts may be altered, but are typically unaffected. An elevated LDH level at the time of diagnosis is associated with an increased risk of disease recurrence (normal LDH level = 9%; elevated LDH level = 50%).[11] LDH level has also been shown to be a marker of recurrent disease.[12] The alkaline phosphatase level can be elevated as well, and is an indicator of upregulated bone turnover.

Local staging studies are important for the successful diagnosis and treatment of Ewing sarcoma. Plain radiographs are not necessarily replaced by other axial imaging techniques. MRI is a sensitive method for determining tumor size, the extent of tumor spread both inside and outside the bone, and the relationship of tumor to

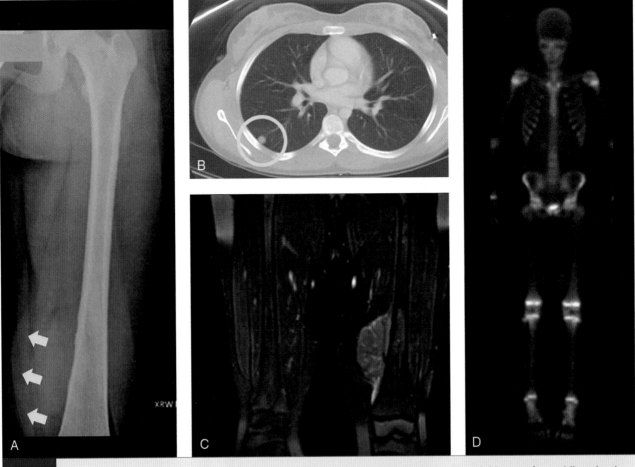

Figure 1 A metastatic presentation of Ewing sarcoma is shown. A 13-year-old girl had a 6-week history of a rapidly enlarging, painful mass in the left distal femur. **A,** Plain radiographs demonstrated a subtle lytic lesion with associated soft-tissue mass (arrows). **B,** A solitary pulmonary metastasis was evident on chest CT (circle). **C,** MRI demonstrated a large soft-tissue mass emanating from the intramedullary canal of the distal femur. **D,** Increased uptake can be seen in the left distal femur and medial thigh soft tissue. No bone metastases were evident.

adjacent anatomic structures. MRI should be performed with and without contrast whenever possible (**Figure 3**). MRI of the entire affected bone is also recommended to identify skip metastases. Ewing sarcoma appears isointense to muscle on T1-weighted sequences and is hyperintense on T2-weighted sequences. Strong contrast enhancement is typical, and can be either homogeneous or heterogeneous depending on the degree of necrosis. Edema is often present in the adjacent soft tissues and marrow space. Although MRI is capable of demonstrating changes in tumor volume following neoadjuvant chemotherapy, data confirm a low to moderate correlation between tumor shrinkage and histologic necrosis. The role of fluorodeoxyglucose positron emission tomography (FDG PET) in determining treatment response is currently under investigation. A standardized uptake value of less than 2.5 following neoadjuvant chemotherapy was shown to be predictive of progression-free survival independent of stage.[13]

Systemic staging studies are undertaken to screen target organs for metastasis, and are the basis of risk-adapted therapy strategies. The primary site of Ewing sarcoma metastasis is the lung, followed by bone. Unusual sites of metastasis such as the brain, the abdominal viscera, and subcutaneous locations have been reported but are rare. Chest CT is sensitive for pulmonary metastasis. Chest CT has high specificity but often fails to distinguish reactive subcentimeter pulmonary nodules from early metastatic lesions. Whole-body technetium bone scanning is sensitive for distant bone metastases and skip metastases. FDG PET is an important aspect of staging for Ewing sarcoma. A recent meta-analysis of whole-body FDG PET demonstrated high sensitivity (96%; 95% confidence interval, 91% to 99%) and specificity (92%; 95% confidence interval, 87% to 96%) in assigning stage for Ewing sarcoma.[14] Data also support the use of whole-body MRI; comparative analyses favor MRI over whole-body bone scanning.[15] Bone marrow assessment, usually via iliac crest aspiration, is performed to determine whether microscopic evidence of marrow metastasis exists. Patients with marrow involvement at presentation have a poor prognosis. Conventional methods for detecting Ewing sarcoma in marrow are based on morphologic

3: Malignant Primary Bone Tumors

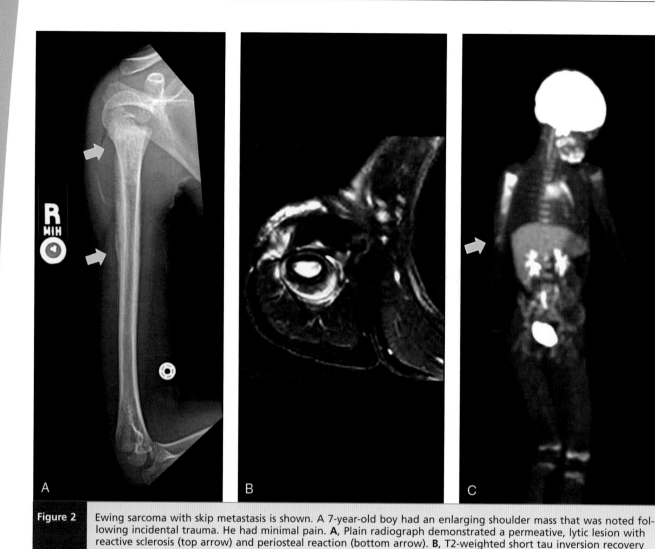

Figure 2 Ewing sarcoma with skip metastasis is shown. A 7-year-old boy had an enlarging shoulder mass that was noted following incidental trauma. He had minimal pain. **A**, Plain radiograph demonstrated a permeative, lytic lesion with reactive sclerosis (top arrow) and periosteal reaction (bottom arrow). **B**, T2-weighted short tau inversion recovery MRI demonstrated a hyperintense soft-tissue mass expanding outside of the humeral cortex. **C**, Whole-body fluorodeoxyglucose positron emission tomography scan identified a skip metastasis in the distal humerus (arrow).

criteria and/or immunohistochemical staining. A highly sensitive and specific polymerase chain reaction (PCR)-based method also exists, and is capable of detecting fusion transcripts in microscopically normal marrow. The clinical significance of molecularly detectable metastasis in morphologically normal bone marrow has yet to be determined.

Histology and Molecular Pathology

Methods for obtaining tissue diagnosis for Ewing sarcoma are similar to those for other bone malignancies. Biopsy accuracy varies by institution and requires a coordinated effort between the treating surgeon, pathologist, and radiologist. The three biopsy techniques for bone malignancy are open biopsy, core biopsy, and fine-needle aspiration biopsy and are discussed in detail in chapter 3, Biopsy. In addition to a thorough histologic analysis, cytogenetic testing is critical for differentiating Ewing sarcoma from other small round blue cell tumors. Early methods for identifying putative Ewing sarcoma translocations required ample amounts of fresh, sterile tumor tissue that could be expanded in tissue culture for karyotype analysis. With the development of commercially available laboratory techniques that can be applied to smaller amounts of fixed tissues, such as fluorescence in situ hybridization ("break-apart probes") or PCR-based identification methods, cytogenetic yields from core biopsy specimens are nearing equivalence with those of open biopsy techniques. Obtaining reliable cytogenetic information from fine-needle aspiration cytology specimens is challenging, but recent successful demonstrations are encouraging.

Ewing sarcoma histology consists of a monotonous population of small round blue cells that exhibit a high nuclear to cytoplasmic ratio (**Figure 4**). Fields of loosely aggregated cells typically have little intervening stroma. Nucleolar definition is often obscured because the nuclei are intensely hyperchromatic. The cytoplasm contains a large amount of glycogen that is demonstrable on a periodic acid-Schiff stain. On the basis of mor-

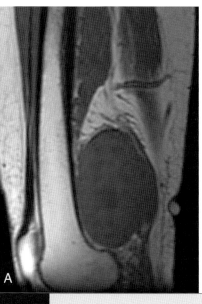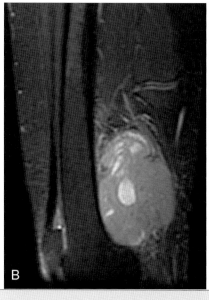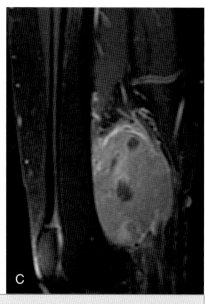

Figure 3   MRI studies show extraosseous Ewing sarcoma in a 56-year-old woman. T1-weighted sequences (A) demonstrate a large mass of intermediate signal intensity in the soft tissues of the posterior thigh. Corresponding T2-weighted (B) and T1 fat-suppressed sequences with gadolinium contrast (C) demonstrate typical signal hyperintensity and contrast enhancement, respectively. Staging workup for this patient was negative.

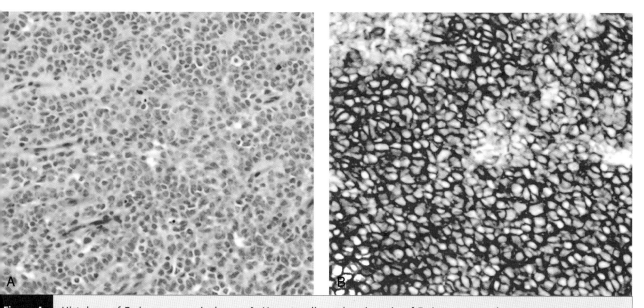

Figure 4   Histology of Ewing sarcoma is shown. A, Hematoxylin and eosin stain of Ewing sarcoma demonstrates a monotonous population of small round blue cells with increased nuclear-to-cytoplasmic ratio, little intervening stroma, and small branching vessels. B, Properly controlled CD99 stain with hematoxylin counterstain demonstrates a strong membranous staining pattern.

phology alone, Ewing sarcoma closely resembles other neoplastic conditions such as hematologic malignancies, histiocytic disorders, metastatic neuroblastoma, rhabdomyosarcoma, and monophasic synovial sarcoma, as well as chronic infection. Immunohistochemistry provides important specificity to routine morphologic observations. Ewing sarcoma tumors strongly express CD99 antigen, or MIC2 (Figure 4). CD99 antigen is a cell-surface glycoprotein transcribed by a pseu-

doautosomal gene located on the short arms of the X and Y chromosomes. CD99 antigen is generally considered to be a sensitive and specific marker for Ewing sarcoma; however, it is also found in synovial sarcoma, non-Hodgkin lymphoma, and gastrointestinal stromal tumor. Concurrent membrane positivity for FLI1, the product of the most common fusion partner in the putative Ewing translocation, offers strong evidence in support of Ewing sarcoma. S-100 is a marker of neural

3: Malignant Primary Bone Tumors

Table 1

Prognostic Factors for Ewing Sarcoma

Prognostic Factor	Effect on Outcome
Site	Outcomes range from better to worse for sites as follows: distal extremities, proximal extremities, pelvis/trunk, and sacrum
Size	Tumor volume greater than 100 mL or greater than 200 mL associated with adverse outcome; size correlates with proximal location
Age	Best outcome in infants and children younger than 15 years; worst outcome in patients older than 15 years
Sex	Better outcome in females than in males
Serum LDH level	Elevated LDH level correlates with diminished survival, tumor size, presence of metastases
Metastatic disease	Single most powerful predictor of a poor outcome (standard imaging or bone marrow aspirate)
Standard cytogenetics	Worse prognosis with a complex karyotype (more than five chromosomal abnormalities) or modal chromosome number less than 50
Detectable fusion transcripts	PCR detection of fusion transcripts in morphologically normal bone marrow aspirate associated with relapse
Biologic factors	Overexpression of p53, expression of Ki-67, loss of 16q, microsomal glutathione S-transferase overexpression (chemoresistance)
Treatment response	Minimal or no residual viable tumor associated with improved survival and local control. Decreased PET uptake following neoadjuvant chemotherapy (good histologic response)

LDH = lactate dehydrogenase, PCR = polymerase chain reaction, PET = positron emission tomography.

differentiation that is often absent in Ewing sarcoma. S-100 positivity, along with the identification of Homer Wright rosettes or pseudorosettes, is often used as a rationale for assigning the diagnosis of PNET. Ewing sarcoma is a mesenchymal neoplasm and expresses vimentin; however, 20% of Ewing sarcomas exhibit local or diffuse staining for epithelial markers, such as pancytokeratin, CAM5.2, and AE1/AE3.[16]

Ewing sarcoma is defined genetically by the presence of a balanced translocation involving the *EWS* locus at chromosome band 22q12 and another member of the ETS family of transcription factors. In approximately 90% of patients,[17] the N terminal of *EWS* is fused with the C terminal of *FLI1*, resulting in a transcriptionally active fusion protein. In addition to *FLI1*, a variety of unique ETS family translocation partners are encountered clinically, including *ERG*, *E1AF*, *FEV*, *ETV1*, and *ETV4*. The 22q12 *EWS* breakpoint is a common site of translocation and has been implicated in · desmoplastic small round cell tumor [*EWS-WT1*; t(11,22)(p13:q12)], myxoid liposarcoma [*FUS-DDIT3*; t(12;22)(q13;q12)], clear cell sarcoma [*EWS-ATF1*; t(12;22)(q13;q12)], extraskeletal myxoid chondrosarcoma [*EWS-CHN*; t(9;22)(q22;q12)], and angiomatoid fibrous histiocytoma [*EWS-ATF1*; t(12; 22)(q13;q12)]. Other numeric and structural chromosomal aberrations have been associated with adverse outcomes; however, their role in facilitating diagnosis is limited.

Prognosis and Treatment

Systemic chemotherapy for primary bone malignancies was originally introduced in the 1970s and resulted in a steady increase in survival for patients with nonmetastatic Ewing sarcoma. Data from the prechemotherapy era confirm that amputation of extremity sarcomas cured fewer than 20% of individuals with localized presentations. Hence, without chemotherapy, occult metastatic disease was able to flourish following definitive local control. Over the past 30 years, the 5-year overall survival rate has improved from 59% to 76% for children younger than 15 years and from 20% to 49% in adolescents. Nearly 25% of patients have detectable evidence of metastasis at presentation. Metastatic disease remains the strongest indicator of a poor prognosis. Pathologic fractures are not considered to significantly affect survival; however, the morbidity of local control is increased. Other prognostic factors for Ewing sarcoma[18,19] are outlined in Table 1.

Durable local control of Ewing sarcoma has been reported using radiation therapy, surgical resection, or both. Many attempts have been made to compare these treatment modalities in terms of local recurrence rate, survival, and late effects. These comparative analyses are confounded by several issues, including the inclusion of multiple anatomic sites within individual cohorts, inconsistent reporting of adjuvant chemotherapy regimens, and a bias toward using radiation therapy in larger tumors where resection is not possible or deemed excessively morbid. Adequately controlled studies confirm an increased risk of local control failure with radiation therapy alone in localized Ewing sarcoma, as well as an increased incidence of secondary malignancy.[20] In a series of 53 patients treated with radiation therapy (30 patients) or with surgery with or without radiation therapy (23 patients), the 15-year actuarial local control rates were 68% and 100%, respectively. No differences in overall survival were demonstrated.[21] In a separate report, 5-year event-free survival (EFS) and local control were significantly lower in patients treated with radiation therapy than in patients treated with surgery with or without radiation therapy (48% versus 66% EFS; 80% versus 94% local control).[22] Of the 1,058 patients treated in the CESS 81, CESS 86, and EICESS 92 treatment trials, the rate of local control failure was 7.5% following complete surgical resection and radiation therapy, compared to 26.3% with radiation therapy as definitive treatment. Overall, radiation therapy was shown to improve local control in both resectable Ewing presentations, and in cases where intralesional or marginal resections were performed.[23] Patients with nonmetastatic pelvic Ewing sarcoma also fared better with surgical resection in terms of local control (surgery 82.6% versus radiation therapy 66.7%) and 5-year EFS (surgery 73.9% versus radiation therapy 30.3%).[24]

The decision to perform limb salvage versus amputation in Ewing sarcoma is based on a variety of patient-related and treatment-related factors. SEER data confirm that 73.9% of Ewing sarcoma patients underwent limb salvage instead of amputation from 1988 to 2007.[25] In the same study, limb salvage was associated with improved survival (71.8%) versus amputation (63.1%) following multivariable adjustment. Similar to other primary bone malignancies, limb salvage in Ewing sarcoma is associated with good functional outcomes, patient satisfaction, and an acceptable rate of ultimate limb preservation. The wide variety of limb salvage options is reviewed in great detail in section 6 of this book.

Chemotherapy regimens differ between institutions but typically include a backbone of vincristine, doxorubicin, and cyclophosphamide alternating with ifosfamide and etoposide (VDC/IE) with myeloid growth factor support.[26] Recent investigations have focused on the effectiveness of dose intensification strategies and on the avoidance of drug-related toxicity. In a completed trial, patients with localized Ewing sarcoma were randomized to receive VDC/IE chemotherapy either every 3 weeks or every 2 weeks.[27] EFS was improved in the more frequent dosing arm (76% versus 65% EFS). The increase in survival was not associated with increased drug toxicity. In another dose intensification approach, patients with localized Ewing sarcoma were randomized to receive standard doses of VDC/IE over 48 weeks or 30 weeks. There was no difference in 5-year EFS between the standard and intensified regimens (72.1% EFS for the 48-week regimen versus 70.1% EFS for the 30-week regimen).[28] A higher incidence of toxicities, including the development of secondary malignancies, impairment of growth and development, and a variety of organ dysfunctions, was reported in the time-compressed regimen. Results of an evaluation of chemotherapy with stem cell rescue in patients with a poor initial response demonstrated improved EFS when high-dose therapy (HDT) was combined with stem cell support (5-year EFS was 72% for patients with poor response who were treated with HDT and stem cell support versus 33% for patients with poor response who did not receive HDT).[29]

Novel therapy targets continue to emerge. Receptor tyrosine kinases are primary regulators of cellular growth, survival, and proliferation. These key regulatory proteins are located on the cell surface and are accessible to both antibody-based and small molecule inhibitors. Insulin-like growth factor 1 receptor (IGF1R) is a prototypical receptor tyrosine kinase and is currently the subject of intensive therapeutic development for a variety of malignancies. Several completed phase 2 trials of IGF1R-targeted therapies in Ewing sarcoma demonstrated antitumor activity and favorable side effect profiles. Ganitumab, a fully human monoclonal antibody against IGF1R, was well tolerated and achieved partial response in 6% and stable disease in 49% of patients; four patients had stable disease for more than 24 weeks.[30] Phase 1/phase 2 trial results regarding cixutumumab activity in Ewing sarcoma were recently reported.[31] Treatment was well tolerated, and only two patients experienced dose-limiting toxicities. Treatment response was assessed in dose-specific cohorts with 10% partial response in each. R1507, a humanized monoclonal IGF1R antibody, was evaluated in recurrent or refractory Ewing sarcoma with 10% of patients having complete or partial response.[32] Of those who had complete or partial response, 10 of 11 patients had initial presentation in bone. Inhibitors of intracellular signaling molecules, such as the PI3K-AKT-mTOR pathway, are also in phase 1 and phase 2 trials for Ewing sarcoma and other pediatric solid tumors.

Molecular Pathogenesis

Ewing sarcoma is defined by the presence of a nonrandom, balanced translocation involving the *EWS* (also known as *EWSR1*) gene and a member of the ETS family of transcription factors, most commonly *FLI1* (approximately 90%). *EWS* belongs to the TET family of RNA-binding proteins. TET proteins contain an 87–amino acid RNA recognition motif that facilitates direct binding of RNA, and RNA-protein interactions. Upstream of this region is a strong transactivation domain that is driven by an active *EWS* promoter. The chimeric EWS-FLI1 protein is the product of an "in-frame" fusion that combines the strong transactivation domain of *EWS* and the DNA-binding domain of *FLI1*. Cell-autonomous EWS-FLI1 expression results in malignant transformation in a variety of experimental systems. Importantly, EWS-FLI1 is considered to be necessary for Ewing sarcoma oncogenesis and hence is a bona fide therapeutic target.

The mechanism whereby EWS-FLI1 induces malignant transformation is an area of intense investigation. Early attempts to identify the downstream effectors of EWS-FLI1 consisted of inducing EWS-FLI1 overexpression in a variety of human cell lines, and subsequently comparing changes in the genetic profiles. As one might expect given the debate regarding the cell of origin for Ewing sarcoma, induced overexpression of EWS-FLI1 in heterologous but relevant human cell lines, such as fibroblasts and neuroblastoma, rhabdomyosarcoma, and mesenchymal stem cell lines, were informative but produced broadly different expression profiles, few of which accurately reflected human disease. Alternative approaches using native Ewing sarcoma tumor samples were sought. Recent studies using strategic inhibitory RNA (RNAi) knockdown of EWS-FLI1 in human tumors have expanded the understanding of its oncogenic mechanisms and, importantly, demonstrated that cellular proliferation, survival, and other phenotypic aspects of disease progression are mitigated by inhibiting EWS-FLI1 function.

Several downstream effectors of EWS-FLI1 have emerged from these studies. NKX2.2 is a key regulator of the Sonic Hedgehog pathway, and is indirectly upregulated in Ewing sarcoma by a GLI1-dependent mechanism through direct binding of EWS-FLI1 to the GLI1 promoter. NKX2.2 is primarily a transcriptional repressor and is necessary for EWS-FLI1–mediated transformation. Demonstrated protein-protein interactions between NKX2.2 and regulators of histone deacetylase (HDAC) function suggest that HDAC inhibitors may be effective in inhibiting NKX2.2-dependent transformation. IGF binding protein 3 (IGFBP3) is a secreted inhibitor insulin-like growth factor 1 ligand, and is significantly downregulated by EWS-FLI1. The therapeutic strategy of inhibiting ligand-dependent IGF1R activation, discussed previously, may be relevant to an autocrine or paracrine activation of IGF1R. Recent studies demonstrate that the EWS-FLI1 transcription factor also binds to GGAA microsatellite regions throughout the human genome. Chromatin immunoprecipitation sequencing (ChIP-seq) studies demonstrating EWS-FLI1 binding to GGAA microsatellite repeats in both promoter regions of coding DNA and intergenic regions suggest possible higher-order regulation of EWS-FLI1 response elements. The array of target genes is currently being analyzed but will likely reveal novel regulatory mechanisms and therapeutic targets.

Interestingly, EWS-FLI1 was recently identified as a biomarker for drug sensitivity to the poly ADP-ribose polymerase (PARP) inhibitors olaparib and AG-014699.[33] This important observation may be relevant to other malignancies with *EWS*-based translocations and is the basis for emerging PARP inhibitor trials in Ewing sarcoma. The action of PARP inhibitors is to prevent PARP-mediated repair of single-stranded breaks in DNA that, if left unrepaired, would normally induce apoptosis during cell division. This effect, known as synthetic lethality, is traditionally thought to occur when an additional double-stranded DNA damage repair mechanism is dysfunctional, such as in the cases of breast cancer in individuals with *BRCA1* or *BRCA2* mutation. In terms of mechanistic relevance in Ewing sarcoma, EWS-FLI1 and EWS-ERG were recently shown to potentiate DNA damage in the context of PARP1 inhibition, and work in a positive feedback loop to maintain PARP1 expression.[34]

Summary

The diagnosis, staging, and treatment of Ewing sarcoma continue to evolve. Despite historical trends demonstrating improved survival over the past three decades, treatment advances are still greatly needed. Understanding of the molecular pathogenesis, epidemiology, and pharmacogenomics of Ewing sarcoma is sure to be enhanced by the application of sequencing technology. Large-scale genomic profiling efforts are already under way to identify new markers of treatment response, risk-stratified treatment strategies, and novel therapeutic targets. Trials aimed at limiting the short-term and long-term effects of treatment-related toxicity also offer hope for patients with Ewing sarcoma.

Annotated References

1. Huvos AG: James Ewing: Cancer man. *Ann Diagn Pathol* 1998;2(2):146-148.

2. Ewing J: Further report on endothelial myeloma of bone. *Proc NY Pathol Soc* 1924;24:93-100.

3. Pinto A, Dickman P, Parham D: Pathobiologic markers of the ewing sarcoma family of tumors: State of the art and prediction of behaviour. *Sarcoma* 2011;2011:856190.

   This review article provides an overview of biomarkers in Ewing sarcoma as they relate to diagnosis and prognosis.

4. Askin FB, Rosai J, Sibley RK, Dehner LP, McAlister WH: Malignant small cell tumor of the thoracopulmonary region in childhood: A distinctive clinicopathologic entity of uncertain histogenesis. *Cancer* 1979;43(6):2438-2451.

5. Fraser CJ, Weigel BJ, Perentesis JP, et al: Autologous stem cell transplantation for high-risk Ewing's sarcoma and other pediatric solid tumors. *Bone Marrow Transplant* 2006;37(2):175-181.

6. Esiashvili N, Goodman M, Marcus RB Jr: Changes in incidence and survival of Ewing sarcoma patients over

the past 3 decades: Surveillance Epidemiology and End Results data. *J Pediatr Hematol Oncol* 2008;30(6): 425-430.

SEER data provide a comprehensive look at disease-specific trends in management and treatment outcomes. Ewing sarcoma survival has improved over the past 30 years but remains challenging in certain age groups and for patients with metastatic disease. Level of evidence: III.

7. Levine RG, Bono CM, Hameed M, et al: Ewing sarcoma in an octogenarian: A case report. *J Bone Joint Surg Am* 2002;84-A(3):445-448.

8. Postel-Vinay S, Véron AS, Tirode F, et al: Common variants near TARDBP and EGR2 are associated with susceptibility to Ewing sarcoma. *Nat Genet* 2012; 44(3):323-327.

This landmark genome-wide association study is a first look at the population genetics of Ewing sarcoma. The two genes associated with Ewing sarcoma development in individuals of European descent, *TARDBP* and *EGR2*, offer insight into the fundamental processes that contribute to Ewing sarcoma development. Level of evidence: I.

9. Enneking WF, Spanier SS, Goodman MA: A system for the surgical staging of musculoskeletal sarcoma. *Clin Orthop Relat Res* 1980;153 :106-120.

10. Biermann JS, Adkins DR, Benjamin RS, et al; National Comprehensive Cancer Network Bone Cancer Panel: Bone cancer. *J Natl Compr Canc Netw* 2010;8(6):688-712.

National Comprehensive Cancer Network guidelines are routinely updated and provide a useful reference for the diagnosis, staging, and treatment of primary bone malignancies.

11. Bacci G, Ferrari S, Longhi A, et al: Prognostic significance of serum LDH in Ewing's sarcoma of bone. *Oncol Rep* 1999;6(4):807-811.

12. Farley FA, Healey JH, Caparros-Sison B, Godbold J, Lane JM, Glasser DB: Lactase dehydrogenase as a tumor marker for recurrent disease in Ewing's sarcoma. *Cancer* 1987;59(7):1245-1248.

13. Hawkins DS, Schuetze SM, Butrynski JE, et al: [18F]Fluorodeoxyglucose positron emission tomography predicts outcome for Ewing sarcoma family of tumors. *J Clin Oncol* 2005;23(34):8828-8834.

14. Treglia G, Salsano M, Stefanelli A, Mattoli MV, Giordano A, Bonomo L: Diagnostic accuracy of ^{18}F-FDG-PET and PET/CT in patients with Ewing sarcoma family tumours: A systematic review and a meta-analysis. *Skeletal Radiol* 2012;41(3):249-256.

This small but compelling meta-analysis confirms a high degree of sensitivity and specificity for ^{18}F-FDG PET and PET-CT for staging of Ewing sarcoma. Level of evidence: I.

15. Mentzel HJ, Kentouche K, Sauner D, et al: Comparison of whole-body STIR-MRI and 99mTc-methylene-diphosphonate scintigraphy in children with suspected multifocal bone lesions. *Eur Radiol* 2004;14(12):2297-2302.

16. Gu M, Antonescu CR, Guiter G, Huvos AG, Ladanyi M, Zakowski MF: Cytokeratin immunoreactivity in Ewing's sarcoma: Prevalence in 50 cases confirmed by molecular diagnostic studies. *Am J Surg Pathol* 2000; 24(3):410-416.

17. de Alava E, Kawai A, Healey JH, et al: EWS-FLI1 fusion transcript structure is an independent determinant of prognosis in Ewing's sarcoma. *J Clin Oncol* 1998; 16(4):1248-1255.

18. O'Connor MI, Pritchard DJ: Ewing's sarcoma: Prognostic factors, disease control, and the reemerging role of surgical treatment. *Clin Orthop Relat Res* 1991; 262:78-87.

19. Wunder JS, Paulian G, Huvos AG, Heller G, Meyers PA, Healey JH: The histological response to chemotherapy as a predictor of the oncological outcome of operative treatment of Ewing sarcoma. *J Bone Joint Surg Am* 1998;80(7):1020-1033.

20. Kuttesch JF Jr , Wexler LH, Marcus RB, et al: Second malignancies after Ewing's sarcoma: Radiation dose-dependency of secondary sarcomas. *J Clin Oncol* 1996;14(10):2818-2825.

21. Indelicato DJ, Keole SR, Shahlaee AH, et al: Long-term clinical and functional outcomes after treatment for localized Ewing's tumor of the lower extremity. *Int J Radiat Oncol Biol Phys* 2008;70(2):501-509.

The investigators reported an increased risk of relapse and local control failure in Ewing sarcoma patients treated with radiation therapy alone. No difference in functional outcomes or survival could be demonstrated. Level of evidence: III.

22. Bacci G, Ferrari S, Longhi A, et al: Role of surgery in local treatment of Ewing's sarcoma of the extremities in patients undergoing adjuvant and neoadjuvant chemotherapy. *Oncol Rep* 2004;11(1):111-120.

23. Schuck A, Ahrens S, Paulussen M, et al: Local therapy in localized Ewing tumors: Results of 1058 patients treated in the CESS 81, CESS 86, and EICESS 92 trials. *Int J Radiat Oncol Biol Phys* 2003;55(1):168-177.

24. Donati D, Yin J, Di Bella C, et al: Local and distant control in non-metastatic pelvic Ewing's sarcoma patients. *J Surg Oncol* 2007;96(1):19-25.

These data support the role of surgery in achieving durable local control of pelvic Ewing sarcoma, but also identify a high-risk cohort of patients whose tumors grew during chemotherapy, all of whom died. Level of evidence: III.

25. Schrager J, Patzer RE, Mink PJ, Ward KC, Goodman

M: Survival outcomes of pediatric osteosarcoma and Ewing's sarcoma: A comparison of surgery type within the SEER database, 1988-2007. *J Registry Manag* 2011;38(3):153-161.

This study compared survival between Ewing patients who underwent limb salvage and those who underwent amputation over a 19-year period. A survival advantage was noted for those undergoing limb salvage; however, the reasons for this trend are unclear. The study also confirmed that most patients with Ewing sarcoma in the United States undergo limb-preserving surgery. Level of evidence: II.

26. Grier HE, Krailo MD, Tarbell NJ, et al: Addition of ifosfamide and etoposide to standard chemotherapy for Ewing's sarcoma and primitive neuroectodermal tumor of bone. *N Engl J Med* 2003;348(8):694-701.

27. Womer RB, West DC, Krailo MD, et al: Abstract: Randomized comparison of every-two-week v. every-three-week chemotherapy in Ewing sarcoma family tumors (ESFT). J Clin Oncol *2008 ASCO Annual Meeting Proceedings* 2008;26(15S):10504.

In a completed trial, patients with localized Ewing sarcoma were randomized to receive VDC/IE chemotherapy either every 3 weeks or every 2 weeks. EFS was improved in the more frequent dosing arm (76% versus 65%). The increase in survival was not associated with increased drug toxicity. Level of evidence: I.

28. Granowetter L, Womer R, Devidas M, et al: Dose-intensified compared with standard chemotherapy for nonmetastatic Ewing sarcoma family of tumors: A Children's Oncology Group Study. *J Clin Oncol* 2009; 27(15):2536-2541.

Patients with localized Ewing sarcoma were randomized to receive standard doses of VDC/IE over 48 weeks or 30 weeks. There was no difference in 5-year EFS between the standard and intensified regimens (72.1% versus 70.1%). A higher incidence of toxicities was reported in the time-compressed regimen, including the development of aggressive secondary malignancies, impairment of growth and development, and a variety of organ dysfunctions. Level of evidence: I.

29. Ferrari S, Sundby Hall K, Luksch R, et al: Nonmetastatic Ewing family tumors: High-dose chemotherapy with stem cell rescue in poor responder patients. Results of the Italian Sarcoma Group/Scandinavian Sarcoma Group III protocol. *Ann Oncol* 2011;22(5): 1221-1227.

Results of this evaluation of chemotherapy with stem cell rescue in patients with a poor initial response demonstrated improved EFS when HDT was combined with stem cell support (5-year EFS was 72% for patients with poor response who were treated with HDT and stem cell support versus 33% for patients with poor response who did not receive HDT). Level of evidence: I.

30. Tap WD, Demetri G, Barnette P, et al: Phase II study of ganitumab, a fully human anti-type-1 insulin-like growth factor receptor antibody, in patients with metastatic Ewing family tumors or desmoplastic small round cell tumors. *J Clin Oncol* 2012;30(15):1849-1856.

Patients older than 16 years with relapsed or refractory Ewing sarcoma or desmoplastic small round cell tumors were administered ganitumab every 2 weeks. No grade 4 or 5 treatment-related events were noted, and four patients had stable disease beyond 24 weeks. Level of evidence: I.

31. Malempati S, Weigel B, Ingle AM, et al: Phase I/II trial and pharmacokinetic study of cixutumumab in pediatric patients with refractory solid tumors and Ewing sarcoma: A report from the Children's Oncology Group. *J Clin Oncol* 2012;30(3):256-262.

Three patients with Ewing sarcoma demonstrated partial responses with single-agent cixutumumab. Doses were well tolerated. Level of evidence: I.

32. Pappo AS, Patel SR, Crowley J, et al: R1507, a monoclonal antibody to the insulin-like growth factor 1 receptor, in patients with recurrent or refractory Ewing sarcoma family of tumors: Results of a phase II Sarcoma Alliance for Research through Collaboration study. *J Clin Oncol* 2011;29(34):4541-4547.

Single-agent R1507 achieved partial or complete responses in 10% of enrolled patients. Nearly all responders had a primary bone Ewing sarcoma as opposed to extraskeletal Ewing sarcoma. The drug was well tolerated at the administered dosage. Level of evidence: I.

33. Garnett MJ, Edelman EJ, Heidorn SJ, et al: Systematic identification of genomic markers of drug sensitivity in cancer cells. *Nature* 2012;483(7391):570-575.

In an unbiased drug screen, the EWS-FLI1 translocation was established as a biomarker for sensitivity to PARP inhibitors.

34. Brenner JC, Feng FY, Han S, et al: PARP-1 inhibition as a targeted strategy to treat Ewing's sarcoma. *Cancer Res* 2012;72(7):1608-1613.

A PARP1 inhibition strategy is examined in Ewing sarcoma. Responses to combination PARP1 inhibitor/temozolomide therapy are demonstrated in a mouse xenograft model.

Chapter 17

Chondrosarcoma of Bone

Richard L. McGough III, MD

Introduction

Chondrosarcoma is an uncommon primary malignant neoplasm of bone. The disease occurs in adults and older individuals and is different from most malignant bone tumors in symptomatology, age distribution, anatomic locale, and natural history.

Conventional chondrosarcoma is a tumor that generally develops in the medullary space and proliferates centrifugally. It is composed of malignant chondrocytes of various grades. Depending on the grade, these cells may produce hyaline cartilage, myxoid cartilage, or a fibromyxoid matrix. The highest grade of chondrosarcoma may produce very little matrix and can be difficult to distinguish from other high-grade malignancies.

The most important aspect of chondrosarcoma is possibly the variability of the disease from indolent to extremely fulminant. Clinical symptoms, radiographic findings, and histology vary along a continuum, and accurate diagnosis can rarely be made with only one of these components. Although diagnosis in musculoskeletal oncology frequently requires a clinical-radiographic-pathologic correlation, this diagnostic acumen is mandatory in chondrosarcoma because of the wide variations involved.

Chondrosarcoma is resistant to most chemotherapy modalities and has very low radiosensitivity. Treatment is therefore almost exclusively surgical.

Spectrum of Disease

Although most bone sarcomas present with a rapidly progressive, fulminant course, this progression is uncommon in chondrosarcoma. The slower progression of chondrosarcoma is explained by the prevalence of low- or intermediate-grade bone sarcomas in this disease, compared to their paucity or absence in other tissue types such as osteosarcoma or Ewing sarcoma. In general, high-grade bone sarcomas occur with severe, unremitting pain, rapidly increasing associated soft-tissue masses, and occasionally pathologic fractures.

Neither Dr. McGough nor any immediate family member has received anything of value from or has stock or stock options held in a commercial company or institution related directly or indirectly to the subject of this chapter.

Unless chondrosarcoma is of high grade, it tends to occur with a long-standing history of pain, mild swelling, and progressive inability to perform sporting or daily activities.[1] Chondrosarcoma is also much more prevalent in adults in their third through seventh decades of life, and is rare in children and adolescents.[2]

The anatomic distribution of chondrosarcoma strongly favors the axial and proximal appendicular skeleton. Chondrosarcoma in the distal extremities is extremely rare, and chondrosarcoma of the hand or foot, although reported, is exceedingly uncommon. Great care must be taken in diagnosing benign cartilage tumors of the axial skeleton because most central or axial cartilage neoplasms behave in a more aggressive manner than their appendicular counterparts.

The natural history of chondrosarcoma varies depending on grade and subtype. Grade 1 chondrosarcomas are generally slow growing and occur with an insidious onset of pain with activity. The pain will progress, sometimes over the course of years, to pain at night. Patients often assume that the pain is caused by a more common, benign condition, such as sciatica, low back pain, rotator cuff disorders, or arthritis. Presence of a palpable soft-tissue mass is rare, but a bony deformity may be palpable if remodeling has occurred. Pathologic fracture can occur, but is unusual in the absence of a traumatic event unless the patient has lived with pain for months to years.

Low-grade chondrosarcoma has the ability to dedifferentiate. Dedifferentiation is the capacity for a low-grade neoplasm to undergo conversion to a high-grade neoplasm. This conversion may occur after a substantial lag period, with the initial tumor remaining fairly indolent for months or years and then rapidly changing into a high-grade tumor. This change is accompanied by relatively rapid increases in tumor size and correspondingly severe symptoms. The dedifferentiation phenomenon is thought to be a characteristic of low-grade malignant neoplasms and is absent in benign chondromas (either enchondromas or periosteal chondromas). Although it has the capability to dedifferentiate and recur locally, grade 1 chondrosarcoma of the extremities has limited capacity for metastasis. Because of this distinction and the social and financial stigma of a sarcoma diagnosis, it may be more appropriate to classify these tumors as low-grade cartilage neoplasms, omitting the sarcoma diagnosis. Axial grade 1 chondrosarcomas, however, have the capacity for distant metas-

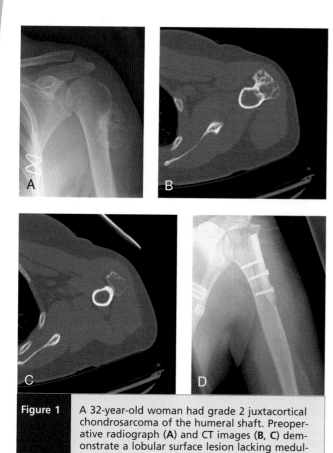

Figure 1 A 32-year-old woman had grade 2 juxtacortical chondrosarcoma of the humeral shaft. Preoperative radiograph (**A**) and CT images (**B, C**) demonstrate a lobular surface lesion lacking medullary continuity. A small soft tissue mass can be seen. Wide resection with cortical allograft reconstruction (**D**) yielded excellent functional results and no evidence of disease at 4 years postoperatively.

tasis and are generally considered to be true malignancies.[2]

Grade 2 chondrosarcomas may occur with a course similar to that of grade 1 chondrosarcoma, especially if the tumor has no substantial myxoid component. Tumors that are more myxoid may demonstrate more rapid growth and a soft-tissue mass. Pain and disability progress more rapidly, with few patients maintaining these tumors for years before diagnosis.

Grade 3 chondrosarcoma, along with dedifferentiated chondrosarcoma, often occurs with a more fulminant course. Within weeks or months, symptoms can progress rapidly from vague night pain to severe pain with functional difficulty. In the case of dedifferentiated chondrosarcoma, vague, indolent symptoms may have been present for months to years before the more severe symptoms occur. A soft-tissue mass is often evident and can grow sizably, especially in pelvic chondrosarcomas. Instead of respecting surrounding anatomic boundaries, high-grade chondrosarcomas may invade through surrounding structures, causing changes to skin and surrounding neural or vascular structures.

Multiple chondrosarcoma variants are known to ex-

ist. Variants include juxtacortical chondrosarcoma, mesenchymal chondrosarcoma, clear cell chondrosarcoma, dedifferentiated chondrosarcoma, secondary chondrosarcoma, and extraskeletal myxoid chondrosarcoma. All of these entities are rare, most appearing only in small case series in the literature. Juxtacortical chondrosarcoma is a chondrosarcoma occurring on the periosteal surface of the bone, in contradistinction to conventional chondrosarcoma, which is a medullary or endosteal process. Juxtacortical chondrosarcomas account for less than 5% of chondrosarcomas (**Figure 1**). These tumors occur in the bone, and are not generally parosteal because they do not surround and entrap the subjacent periosteum. This distinction is useful because the differential diagnosis of juxtacortical chondrosarcoma often includes parosteal osteosarcoma and enchondroma protuberans. Because of their juxtacortical location, these tumors much more readily occur with a palpable mass or functional limitation, even as low-grade lesions.

Mesenchymal chondrosarcoma is an extremely rare, high-grade chondrosarcoma variant that accounts for less than 1% of all chondrosarcomas. The course of this disease is fulminant, with rapidly progressive pain, dysfunction, and soft-tissue mass formation. Mesenchymal chondrosarcoma has a significant round cell component and the uncommon ability to form skip metastases or to metastasize to other bones. Skeletal surveillance is necessary to screen for recurrence in this disorder. Treatment is difficult, and a 40% mortality rate has been reported.[3]

Clear cell chondrosarcoma is an extremely rare variant, one of a very few types of epiphyseal tumors, and has therefore been dubiously correlated with chondroblastoma. This lesion occurs as a slow-growing, painful joint process. Progressive pain, occasionally coupled with a joint effusion, is a hallmark of this disease.

Dedifferentiated chondrosarcoma is a high-grade chondrosarcoma developed from a low-grade tumor (either conventional grade 1 chondrosarcoma or a secondary chondrosarcoma). These tumors demonstrate a rapid change in clinical course from indolent to fulminant symptoms.

Secondary chondrosarcoma is a chondrosarcoma arising from a previously benign lesion. Originally described as a malignant transformation from a previous osteochondroma, this lesion has also been described as developing from chondromas (either enchondromas or periosteal chondromas), synovial chondromatosis, or fibrous dysplasia.[2] This transformation produces a low-grade neoplasm, with slow growth and an insidious increase in symptoms from a previous baseline.[4] In very rare circumstances, a secondary chondrosarcoma may be grade 2 or higher, but most are low-grade lesions.

Extraskeletal myxoid chondrosarcoma is a high-grade, soft-tissue sarcoma. It differs from bone chondrosarcoma in all aspects, and is discussed in detail in chapter 29.

Radiographic Characteristics

Careful consideration of radiographs is critical in the diagnosis and appropriate treatment of cartilage neoplasms. These diseases exist on a continuum, and the radiographs reflect this. Because of the microscopic heterogeneity inherent in these tumors, accurate interpretation of radiographs can be more beneficial in determining treatment than a limited histologic sample via biopsy. Anatomic locale matters in these diseases: central lesions behave much more aggressively than appendicular or distal lesions, and should be treated in a more aggressive manner.

Care must be taken when choosing diagnostic studies. The radiographic evaluation should begin with high-quality plain radiographs. Although other modalities can yield useful information and may alter the diagnostic and treatment plan, routine plain radiographs are the preferred method for determining the interaction between tumor biology and bone biology. This interaction, when combined with the clinical findings, helps determine tumor grade. Plain radiographs allow the diagnostician to determine whether the bone growth is keeping pace with that of the tumor, or whether the tumor is growing at such a rapid rate that the biologic process is unable to maintain the bone's structure.[1,5]

Beyond plain radiography, the choice of diagnostic study becomes more complex. MRI is often used as a follow-up to an abnormal plain radiograph. Unfortunately, because of both the high water content of cartilage tumors and the fact that bone is seen as black on all MRI sequences, MRI often obscures the fine changes at the endosteal surface and overestimates the aggressiveness of the lesion. It is, however, the best study in determining the marrow extent and soft-tissue extent of any bone tumor. CT yields the finest detail of cortical integrity and is therefore a superior study for lower-grade cartilage neoplasms. In determining endosteal scalloping or cortical penetration, CT yields the highest-quality images.

Other imaging modalities have limited usefulness with chondrosarcoma, especially in low-grade lesions. Although necessary for skeletal or chest screening, other imaging techniques add little to the diagnosis and treatment of any local disease.

Because approximately 60% of all chondrosarcomas are grade 1, distinguishing between a low-grade chondrosarcoma and an enchondroma is of primary importance. Generally, enchondromas cause little pain, are found incidentally, and are Enneking stage 1 (or at most stage 2) lesions. Although they can grow and fill the medullary space, they cause minor endosteal scalloping (>50%) and do not cause substantial cortical expansion. Endosteal scalloping is the phenomenon whereby a medullary tumor expands into the endosteum of the bone. The cortex often remodels around this tumor expansion, and a small pit is formed in the cortex. This occurrence is not true bony invasion, but is

an application of Wolff's law that demonstrates the interaction between the biology of the tumor and the biology of the bone. Tumors that grow more rapidly are able to push deeper into the bone, and the bone cannot remodel quickly enough to respond to the tumor's pressure. Deeper scallops are therefore a hallmark of more active tumors and help distinguish enchondromas and low-grade cartilage neoplasms. As the lesions age, they progressively calcify and demonstrate the typical radiographic characteristics of cartilage tumors (punctate calcifications, rings and arcs, and a "popcorn" appearance). More active tumors cause endosteal scalloping, and the surrounding bone may be expanded by the tumor. The cortices are generally intact circumferentially, unless a fracture has occurred, but may be thinned. These active findings should be regarded with caution, and a careful search for extraosseous tumor should be undertaken because its presence has diagnostic, treatment, and prognostic implications[6] (**Figure 2**).

Grade 2 chondrosarcoma demonstrates a much more aggressive behavior pattern. These tumors often breach the cortex (Enneking stage 1B) and cause substantial bony destruction. Changes may occur on the periosteal surface as the tumor invades the cortex, and periosteal new bone formation can occur. Mineralization is decreased or absent, but the lobular pattern of tumor growth is often preserved. Pathologic fracture or joint disruption may occur more frequently than in low-grade neoplasms.

Because treatments often differ between grade 1 and grade 2 chondrosarcoma, an accurate radiographic diagnosis is important. Although grade 1 chondrosarcomas are often active lesions, they typically do not produce extensive extraosseous tumor, do not permeate the cortex, and reflect a bone-tumor relationship that is compensated, meaning that the bone biology can remodel and respond to the tumor biology, maintaining the bone's structural integrity. The appearance of grade 2 chondrosarcoma often uncompensated, meaning that the bone cannot respond adequately to the tumor. Periosteal reactions, extraosseous tumor, and substantial cortical changes can occur. These occurrences should be regarded with extreme caution because limited intralesional surgical techniques are not sufficient for the treatment of this grade of disease (**Figure 3**).

Grade 3 chondrosarcoma appears radiographically as a high-grade tumor, with substantial bony destruction, cortical disruption, associated soft-tissue masses, and substantial periosteal changes. The differential diagnosis includes osteosarcoma, Ewing sarcoma, and fibrosarcoma of bone. Unless a dedifferentiated lesion exists, calcification is rare and not prominent. MRI is likely to show increased soft-tissue mass formation (sometimes massive), and the internal characteristics lack resemblance to typical cartilage neoplasms.[7] Positron emission tomography (PET), although increasingly used for certain carcinomas and hematologic malignancies, is unproved in the diagnosis of sarcoma. PET may, however, show differential signal characteristics be-

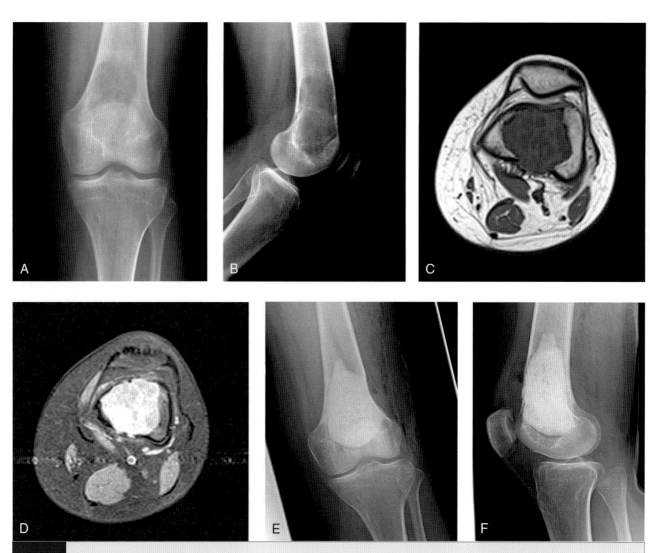

Figure 2 A 52-year-old man had grade 1 intramedullary chondrosarcoma (low-grade cartilage neoplasm) with active features in the distal femur. Preoperative AP (**A**) and lateral (**B**) radiographs demonstrate a lytic distal femoral lesion. The lateral view demonstrates active features, with potential cortical perforation anteriorly. The differential diagnosis includes giant cell tumor, metastatic disease, plasmacytoma, and chondrosarcoma because lobular architecture can be distinguished. T1-weighted (**C**) and T2-weighted (**D**) MRIs show a water signal intensity lesion with cortical thinning that is suggestive of internal matrix formation. Biopsy revealed a low-grade cartilage neoplasm. The patient underwent curettage and cementation (**E**, **F**). He remains free of disease at 6 years.

tween low-grade and high-grade cartilage tumors, and may therefore be of diagnostic benefit.[8]

Juxtacortical chondrosarcoma may appear similar to a large periosteal chondroma. With lower-grade juxtacortical chondrosarcoma, calcification may be present and may be prominent. Because the tumor does not have the surrounding cortex to contain its growth, the tumor's lobular architecture is usually apparent. In contrast to periosteal chondroma, substantial saucerization and shouldering of the subjacent cortex is rarely present because the tumor invades that cortex rather than pushing upon it. The bone's inability to contain the lesion, along with the size of the lesion, are the most important clues that a surface cartilage neoplasm is malignant.

Mesenchymal chondrosarcoma demonstrates imaging characteristics similar to Ewing sarcoma, befitting the small cell nature of its development. Lytic bone destruction with permeation and periosteal "sunburst" may occur. Because of this disease's propensity for skeletal metastasis and multifocal disease, skeletal scanning with either standard bone scan or PET is advantageous for staging purposes.

Because of its biphasic nature, dedifferentiated chondrosarcoma often has the radiographic characteristics of both grade 1 and grade 3 chondrosarcoma. The diagnosis can be made when the radiographs show two distinct, apposed areas, one heavily calcified and appearing more benign, and the other having the radiographic characteristics of a high-grade bone sarcoma.

The imaging characteristics of secondary chondrosarcoma depend on the primary lesion. In a secondary chondrosarcoma arising from a prior osteochondroma, the stalk of the initial lesion may appear eroded or perforated, with a large (> 10 mm) cartilage cap destroying either the stalk or the surrounding bony cortex. Care must be taken in interpreting the thickness of a cartilage cap. In children, adolescents, and young adults, the cap may be as thick as 20 mm without concern for secondary transformation. In older adults, the cap should be less than 10 mm and is often much thinner. Imaging of the secondary transformation of an intraosseous enchondroma demonstrates findings similar to those described for grade 1 chondrosarcoma.[4]

Histologic Characteristics

The histologic characteristics of chondrosarcoma are as varied as clinical and radiographic findings. The overarching theme of chondrosarcoma histology is heterogeneity: lesions demonstrate not only cellular heterogeneity but also areas of varying grades within the tumor. This heterogeneity causes several problems. In diagnosis, limited biopsy techniques (fine-needle aspiration, core needle, or even limited open biopsy) may not accurately reflect the final diagnosis. Furthermore, the treatment (as detailed later) reflects not only the suspected grade of the tumor but also the amount of damage that the surrounding bone has sustained. Determination of the grade depends on anatomic locale: a histologically low-grade lesion in the finger will be a benign enchondroma, whereas an identical lesion in the pelvis will be a grade 1 or 2 chondrosarcoma and act accordingly. Accurately determining the final grade of any cartilage neoplasm therefore demands examination of the clinical, radiographic, and histologic characteristics by an experienced, multidisciplinary musculoskeletal team.[9]

Grade 1 chondrosarcoma often appears similar to an enchondroma. The cartilage will be hyaline, with all cells residing within the lacunae and minimal myxoid changes. Classic histologic changes in low-grade chondrosarcoma include hypercellularity, disorganization, increased nuclear detail (often the presence of a nuclear membrane), and more-than-occasional binucleate cells.[5] In certain circumstances, such as distal extremity lesions or synovial chondromas, all of these characteristics may be present without any concrete diagnosis of malignancy. Anatomic locale is therefore of paramount importance in rendering an accurate diagnosis.

Grade 2 chondrosarcoma generally is more distinctive than grade 1; the typical characteristics of benign cartilage disappear. The overall architecture remains lobular, but hyaline matrix gives way to a myxoid background. The cells appear more disorganized, and the cytologic features of sarcoma such as the presence of nucleoli and mildly pleomorphic forms, become more evident.

Histologically, grade 3 chondrosarcoma can be difficult to distinguish from cartilage. Minimal calcification is present, and the lacunar structure found in hyaline

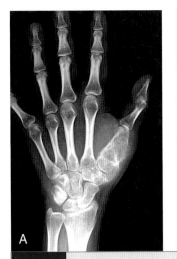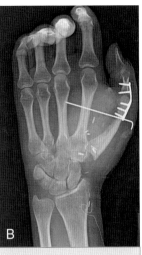

Figure 3 A 23-year-old woman had grade 2 chondrosarcoma of the first metacarpal. A preoperative radiograph (**A**) demonstrates the bony hallmarks of malignancy in cartilage neoplasms, with cortical perforation, permeative changes, and a large soft-tissue mass. Because of these findings, aggressive surgical treatment consisting of metacarpal resection, vascularized fibula reconstruction, metacarpal-phalangeal fusion, and basal joint reconstruction was performed (**B**).

cartilage may be completely absent. The overall architecture remains lobular, but substantial pleomorphism and nearly complete anaplasia mark the tumor as high grade. Mitoses, which are generally not present in lower-grade chondrosarcoma, are prominent and more abnormal. Because high-grade chondrosarcoma is quite rare and the features of grade 3 chondrosarcoma and chondroblastic osteosarcoma overlap substantially, the diagnosis of grade 3 chondrosarcoma requires a careful search for malignant osteoid. This distinction has treatment and prognostic implications, and should not be overlooked.

Chondrosarcoma variants have interesting histopathologic features (**Figure 4**). Mesenchymal chondrosarcoma is a biphasic tumor in which the features of a low-grade chondrosarcoma are juxtaposed with (and sometimes superimposed on) those of a small, round blue cell tumor. Lobules of hyaline cartilage containing areas of disorganization and binucleate cells are interspersed with areas of monotonous, small blue cells similar to those of Ewing sarcoma. At times, these features exist in the same field, with the small cell, high-grade component seen within the hyaline matrix.

Clear cell chondrosarcoma, a rare epiphyseal sarcoma, maintains the lobular architecture characteristic of all cartilage neoplasms. Unlike hyaline chondrocytes, the cells in this entity are large, vacuolated cells with clear cytoplasm. Highly malignant features, such as bizarre mitoses, marked nucleoli, and open chromatin, are generally absent, and the cellular grade is usually

3: Malignant Primary Bone Tumors

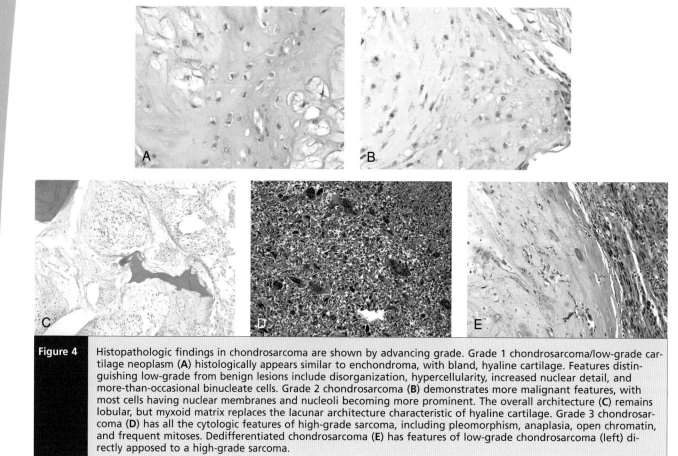

Figure 4 Histopathologic findings in chondrosarcoma are shown by advancing grade. Grade 1 chondrosarcoma/low-grade cartilage neoplasm (**A**) histologically appears similar to enchondroma, with bland, hyaline cartilage. Features distinguishing low-grade from benign lesions include disorganization, hypercellularity, increased nuclear detail, and more-than-occasional binucleate cells. Grade 2 chondrosarcoma (**B**) demonstrates more malignant features, with most cells having nuclear membranes and nucleoli becoming more prominent. The overall architecture (**C**) remains lobular, but myxoid matrix replaces the lacunar architecture characteristic of hyaline cartilage. Grade 3 chondrosarcoma (**D**) has all the cytologic features of high-grade sarcoma, including pleomorphism, anaplasia, open chromatin, and frequent mitoses. Dedifferentiated chondrosarcoma (**E**) has features of low-grade chondrosarcoma (left) directly apposed to a high-grade sarcoma.

low to intermediate. Giant cells, either individually or in clusters, are prominent and assist with the diagnosis.

Dedifferentiated chondrosarcoma is a biphasic tumor with a specialized pattern. One portion is a typical low- or intermediate-grade chondrosarcoma with the characteristics described previously. The other is a high-grade sarcoma, with the tissue types being high-grade chondrosarcoma, chondroblastic osteosarcoma, or high-grade fibrosarcoma. An abrupt change from one tumor type to the other is evident, sometimes within one high-powered field. This change generates the appearance of two completely different tumors pressed together, with an abrupt transition from one to the other.

Treatment and Treatment Decisions

Not surprisingly, the treatment of chondrosarcoma is as varied as its clinical, radiographic, and histologic characteristics. A few principles remain constant throughout this spectrum of disease. First and foremost, chondrosarcoma requires surgical treatment. Because of multiple factors, chondrosarcoma is resistant to chemotherapy and radiation therapy, and any treatment relies primarily or solely on surgery. Surgical treatment of this disease varies and depends on the clinical-

radiographic-pathologic diagnosis. Unfortunately, the diagnosis of chondrosarcoma is quite complex, and misidentification of the final grade of a chondrosarcoma remains possible even when a diligent diagnostic workup has been conducted.

Although little doubt exists that most grade 1 chondrosarcomas should be treated, accurately distinguishing a grade 1 chondrosarcoma from an enchondroma may be impossible preoperatively. The first consideration is symptomatology: if the lesion is causing pain, it should be treated. The pain may begin as activity-related pain but may progress to nonactivity-related or night pain. This symptom is often more important than any radiographic or biopsy findings. Radiographic signs of aggressiveness include deep endosteal scalloping, periosteal changes, bony remodeling, and cortical disruption. Substantial clinical judgment is required in the treatment of asymptomatic patients. Because many benign enchondromas have endosteal activity, endosteal scalloping is a relative, but not absolute, indication for surgery. Unless cortical disruption has occurred, endosteal scalloping can be monitored radiographically in patients without symptoms. Unfortunately, biopsy is not useful in the decision to treat chondrosarcoma. Chondrosarcomas are extremely heterogeneous histologically, so core biopsy may yield only hyaline cartilage. Biopsy in this circumstance is more

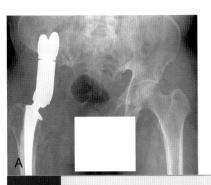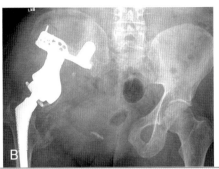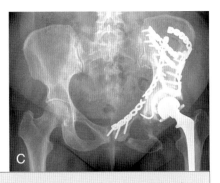

Figure 5 Some options for pelvic reconstruction after periacetabular resection for chondrosarcoma are shown. Functional ambulation after acetabular resection frequently requires reconstruction. Options for this include a saddle prosthesis (**A**), which provides a stable fulcrum for a hip prosthesis against the remaining ilium; a custom acetabular prosthesis (**B**), which attaches rigidly to the remaining ilium; or an alloprosthetic composite (**C**), which attempts to reconstruct the native pelvic ring. Other options include arthrodesis, creation of a pseudarthrosis, osteoarticular allograft, or interposition arthroplasty.

frequently used for confirmation of a chondroid neoplasm, and the choice to treat is made regardless of this information. Any tumor that has radiographic characteristics of greater concern, such as those detailed for grades 2 and 3 chondrosarcoma; should undergo biopsy because this finding may substantially change the surgical treatment plan. For a biopsy performed via intraoperative frozen section, this finding may necessitate abandoning a planned intralesional procedure until the final diagnosis is established.

Once the decision to treat has been made, the surgeon needs to decide on the type of treatment. Historically, all chondrosarcomas were treated with wide resection with the intent to achieve negative bony margins. This treatment required bony reconstruction in many patients and caused substantial functional disability. As data accrued regarding the relatively benign nature of grade 1 chondrosarcoma (prompting many physicians to abstain from the sarcoma designation and, instead, term this condition low-grade cartilage neoplasm), clinical studies demonstrated that the metastatic rate from grade 1 chondrosarcoma of the extremities approached 0%. In situations in which a later, wide resection could be performed in case of recurrence, multiple authors recommended intralesional curettage instead of wide resection.[10] Subsequent clinical series demonstrated that intralesional curettage was safe, effective, and yielded a functional result superior to that of wide bony resection.[10-14] Although local recurrences after this more limited treatment have occurred and necessitated either revision curettage or wide resection, adverse oncologic outcomes (metastasis or death by disease) have rarely occurred, and recurrence with dedifferentiation has not been common. Intralesional treatment has therefore become more common than bony resection for this disease.[15]

Choosing limited, intralesional surgery for grade 1 chondrosarcoma has some caveats. Although the results in series of extremity lesions have been excellent, the treatment of pelvic lesions has been much less satisfactory.[16,17] There are several reasons for this difference.

Pelvic lesions are less accessible in general, particularly in a revision setting. Pelvic lesions are also more likely to be of higher grade than appendicular lesions, and the grade may not be determined by core biopsy. In addition, grade 1 chondrosarcoma of the pelvis is similar to a higher-grade chondrosarcoma: it has a higher risk of local recurrence and a risk of metastasis. For this reason, most authors do not recommend limited curettage of axial lesions. In treating appendicular grade 1 chondrosarcoma intralesionally, the approach should be similar to that undertaken for giant cell tumor of bone, which is another benign but locally aggressive lesion. The tumor should be thoroughly exteriorized so that all portions of the cavity are visible. Meticulous curettage should be performed and a high-speed burr should be used, with great care taken to ensure that the tumor does not contaminate the surrounding tissues. Adjuvant therapy, similar to that used in the treatment of giant cell tumor, has been described[18,19] and is used widely in this setting, although efficacy has not been conclusively demonstrated when compared to intralesional treatment without adjuvant therapy. Finally, intralesional treatment should be avoided when substantial extraosseous tumor is present.[20] The presence of extraosseous tumor usually indicates a higher grade. Controlling the margin in a curettage with extraosseous tumor is also technically more difficult, and the risk of local recurrence may be higher.

The treatment of grade 2 chondrosarcoma is less controversial. Because most grade 2 chondrosarcomas display substantial bony changes and extracompartmental tumor, they are less technically amenable to adequate curettage. Although intralesional treatment has been successful in some situations,[21] complete resection, in the form of either wide or marginal resection, is preferable[22] (**Figure 5**). Margin distance has been discussed and debated, but no clear acceptable distance has become available. Data seem to indicate that as long as all tumor is removed in a controlled manner, a positive oncologic outcome can be expected.[23] This finding is especially important because, as a result of the previously

3: Malignant Primary Bone Tumors

mentioned histologic heterogeneity in cartilage tumors, an aggressive grade 1 chondrosarcoma may in fact be of higher grade.[20] Although this finding was of prognostic importance, successful en bloc removal of all tumor is likely adequate for treatment. Local recurrence may have more importance in grade 2 chondrosarcoma because this tumor has some ability to metastasize, and the rate of dedifferentiation is higher than in low-grade cartilage neoplasms.

Grade 3 chondrosarcoma is a difficult disease to treat. Diagnosis is difficult because bone fibrosarcoma can be confused with chondroblastic osteosarcoma. With osteosarcoma, treatment protocols may differ dramatically and depend more on successful chemotherapy. Chondrosarcoma is generally resistant to chemotherapy and radiation therapy, and all surgical treatments should therefore be as complete as possible to attain a wide margin. Although wide surgical margins provide little guarantee against metastasis, local recurrence of grade 3 chondrosarcoma has dire prognostic implications. In both high-grade and dedifferentiated chondrosarcoma, the role of chemotherapy is still debated. Because of its high-grade small cell component, chemotherapy has also been advocated for treatment of mesenchymal chondrosarcoma, with some success.[24] Some studies have demonstrated a survival benefit, whereas other authors have recommended against systemic therapy. Clearly, decisions must be individualized given that all series of chemotherapy for this disease are hindered by low numbers and poor statistical validity.

Prognosis

The prognosis in chondrosarcoma is, not surprisingly, as varied as its clinical and radiographic spectrum. Anatomic locale also plays a role in prognosis: axial lesions generally have a poorer prognosis than appendicular lesions. In this regard, distinguishing biology from treatment is difficult. Many authors have reported poorer prognoses per grade in spinopelvic tumors than in lesions of the extremities. These findings may be tainted by selection bias against tumors that were considered unresectable. With advances in anesthesia and improved surgical techniques, the definition of an unresectable chondrosarcoma has diminished substantially, and techniques have been developed to remove many spinal or pelvic tumors with at least marginal resection. The ability to perform en bloc resection on these axial lesions may improve outcomes and align their prognoses with those of extremity lesions of the same grade.[25] Further study is required, however, to know whether central or axial tumors indeed differ biologically from appendicular lesions.

In grade 1 chondrosarcoma, the systemic consequences of the disease are minimal. Even in central lesions, metastasis is extremely rare without dedifferentiation. Metastasis from an appendicular grade 1 chondrosarcoma is reportable. Unlike enchondromas,

low-grade cartilage neoplasms have the capacity to dedifferentiate, and do so at a rate that depends on size, location, and prior failed treatments. The overall rate, however, is less than 5%.

Regardless of treatment, grade 1 chondrosarcoma can recur locally. Local recurrence after wide resection with negative margins is rare at best unless substantial contamination has occurred. The recurrence rate after intralesional treatment is much higher; the best series reported a risk of slightly less than 5% and most studies reported recurrence rates between 5% and 15%. No substantial difference was noted irrespective of technique; some authors preferred cryosurgery or other adjuvant treatments. The available data demonstrated no difference among these adjuvant treatments, however. As with giant cell tumor of bone, the thoroughness of exposure and curettage is likely the most important determinant of local success or failure.[26]

Grade 2 chondrosarcoma has a much more serious prognosis than grade 1. Its rate of local recurrence depends on both biology and surgical technique. Although some authors have extended intralesional treatment to grade 2 chondrosarcoma,[21] most have found an unacceptably high rate of local recurrence if resection with a negative margin is not attempted. This tumor can also metastasize, with rates from 5% to 15% being reported. Dedifferentiation can also occur, but the exact risk of this phenomenon in grade 2 chondrosarcoma is unknown.

Grade 3 chondrosarcoma is a high-grade malignancy. Both local and distant recurrence rates are higher, with a local recurrence rate of approximately 25% and a distant metastasis rate of greater than 30%.[25] Local recurrence and distant metastasis have been positively correlated in multiple studies; one large series reported a 73% correlation between local recurrence and distant metastasis. The cause of the correlation has been debated: some authors have implicated local recurrence as a direct factor in the development of distant metastasis, whereas others have hypothesized that both represent biologic aggressiveness and thus exhibit covariation.[27] Although cytotoxic chemotherapy is not widely used, its effect on prognosis is debated, with some authors arguing that it improves survival[23] and other studies demonstrating no effect.[28]

Grade 2 and grade 3 chondrosarcomas are entirely different from grade 1 chondrosarcomas. Grade 2 and grade 3 chondrosarcomas are true malignancies, with resultant risks of metastasis and death. The metastatic rate of these grades is approximately 30%. A study that analyzed Surveillance, Epidemiology and End Results (SEER) data demonstrated significant differences between low-grade and high-grade tumors. Overall survival was 70% at 5 years for conventional chondrosarcoma (all grades). Certain subtypes did fare differently, however, with 48% survival for mesenchymal chondrosarcoma, 100% survival for clear cell chondrosarcoma, and 0% survival for dedifferentiated chondrosarcoma.[29] Other authors have confirmed the dismal prognosis in dedifferentiated chondrosarcoma,[30,31] and have recommended against aggressive surgical treatment in metastatic high-grade or dedifferentiated chondrosarcoma, because the survival rate approaches 0%.[31]

Recent Advances

Perhaps the most interesting, and troubling, finding from the SEER study was the lack of change in prognosis over a 30-year period. The authors demonstrated no improvement in disease-specific survival during this period, and concluded that current treatment algorithms have not yielded any survival benefit.[29] Chondrosarcoma remains insensitive to current cytotoxic chemotherapy and is relatively resistant to radiation therapy.

Although a statistically proven survival benefit has not been demonstrated, surgical advances have allowed individuals with certain axial tumors to survive their diseases. Because of improvements in anesthesia, surgical technique, and critical care medicine, many patients are able to undergo large pelvic and spinal resections for cure. The definition of an unresectable tumor has changed, and many tumors that were initially thought to be too aggressive for surgical management can now be removed safely.[32] Although it was initially believed that pelvic chondrosarcoma was biologically more aggressive than its appendicular counterparts by grade, large series have failed to demonstrate differences between pelvic and appendicular tumors when controlled for margin status.[25]

With improvements in spinal reconstruction hardware, the safety of en bloc spinal resection has improved, and reconstruction for primary spinal malignancies has become possible. Applying musculoskeletal oncologic concepts to this area has been difficult because of both the technical difficulty of attaining negative margins in this area and the lack of oncology training among surgeons who manage most spinal diseases. Case series of spinal malignancies with intent to resect with negative margins have become available and have demonstrated results far better than those achieved with piecemeal or intralesional resection.[33,34] Adverse events are not uncommon with procedures of this extent and difficulty, but oncologic results have improved enough to warrant these procedures in patients with a suitable stage and medical comorbidity profile.[34]

As stated previously, chondrosarcoma is resistant to many if not most chemotherapeutic agents. Investigators have therefore searched for other therapeutic targets to offer some hope of systemic therapy for high-grade or metastatic lesions. Multiple studies have demonstrated a profound difference between the microvascularity of low-grade chondrosarcoma and that of intermediate or high-grade tumors.[35,36] This finding has led to studies that have demonstrated that one hallmark of "biologically dangerous" chondrosarcoma is angiogenesis.[36] Throughout oncology, angiogenesis is being investigated as a therapeutic target, and it may represent one of the few targets available in chondrosarcoma.

Angiogenic chondrosarcomas have demonstrated notable increases in vascular endothelial growth factor (VEGF), a potent pro-angiogenesis cytokine.[36] This increase is thought to be directed by *EPAS1* (also known as *HIF2A*), a physiologic gene responsible for angiogenesis in response to hypoxemia.[37,38] A switch to this angiogenic phenotype via hypoxia-inducible factor 2α (HIF-2α) seems to occur in higher-grade chondrosarcomas, along with dysregulation of other factors including histone deacetylase 4 (HDAC4), RUNX2, and Beclin 1.[37,39] Aside from any prognostic information that might be gathered from changes in these factors, they may provide future therapeutic targets.

Mutations in isocitrate dehydrogenase 1 (IDH1) and IDH2 have recently been identified in cartilaginous tumors and represent the first common genetic abnormalities to be identified these neoplasms.[40] This finding is clinically important for two reasons. Diagnostically, the pathologist now has a new tool in distinguishing primary cartilage tumors in difficult cases. Therapeutically, monoclonal antibodies that have been developed against these mutations suggest that perhaps targeted therapies may one day be possible for chondrosarcoma treatment. One xenograft model demonstrated tumor necrosis when the antiangiogenic factor ET-743 was combined with cytotoxic chemotherapy, suggesting that combination therapy may hold promise in chondrosarcoma treatment.[41] Although no current regimen has demonstrated definite efficacy in treating disseminated chondrosarcoma, treatment using these nonconventional agents may have promise.

Summary

Chondrosarcoma is a malignant primary bone tumor composed of chondrocytes with various degrees of malignancy. It therefore produces clinical, radiographic, and prognostic pictures that vary from minimally symptomatic conditions to rapidly progressive malignancy. To safely and adequately diagnose and treat this condition, the musculoskeletal oncologist must use the entire armamentarium of clinical judgment with radiographic and pathologic assistance. Even the decision whether to treat chondrosarcoma is not straightforward. Because both overtreatment and undertreatment are possible, a clinical, radiologic, and pathologic decision regarding the most accurate assessment of the grade of the tumor gives the best guidance for treatment. At its root, this disease requires surgical treatment, and assistance from medical and radiation oncology is rarely advantageous. Individualized treatment of cartilage neoplasms is mandatory to improve both oncologic and functional patient outcomes.

Acknowledgment

The author would like to thank Uma Rao, MD, Professor of Pathology at the University of Pittsburgh, for her assistance with photomicrographs.

Annotated References

1. Marco RA, Gitelis S, Brebach GT, Healey JH: Cartilage tumors: Evaluation and treatment. *J Am Acad Orthop Surg* 2000;8(5):292-304.

2. Unni KK: *Dahlin's Bone Tumors: General Aspects and Data on 11,087 Cases*. Philadelphia, PA, Lippincott-Raven, 1996, pp 71-108.

3. Shakked RJ, Geller DS, Gorlick R, Dorfman HD: Mesenchymal chondrosarcoma: Clinicopathologic study of 20 cases. *Arch Pathol Lab Med* 2012;136(1):61-75.

   This series presents 20 cases of mesenchymal chondrosarcoma. Radiographic and histopathologic characteristics are reviewed. A mortality rate of 40% is reported with a trend toward better results in patients who were able to undergo surgical resection. Level of evidence: IV.

4. Lin PP, Moussallem CD, Deavers MT: Secondary chondrosarcoma. *J Am Acad Orthop Surg* 2010; 18(10):608-615.

   This article reviews secondary chondrasarcoma, describing its pathogenesis, clinical, radiographic, and histologic characteristics. Level of evidence: V.

5. Brien EW, Mirra JM, Kerr R: Benign and malignant cartilage tumors of bone and joint: Their anatomic and theoretical basis with an emphasis on radiology, pathology and clinical biology. I: The intramedullary cartilage tumors. *Skeletal Radiol* 1997;26(6):325-353.

6. Parlier-Cuau C, Bousson V, Ogilvie CM, Lackman RD, Laredo JD: When should we biopsy a solitary central cartilaginous tumor of long bones? Literature review and management proposal. *Eur J Radiol* 2011; 77(1):6-12.

   The authors of this study proposed radiographic criteria for biologic aggressiveness in long bone cartilaginous lesions: cortical destruction, permeative osteolysis, fracture, edema, or soft-tissue mass. Biologic *activity* was defined by deep endosteal scalloping, extensive endosteal scalloping, cortical thickening, and medullary expansion. If two or more active criteria were present, biopsy was recommended. More quiescent lesions could be safely followed. Level of evidence: IV.

7. Yoo HJ, Hong SH, Choi JY, et al: Differentiating high-grade from low-grade chondrosarcoma with MR imaging. *Eur Radiol* 2009;19(12):3008-3014.

   The authors of this study defined MRI characteristics that distinguish low- from high-grade cartilage neoplasms. In a multivariate analysis, the formation of a soft-tissue mass favored a high-grade diagnosis, whereas entrapped fat signal within the lesion predicted a low grade. Level of evidence: III.

8. Lee FY, Yu J, Chang SS, Fawwaz R, Parisien MV: Diagnostic value and limitations of fluorine-18 fluorodeoxyglucose positron emission tomography for cartilaginous tumors of bone. *J Bone Joint Surg Am* 2004;86-A(12):2677-2685.

9. Evans HL, Ayala AG, Romsdahl MM: Prognostic factors in chondrosarcoma of bone: A clinicopathologic analysis with emphasis on histologic grading. *Cancer* 1977;40(2):818-831.

10. Bauer HC, Brosjö O, Kreicbergs A, Lindholm J: Low risk of recurrence of enchondroma and low-grade chondrosarcoma in extremities: 80 patients followed for 2-25 years. *Acta Orthop Scand* 1995;66(3): 283-288.

11. Aarons C, Potter BK, Adams SC, Pitcher JD Jr, Temple HT: Extended intralesional treatment versus resection of low-grade chondrosarcomas. *Clin Orthop Relat Res* 2009;467(8):2105-2111.

    The authors presented a retrospective series of low-grade chondrosarcoma of the extremities treated with extended curettage. One of 17 patients treated intralesionally demonstrated a local recurrence, and no cases of metastasis or dedifferentiation were reported. Functional scores were higher in the intralesional group than in the wide resection group. Level of evidence: IV.

12. Donati D, Colangeli S, Colangeli M, Di Bella C, Bertoni F: Surgical treatment of grade I central chondrosarcoma. *Clin Orthop Relat Res* 2010;468(2): 581-589.

    In this study, 15 patients with low-grade chondrosarcoma of the extremities underwent curettage and were compared with 16 matched control patients undergoing wide resection. Two recurrences occurred in the intralesional group, both of which were salvaged with wide resection. No metastases occurred. Both patients who experienced local recurrence had more aggressive radiographic characteristics. Level of evidence: IV.

13. Hanna SA, Whittingham-Jones P, Sewell MD, et al: Outcome of intralesional curettage for low-grade chondrosarcoma of long bones. *Eur J Surg Oncol* 2009;35(12):1343-1347.

    In this study, 39 patients underwent curettage and cementation for low-grade chondrosarcoma. Two local recurrences were treated with repeat intralesional treatment. No systemic disease was noted. Musculoskeletal Tumor Society (MSTS) scores were excellent (94%). Level of evidence: IV.

14. van der Geest IC, de Valk MH, de Rooy JW, Pruszczynski M, Veth RP, Schreuder HW: Oncological and functional results of cryosurgical therapy of enchondromas and chondrosarcomas grade 1. *J Surg Oncol* 2008;98(6):421-426.

    This study grouped patients with grade 1 chondrosarcoma and enchondroma, and both were treated with intralesional cryosurgery. No recurrences occurred in the chondrosarcoma group, whereas two occurred in the enchondroma group. Level of evidence: III.

15. Hickey M, Farrokhyar F, Deheshi B, Turcotte R, Ghert M: A systematic review and meta-analysis of intralesional versus wide resection for intramedullary grade I chondrosarcoma of the extremities. *Ann Surg Oncol* 2011;18(6):1705-1709.

    The authors of this meta-analysis of five studies comprising 78 chondrosarcomas treated by curettage concluded that intralesional treatment did not greatly increase the risk for local recurrence or metastasis. Level of evidence: I.

16. Normand AN, Cannon CP, Lewis VO, Lin PP, Yasko AW: Curettage of biopsy-diagnosed grade 1 periacetabular chondrosarcoma. *Clin Orthop Relat Res* 2007;(459):146-149.

    The authors reported on eight patients who underwent intralesional treatment of periacetabular low-grade chondrosarcoma. Final pathology revealed grade 2 chondrosarcoma in two patients and dedifferentiated chondrosarcoma in one. Only three patients remained disease free, two low-grade lesions recurred as high-grade tumors, and three deaths from disease were reported. Curettage of pelvic lesions was not recommended. Level of evidence: IV.

17. Streitbürger A, Ahrens H, Balke M, et al: Grade I chondrosarcoma of bone: The Münster experience. *J Cancer Res Clin Oncol* 2009;135(4):543-550.

    The authors of this study demonstrated no difference in overall survival or recurrence between intralesional and wide resection margins in the extremities. Curettage of pelvic lesions, however, did result in a recurrence rate of 100%. No survival difference was noted. Level of evidence: IV.

18. Di Giorgio L, Touloupakis G, Vitullo F, Sodano L, Mastantuono M, Villani C: Intralesional curettage, with phenol and cement as adjuvants, for low-grade intramedullary chondrosarcoma of the long bones. *Acta Orthop Belg* 2011;77(5):666-669.

    The author of this study reported on 23 patients with low-grade chondrosarcoma who underwent extended curettage with phenol as an adjuvant. One local recurrence was noted and treated with resection and megaprosthetic reconstruction. Three fractures occurred. The final mean MSTS score was 89.8%. Level of evidence: IV.

19. Mohler DG, Chiu R, McCall DA, Avedian RS: Curettage and cryosurgery for low-grade cartilage tumors is associated with low recurrence and high function. *Clin Orthop Relat Res* 2010;468(10):2765-2773.

    The authors of this study followed 46 patients who underwent curettage and cryosurgery for low-grade chondrosarcoma. Two local recurrences were found, both of which were salvaged with wide resection. No cryosurgery complications were noted. Level of evidence: IV.

20. Leerapun T, Hugate RR, Inwards CY, Scully SP, Sim FH: Surgical management of conventional grade I chondrosarcoma of long bones. *Clin Orthop Relat Res* 2007;463(463):166-172.

    The authors of this study compared 13 patients who underwent intralesional treatment of grade 1 chondrosarcoma with 57 patients who underwent resection. One patient in each group experienced both a local recurrence and a metastatic event. The patients in the intralesional treatment group were carefully selected for low radiographic aggressiveness. Level of evidence: III.

21. Cho WH, Song WS, Jeon DG, et al: Oncologic impact of the curettage of grade 2 central chondrosarcoma of the extremity. *Ann Surg Oncol* 2011;18(13):3755-3761.

    The authors reported on 15 patients with nonmetastatic grade 2 chondrosarcoma who underwent intralesional treatment. None of the tumors had aggressive characteristics on imaging, and all were intracompartmental lesions. Event-free survival was similar for this group and a control group who underwent conventional wide resection. Careful selection of tumors with nonaggressive radiographic characteristics was emphasized. Level of evidence: IV.

22. de Camargo OP, Baptista AM, Atanásio MJ, Waisberg DR: Chondrosarcoma of bone: Lessons from 46 operated cases in a single institution. *Clin Orthop Relat Res* 2010;468(11):2969-2975.

    The authors described the outcomes for patients with grade 1 and grade 2 chondrosarcoma. Twenty-five of 46 patients underwent curettage as the definitive treatment. The overall survival was 94%. Of 16 local recurrences, 10 occurred in the grade 2 group. Of these, three patients experienced metastasis and died. Resection was recommended for grade 2 tumors. Level of evidence: III.

23. Andreou D, Ruppin S, Fehlberg S, Pink D, Werner M, Tunn PU: Survival and prognostic factors in chondrosarcoma: Results in 115 patients with long-term follow-up. *Acta Orthop* 2011;82(6):749-755.

    In this study, the authors reviewed 115 patients, 47 of whom had axial tumors. Fifty-nine of 115 tumors were intermediate or high grade. Tumor grade and location were significant prognostic factors. The quality of the surgical margins did not influence survival. Patients with metastases who underwent chemotherapy, radiation therapy, or surgery did better than patients who received palliative care. Level of evidence: IV.

24. Dantonello TM, Int-Veen C, Leuschner I, et al; CWS study group; COSS study group: Mesenchymal chondrosarcoma of soft tissues and bone in children, adolescents, and young adults: Experiences of the CWS and COSS study groups. *Cancer* 2008;112(11):2424-2431.

    The authors of this study presented a series of 15 patients with mesenchymal chondrosarcoma. With excellent outcomes and a minimal rate of metastasis, this study differs from many previous reports. Multimodal treatment was thought to yield this result. Level of evidence: IV.

3: Malignant Primary Bone Tumors

25. Fiorenza F, Abudu A, Grimer RJ, et al: Risk factors for survival and local control in chondrosarcoma of bone. *J Bone Joint Surg Br* 2002;84(1):93-99.

26. McGough RL, Rutledge J, Lewis VO, Lin PP, Yasko AW: Impact severity of local recurrence in giant cell tumor of bone. *Clin Orthop Relat Res* 2005;(438): 116-122.

27. Schwab JH, Wenger D, Unni KK, Sim FH: Does local recurrence impact survival in low-grade chondrosarcoma of the long bones? *Clin Orthop Relat Res* 2007; (462):175-180.

    The authors reviewed 164 patients treated for grade 1 chondrosarcoma. Twenty-one sustained local recurrences, and of these, four had progression of grade and seven experienced metastasis. Six of the 21 patients died of disease. The authors concluded that recurrence predicts an aggressive behavior pattern. Level of evidence: IV.

28. Grimer RJ, Gosheger G, Taminiau A, et al: Dedifferentiated chondrosarcoma: Prognostic factors and outcome from a European group. *Eur J Cancer* 2007; 43(14):2060-2065.

    The authors of this report reviewed 337 patients with dedifferentiated chondrosarcoma. Those with metastases had a median survival of 5 months. Regardless of chemotherapy, the survival rate was 24% at 5 years. Level of evidence: IV.

29. Giuffrida AY, Burgueno JE, Koniaris LG, Gutierrez JC, Duncan R, Scully SP: Chondrosarcoma in the United States (1973 to 2003): An analysis of 2890 cases from the SEER database. *J Bone Joint Surg Am* 2009;91(5): 1063-1072.

    The authors of this analysis of the SEER database investigated 2,890 cases of chondrosarcoma. Over a 30-year period, no measurable improvements in survival occurred. Tumor grade and stage were independent prognostic factors. At 10 years after treatment, the likelihood of death from another cause is greater than the risk of death from disease, and a discontinuance of surveillance may be considered. Level of evidence: I.

30. Mitchell AD, Ayoub K, Mangham DC, Grimer RJ, Carter SR, Tillman RM: Experience in the treatment of dedifferentiated chondrosarcoma. *J Bone Joint Surg Br* 2000;82(1):55-61.

31. Streitbuerger A, Ahrens H, Gosheger G, et al: The treatment of locally recurrent chondrosarcoma: Is extensive further surgery justified? *J Bone Joint Surg Br* 2012;94(1):122-127.

    The authors of this study attempted to define the treatment criteria for patients with recurrent chondrosarcoma. Metastatic disease occurred in 41 of 77 patients with recurrent chondrosarcoma, synchronously in one half. Type of surgery did not affect overall survival. Because the survival rate was 0%, extensive surgery was not recommended in patients with recurrent grade 3 or dedifferentiated chondrosarcoma. Level of evidence: IV.

32. Donati D, El Ghoneimy A, Bertoni F, Di Bella C, Mercuri M: Surgical treatment and outcome of conventional pelvic chondrosarcoma. *J Bone Joint Surg Br* 2005;87(11):1527-1530.

33. Hu Y, Xia Q, Ji J, Miao J: One-stage combined posterior and anterior approaches for excising thoracolumbar and lumbar tumors: Surgical and oncological outcomes. *Spine (Phila Pa 1976)* 2010;35(5):590-595.

    The authors described the results of one-stage total spondylectomy for primary spinal neoplasms. Fifteen patients underwent the procedure with acceptable complications, good oncologic results, and decreased surgical time when compared to multistage procedures. Level of evidence: IV.

34. Yamazaki T, McLoughlin GS, Patel S, Rhines LD, Fourney DR: Feasibility and safety of en bloc resection for primary spine tumors: A systematic review by the Spine Oncology Study Group. *Spine (Phila Pa 1976)* 2009;34(Suppl 22):S31-S38.

    The authors performed a systematic review of all literature relating to en bloc vertebrectomy for primary spinal tumors. Eight articles met the final selection criteria. Correct biopsy techniques are emphasized, and complication rates are high, even in experienced centers. Level of evidence: IV.

35. Kalinski T, Sel S, Kouznetsova I, Röpke M, Roessner A: Heterogeneity of angiogenesis and blood vessel maturation in cartilage tumors. *Pathol Res Pract* 2009; 205(5):339-345.

    The authors of this study investigate the proliferating capillary index in cartilage tumors. A distinct difference was found between grades 2 and 3 chondrosarcoma and other cartilage neoplasms. Level of evidence: III.

36. McGough RL, Lin C, Meitner P, Aswad BI, Terek RM: Angiogenic cytokines in cartilage tumors. *Clin Orthop Relat Res* 2002;397:62-69.

37. Chen C, Ma Q, Ma X, Liu Z, Liu X: Association of elevated HIF-2α levels with low Beclin 1 expression and poor prognosis in patients with chondrosarcoma. *Ann Surg Oncol* 2011;18(8):2364-2372.

    The authors reported that levels of HIF-2α, a potent intranuclear pro-angiogenesis factor, were increased in chondrosarcoma when compared to nontumor tissues. Beclin 1 demonstrated an inverse relationship and was a factor in survival. This finding may yield prognostic and diagnostic information. Level of evidence: III.

38. Kubo T, Sugita T, Shimose S, Matsuo T, Arihiro K, Ochi M: Expression of hypoxia-inducible factor-1alpha and its relationship to tumour angiogenesis and cell proliferation in cartilage tumours. *J Bone Joint Surg Br* 2008;90(3):364-370.

    The authors of this study investigated hypoxia-inducible factor 1α (HIF-1α), HIF-2α, and microvessel density in cartilage neoplasms. HIF-1α expression correlated significantly with a shorter, disease-free survival. This factor may be a substantial prognostic factor. Level of evidence: III.

39. Sun X, Wei L, Chen Q, Terek RM: HDAC4 represses vascular endothelial growth factor expression in chondrosarcoma by modulating RUNX2 activity. *J Biol Chem* 2009;284(33):21881-21890.

   The authors demonstrated that decreased HDAC4 expression may lead to increased expression of VEGF. This increase in VEGF had been implicated as one of the aggressive genetic traits of high-grade chondrosarcoma. Level of evidence: III.

40. Morioka H, Weissbach L, Vogel T, et al: Antiangiogenesis treatment combined with chemotherapy produces chondrosarcoma necrosis. *Clin Cancer Res* 2003;9(3):1211-1217.

41. Amary MF, Bacsi K, Maggiani F, et al: IDH1 and IDH2 mutations are frequent events in central chondrosarcoma and central and periosteal chondromas but not in other mesenchymal tumours. *J Pathol* 2011; 224(3):334–343.

   The authors studied somatic mutations in patients with multiple enchondromas. It appears that a mosaic pattern of IDH-mutation-bearing cells is responsible for diverse tumors in the same patient.

3: Malignant Primary Bone Tumors

Chapter 18

Miscellaneous Malignant Primary Bone Tumors

David McKeown, MD   Patrick J. Boland, MD

Introduction

Analysis of data collected by the National Cancer Institute's Surveillance, Epidemiology, and End Results (SEER) Program from 1973 to 1987 shows that osteogenic sarcoma, chondrosarcoma, and Ewing sarcoma account for 77% of all primary bone tumors.[1] Rare bone tumors, which are discussed in this chapter, include chordoma, undifferentiated pleomorphic sarcoma (previously known as malignant fibrous histiocytoma), fibrosarcoma, malignant vascular tumors, and adamantinoma. Diagnostic modalities, staging, and treatment of fibrosarcoma, malignant vascular tumors, and adamantinoma follow the same principles as those for the more common tumors.

Chordoma

Chordoma is a slow-growing, locally destructive, malignant bone tumor thought to arise from vestigial or ectopic notochordal tissue.[2,3]

Epidemiology

Analysis of the SEER database indicates that chordoma accounts for 8.4% of all primary bone tumors, making it the fourth most common.[1] Although chordoma occurs almost exclusively in the axial skeleton, rare cases are reported in the appendicular skeleton and soft tissues. Anatomically, the sacrococcygeal, spheno-occipital, and mobile spine are involved, in that order of frequency.[3]

Chordoma is rare in children and adolescents. The overall incidence increases with age, and the median age at diagnosis is 58 years.[1,2] Spheno-occipital tumors are more common in younger patients, whereas sacral involvement predominates in older age groups. Like Ewing sarcoma, chordoma is extremely rare among populations of African origin globally.[1,3] A familial form has been described. The association between intraosseous benign notochordal tumors (IOBNCTs) and chordoma is currently under debate. The literature includes several reports of the two entities coexisting in the spine, but definitive transformation of IOBNCTs to chordoma has not been confirmed.[4,5]

Patients with spheno-occipital lesions may have headaches, cranial nerve palsies, dysphagia, and secondary endocrinopathies from pituitary destruction. Long-standing low back pain is common in sacrococcygeal tumors; however, sciatica and bowel or bladder dysfunction usually indicate advanced disease.[2,3] Metastases to the lungs, bone, and subcutaneous tissues are late manifestations of chordoma and occur in 30% of patients.[6]

Imaging

Radiographically, chordomas are lytic, with an epicenter in the midvertebral body. Sacrococcygeal tumors are difficult to see on plain radiographs and thus are frequently overlooked. Bone scintigraphy may show reduced or normal radioisotope uptake.

MRI is the most useful imaging modality. In addition to central vertebral body lysis, anterior and posterior cortical destruction is a common feature in chordoma, but is rarely seen in IOBNCTs (**Figure 1**). In sacral lesions, extension into the piriformis muscles and sacroiliac ligaments is common and important to note when planning for surgery. CT scans show bone lysis and bone destruction in chordoma, whereas sclerosis and no cortical destruction are more common radiographic features of IOBNCTs[4,5] (**Figure 2**).

Pathology

Diagnosis can usually be made with a carefully planned core biopsy. Histologically, three types of chordoma are observed: classic, chondroid, and dedifferentiated.[2,3]

In classic chordoma, lobules containing cells arranged in cords or nests in myxoid stroma are identified (**Figure 3**). The cells typically have vacuolated cytoplasm (physaliferous cells). Mitotic figures and pleomorphism are present. Myxoid stroma, mitotic figures, and pleomorphism are features not seen in IOBNCTs.[4,5]

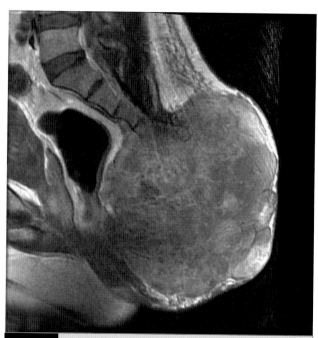

Figure 1 Sagittal MRI view of the sacrum shows typical chordoma with bony destruction and soft-tissue extension both anteriorly and posteriorly.

The chondroid variant comprises 15% of chordomas. They occur in the spheno-occipital area, and patients with these tumors have a better prognosis than those with other chordoma types. The features of chondroid chordomas overlap with those of chondrosarcoma. Dedifferentiated chordomas contain areas of high-grade malignant spindle cells and have a poor prognosis.[3]

Immunohistochemical staining for S-100 and epithelial markers is positive. Recently, staining for Brachyury, a T-box transcription factor expressed by notochordal cells, has become routine in the diagnosis of all notochordal tumors. This immunoprofile helps distinguish chordoma from chondrosarcoma and most other tumors.[2,4,5,7]

Treatment

It is important to distinguish benign notochordal tumors from chordomas. In addition to the radiographic and histologic distinctions discussed previously, the benign tumors typically exhibit asymptomatic, incidental clinical findings that require no further treatment. The rare symptomatic lesion may be treated with intralesional excision.

Chordomas, however, require more aggressive treatment. Surgery is the mainstay. Several series report significant improvement in local control and survival with wide resection when compared to intralesional or marginal excision.[2] For sacrococcygeal tumors, complete resection is usually possible.

Wide resection of chordomas of the mobile spine is preferred but is not always possible, in which case in-

complete resection and radiation therapy are recommended. Complete surgical resection of spheno-occipital tumors is rarely possible, but good results have been reported using marginal or intralesional surgery combined with radiation therapy. Endoscopic resection is commonly used for these lesions.[2]

Advances in radiation oncology using image-guided photons have facilitated the administration of effective, high-dose radiation therapy in spinal tumors.[2] More recently, the use of protons and carbon ions (hadron therapy) has provided means of administering greater biologic doses of radiation therapy to chordomas while sparing sensitive neural or visceral structures.[8] Early results from the use of these modalities in addition to surgery have been encouraging. Chordomas are resistant to conventional chemotherapy, and new agents that target known molecular pathways are being investigated.[2,3,7]

Undifferentiated Pleomorphic Sarcoma of Bone

Undifferentiated pleomorphic sarcoma (UPS) (previously known as malignant fibrous histiocytoma) represents 3% to 8% of all primary bone tumors. Approximately 70% to 75% of these bony tumors arise in the appendicular skeleton. Skeletal UPS is usually high grade.[9]

Epidemiology

Males are affected more commonly than females, and the incidence rises in patients older than 40 years. These malignant lesions can arise de novo in bone or can occur secondary to irradiation, bone infarct, Paget disease, or chronic osteomyelitis.[10-12] Rare cases associated with orthopaedic prostheses have been reported.[13,14]

The appendicular skeleton of the lower limb is the most frequent site of involvement, with a predilection for the distal femur and proximal tibial metaphysis.[10]

Clinical Features

Pain is the most common presenting symptom, and patients may have a pathologic fracture. Pulmonary metastases are reported in up to 46% of patients. Radiographically, the tumors are typically lytic, with ill-defined margins and a permeative moth-eaten appearance. Periosteal reaction is not a prominent feature.[10,15]

Pathology

UPS is characterized by a mixture of spindle cells arranged in a storiform pattern. Histiocytoid and pleomorphic cells can also be present. Unlike osteogenic sarcoma, osteoid is not elaborated by the malignant cells.[10]

Most authors categorize UPS as either high or low grade on the basis of histology, but the prognostic significance of this distinction is unclear. The differential

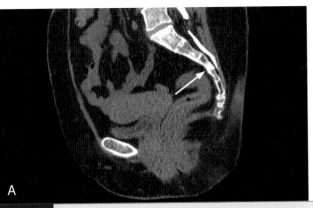
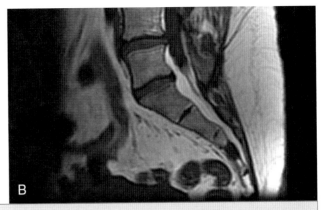

Figure 2 A, Sagittal CT scan of the sacrum demonstrates a sclerotic intraosseous benign notochordal tumor (arrow). B, MRI of the same patient shows no cortical destruction.

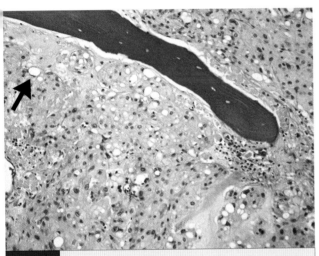

Figure 3 Photomicrograph showing classic chordoma, with typical vacuolated physaliferous cells (arrow).

diagnosis includes osteogenic sarcoma, fibrosarcoma, and leiomyosarcoma. Metastatic carcinomas such as sarcomatoid renal cell carcinoma and malignant melanoma can also mimic UPS.

Treatment

Treatment of high-grade UPS of bone usually consists of chemotherapy and wide surgical resection. Chemotherapy for UPS in the pediatric and young adult age group is similar to that used in osteogenic sarcoma. Neoadjuvant chemotherapy followed by surgery and postoperative adjuvant chemotherapy is typical.[9]

A small percentage of patients with resectable pulmonary metastases can be successfully treated with chemotherapy, local tumor resection, and metastasectomy.

Prognostic factors include grade of tumor and clinical stage at presentation. The authors of a 1986 study reported decreased survival in older patients with high-grade tumors and secondary UPS.[15] In a 2010 report, researchers showed no difference in 5-year survival between primary and secondary UPS.[11] A 2011 study reported a 5-year disease-free survival of 61% among patients without metastases who were treated with chemotherapy and adequate surgery. Histologic response to neoadjuvant chemotherapy was a predictor of survival.[9]

Fibrosarcoma

Fibrosarcoma of bone accounts for fewer than 5% of primary bone tumors. As with UPS, it may arise de novo or be secondary to irradiation, fibrous dysplasia, Paget disease, or chronic osteomyelitis. Some reports exist of fibrosarcoma developing in irradiated giant cell tumors and, rarely, in nonirradiated recurrent giant cell tumors of bone.[12,16]

Clinical Features

Fibrosarcoma occurs more commonly in males. Its incidence peaks in the second to sixth decades; however, this lesion has been described in infancy. Fibrosarcoma has a skeletal distribution similar to that of UPS. Typically, pain is the presenting symptom. Some series report a high incidence of pathologic fractures. Radiographs show lytic, permeative lesions, often with soft-tissue extension.

Pathology

Typically the tumor is composed of spindle-shaped cells arranged in a herringbone pattern with varied amounts of collagen and myxoid tissue. Higher-grade tumors have less collagen and more mitotic figures. Low-grade lesions can be distinguished from a benign desmoplastic fibroma, which has little or no cellular atypia and fewer mitoses.[16]

Treatment and Prognosis

Patients with low-grade lesions are treated with wide resection and have a good prognosis with a 10-year disease-free survival rate of 83%, whereas the survival

3: Malignant Primary Bone Tumors

rate for those with high-grade lesions is 34%. High-grade tumors are managed with chemotherapy and surgery using the same protocol as that for high-grade UPS.[16]

Leiomyosarcoma of Bone

Leiomyosarcoma of bone is a rare spindle cell malignancy with smooth muscle cell differentiation. Primary leiomyosarcoma of bone must be distinguished from the more common metastatic leiomyosarcoma, where the primary tumor is usually located in the uterus or gastrointestinal tract.

Clinical Features
In patients who have undergone hysterectomy, the possibility of metastatic tumor must be considered. Primary leiomyosarcoma is most commonly located in the pelvis or in the metaphysis of lower limb bones. Pain and pathologic fractures are common presentations. Radiographic features are nonspecific but usually show an aggressive lytic lesion with cortical disruption. The mean age at the time of presentation is mid 40s. Pulmonary metastases develop in 50% of patients.[17,18]

Pathology
Leiomyosarcoma consists of pleomorphic, plump spindle cells, with frequent mitoses, arranged in fascicles intersecting at 90°. Positive immunohistochemical staining for both smooth muscle actin and desmin confirms the diagnosis.[17,18]

Treatment and Prognosis
Wide surgical excision is the only treatment that has proved effective. The role of chemotherapy is debated. A 1997 study showed no survival benefit with its use.[18] However, a recent publication suggested a benefit in patients who showed a histologically favorable response to neoadjuvant chemotherapy. In the same report, prognosis was related to the stage of disease at presentation. Low-grade tumors had an excellent outcome with surgery, whereas patients with intermediate- to high-grade lesions had a 60% survival rate at 5 years and a 45% survival rate at 10 and 15 years.[17]

Malignant Vascular Tumors

Epithelioid Hemangioendothelioma of Bone
Epithelioid hemangioendothelioma (EHE) is a well-differentiated malignant endothelial tumor with metastatic potential. These tumors occur more commonly in the liver and lung and are rarely seen in bone. The tibia is the most frequently involved bone. Involvement of other bones in the same extremity is not uncommon. In 2002, the World Health Organization's Sarcoma Working Group updated the classification of bone EHE, making it consistent with soft-tissue EHE. Two different terms are used, depending on the degree of cytologic atypia: classic or conventional EHE and malignant EHE.[19]

Clinical Features
The peak age of incidence of these malignant tumors is reported to be 32 years. Pain is the usual presenting symptom. Patients with spine involvement may have back pain, radiculopathy, or myelopathy. Radiographic features include solitary or multiple, often well-defined lytic lesions. The rate of metastasis in conventional EHE is approximately 10%, whereas in malignant EHE it is reported to be approximately 30%.[20]

Pathology
Classic EHE is more common and is composed of anastomosing cords, solid nests, and strands of endothelial cells with eosinophilic cytoplasm. The cells are bland, and the nuclei show little or no mitotic activity or cellular pleomorphism.[19,21]

Malignant EHE shows increased nuclear atypia, mitotic activity, and cellular pleomorphism. These tumors are more aggressive and have a higher rate of recurrence and metastasis following surgery than the classic form.[19,21]

Genetics
A translocation involving chromosomes 1 and 3 has been described.[22]

Treatment
Wide resection is recommended. In patients with multifocal or spinal tumors, partial resection and radiation therapy may be the treatment of choice.

Angiosarcoma
Angiosarcoma of bone is a very rare high-grade malignant vascular endothelial tumor. These tumors occur most commonly in long bones and are sometimes multifocal. They have been noted anecdotally to develop in a previously irradiated benign hemangioma.[21,23]

Clinical Features
Patients can have pain or a pathologic fracture. Spinal tumors cause neurologic signs and symptoms secondary to spinal cord compression or fracture. The radiographic features demonstrate lytic destructive lesions with cortical breakthrough.[21,23]

Pathology
Tumors consist of highly atypical endothelial cells with vasoformative features. However, some tumors lack these classic features and demonstrate pleomorphism and high mitotic activity. An epithelioid form has been described and can be confused with metastatic carcinoma because of its reactivity for epithelial markers by immunohistochemistry.[21,23]

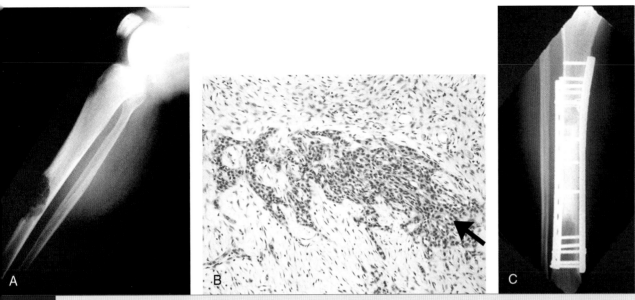

Figure 4 **A**, Lateral view of the tibia shows extensive destructive changes consistent with classic adamantinoma. **B**, Islands of malignant epithelial cells (arrow) in fibrous stroma are typical in adamantinoma. **C**, Intercalary allograft reconstruction following wide resection of classic adamantinoma is shown.

Treatment

Most angiosarcomas are extremely aggressive and have a poor prognosis. Radical resection or amputation should be performed when possible. Adjuvant radiation therapy and chemotherapy may be used, but no strong data support this.[21]

Adamantinoma

Adamantinoma is a low-grade, malignant epithelial tumor of bone. Typically, it has a biphasic histology consisting of a malignant epithelial component surrounded by a band of fibro-osseous proliferation. Two types are described: classic adamantinoma and osteofibrous dysplasia (OFD)-like adamantinoma, also known as differentiated adamantinoma.[24-26]

Clinical Features

The anterior tibial diaphysis is primarily involved in more than 90% of patients.[26] Synchronous involvement of the ipsilateral fibula is common. Rarely, the tumor has been reported in other bones. Classic adamantinoma is extremely rare in patients younger than age 20 years and occurs most commonly in the third and fourth decades. OFD-like adamantinoma typically occurs in the second decade.

Tibial pain with anterior tibial bowing is a common presenting feature. Hypercalcemia has been reported as a paraneoplastic feature in some patients. Metastases to lung or other bones are reported in 30% of patients with classic adamantinoma.[27]

Radiographic Features

Plain radiographs may show multifocal lytic intracortical lesions, or, in more aggressive forms, a large lytic lesion with anterior cortical destruction and medullary invasion (**Figure 4, A**).[26]

OFD-like adamantinoma cannot be distinguished from benign OFD radiographically. In OFD-like adamantinoma, the lesions are usually intracortical. Although MRI is not diagnostic, it helps outline the anatomic extent of the tumor and can show features suggestive of an aggressive form of disease. This diagnostic tool helps with surgical planning.[24]

Pathology

Most orthopaedic oncologists recommend an open biopsy for definitive diagnosis, especially when one needs to differentiate OFD-like adamantinoma from primary OFD.[27]

Classic adamantinoma is composed of islands or nests of malignant epithelial cells in a bland fibrous stroma (**Figure 4, B**). Morphology varies throughout the tumor. Four different patterns are described: basaloid, spindle/sarcomatoid, squamoid, and tubular.[25,26]

The OFD-like variant of adamantinoma is characterized by a predominance of osteofibrous tissue containing small nests of epithelial cells, which may require careful examination to detect and demonstrate cytokeratin positivity, unlike OFD cells, which are negative.[24,26]

Cytogenetic studies have demonstrated trisomy of chromosomes 7, 8, 12, and 19. Similar abnormalities have been demonstrated in OFD. These findings, together with similarities in anatomic location, radiographic appearance, and some histologic features, suggest a relationship among OFD, OFD-like adamantinoma, and classic adamantinoma. Whether one condition can progress or regress to another is unclear.[24-26]

Treatment

Classic adamantinoma requires wide surgical resection, usually followed by reconstruction (**Figure 4, C**). Marginal or intralesional excision can result in local recurrence and distant metastases. Neither chemotherapy nor radiation therapy has been shown to be effective. Ten-year survival rates of 87% have been reported following wide resection. Several authors stress the importance of long-term follow-up, because local recurrence and metastases have been reported up to 30 years following resection. Pulmonary metastases should be resected if possible.[21,24]

Management of OFD-like adamantinoma is controversial. Metastases have never been reported in OFD-like adamantinoma, and because progression to classic adamantinoma is unlikely, most authorities recommend careful observation, especially before skeletal maturity. If progression is noted, surgical resection is appropriate.

Summary

Osteogenic sarcoma, Ewing sarcoma, and chondrosarcoma account for more than 70% of malignant bone tumors. The rarity of the tumors discussed in this chapter does not diminish their importance to physicians involved in the management of bone tumors. Recent changes in nomenclature and classifications introduced by the World Health Organization's Sarcoma Working Group have been outlined and should be adopted.

Annotated References

1. Dorfman HD, Czerniak B: Bone cancers. *Cancer* 1995; 75(Suppl 1):203-210.

2. Walcott BP, Nahed BV, Mohyeldin A, Coumans JV, Kahle KT, Ferreira MJ: Chordoma: Current concepts, management, and future directions. *Lancet Oncol* 2012;13(2):e69-e76.

   The authors of this comprehensive review discuss the pathogenesis, clinical features, and management strategies for chordoma. Level of evidence: V.

3. Chugh R, Tawbi H, Lucas DR, Biermann JS, Schuetze SM, Baker LH: Chordoma: The nonsarcoma primary bone tumor. *Oncologist* 2007;12(11):1344-1350.

   The authors of this review briefly discuss the genetic characteristics of chordoma and summarizes surgical, radiation, and medical therapies, as well as their associated outcomes. Level of evidence: V.

4. Kyriakos M: Benign notochordal lesions of the axial skeleton: A review and current appraisal. *Skeletal Radiol* 2011;40(9):1141-1152.

   This article provides an up-to-date description of the nomenclature, embryogenesis, and clinical features of tumors thought to be of notochordal origin. Level of evidence: V.

5. Amer HZ, Hameed M: Intraosseous benign notochordal cell tumor. *Arch Pathol Lab Med* 2010;134(2):283-288.

   The authors of this article discuss the relationship between benign notochordal tumors and chordoma. Differences between the two entities are outlined based on clinical, radiographic, and histologic factors.

6. Chambers PW, Schwinn CP: Chordoma: A clinicopathologic study of metastasis. *Am J Clin Pathol* 1979; 72(5):765-776.

7. Schwab JH, Boland PJ, Agaram NP, et al: Chordoma and chondrosarcoma gene profile: Implications for immunotherapy. *Cancer Immunol Immunother* 2009; 58(3):339-349.

   The authors evaluated gene expression profiles of chordoma and chondrosarcoma to identify potential molecular therapeutic targets. The profiles were compared to other sarcomas and normal tissues of similar mesenchymal lineage to determine whether they express unique gene signatures. Specific immunotherapy targets were identified. Level of evidence: V.

8. Braccini S: Photons and hadrons for health. *Acta Physica Polonica B* 2006;37(3):961-967.

9. Jeon DG, Song WS, Kong CB, Kim JR, Lee SY: MFH of bone and osteosarcoma show similar survival and chemosensitivity. *Clin Orthop Relat Res* 2011;469(2):584-590.

   The authors described a retrospective study comparing the outcomes of 27 patients with malignant fibrous histiocytoma of bone with the outcomes of 38 patients with osteogenic sarcoma of similar stage. Similar survival rates and response to chemotherapy were found. Level of evidence: III.

10. Huvos AG, Heilweil M, Bretsky SS: The pathology of malignant fibrous histiocytoma of bone: A study of 130 patients. *Am J Surg Pathol* 1985;9(12):853-871.

11. Koplas MC, Lefkowitz RA, Bauer TW, et al: Imaging findings, prevalence and outcome of de novo and secondary malignant fibrous histiocytoma of bone. *Skeletal Radiol* 2010;39(8):791-798.

    In this retrospective review, the demographics, outcomes, and imaging features of 28 patients with primary and secondary malignant fibrous histiocytoma (MFH) were presented. Five-year survival was 53%. Metastases, mostly pulmonary and osseous, occurred in 46% of patients. Secondary and primary MFH had similar prognoses. Level of evidence: IV.

12. Mavrogenis AF, Pala E, Guerra G, Ruggieri P: Postradiation sarcomas: Clinical outcome of 52 patients. *J Surg Oncol* 2012;105(6):570-576.

    In this retrospective study of 52 patients with postirradiation sarcoma, 45 had bone sarcomas. The risk of postirradiation sarcoma was 0.06% at a mean latency of 15 years. Five-year survival was 45%. Sarcoma type was the only significant variable for survival. Level of evidence: IV.

13. Lucas DR, Miller PR, Mott MP, Kronick JL, Unni KK: Arthroplasty-associated malignant fibrous histiocytoma: Two case reports. *Histopathology* 2001;39(6): 620-628.

14. Yoon PW, Jang WY, Yoo JJ, Yoon KS, Kim HJ: Malignant fibrous histiocytoma at the site of an alumina-on-alumina-bearing total hip arthroplasty mimicking infected trochanteric bursitis. *J Arthroplasty* 2012;27(2): e9, e12.

   The authors reported a case of malignant fibrous histiocytoma at the site of a total hip arthroplasty in an older patient. Level of evidence: V.

15. Huvos AG, Woodard HQ, Heilweil M: Postradiation malignant fibrous histiocytoma of bone: A clinicopathologic study of 20 patients. *Am J Surg Pathol* 1986;10(1):9-18.

16. Kahn LB, Vigorita V: Fibrosarcoma of bone, in Fletcher CDM, Unni KK, Mertens F (eds): *Pathology and Genetics of Tumours of Soft Tissue and Bone: World Health Organization Classification of Tumours.* Lyon, France, IARC Press, 2002, pp 289-290. http:// www.iarc.fr/en/publications/pdfs-online/pat-gen/bb5/ BB5.pdf. Accessed August 1, 2012.

17. Brewer P, Sumathi V, Grimer RJ, et al: Primary leiomyosarcoma of bone: Analysis of prognosis. *Sarcoma* 2012;2012:636849.

   This report analyzed a database of 3,364 patients with primary bone sarcomas. Only 31 patients had leiomyosarcoma. Twenty-eight patients underwent surgery. Fifty percent developed local recurrence. The disease-specific survival rate was 53% at 5 years and 44% at 10 years. Level of evidence: IV.

18. Antonescu CR, Erlandson RA, Huvos AG: Primary leiomyosarcoma of bone: A clinicopathologic, immunohistochemical, and ultrastructural study of 33 patients and a literature review. *Am J Surg Pathol* 1997; 21(11):1281-1294.

19. Adler CP, Wold L: Haemangioma and related lesions, in Fletcher CDM, Unni KK, Mertens F (eds): *Pathology and Genetics of Tumours of Soft Tissue and Bone: World Health Organization Classification of Tumours.* Lyon, France, IARC Press, 2002, pp 320-321. http:// www.iarc.fr/en/publications/pdfs-online/pat-gen/bb5/ BB5.pdf. Accessed August 1, 2012.

20. Deyrup AT, Tighiouart M, Montag AG, Weiss SW: Epithelioid hemangioendothelioma of soft tissue: A proposal for risk stratification based on 49 cases. *Am J Surg Pathol* 2008;32(6):924-927.

21. Weiss SW, Ishak KG, Dail DH, Sweet DE, Enzinger FM: Epithelioid hemangioendothelioma and related lesions. *Semin Diagn Pathol* 1986;3(4):259-287.

22. Errani C, Zhang L, Sung YS, et al: A novel WWTR1-CAMTA1 gene fusion is a consistent abnormality in epithelioid hemangioendothelioma of different anatomic sites. *Genes Chromosomes Cancer* 2011;50(8): 644-653.

   This article describes a molecular analysis of 12 cases of EHE that demonstrated unique chromosomal translocations. These findings differentiate EHE from endothelial hemangioma and angiosarcoma. Level of evidence: IV.

23. Roessner A, Boehling T: Angiosarcoma, in Fletcher CDM, Unni KK, Mertens F (eds): *Pathology and Genetics of Tumours of Soft Tissue and Bone: World Health Organization Classification of Tumours.* Lyon, France, IARC Press, 2002, pp 322-323. http:// www.iarc.fr/en/publications/pdfs-online/pat-gen/bb5/ BB5.pdf. Accessed August 1, 2012.

24. Most MJ, Sim FH, Inwards CY: Osteofibrous dysplasia and adamantinoma. *J Am Acad Orthop Surg* 2010; 18(6):358-366.

   The authors discussed the possible relationship between OFD and OFD-like adamantinoma. Management strategies also were discussed. Level of evidence: V.

25. Czerniak B, Rojas-Corona RR, Dorfman HD: Morphologic diversity of long bone adamantinoma: The concept of differentiated (regressing) adamantinoma and its relationship to osteofibrous dysplasia. *Cancer* 1989;64(11):2319-2334.

26. Kahn LB: Adamantinoma, osteofibrous dysplasia and differentiated adamantinoma. *Skeletal Radiol* 2003; 32(5):245-258.

27. Papagelopoulos PJ, Mavrogenis AF, Galanis EC, Savvidou OD, Inwards CY, Sim FH: Clinicopathological features, diagnosis, and treatment of adamantinoma of the long bones. *Orthopedics* 2007;30(3):211-215, quiz 216-217.

   This article describes the radiographic and histologic features of adamantinoma of the long bones as well as current treatment modalities. Survival rates range from 82% to 87% following wide resection, limb salvage, or amputation. Level of evidence: V.

3: Malignant Primary Bone Tumors

Chapter 19

Lymphoma and Myeloma

Wakenda K. Tyler, MD, MPH   Adam S. Levin, MD

Introduction

Lymphoma and multiple myeloma are both malignancies of the hematopoietic cell lineage. More specifically, both conditions derive from cells of varied stages of development within the lymphocytic cell line. Myeloma is derived from mature B lymphocytes, whereas lymphoma is derived from either T or B lymphocytes or natural killer lymphocytic cells at a variety of stages of maturation. Because both malignancies derive from the hematopoietic cell lines, there is a strong tendency for bone marrow involvement. This marrow involvement can lead to remodeling of both the medullary and cortical trabeculae, which can eventually lead to weakening of the bone and pathologic fracture. Aside from their common cell lineage, lymphoma and myeloma differ in their classification, presentation, and response to treatments. Their bony involvement often differs as well, with myeloma having a distinct radiographic appearance. Lymphoma can present with a variety of radiographic appearances within the bone, but also tends to have classic features that differ from myeloma.

This chapter discusses the relevant biology, epidemiology, clinical presentation, and treatment considerations that orthopaedic surgeons need to be aware of for both of these malignant conditions of the bone marrow.

Lymphoma

Lymphoma is the terminology used to describe a broad category of malignancies that are thought to be derived from the lymphocytes of the normal human immune system. Lymphocytes are white blood cells that function to regulate and modulate the immune system. There are three main types of lymphocytes: T cells, B cells, and natural killer cells. Lymphomas are divided into two categories based on specific histologic and cytogenetic features: Hodgkin lymphoma and non-Hodgkin lymphoma.[1] The non-Hodgkin lymphomas are then further characterized based on their presumed lymphocytic cell of origin. These are often further subclassified based on prognostic factors and location of involvement.[2]

Epidemiology and Prognosis

Hodgkin lymphoma is thought to be of the B cell lineage and is most notable on histologic analysis for its large Reed-Sternberg cells. It has an incidence in the United States of 2.7 per 100,000, with 7,400 new cases diagnosed each year. It has a bimodal age distribution with a peak at age 25 years and then a smaller peak again at age 75 to 80 years.[3] It occurs across all nationalities and races. Most patients present with painless lymphadenopathy. They may also have fever, chills, night sweats, and weight loss. Hodgkin lymphoma, unlike non-Hodgkin lymphoma, does not typically present with primary bony involvement. Bony involvement indicates widely metastatic stage IV disease. Patients with stage IV disease can often have bone pain and impending pathologic fractures.

The prognosis for Hodgkin lymphoma has improved greatly over the past several decades. With modern combined modality treatment, patients with stage I or II disease have a 5-year survival rate of 90% or greater.[3] Even patients with advanced disease can still have a 5- to 10-year survival rate of 65% or greater.[3] The high rate of remission in this lymphoma means that treatment of bony involvement should be durable and potentially capable of lasting for 20+ years. Most cases of bony disease are treated with both systemic chemotherapy and local radiation therapy to the involved bone. Many patients also undergo autologous stem cell transplantation. Hodgkin lymphoma is extremely sensitive to radiation and it is expected that local control of bone sites will be accomplished solely with radiation. Patients typically show significant bone reconstitution and remodeling posttherapy. As with radiation of bone in other diseases, high doses of radiation given either before or after treatment can lead to a high rate of fracture nonunion if a fracture is present at the time of treatment.

Non-Hodgkin lymphomas are a group of hematologic malignancies that share a common T or B cell lineage, but otherwise differ greatly in their response to

3: Malignant Primary Bone Tumors

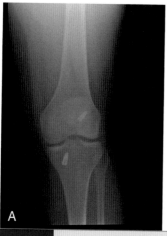
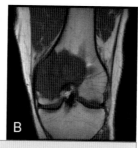

Figure 1 Three years after anterior cruciate ligament (ACL) reconstruction, an 18-year-old man reported left knee pain and a sense of "instability." A plain radiograph (**A**) was obtained, which was read as normal, and MRI was performed to assess ACL integrity. T1 MRI (**B**) showed geographic edema in the distal femur. The patient was referred to an orthopaedic oncologist for evaluation and biopsy. The biopsy revealed diffuse large B-cell lymphoma.

treatment and long-term cure rates. The incidence of non-Hodgkin lymphoma is increasing throughout the world, at a rate of approximately 4% per year.[4] In the United States, approximately 70,000 new cases were diagnosed in the year 2012, making non-Hodgkin lymphoma the seventh most common malignancy among adults.[5] The median age at diagnosis is 66 years and the incidence dramatically increases with increasing age; however, non-Hodgkin lymphoma is reported in all age groups.[5] Males have a slightly higher incidence than females. Diffuse large B-cell and follicular lymphoma (also B cell origin) are the two most common types of non-Hodgkin lymphoma, making up approximately two thirds of all cases. Follicular lymphoma is considered an indolent form of lymphoma, which is often but not always incurable with a very slow progression of disease. Diffuse large B-cell lymphoma tends to be more aggressive, but is considered curable and has a fairly good prognosis when treated with modern chemotherapy and radiation modalities.

As with Hodgkin lymphoma, patients with non-Hodgkin lymphoma often present with systemic signs, such as fever, chills, weight loss, and lymphadenopathy. Unlike patients with Hodgkin lymphoma, patients with non-Hodgkin lymphoma frequently present with bone involvement and even pathologic fracture. Approximately 25% to 30% of all non-Hodgkin lymphomas will have bone marrow involvement at presentation.[6,7] Only a fraction of these will develop or present with pathologic fracture, but bone or joint pain in a patient with non-Hodgkin lymphoma is cause for concern. Some of these patients will present with the initial report of musculoskeletal pain and in these cases, the or-

thopaedic surgeon will make the initial discovery and diagnosis (**Figure 1**). In a study of 238 patients with presumed osteoporotic vertebral compression fractures who presented to the orthopaedic surgeon for treatment of their compression fractures, it was found that 1.3% of patients had an underlying undiagnosed lymphoma. In this small group of patients, the compression fracture and back pain were the initial presenting symptoms for their lymphomas.[8]

The overall relative 5-year survival of patients with non-Hodgkin lymphoma is approximately 68%. Those with isolated localized disease have a 5-year survival of greater than 80%, whereas those with distant metastasis and stage IV disease still have a 5-year relative survival of approximately 60%.[5] Prognosis can vary greatly depending on the type of lymphoma. For instance, the 5-year relative survival of patients with stage IV disease of T cell origin lymphoma is only 37% compared to 60% for B-cell origin lymphoma.[5] Much like Hodgkin lymphoma, many patients with non-Hodgkin lymphoma have a long life span and will ultimately be cured of their cancers, even with significant bony involvement. Non-Hodgkin lymphoma is well controlled with systemic treatment (chemotherapy, steroids, and NSAIDs) and radiation treatment, and it is often the combination of these that is used by the oncology team to treat patients. Prophylactic fixation before fracture occurrence is the ideal treatment of patients with impending fractures.

Primary lymphoma of bone is a distinct pathologic entity defined as lymphoma involving a single bony site plus or minus a single regional lymph node without any other sites of involvement for 6 months from diagnosis. Because of the small disease burden, these patients often lack systemic symptoms of disease. Most instances of primary lymphoma of bone are diffuse large B cell type. Primary lymphoma of bone accounts for less than 2% of all lymphomas and approximately 3% of all primary malignancies of bone.[9,10] There is a slight male predominance and the median age at diagnosis is approximately 60 years.[10] Although primary lymphoma of bone tends to occur in middle-aged males, young adults and even children can present with this form of lymphoma. The axial skeleton is a common site of involvement.[10] Primary lymphoma of bone is also frequently seen in the metaphyseal region of long bones, such as the femur, humerus, and tibia. In general, the skeletal distribution tends to follow areas of increased hematopoietic activity. Patients with early-stage primary lymphoma of bone usually have an excellent prognosis, with up to a 90% 5-year survival rate when chemotherapy can be given. That prognosis decreases with increasing stage of disease, as with the other forms of lymphoma.

Clinical Presentation

Most patients who present with lymphoma involvement of bone also have significant pain during activity and at rest. The patient will often report night pain that

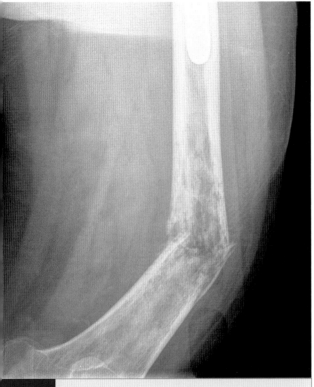

Figure 2 Plain radiograph shows pathologic fracture of the left femur in a 70-year-old patient, who developed this fracture through primary lymphoma of bone in the femur when rising from a sitting position in a chair.

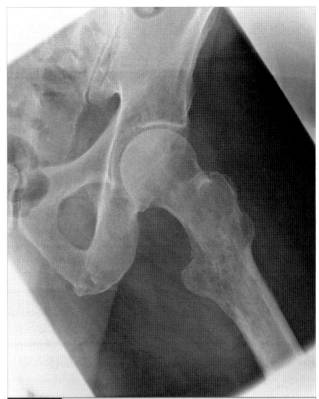

Figure 3 Plain radiograph shows the left proximal femur of a 78-year-old man with newly diagnosed non-Hodgkin lymphoma. Note the permeative pattern of bone destruction in a poorly marginated lesion of the proximal femur.

keeps him or her from falling asleep or wakes him or her up from sleep. Patients will sometimes report that the pain is relieved with NSAIDs or corticosteroids, but this relief is usually short lived or only a partial response. This occurs because the lymphoma cells (B cells and T cells) are often extremely responsive to agents that inhibit the normal inflammatory cascade. Some patients will present with pathologic fracture (**Figure 2**) after normal activity. It is not uncommon for patients to also present with abnormal MRI findings when imaging is obtained for what is thought to be a different diagnosis, such as meniscal tear or rotator cuff pathology.

It is important in patients in whom any type of malignancy is expected or who are being evaluated for an abnormality on imaging that questions regarding constitutional systems are asked. For lymphoma, a history of night sweats, fever, weight loss, and/or prolonged swollen lymph nodes is concerning for lymphoma or some other systemic process. Patients with isolated primary lymphoma of bone are less likely to have these symptoms, but will still present with isolated bone pain and findings on imaging to suggest an abnormal process within the bone marrow.

Imaging Characteristics

The plain radiograph presentation for lymphoma involvement of bone can vary. Because lymphoma is an infiltrative process of the marrow space, the lesion of interest is often poorly defined in its geographic borders. It is extremely rare to find a well-defined border around lymphoma lesions on both plain film and MRI. Plain radiographs can be completely normal in a patient with early lymphoma of bone (**Figure 1**, A), but when greater than 30% of the bone's mineral component is lost, a permeative pattern of bone lysis is often seen (**Figure 3**). The tumor will often permeate through the cortex and cause extreme weakening of the bone. Often, once treatment is started, the lytic areas will undergo remodeling and become more sclerotic with time. Some lymphomas present with a mixed lytic-sclerotic process before treatment or even an all-sclerotic process, although these lymphomas are seen much less frequently. It has been shown in the setting of lymphocyte-induced bone resorption that receptor activator nuclear factor kappa (RANK) is activated on the osteoclast.[11] There is also evidence that the tumor cells suppress the production of osteoprotegerin, which is the primary inhibitor of RANK ligand (RANKL) binding to RANK. The net result is a state of bone resorption by osteoclasts likely mediated by RANKL binding to RANK.

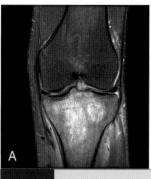
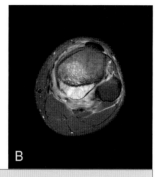

| Figure 4 | T2-weighted MRI of the left knee is shown in coronal (**A**) and axial (**B**) sections. Note the poorly defined edema pattern in the proximal tibia on the coronal imaging, as well as the posterior soft-tissue component noted in the posterior aspect of the tibia on the axial image. Biopsy confirmed lymphoma of bone. |

Osteoclast-stimulating proteins, such as parathyroid hormone-related protein and macrophage inflammatory protein-1α (MIP-1α) have been shown to be upregulated in the malignant lymphocytes and could be the secreted factors that lead to RANKL/RANK-mediated activation of the osteoclasts.[11]

MRI is often necessary in identifying the extent of bony involvement and in many cases the actual lesion itself will be first identified on MRI. The lesions seen on MRI usually have a poorly defined border with extensive marrow edema (**Figure 4, A**). The lesions are usually high signal on T2-weighted images and low signal on T1-weighted images, and can show varying amounts of cortical destruction and periosteal reaction. It is common for lymphoma involvement of bone to show a soft-tissue component, which can sometimes be greater than the bony component (**Figure 4, B**).

On both fluorodeoxyglucose positron emission tomography (FDG PET) and bone scan, the areas of bony involvement from lymphoma will have avid uptake of the radionuclide (**Figure 5**). Unfortunately, these findings are nonspecific, as most bony processes with high levels of bone turnover will have pronounced uptake on these scans. The PET scan, especially when combined with a CT of the chest, abdomen, and pelvis, can be extremely helpful in identifying other sites of involvement, both in the bone and in the other organs of the body. Although there is not a role for PET-CT in establishing the diagnosis of the bone lesion as lymphoma, subsequent to diagnosis, medical oncologists will likely obtain a PET-CT as part of the staging workup for lymphoma before treatment.

Diagnosis

The most definitive method for determining the diagnosis of lymphoma is through tissue acquisition via biopsy. In many cases, where there is lymph node or other organ involvement, the oncologist obtains the biopsy, often using image-guided techniques offered by the interventional radiology team. However, if the only

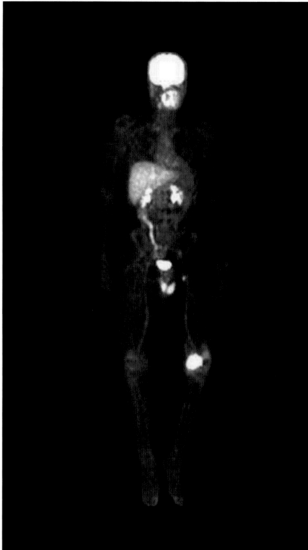

| Figure 5 | Fluorodeoxyglucose positron emission tomography (FDG PET) scan shows a patient with isolated lymphoma of bone of the left proximal tibia. Note the marked uptake of the radioactively labeled glucose in the left proximal tibia and knee region. Although PET scanning is rarely used to establish the diagnosis, it has considerable utility in staging to determine optimal treatment. |

site of involvement is bone, as in the case of primary lymphoma of bone, or the least difficult site to biopsy is bone, the orthopaedic surgeon is often consulted to help obtain an adequate specimen. Lymphoma tissue is sensitive to crush artifact and needs to be handled delicately. Furthermore, an adequate amount of tissue must be obtained for ancillary techniques including immunophenotyping, flow cytometry, fluorescent in situ hybridization, and polymerase chain reaction. The biopsy specimen should be placed in normal saline, not formalin, because formalin interferes with the ability to obtain accurate ancillary studies, which are necessary for prognostic and therapy determination. This can be accomplished via multiple passes with a core needle biopsy to ensure adequate volume and attention to proper tissue handling.

Because of the challenges of tissue sensitivity and the need to perform multiple tests on the specimen, some centers advocate open biopsy over needle biopsy despite the additional costs and requirements for anesthesia. Obtaining adequate specimens for the diagnosis of lymphoma even with open biopsy can be challenging. The malignant lymphoma cells are extremely sensitive to both mechanical and pharmacologic manipulation. The cells are easily crushed by what may seem like gentle grasping with forceps by the surgeon. These crushed cells can make diagnosis by the cytopathology team nearly impossible. Therefore, it is recommended when attempting an open biopsy that meticulous care of the tissues be undertaken. A small pituitary rongeur can be used to gently grasp tissue, or even better, a curet can allow for scooping up of tumor material without crushing the sample. The operating room technician or resident must be forewarned that they are not to grab or pinch the specimen between the fingers when taking it from the surgeon. The samples should be very gently placed in saline and formalin with the least amount of manipulation. A frozen section is obtained to ensure diagnostic tissue is present.

Lymphoma cells are extremely sensitive to steroids and NSAIDs. It is not uncommon for lymphoma lesions to almost "melt away" with just a single dose of prednisone. Because of the exquisite sensitivity of lymphoma cells, repeat biopsies are not uncommon to firmly establish a diagnosis.

Histologically, lymphoma appear similar to other round blue cell tumors (**Figure 6**). The cells vary in size and are often larger than those seen in Ewing sarcoma, but without a size reference on the slide, this finding can be difficult to appreciate. The cells often vary in shape, darkness of staining, and presence of nucleoli (pleomorphic in nature). Hodgkin lymphoma has pronounced cellular atypia and the diagnostic Reed-Sternberg cells. Both Hodgkin lymphoma and non-Hodgkin lymphoma show a high level of mitotic activity. If present within the bone marrow, both will show an infiltrative nature to the growth of the tumor, often replacing the normal fatty marrow with sheets of small, round, blue cells. Immunohistochemical staining, flow cytometry, and fluorescent in situ hybridization analysis are often used in combination to definitively determine the diagnosis of lymphoma and to specifically determine the histologic subtype of the lymphoma. A marker used by pathologists to distinguish lymphoma from other small, round blue cell tumors is CD20, which is a common B cell-specific lymphocyte marker and is usually not positive in tumors such as Ewing sarcoma or rhabdomyosarcoma.

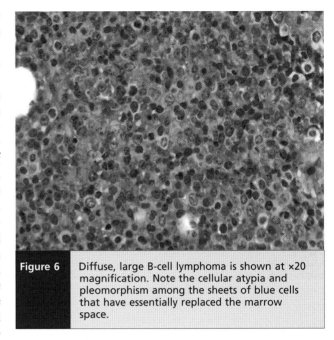

Figure 6 Diffuse, large B-cell lymphoma is shown at ×20 magnification. Note the cellular atypia and pleomorphism among the sheets of blue cells that have essentially replaced the marrow space.

Surgical Management

The main surgical indications for patients with lymphoma are to establish a diagnosis or treat impending or actual pathologic fractures. Patients often respond rapidly to steroids and chemotherapy, and in areas where pathologic fracture is either not likely or will not greatly affect functional status, surgery can be avoided. In weight-bearing long bones, the morbidity of fracture is high and therefore these areas need to be carefully assessed for risk of fracture. Many classification systems have been devised in the past to try to predict the risk of pathologic fracture, and these can be useful for communicating the risk of fracture between physicians or as a guideline for determining when to move forward with surgery.[12,13] The ultimate goal of the surgeon is to stabilize those lesions at risk for fracture before an actual fracture occurs. When a fracture occurs, treatment and recovery from surgery become much more difficult in this patient population.

Because lymphoma tends to be predominantly lytic when bone is involved, large infiltrative lesions pose a high risk for fracture and are mainly treated in a manner similar to metastatic epithelial cancers of bone. Lesions in the flat bones of the axial skeleton, such as the pelvis, scapula, and clavicle, should be treated nonsurgically with activity modification and assistive devices, such as crutches or a walker, until systemic treatment and/or radiation is initiated and pain resolves. Using pain as a guide for when to resume activity or discontinue use of assistive devices is generally an acceptable method of moving these patients toward normal functional status.

For lesions in the long bones requiring surgical stabilization, basic orthopaedic oncologic principles, which are covered in great detail in chapters 33 and 34, should be used. The entire involved bone should be

3: Malignant Primary Bone Tumors

addressed at the time of surgery. The goal of surgery is to allow for immediate weight bearing. Destructive lesions of the proximal femur are best treated with prosthetic devices. Midshaft fracture of the long bones can be adequately addressed with intramedullary devices. Destructive lesions of the proximal humerus can often be treated nonsurgically, because systemic treatment likely leads to adequate healing if activity modification can be accomplished. Periacetabular lesions are challenging and require considerable thought as to a surgical versus a nonsurgical approach. When surgery is performed for pelvic fractures, supplementation with mechanisms such as polymethyl methacrylate (PMMA), Steinman pins, or protrusio cages may be required.

The decision for surgical management of lymphoma in bone is tempered by understanding the rapid regenerative response of bone once chemotherapy is initiated. This response can be dramatic, and lymphoma differs greatly from bone metastatic disease in this regard. Additionally, the systemic therapies generally available for lymphoma are considerably more efficacious than those for most epithelial tumors, and the decision for surgery must be made in the context of understanding that this delays administration of what are usually highly effective systemic agents. Additionally, the likelihood of long-term survival in lymphoma is usually considerably greater, with cure (rather than disease progression control) possible. The decision to operate and the choice of implants also should reflect this understanding. Once treatment is initiated, the bone in these well-vascularized and muscle-engulfed bones regenerates at a surprisingly fast rate. Surgery at a later date, when the bone has regenerated in these areas, is much easier than when tumor has compromised the bone quantity and quality. As with metastatic disease, the bone will likely undergo radiation as part of the treatment after surgery, and surgical plans must take this into account. Using bone ingrowth devices, such as press-fit implants, can lead to early catastrophic failures. However, there have been some early reported successes in using tantalum metal implants in late reconstruction for irradiated bone.[14-16]

Medical Management

Medical therapy for lymphoma is complex and depends on a host of factors such as tumor genetics, molecular staging, and patient comorbidities. Traditional therapy for more aggressive non-Hodgkin lymphoma, such as diffuse large B-cell lymphoma, has consisted of systemic chemotherapy regimens with prednisone (cyclophosphamide, doxorubicin, vincristine and prednisone [CHOP]). More recently, an immune modulating antibody known as rituximab has been added to the standard protocol. Rituximab is a monoclonal chimeric antibody directed at the B cell antigen CD20, which is expressed in 95% of non-Hodgkin lymphomas.[17] Clinical studies have shown both an early and late improved overall survival rate in patients treated with rituximab in addition to the traditional CHOP therapy

(known as R-CHOP).[17] For Hodgkin lymphoma, traditional cytotoxic chemotherapeutic agents are still used (adriamycin, bleomycin, vincristine and dacarbazine). Several second-line therapies are available for relapsed patients.

One of the biggest concerns for orthopaedic surgeons regarding patients treated with R-CHOP or other chemotherapy protocols is risk of infection; all of the aforementioned agents alter the immune system and increase infection risk. Orthopaedic consultation for septic joints and osteomyelitis may be requested. If patients are placed on these regimens shortly after surgery, the risk of infection of metallic implants is a concern. Patients should be monitored closely during the early wound healing if they are receiving chemotherapy.

Patients with lymphoma are a complex group with varying disease processes that have been categorized under one heading. They have in common only that their malignant cells are thought to originate from lymphocytes. Long-term survival and overall outcome varies for each patient. Patients of all ages with lymphoma have the potential to be cured of disease or enter a long-term remission. The role of the orthopaedic surgeon in diagnosis and treatment of patients with lymphoma involvement of bone can be complex. The surgeon's main goal should be restoring function and controlling pain. This can be done using specific assistive devices and splints or with surgical stabilization or reconstruction of the bone. The surgeon may also be asked to assist in the initial diagnosis of lymphoma and should therefore understand the basic principles of obtaining an adequate tissue sample.

Myeloma

Multiple myeloma is a malignancy composed of neoplastic plasma cells, representing the end of a spectrum of plasma cell dyscrasias of increasing clinical significance. In most patients, this disease is thought to progress from monoclonal gammopathy of undetermined clinical significance (MGUS) to smoldering or asymptomatic myeloma, and ultimately developing into symptomatic myeloma.[18] A diagnosis of MGUS confers a small but persistent risk of progression to multiple myeloma, which ranges from 5% to 58% over 20 years, depending on various disease-specific factors.[19] Approximately 70% of patients with smoldering myeloma will establish symptomatic myeloma within 15 years.[20] Because the progression of MGUS to myeloma results in a change in management, musculoskeletal complaints in patients with MGUS should be evaluated with plain films, with a low threshold for cross-sectional imaging and/or biopsy as needed.

One of the hallmarks of multiple myeloma, and perhaps the primary concern for the orthopaedic surgeons, is lytic bone disease. In skeletal lesions, increased production of multiple cytokines (interleukin [IL]-1β, IL-3, and IL-6) help promote osteoclastic differentiation, whereas additional factors (tumor necrosis factor-α, hepatocyte growth factor, and vascular endothelial growth factor) further support osteoclast survival and bone resorption.[21] Myeloma cells produce MIP-1α, a chemokine involved in cell adhesion and migration, which stimulates survival, proliferation, and migration of myeloma cells.[22] MIP-1α-induced expression of IL-6 and RANKL by local marrow cells could play a significant role in osteoclastogenesis and the development of skeletal lesions.[23]

Although many tumor-related osteolytic processes are accompanied by a compensatory attempt at remodeling via osteoblastic bone formation, in myeloma bone disease, this action is characterized by a combination of increased osteoclastic resorption and suppressed bone formation. Patients with multiple myeloma have increased expression of Dickkopf-related protein-1 (DKK1) and soluble frizzled-related protein-2 (sFRP-2), both of which are inhibitors of Wnt signaling, the key pathway for osteoblast differentiation.[24] The enhanced osteoclastic bone resorption, together with the inhibition of osteoblastic bone formation, strongly favors osteolysis in the skeletal lesions, as manifested by the typical radiologic findings of skeletal lesions. Novel drug design is currently under way in attempts to affect each of these pathways.

Incidence/Prevalence

Multiple myeloma is the most common primary malignancy of bone, representing approximately 1% of all malignancies. The diagnosis of multiple myeloma is made in more than 20,000 patients each year in the United States, equating to an annual age-adjusted incidence of approximately 61 cases per million.[5] Although the incidence has not significantly changed over recent decades, modest improvements in survival have increased the overall prevalence of myeloma over the past 20 years.[25] This disease has a slight male predominance, and is nearly twice as common in those of African descent.[5] The median age is approximately 70 years, although 37% are older than 75 years and 37% are younger than 65 years at diagnosis.[26]

Clinical Presentation

Painful bony symptoms are common in patients with multiple myeloma. Given the overlap in age distribution, myeloma is consistently included with metastatic carcinoma and lymphoma in the differential diagnosis for a bone lesion of unknown origin, in patients older than 55 years. Routine testing of complete blood count (CBC), erythrocyte sedimentation rate (ESR), or bleeding time may provide the impetus for evaluation in asymptomatic patients. Myeloma bone disease or spinal cord compression, however, are likely to direct a patient toward orthopaedic care, as bony lesions develop in nearly 80% of cases.[27] It is important to recognize that the presenting clinical features can vary widely, including renal dysfunction, anemia, infection, hyperviscosity, bleeding, or hypercalcemia. The prompt recognition of these, particularly with regard to spinal cord compression, renal dysfunction, and hypercalcemia, may be critical, as emergent treatment can prevent severe or life-threatening complications.

Diagnostic Workup

Evaluation of a patient suspected of having myeloma, including adults with a lytic bone lesion of unknown etiology, involves a complete history and physical examination and a standard battery of screening studies, before attempted histologic analysis. Laboratory blood tests include CBC, ESR, coagulation times, and serum chemistries (blood urea nitrogen, creatinine, serum calcium, serum albumin). Serum protein electrophoresis should be performed, with immunofixation for identification and typing of M-protein.[28] Additional quantification of M-protein is determined by densitometry. Concentrated urine protein electrophoresis or screening urine for Bence-Jones proteinuria will capture those patients with light chain disease, which often does not appear in routine serum analysis. In patients with strong clinical suspicion of myeloma or a diagnosis of solitary plasmacytoma, where routine serum protein electrophoresis and urine protein electrophoresis are negative, a serum-free light chain assessment increases sensitivity for detection of light-chain-only myeloma.

In addition to detection of M-protein, the diagnosis of myeloma requires histopathologic demonstration of monoclonal or abnormal plasma cells. This is usually evaluated on a bone marrow aspirate, which is ideally performed using a 20-mm trephine biopsy device. Confirmation can be made by biopsy of a skeletal lesion, so radiographs of symptomatic lesions should be performed before marrow aspiration. In some cases in which histologic features may be equivocal, flow cytometry or immunohistochemical staining for CD138 can be useful. Conventional karyotyping and fluorescence in situ hybridization are becoming standard of care, as they demonstrate prognostic and potential therapeutic significance.[28]

Diagnostic Criteria

To support a diagnosis of multiple myeloma, M-protein must be present in the serum or urine, as well as either clonal plasma cells in the bone marrow or a histologically proved plasmacytoma. The primary factor to distinguish symptomatic myeloma from asymptomatic myeloma is the presence of myeloma-related organ or tissue impairment. On rare occasion, the patient may have biopsy-proven clonal plasma cells and myeloma-related organ or tissue impairment in the absence of detectable M-protein in the serum or urine, a true nonsecretory multiple myeloma. End-organ damage often goes by the mnemonic CRAB: hypercalcemia (serum calcium > 10.5 mg/dL), renal insufficiency (creatinine > 2mg/dL), anemia (Hgb < 10 g/dL), or bone lesions, although any other sign or symptom of organ dysfunction related to plasma cell proliferation can qualify as a diagnostic criterion.[28]

<table>
<tr><td colspan="3">Table 1</td></tr>
</table>

International Staging System for Multiple Myeloma

Stage	Serum Beta-2 Microglobulin (mg/L)	Serum Albumin Level (g/dL)
Stage 1	< 3.5	≥ 3.5
Stage 2	< 3.5 or 3.5-5.5	< 3.5 or Any albumin level
Stage 3	> 5.5	Any albumin level

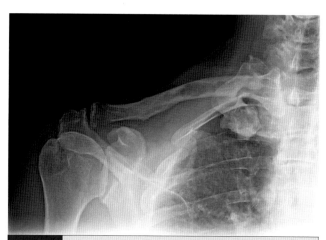

<table>
<tr><td>Figure 7</td><td>Plain radiograph shows a clavicle with significant involvement from multiple myeloma, characterized by well-demarcated "punched out" lytic lesions throughout the bone.</td></tr>
</table>

Staging

Once a diagnosis of multiple myeloma has been established, staging studies should be performed to assess tumor burden, prognosis, and myeloma-related organ and tissue impairment. A skeletal survey provides useful information, as severity of bone involvement demonstrates prognostic significance.[29] Similarly, markers of bone resorption (C-telopeptide, N-telopeptide, pyridinoline, deoxypyridinoline) and bone formation (alkaline phosphatase, osteocalcin) have been correlated with skeletal-related events, progression, and survival.[30] Other prognostic factors, such as M-protein quantity and serum levels of hemoglobin, calcium, and creatinine, were included in the Durie-Salmon staging system for multiple myeloma.[29] Serum albumin, and β2-microglobulinemia are additional independent prognostic indicators, which determine the widely used International Staging System (ISS)[31] (**Table 1**)

Prognosis

Among patients with symptomatic myeloma, the prognosis can vary widely, with duration of survival ranging from weeks to decades. Overall, the 5-year survival rate is approximately 35%, although recent advances in treatment, particularly in patients younger than 60 years, have resulted in improvements in long-term survival.[26] In addition to age, the ISS staging system has prognostic significance. Patients with ISS stage I disease have a median survival of 62 months, as compared to 44 months for stage II and 29 months for stage III.[31] More recent efforts have incorporated fluorescent in situ hybridization and conventional karyotyping for risk stratification, as well as risk-adapted therapeutic strategies. Those with hyperdiploidy, t(11;14), or t(6,14), comprise the standard risk cohort, with a median survival of 65 months. In contrast, tumors bearing 17p deletions, t(4;14), t(14;16), t(14;20), chromosome 13 deletion, or hypodiploidy represent high-risk cytogenetic features, with a median survival of 37 months.[32]

Imaging

Radiologically, the appearance of multiple myeloma is dictated by the pathophysiology responsible for the skeletal lesions. The disease primarily involves the red marrow, with subsequent trabecular bone resorption. As a result, the most common sites of disease are those rich in red marrow in the adult population: spine, skull, pelvis, ribs, proximal femur, and proximal humerus. With progression of disease and increasing marrow replacement, additional long bone involvement often follows. Also, in light of the biologic process of osteoclastic bone resorption, with a relative paucity of osteoblastic bone formation on histopathology, the radiographic findings are most often characterized by focal, osteolytic lesions without a sclerotic rim. These lesions generally begin centrally in the marrow, but with enlargement of the tumors, bone lesions can develop endosteal scalloping, cortical destruction, fracture, and the formation of a soft-tissue mass. Osteolytic foci are often well circumscribed, with a sharp zone of transition (**Figure 7**). In the skull, they are described as punched-out lesions. In some patients, myeloma may produce a more diffuse pattern of osteolysis, which can mimic senile osteoporosis.

The typical radiologic workup of a skeletal lesion suspicious for metastatic carcinoma involves a technetium bone scan to identify additional sites of disease. Because a bone scan uses Tc-99m-labeled methylene diphosphonate, it is a marker of bone formation, which is not a hallmark of myeloma bone disease. This modality detects only 35% to 60% of skeletal lesions from myeloma, with a sensitivity and specificity less than that of a skeletal survey.[33] Technetium bone scanning, therefore, is not generally used in the evaluation of the extent of bone involvement for multiple myeloma. Instead, a skeletal survey involving: AP and lateral views of the cervical, thoracic, and lumbar spine, both humeri, both femora, and the skull; PA view of the chest; and AP view of the pelvis. Additional areas should be imaged based upon symptomatic involvement. Approximately 80% of patients in whom multiple myeloma is newly diagnosed will have a lesion detectable on skeletal survey.[34]

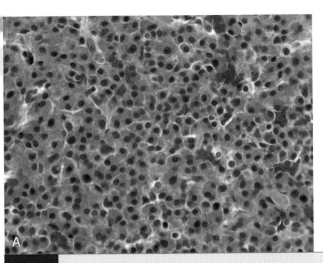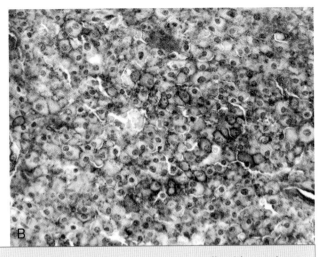

Figure 8 **A**, Hematoxylin-eosin stain of multiple myeloma is shown at ×20 magnification. Large plasma cells with prominent nuclei and abundant cytoplasm, with a lack of stroma, characterize this lesion. **B**, The tissue stains positive for CD138+ immunohistochemical stain, frequently used to confirm the diagnosis of multiple myeloma.

To identify an osteolytic lesion radiographically, 30% of the trabecular bone must be devoid of calcium, impairing detection of early bone resorption.[35] Combined with difficulties in identifying lytic lesions in certain anatomic locations of interest, and poor assessment of treatment response, the utility of skeletal radiographs for following disease progression has been limited. Using radiographs alone, one cannot be certain whether a skeletal complication is the result of disease progression, rather than the failure to remodel a cortical erosion after significant treatment response. As a result, the role of advanced imaging has played an increasingly important role in the management of myeloma bone disease.

If radiographs are equivocal, CT can provide greater clarification, particularly in anatomic areas that are difficult to evaluate radiographically. A CT scan is more sensitive than radiographs in determining the presence of a lesion, and may provide improved ability to determine risk of fracture or the presence of a lung or abdominal mass.[34] Although the radiation exposure is greater than that of radiography, CT may be beneficial in limiting the need to reposition a patient with painful lesions for complete and adequate imaging. These studies can be adequately performed without contrast, which is preferable considering that these patients may have renal compromise. Skeletal lesions are usually lytic, with attenuation similar to soft tissues. Although rare, a sclerotic rim can sometimes be seen after treatment response or in the setting of polyneuropathy, organomegaly, endocrinopathy, monoclonal-protein, and skin abnormalities.

The determination of smoldering versus symptomatic myeloma has significant prognostic and treatment implications and is made on the presence of a bone lesion. In patients with a negative skeletal survey, one half will have a lesion detectable by MRI.[36] When comparing imaging modalities, MRI is significantly better

at identifying lesions in the spine, pelvis, and sternum. However, radiographs were at least as effective as MRI for identifying lesions in the skull, shoulders, ribs, and long bones.[36] In addition to discrete lesions and tumors, MRI is capable of detecting marrow infiltration, and is ideal for evaluating soft-tissue tumors. Many patients with myeloma are treated for anemia with erythropoiesis-stimulating agents. Distinguishing between marrow involvement and the effects of granulocyte colony-stimulating factor treatment remains difficult, with reports estimating up to 40% mimicry of imaging features.[37]

With a sensitivity and specificity of approximately 85% and 90%, respectively, FDG-PET/CT is better at identifying skeletal lesions than radiographs in 46% of patients.[38] The detection of lesions smaller than 1 cm is limited with FDG-PET/CT, and this modality failed to detect a lesion identified on MRI in 30% of patients, most commonly in those with diffuse marrow involvement. However, FDG-PET/CT was able to detect lesions that were out of the MRI field of view in 35% of patients, suggesting value in whole-body evaluation.[39]

Histology

Neither MGUS nor smoldering myeloma exhibit myeloma-related organ or tissue impairment, including identifiable bone changes. For symptomatic myeloma, no discrete numbers are used for the diagnosis, but rather the presence of end-organ damage. In the setting of a plasmacytoma or marrow replacement, the histologic appearance includes nodules or sheets of plasma cells that displace normal marrow elements. Most plasma cells may appear normal in histologic appearance—a basophilic round cell with a prominent perinuclear halo. Large, peripheral clumps of heterochromatin give the nucleus the appearance of a clock face or cartwheel (**Figure 8**). Despite the typical histologic appearance of most cells, flow cytometric analysis demonstrates that more than 90% will have a neoplastic phenotype.[40] Other more atypical features include dysplastic plasmablasts with large nucleoli, binucleation, or intracellular inclusions and Russell bodies. Cells with abundant immunoglobulin AA production may exhibit a bright red staining cytoplasm (flame cell).

Despite its origination as a terminally differentiated B-lymphocyte, the cells in plasmacytomas generally do not express the typical B cell antigens CD19 and CD20, which helps distinguish them from normal plasma cells. Expression of CD38, CD56, CD79, and CD138 is common in myeloma cells, and can be used in flow cytometry or immunohistochemistry for diagnostic confirmation, particularly in bone marrow biopsies.[40]

Medical Treatment

Patients with MGUS or smoldering myeloma are treated with clinical observation because chemotherapy has not been shown to be beneficial. Those patients with a solitary plasmacytoma, without evidence of elevated M-protein, may be treated with local therapy for the tumor with continued observation for progression of disease. However, for symptomatic myeloma, systemic treatment should be started promptly upon diagnosis. Induction regimens currently consist of treatment with at least one of the novel chemotherapeutic agents for myeloma, such as thalidomide, lenalidomide, or bortezomib. These are usually combined with a corticosteroid, and often with a cytotoxic agent, such as cyclophosphamide, doxorubicin, or melphalan.[26]

The management of multiple myeloma is largely dependent on the patient's age and medical comorbidities. In patients older than 75 years or with substantial coexisting conditions, reduced dosage of chemotherapy may be required to limit toxicity.[26] For patients younger than 65 years in whom multiple myeloma has been newly diagnosed, without precluding heart, lung, liver, or renal dysfunction, high-dose induction therapy with autologous stem cell transplant should be considered.[28] Although some centers perform tandem autologous stem cell transplants, no conclusive data exist to support an improvement over a single transplant in treatment-naïve patients.

Bisphosphonates

Given their potent antiosteoclastic activity, bisphosphonates have been studied extensively in the management of myeloma bone disease. A recent Cochrane review concluded that bisphosphonates reduced pain and vertebral fractures in myeloma, but did not improve survival.[41] Several high-quality randomized control trials have helped solidify the role of bisphosphonates as part of the medical treatment of myeloma. Clodronate is the only oral bisphosphonate to demonstrate a clinical benefit, with reductions in development of new osteolytic lesions, hypercalcemia, and vertebral and nonvertebral fractures.[42] More recently, intravenous zoledronic acid has been shown to have superior efficacy over oral clo-

dronate in reducing skeletal-related events, and had a small yet significant improvement in progression-free and overall survival.[43] Infusion of pamidronate has efficacy similar to that of zoledronic acid with regard to preventing skeletal-related events.[44] Zoledronic acid demonstrates greater improvement in normalization of markers of bone turnover than pamidronate, and has proved superior in the management of hypercalcemia of malignancy, thus becoming the bisphosphonate of choice for patients with multiple myeloma.[28]

The use of bisphosphonates should involve consideration of potential adverse effects from bisphosphonate treatment, notably osteonecrosis of the jaw and atypical subtrochanteric fractures. No study or guidelines have yet been published to definitively establish the optimal treatment duration, although some have supported stopping the medication after 2 to 5 years, or in patients achieving a posttransplant complete response or very good partial response, in the absence of bone lesions.[28] Limited data are available to indicate whether treatment should be initiated in patients with asymptomatic myeloma, although a large study has suggested that zoledronic acid can reduce the number of skeletal-related events at the time of progression.[45] These results, together with extensive in vitro and preclinical data, supports the notion that bisphosphonates may have a direct antimyeloma effect, in addition to their role in inhibiting osteoclasts.[46] Additional agents, such as denosumab, osteoprotegerin, activin-A antagonists, antisclerostin antibodies, Src inhibitors, statins, and Wnt agonists are all in different stages of development for the prevention of skeletal complications from malignancy.

Radiotherapy

As with most hematologic malignancies, plasmacytomas are highly radiosensitive. For a solitary plasmacytoma, external beam radiation at a dose of 4,000 to 4,500 cGy can provide local control in up to 92% of patients.[47] Radiation is used most frequently in the management of cord compression or painful bony lesions, for which radiation doses as low as 800 cGy can provide significant and durable pain relief. Patients with extensive osseous disease can obtain considerable palliation from hemibody radiation or bone-seeking radionuclides (Sm-153, Sr-89, P-32, Re-186).[48] Although the relatively low dose of radiation decreases radiation-associated complications, the use of these modalities is largely limited by myelosuppression from the destruction of red marrow.

Surgical Management

With the exception of the biopsy for diagnosis, the role of surgical treatment in multiple myeloma is palliative. Although spinal cord compression occurs in up to 5% of patients with myeloma, it is most commonly the result of compression from soft-tissue tumor that can be adequately treated by corticosteroids and urgent radiation therapy.[27] For acute structural cord compression, emergent surgical decompression may be necessary. Radiation therapy, while demonstrating excellent tumoricidal activity, does not generally allow for reconstitution of cortical bone. As a result, in the setting of spinal instability, surgical stabilization is necessary regardless of the efficacy of radiation treatment.

Although the use of bisphosphonates has significantly decreased skeletal-related events in multiple myeloma, at least 5% of patients will sustain a vertebral fracture.[43] In properly indicated patients, vertebroplasty and kyphoplasty are effective in relieving pain from vertebral compression fractures in myeloma.[49] These procedures do not relieve cord compression or spinal instability. Caution should be exercised, particularly in the setting of posterior cortical disruption, for the risk of PMMA extravasation into the spinal canal.

The other major role for orthopaedic surgery in patients with multiple myeloma is in the management of fractures and impending pathologic fractures of long bones, which affect approximately 14% of patients with the disease.[41] Fractured bones and those at risk of fracture from normal activity should undergo stabilization and protection of the entire bone. Because multiple myeloma is a systemic disease that is highly sensitive to radiation, complete removal of neoplastic cells from the lesion during fixation is not necessary. After stabilization, typically using either an intramedullary nail or a cortical plate and screws, the affected bone can be effectively treated with radiation therapy. Large skeletal defects often benefit from curettage, with a combination of PMMA and metal used to augment fixation, to allow for immediate weight bearing.

Destructive myeloma lesions in the femoral head and neck are most amenable to joint arthroplasty, which may require a long-stem cemented prosthesis to bypass distal femur lesions if present. Although evidence suggests that arthroplasty gives better results than fixation for peritrochanteric lesions in metastatic carcinoma, myeloma, and lymphoma, additional studies are ongoing to verify these findings.[50] As with metastatic carcinoma, the use of imaging studies and an intraoperative acetabular assessment can determine whether total hip arthroplasty is necessary. Significant periacetabular destruction may require augmentation with a modification of the Harrington hip reconstruction, using cement and metal pins or screws to bridge the pelvic or acetabular defect. Alternatively, recent evidence suggests a potential role for porous metal acetabular augmentation, with bone ingrowth demonstrated even in the setting of radiation therapy.[16] Most other anatomic sites can be adequately treated with surgical fixation, unless articular destruction dictates the necessity of joint arthroplasty.

Perioperative Complications

Multiple myeloma can affect several organ systems, leading to the potential for significant perioperative complications. Myeloma-associated anemia can usually be controlled with erythropoiesis-stimulating agents, but transfusion may be necessary for procedures with moderate volumes of expected blood loss. Thrombotic complications are not uncommon in multiple myeloma, with an incidence of deep vein thrombosis reported at 8.7 per 1,000 patients with multiple myeloma.[51] The risk of venous thromboembolism can be increased further by the use of corticosteroids and chemotherapeutic agents for treatment. Thromboembolic events can be exacerbated by hyperviscosity, which is the result of elevated levels of serum paraprotein. Hyperviscosity syndrome can have a wide range of manifestations, including headaches, blurred vision, or heart failure, which necessitates plasmapheresis or exchange transfusion on occasion.[28] Because of an impaired immune system from both the disease and its chemotherapeutic agents, patients with myeloma have an increased risk of early infection.[49]

Approximately 30% of patients with multiple myeloma will develop hypercalcemia, which can develop into a medical emergency.[28] Potential symptoms include confusion or coma, cardiac arrhythmias, and renal insufficiency. In cases of hypercalcemia resulting from myeloma, urgent hydration and intravenous zoledronic acid treatment should be initiated. In light of the high rate of renal dysfunction in advanced myeloma, dose adjustments of bisphosphonates may be necessary in these patients.

Summary

Orthopaedic surgeons are commonly involved in both the diagnosis and treatment of patients with myeloma and lymphoma. The ultimate goals of orthopaedic care in this patient population are accurate diagnosis, improved function, and decreased pain. Pathologic fractures are common and should be prevented whenever possible. Coordinated care with radiation and medical oncology is also important to the care of patients with myeloma or lymphoma. Thoughtful evaluation of any patient with unexplained bone pain should be undertaken by every orthopaedic surgeon to prevent delayed diagnosis of an underlying malignancy.

Annotated References

1. Swerdlow S, Campo E, Harris N, et al (eds): *WHO Classification of Tumours of Haematopoietic and Lymphoid Tissues*, ed 4. Lyon, France, IARC Press, 2008.

   The World Health Organization (WHO) classification of lymphoid tissue tumors includes the most recent updates on classification criteria for the numerous types of lymphoma and leukemia.

2. Jaffe ES: The 2008 WHO classification of lymphomas: Implications for clinical practice and translational research. *Hematology Am Soc Hematol Educ Program* 2009;523-531.

3: Malignant Primary Bone Tumors

This article nicely summarizes the very extensive WHO classification system for lymphomas and applies the classification system to clinical practice and translational research.

3. Horning SJ: *Abeloff's Clinical Oncology*, ed 4. Philadelphia, PA, Churchill Livingstone/Elsevier, 2008, p 2353.

This chapter summarizes Hodgkin lymphoma, its treatment, and its prognosis.

4. Wilson WH, Armitage JO: Non-Hodgkin's lymphoma, in Abeloff MD, Armitage JO, Niederhuber JE, Kastan MB, McKenna WG (eds): *Abeloff's Clinical Oncology*, ed 4. Philadelphia, PA, Churchill-Livingstone/Elsevier, 2008, p 2371.

This chapter provides an excellent review of the pertinent clinical features, diagnostic criteria, and basic biology of non-Hodgkin lymphoma. It also reviews the treatment protocols for non-Hodgkin lymphoma as of 2008. Because of its publication year, this chapter does not provide much information on rituximab.

5. Howlader N, Noone A, Krapcho M, et al: *SEER Cancer Statistics Review, 1975-2009 (Vintage 2009 Populations)*. Bethesda, MD, National Cancer Institute, 2011. http://seer.cancer.gov/csr/1975_2009_pops09/. Based on November 2011 SEER data submission, posted to the SEER web site, 2012. Accessed June 2012.

Data provided in this chapter were taken from the Surveillance, Epidemiology, and End Results (SEER) database and Website provided by the National Institutes of Health.

6. Kittivorapart J, Chinthammitr Y: Incidence and risk factors of bone marrow involvement by non-Hodgkin lymphoma. *J Med Assoc Thai* 2011;94(Suppl 1):S239-S245.

The authors of this study retrospectively reviewed 320 patients with non-Hodgkin lymphoma at one institution, looking at the rate of bone marrow involvement in patients in whom non-Hodgkin lymphoma was diagnosed and who also underwent bone marrow biopsies.

7. Conlan MG, Bast M, Armitage JO, Weisenburger DD; Nebraska Lymphoma Study Group: Bone marrow involvement by non-Hodgkin's lymphoma: The clinical significance of morphologic discordance between the lymph node and bone marrow. *J Clin Oncol* 1990;8(7):1163-1172.

8. Shindle MK, Tyler W, Edobor-Osula F, et al: Unsuspected lymphoma diagnosed with use of biopsy during kyphoplasty. *J Bone Joint Surg Am* 2006;88(12):2721-2724.

9. Limb D, Dreghorn C, Murphy JK, Mannion R: Primary lymphoma of bone. *Int Orthop* 1994;18(3):180-183.

10. Ramadan KM, Shenkier T, Sehn LH, Gascoyne RD, Connors JM: A clinicopathological retrospective study of 131 patients with primary bone lymphoma: A population-based study of successively treated cohorts from the British Columbia Cancer Agency. *Ann Oncol* 2007;18(1):129-135.

In this retrospective analysis of the British Columbia Agency Lymphoid Cancer Database from 1983 to 2005, the authors noted trends toward improved outcomes in patients treated with cyclophosphamide, doxorubicin, vincristine, and prednisone chemotherapy compared to other older protocols. The authors also noted specific trends in sex, age, and histologic subtype for primary bone lymphoma.

11. Shu ST, Martin CK, Thudi NK, Dirksen WP, Rosol TJ: Osteolytic bone resorption in adult T-cell leukemia/lymphoma. *Leuk Lymphoma* 2010;51(4):702-714.

In this study, researchers co-cultured human adult T cell lymphoma and leukemia cells with murine calvaria under conditioned media conditions. They found RANK-dependent increased osteoclastic activity in these cell culture conditions. They also studied the gene expression of the cell lines.

12. Mirels H: Metastatic disease in long bones: A proposed scoring system for diagnosing impending pathologic fractures. *Clin Orthop Relat Res* 1989;249:256-264.

13. McBroom RJ, Cheal EJ, Hayes WC: Strength reductions from metastatic cortical defects in long bones. *J Orthop Res* 1988;6(3):369-378.

14. Rose PS, Halasy M, Trousdale RT, et al: Preliminary results of tantalum acetabular components for THA after pelvic radiation. *Clin Orthop Relat Res* 2006;453:195-198.

15. Demircay E, Unay K, Sener N: Cementless bilateral total hip arthroplasty in a patient with a history of pelvic irradiation for sarcoma botryoides. *Med Princ Pract* 2009;18(5):411-413.

This article is a case report of a patient treated with bilateral cementless total hip arthroplasty at 38-month follow-up for one hip and 84-month follow-up for the other hip. The patient received high-dose pelvic irradiation as a child at the age of 18 months.

16. Joglekar SB, Rose PS, Lewallen DG, Sim FH: Tantalum acetabular cups provide secure fixation in THA after pelvic irradiation at minimum 5-year followup. *Clin Orthop Relat Res* 2012;470(11):3041-3047.

The authors performed a 5-year follow-up analysis of tantalum cups used in patients with a prior history of pelvic irradiation. Seventeen patients from the authors' previous analysis had 5-year or greater follow-up, and all patients in this analysis maintained a stable, well-fixed implant with the tantalum cup used at this institution.

17. Maloney DG: Anti-CD20 antibody therapy for B-cell lymphomas. *N Engl J Med* 2012;366(21):2008-2016.

This article is an outstanding review and summary of the current literature on the use of rituximab (anti-

CD20) in the treatment of non-Hodgkin lymphoma. Recently performed clinical trials, their outcomes, and the current National Comprehensive Cancer Network recommendations are outlined. An excellent review of the biology behind the mechanism of the action of this immunomodulator is provided.

18. Landgren O, Kyle RA, Pfeiffer RM, et al: Monoclonal gammopathy of undetermined significance (MGUS) consistently precedes multiple myeloma: A prospective study. *Blood* 2009;113(22):5412-5417.

 From a large, population-based cancer screening study, serum samples were analyzed in 71 patients who developed myeloma during the study course. Samples collected 2 to 10 years before diagnosis indicate that an asymptomatic MGUS preceded myeloma in each patient. Level of evidence: II.

19. Rajkumar SV, Kyle RA, Therneau TM, et al: Serum free light chain ratio is an independent risk factor for progression in monoclonal gammopathy of undetermined significance. *Blood* 2005;106(3):812-817.

20. Kyle RA, Remstein ED, Therneau TM, et al: Clinical course and prognosis of smoldering (asymptomatic) multiple myeloma. *N Engl J Med* 2007;356(25):2582-2590.

 A retrospective review of 276 patients with smoldering myeloma over a 25-year period at the Mayo Clinic is presented, and the risk of progression to symptomatic disease is evaluated. Level of evidence: II

21. Dankbar B, Padró T, Leo R, et al: Vascular endothelial growth factor and interleukin-6 in paracrine tumor-stromal cell interactions in multiple myeloma. *Blood* 2000;95(8):2630-2636.

22. Choi SJ, Oba Y, Gazitt Y, et al: Antisense inhibition of macrophage inflammatory protein 1-alpha blocks bone destruction in a model of myeloma bone disease. *J Clin Invest* 2001;108(12):1833-1841.

23. Oyajobi BO, Franchin G, Williams PJ, et al: Dual effects of macrophage inflammatory protein-1alpha on osteolysis and tumor burden in the murine 5TGM1 model of myeloma bone disease. *Blood* 2003;102(1):311-319.

24. Tian E, Zhan F, Walker R, et al: The role of the Wnt-signaling antagonist DKK1 in the development of osteolytic lesions in multiple myeloma. *N Engl J Med* 2003;349(26):2483-2494.

25. Kumar SK, Rajkumar SV, Dispenzieri A, et al: Improved survival in multiple myeloma and the impact of novel therapies. *Blood* 2008;111(5):2516-2520.

 Two cohorts of patients treated for multiple myeloma were evaluated at a single institution. Improvements in survival were suggested for patients in whom a recent diagnosis was made and in patients receiving thalidomide, lenalidomide, or bortezomib. In patients who relapsed following stem cell transplant, those relapsing

after 2000 had improved outcomes. Level of evidence: III.

26. Palumbo AK, Anderson K: Multiple myeloma. *N Engl J Med* 2011;364(11):1046-1060.

 This article provides an outstanding general review of multiple myeloma biology, diagnosis, and management, with a predominant focus on medical treatment regimens.

27. Kyle RA, Gertz MA, Witzig TE, et al: Review of 1027 patients with newly diagnosed multiple myeloma. *Mayo Clin Proc* 2003;78(1):21-33.

28. Bird JM, Owen RG, D'Sa S, et al; Haemato-oncology Task Force of British Committee for Standards in Haematology (BCSH) and UK Myeloma Forum: Guidelines for the diagnosis and management of multiple myeloma 2011. *Br J Haematol* 2011;154(1):32-75.

 This article provides an update of the comprehensive, evidence-based guidelines for the diagnosis and management of multiple myeloma in the United Kingdom. This excellent and current review primarily focused on diagnostic criteria and medical treatment options, with corresponding levels of evidence. Level of evidence: II.

29. Durie BG, Salmon SE: A clinical staging system for multiple myeloma: Correlation of measured myeloma cell mass with presenting clinical features, response to treatment, and survival. *Cancer* 1975;36(3):842-854.

30. Abildgaard N, Brixen K, Kristensen JE, Eriksen EF, Nielsen JL, Heickendorff L: Comparison of five biochemical markers of bone resorption in multiple myeloma: Elevated pre-treatment levels of S-ICTP and U-Ntx are predictive for early progression of the bone disease during standard chemotherapy. *Br J Haematol* 2003;120(2):235-242.

31. Greipp PR, San Miguel J, Durie BG, et al: International staging system for multiple myeloma. *J Clin Oncol* 2005;23(15):3412-3420.

32. Rajkumar SV: Multiple myeloma: 2012 update on diagnosis, risk-stratification, and management. *Am J Hematol* 2012;87(1):78-88.

 This article presents updated clinical results, particularly supporting the role of molecular cytogenetic risk stratification in multiple myeloma. Level of evidence: V.

33. Dimopoulos M, Terpos E, Comenzo RL, et al; IMWG: International myeloma working group consensus statement and guidelines regarding the current role of imaging techniques in the diagnosis and monitoring of multiple myeloma. *Leukemia* 2009;23(9):1545-1556.

 A comprehensive review of the available literature regarding imaging techniques for the diagnosis and staging of multiple myeloma, with consensus guidelines from the International Myeloma Working Group, is presented. Level of evidence: V.

3: Malignant Primary Bone Tumors

34. Terpos E, Mouloupoulos LA, Dimopoulos MA: Advances in imaging and the management of myeloma bone disease. *J Clin Oncol* 2011;29(14):1907-1915.

    The authors presented several clinical trials demonstrating the role of bisphosphonates in preventing skeletal complications in multiple myeloma, as well as providing an excellent assessment of the role of various imaging modalities for evaluation of skeletal lesions. Level of evidence: V.

35. Edelstyn GA, Gillespie PJ, Grebbell FS: The radiological demonstration of osseous metastases: Experimental observations. *Clin Radiol* 1967;18(2):158-162.

36. Walker R, Barlogie B, Haessler J, et al: Magnetic resonance imaging in multiple myeloma: Diagnostic and clinical implications. *J Clin Oncol* 2007;25(9):1121-1128.

    Both MRI and skeletal surveys were available in 611 of 668 patients treated on a uniform autologous stem cell transplant protocol. MRI demonstrated improved detection of focal osseous lesions over skeletal survey. Level of evidence: II.

37. Hartman RP, Sundaram M, Okuno SH, Sim FH: Effect of granulocyte-stimulating factors on marrow of adult patients with musculoskeletal malignancies: Incidence and MRI findings. *AJR Am J Roentgenol* 2004; 183(3):645-653.

38. Bredella MA, Steinbach L, Caputo G, Segall G, Hawkins R: Value of FDG PET in the assessment of patients with multiple myeloma. *AJR Am J Roentgenol* 2005; 184(4):1199-1204.

39. Zamagni E, Nanni C, Patriarca F, et al: A prospective comparison of 18F-fluorodeoxyglucose positron emission tomography-computed tomography, magnetic resonance imaging and whole-body planar radiographs in the assessment of bone disease in newly diagnosed multiple myeloma. *Haematologica* 2007;92(1):50-55.

    In a small series of 46 patients in whom multiple myeloma was newly diagnosed, the authors prospectively evaluated the diagnostic detection of osseous lesions with skeletal survey, MRI, and FDG-PET/CT. FDG-PET/CT was superior to skeletal survey in detecting spine lesions, though was inferior to MRI. FDG-PET/CT was able to detect some lesions that were outside the field of MRI view, and the combination of MRI of the spine and pelvis with FDG-PET/CT was able to detect 92% of all sites of active myeloma lesions. Level of evidence: III.

40. Rawstron AC, Orfao A, Beksac M, et al; European Myeloma Network: Report of the European Myeloma Network on multiparametric flow cytometry in multiple myeloma and related disorders. *Haematologica* 2008;93(3):431-438.

    This paper reviews the European Myeloma Network's recommendations regarding the indications for flow cytometry in multiple myeloma, as well as the recommended panel of markers. Level of evidence: V.

41. Mhaskar R, Redzepovic J, Wheatley K, et al: Bisphosphonates in multiple myeloma: A network meta-analysis. *Cochrane Database Syst Rev* 2012;5: CD003188.

    An update on a previous Cochrane Database review, which evaluated the literature regarding bisphosphonateuse in multiple myeloma, is presented. This report suggested that bisphosphonates decrease skeletal-related events and pain in myeloma. There was no significant difference in toxicity between the various bisphosphonates used. Level of evidence: I.

42. McCloskey EV, Dunn JA, Kanis JA, MacLennan IC, Drayson MT: Long-term follow-up of a prospective, double-blind, placebo-controlled randomized trial of clodronate in multiple myeloma. *Br J Haematol* 2001; 113(4):1035-1043.

43. Morgan GJ, Davies FE, Gregory WM, et al; National Cancer Research Institute Haematological Oncology Clinical Study Group: First-line treatment with zoledronic acid as compared with clodronic acid in multiple myeloma (MRC Myeloma IX): A randomised controlled trial. *Lancet* 2010;376(9757):1989-1999.

    This randomized, controlled trial of 1,970 patients demonstrated improved overall and progression-free survival with intravenous zoledronic acid treatment over oral clodronate. Level of evidence: I.

44. Rosen LS, Gordon D, Kaminski M, et al: Long-term efficacy and safety of zoledronic acid compared with pamidronate disodium in the treatment of skeletal complications in patients with advanced multiple myeloma or breast carcinoma: A randomized, double-blind, multicenter, comparative trial. *Cancer* 2003; 98(8):1735-1744.

45. Musto P, Petrucci MT, Bringhen S, et al; GIMEMA (Italian Group for Adult Hematologic Diseases)/ Multiple Myeloma Working Party and the Italian Myeloma Network: A multicenter, randomized clinical trial comparing zoledronic acid versus observation in patients with asymptomatic myeloma. *Cancer* 2008; 113(7):1588-1595.

    The authors found that monthly use of zoledronic acid in patients with asymptomatic myeloma reduced the incidence of skeletal-related events but did not affect the natural history of the disease.

46. Zwolak P, Manivel JC, Jasinski P, et al: Cytotoxic effect of zoledronic acid-loaded bone cement on giant cell tumor, multiple myeloma, and renal cell carcinoma cell lines. *J Bone Joint Surg Am* 2010;92(1):162-168.

    The authors examined the elution of zoledronic acid from bone cement and assessed its effect on tumor growth.

47. Reed V, Shah J, Medeiros LJ, et al: Solitary plasmacytomas: Outcome and prognostic factors after definitive radiation therapy. *Cancer* 2011;117(19):4468-4474.

    This retrospective review of 84 patients with solitary plasmacytoma demonstrated 92% local control, though 56% of bone solitary plasmacytoma patients progressed to multiple myeloma within 5 years.

48. Yeh HS, Berenson JR: Treatment for myeloma bone disease. *Clin Cancer Res* 2006;12(20 pt 2):6279s-6284s.

49. Snowden JA, Ahmedzai SH, Ashcroft J, et al; Haemato-oncology Task Force of British Committee for Standards in Haematology and UK Myeloma Forum: Guidelines for supportive care in multiple myeloma 2011. *Br J Haematol* 2011;154(1):76-103.

This article presents evidence-based guidelines for the supportive care of myeloma in the United Kingdom. Although it largely focuses on pain and palliative care, it contains a good current review of anemia, bleeding, venous thromboembolism, and infection management.

50. Steensma M, Boland PJ, Morris CD, Athanasian E, Healey JH: Endoprosthetic treatment is more durable for pathologic proximal femur fractures. *Clin Orthop Relat Res* 2012;470(3):920-926.

The authors compared surgical treatment failure rates of intramedullary nailing, endoprosthetic reconstruction, and open reduction/internal fixation and found that endoprosthetic reconstruction led to fewer failures and greater durability of the implant in patients with pathologic fractures of the proximal femur. Level of evidence: III.

51. Kristinsson SY, Fears TR, Gridley G, et al: Deep vein thrombosis after monoclonal gammopathy of undetermined significance and multiple myeloma. *Blood* 2008;112(9):3582-3586.

3: Malignant Primary Bone Tumors

Chapter 20

Surgical Management of Malignant Primary Bone Tumors

Satoshi Kawaguchi, MD   Valerae O. Lewis, MD

General Principles

The primary goal of oncologic surgery is to achieve local cure. Practically, it is to attain negative surgical margins. Toward this goal, surgery aims to remove the whole tumor in one piece, together with a margin of normal osseous and soft tissue around it.[1-3] Margins can be defined as intralesional, marginal, wide, or radical.[4] An intralesional excision is through the tumor. A marginal excision is through the reactive tissue that surrounds the tumor but is not actually part of the tumor. A wide excision is through entirely normal tissues, leaving a cuff of normal tissue on all sides of the tumor. A radical resection is when the entire bony or myofascial compartment or compartments containing the tumor is resected. Malignant tumors are typically excised with wide surgical margins. However, the size of the margin or cuff of the normal tissue surrounding the tumor that should be excised is a controversial topic. Although no specific distance/amount of tissue has been proven to be the ideal amount, conventional teaching has recommended that at least 3 cm of histologically uninvolved bone in the longitudinal direction and at least one named soft-tissue layer in the radial direction from the tumor-bearing bone should be incorporated into the margin. However, the amount of tissue required remains quite controversial, and in the case of sarcoma surgery no particular amount of normal tissue surrounding the tumor has been found to carry prognostic significance.[5] Wide excision of the tumor is the standard procedure for malignant primary bone tumors; however, if a vital neurovascular structure is at risk, because it is intimately associated with the tumor yet not within the tumor, sacrifice of the neurovascular bundle is not necessary. Arteriolysis and/or neurolysis can be

performed, freeing the structures and facilitating removal of the tumor. Although this is technically a marginal excision, passing through the edematous zone immediately adjacent to the tumor, this resection technique has not been associated with increase in recurrence when used in the setting of an effective adjuvant such as chemotherapy or radiotherapy.[6,7]

Once the involved bone has been removed, a preliminary evaluation of surgical margins is often performed. Typically a curettage specimen of the remaining transected bone is examined via frozen section. It is important to maintain meticulous control of the bone contents; for example, bone wax can be placed over the cut surface until the frozen section findings have been confirmed. If the frozen section does not identify tumor, the surgeon may proceed with the planned reconstruction. If the frozen section is positive for tumor cells, additional bone needs to be resected to achieve a negative margin. On occasion, soft-tissue margins may be sent depending on the surgeon's suspicion of a close or contaminated area.

The entire resection specimen is then sent for pathologic analysis to determine final margin status and percentage of tumor necrosis, and procure tissue for research purposes. Margins are assessed by inking the periphery of the specimen and microscopically examining selected inked sections. Tumor touching the ink is called a positive margin, whereas normal tissue touching ink is called a negative margin. For tumors treated with preoperative chemotherapy, the percentage of necrotic tumor is a surrogate for treatment efficacy and hence provides valuable information. The technique of computing percentage of necrosis varies among institutions. Typically specimens are mapped (**Figure 1**), the amount of viable tumor for each section is determined histologically, and the overall extent of necrosis is calculated. In addition to prognostic significance, tumor necrosis can direct additional local control measures for certain tumor types such as Ewing sarcoma.

The secondary goal of oncologic surgery is functional and durable reconstruction. Although postoperative function depends largely on the type of reconstruction, the planned reconstruction should never compromise the extent of the surgical margin. Thus, in practice, surgical management of malignant primary

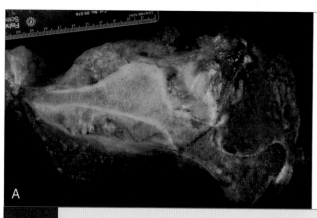
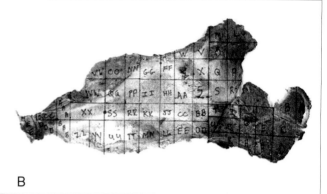

Figure 1 **A,** Gross resection specimen of a pelvic osteosarcoma. **B,** Map of tumor specimen for the purposes of assessing percent necrosis.

bone tumor is composed of two steps: wide excision followed by reconstruction.

Limb salvage surgery is indicated only when both the primary and secondary goals are achievable at a level comparable to or better than amputation. Advances in imaging, chemotherapy, reconstruction techniques, and patient expectations have made it possible to treat most patients with primary malignant bone tumor with limb salvage surgery. Amputation, while still a valuable option, is often relegated to those tumors that have either progressed with chemotherapy or in cases where amputation would yield a superior functional result compared to limb salvage. Examples of the latter scenario would include tumors that require neurovascular or extensive soft-tissue sacrifice resulting in a useless limb, and tumors in anatomic locations without good reconstructive options, such as the calcaneus. The principles of bone cancer management are presented in **Table 1**.

Reconstruction Considerations by Anatomic Site

Pelvis

Resections of the pelvis can be divided into limb-sparing resections (colloquially referred to as internal hemipelvectomy) and hindquarter amputations (also known as external hemipelvectomy). Whether a limb can be salvaged depends on the location of the tumor and its relationship to the structures within the pelvis. There are three essential components for a functional leg: the lumbosacral plexus, the femoral neurovascular bundle, and the hip joint. If the tumor encompasses any two of these three structures, resection of the tumor results in an insensate, useless limb and thus amputation is indicated.

Pelvic resections have been classified to facilitate consistent discussions about resection and reconstruction techniques. The Enneking and Dunham classification is as follows: type I involves resection of all or part of the ilium, sparing the acetabulum; type II involves resection of the periacetabular region; type III involves resection of ischiopubic region; and type IV involves resection of the pelvis and partial or complete sacral resection[8] (**Figure 2**). Once a pelvic resection is chosen/performed, careful thought should be given to whether reconstruction is necessary. Pelvic reconstruction following resection should be considered when one of two structural conditions exists: (1) there is loss of pelvic bony continuity between the acetabulum and the sacrum, or (2) the acetabulum is resected (ie, type II). Partial type I resections and type III resections typically do not require reconstruction. The decision regarding the type of reconstruction to perform should be made by both the physician and the patient and is a complex process that depends on several factors, including patient comorbidities, life expectancy, and patient demands and expectations.

Complete type I resections result in pelvic discontinuity and there are several reconstructive options including strut grafting, vascularized (double barrel versus single barrel) fibular bone grafting, and, if the distance between the remaining ilium and the sacrum is small, direct appositional iliosacral arthrodesis. Reconstruction offers the benefits of leveling and stabilizing the pelvis, thus alleviating the need for shoe lifts and preventing the development of postoperative scoliosis.[9]

However, in this type of resection, not reconstructing the defect is a viable and functional option.

Type II pelvic resections, because of the loss of the hip joint itself, present the greatest challenges to reconstruction. Many reconstructive techniques have been developed to restore the function of the hip joint, including biologic reconstruction with allograft or autograft bone, prosthetic reconstructions with pelvic or saddle prostheses, combinations of biologic and prosthetic reconstructions such as allograft-prosthetic composite (APC) options, or iliofemoral arthrodesis. These types of reconstructions are associated with significant risk of postoperative morbidity. There is a high complication rate with reconstruction of pelvic defects using allografts and endoprosthesis, especially in patients undergoing adjuvant therapy.[10-14]

Table 1

Principles of Bone Cancer Management

Biopsy

Biopsy diagnosis is necessary before any surgical procedure or fixation of primary site.

Biopsy is optimally performed at a center that will do definitive management.

Placement of biopsy is critical.

Biopsy should be core needle or surgical biopsy.

Technique: apply same principles for core needle or open biopsy. Needle biopsy is not recommended for skull base tumors.

Appropriate communication between the surgeon, musculoskeletal radiologist, and bone pathologist is critical.

Fresh tissue may be needed for molecular studies and tissue banking.

In general, failure to follow appropriate biopsy procedures can lead to adverse patient outcomes.

Final pathological evaluation should include assessment of surgical margins and size/dimensions of tumor.

Surgery

Wide excision should achieve histologically negative surgical margins.

Negative surgical margins optimize local tumor control.

Local tumor control can be achieved by either limb-sparing resection or limb amputation (individualized for a given patient).

Limb-sparing resection is preferred to optimize function if reasonable functional expectations can be achieved.

Laboratory Studies

Laboratory studies such as complete blood count, lactate dehydrogenase, and alkaline phosphatase may have relevance in the diagnosis, prognosis, and management of patients with bone sarcoma and should be performed before definitive treatment and periodically during treatment and surveillance.

Treatment

Fertility issues should be addressed with patients prior to commencing chemotherapy.

Care for bone cancer patients should be delivered directly by physicians on the multidisciplinary team (category 1).

Long-Term Follow-up and Surveillance/Survivorship

Patients should have a survivorship prescription to schedule follow-up with a multidisciplinary team.

Lifelong follow-up is recommended for surveillance and treatment of late effects of surgery, radiation, and chemotherapy in long-term survivors.

(Reproduced with permission from Biermann JS, Adkins DR, Agulnik M, et al: Bone Cancer. *J Natl Compr Canc Netw* 2013;11:688-723.)

The presence of numerous reconstructive options reflects a lack of a single superior treatment. In addition, each reconstruction option will eventually fail, and the patient will require revision and further surgeries. Interestingly, despite the loss of the hip joint, patients can do functionally well without reconstruction. When the pelvis is not reconstructed, the gap between the femur and the remaining pelvis is eventually bridged and fortified by scar tissue, and this allows stable weight bearing (**Figure 3**). Although a shoe lift is often required for ambulation, the complication rate is significantly decreased and the need for further surgery is obviated.

Femur

The femur is the most common site for primary malignancy of bone. The reconstruction options include modular and expandable endoprosthesis, APC, osteoarticular allograft, vascularized autograft, amputation, and rotationplasty. The development of modular prosthetic systems that can be easily assembled during a surgical procedure has expanded the utility of the pros-

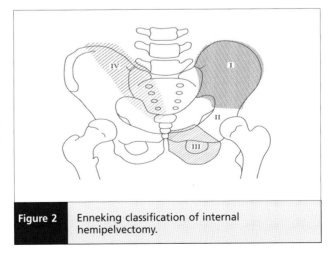

| Figure 2 | Enneking classification of internal hemipelvectomy. |

thetic reconstruction. The benefits of endoprosthetic reconstruction include immediate weight bearing and rapid rehabilitation. However, prosthetic longevity is limited. In recent studies with proximal femoral re-

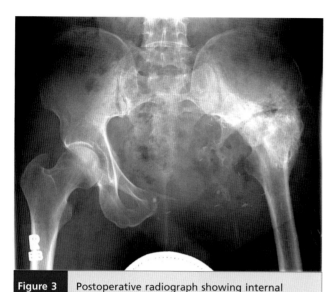

Figure 3 Postoperative radiograph showing internal hemipelvectomy without reconstruction.

placements for tumor reconstruction, 10- and 20-year implant survivorships were 78% to 84%, and 55% to 56%, respectively.[15,16] In the distal femoral reconstructions, 10- and 20-year implant survivorships were 67% to 77% and 42% to 58%, respectively.[17-19] The primary modes of failure are infection, aseptic loosening, and implant fracture.[20]

Although the entire femur is reconstructible with an endoprosthesis, limited options exist for functional muscle reconstruction. A femoral tumor that requires total quadriceps excision to achieve a wide margin represents a contraindication for limb salvage, not because of the difficulty of osseous reconstruction, but because of muscle reconstruction and soft-tissue coverage. Absence of the quadriceps muscles surrounding the endoprosthesis increases biomechanical stress at the host bone-endoprosthesis junction, which leads to eventual failure, increases the susceptibility to infection, and decreases the functionality of the limb.

The methods of reconstruction for proximal femoral bone tumors that are most commonly used include modular prosthetic replacement and allograft-prosthesis composite reconstruction. When the proximal femur is resected, the abductors are released from the femur. The most commonly used proximal femur endoprostheses are designed so that the abductors can be attached to the trochanter either through drill holes or with a device that allows direct fixation to the prosthesis (**Figure 4**). Although endoprosthetic reconstruction allows immediate weight bearing and leads to rapid rehabilitation, this kind of soft-tissue reconstruction might not restore the strength of the gluteal muscles, and can lead to joint instability and an antalgic gait.

APC reconstruction serves as an alternative to megaprosthetic reconstruction in the proximal femur. The advantage of APC over endoprosthetic reconstructions is the potential for reattaching abductors and recon-

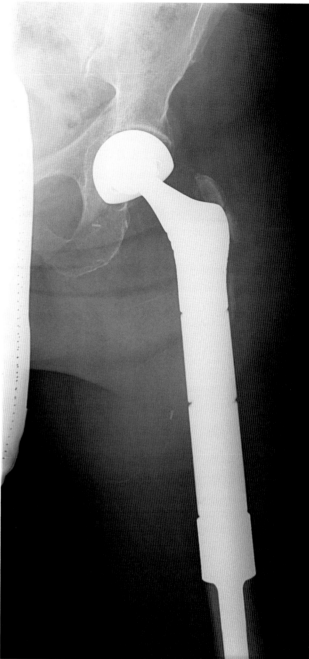

Figure 4 Radiograph showing endoprosthesis of the proximal femur.

structing the soft-tissue attachments about the hip. Attachment and healing of capsule and tendons of the hip adductors, abductors, and iliopsoas muscles to the allograft can prevent dislocation and facilitate function (**Figure 5**). Mechanical gait analysis has found that patients with APC reconstruction have a more efficient muscular recovery and thus more efficient gait. It has been suggested that the consistent restoration of abductor muscle strength, combined with low morbidity and high durability, support the use of APC reconstruction in patients with long life expectancy. The disadvantages

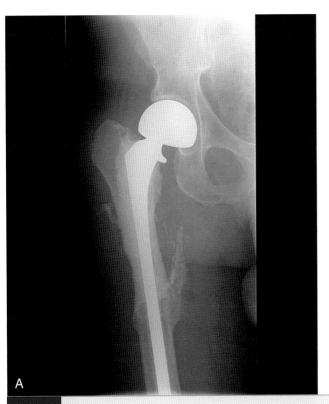 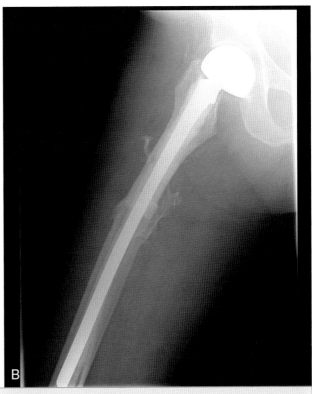

Figure 5 APC reconstruction of the proximal femur. **A,** AP radiographic view. **B,** Lateral radiographic view.

of APC reconstruction are prolonged postoperative non–weight bearing until the osteosynthesis site is healed, and nonunion of the osteosynthesis site. However, to decrease the incidence of nonunion, immediate vascularized fibula fixation and/or compression plating of the osteosynthesis site has been purported.[21]

In the femoral diaphysis, intercalary allografts offer a biologic reconstruction option.[22] However, the midportion of the graft does not become viable and does not offer the same mechanical strength, stability, or durability as normal bone. To augment this, some authors advocate filling the allograft with cement and then plating, fixing the allograft with intramedullary rod fixation, or augmenting the reconstruction with a vascularized fibula. The risks involved in intercalary allografts include late fracture, infection, and nonunion; these risks are more pronounced in those patients receiving chemotherapeutic agents. This was reiterated in a study that found that intercalary allografts had high rates of nonunion and the incidence of nonunion increased in the face of chemotherapy.[23]

The distal femur is the most common location of primary tumors of bone. Reconstruction options for the distal femur include megaprosthesis/endoprosthetic reconstruction and osteoarticular allograft reconstruction. The ease in assembly, insertion, and rehabilitation and excellent functional outcome has made endoprosthetic reconstruction the most popular reconstructive option in the distal femur. However, as in the proximal femur, prosthetic longevity is limited. In recent studies

with distal femoral reconstructions, 10- and 20-year implant survivorships were 67% to 77% and 42% to 58%, respectively[17-19] (**Figure 6**). Osteoarticular allografts in the distal femur are associated with a high complication rate; infection, fracture, and degeneration of the articular surface requiring revision, have made this reconstructive option less desirable.

In the skeletally immature patient, limb-salvage procedures that rely on endoprotheses or allograft present unique challenges that include the small size of the pediatric skeleton, the growth potential of the patient, the ensuing limb-length discrepancy, and the need for correction of the discrepancy. Expandable prostheses have been developed for skeletally immature patients to combat the ensuing limb-length discrepancy. The mechanism of expansion has shifted from modular systems that require open procedures to minimally invasive (telescoping using a gear device) and noninvasive (telescoping using electromagnetic induction) mechanisms. The Repiphysis (Wright Medical Technology) and the Juvenile Tumour System (JTS: Stanmore Implants Worldwide) are noninvasive expandable prostheses that were approved by the Food and Drug Administration in 2002 and 2011, respectively. Lengthening involves placing the limb inside a radiofrequency coil that unlocks the spring in the Repiphysis and spins the motor in the Juvenile Tumour System. Although expandable prostheses provide the skeletally immature patient with the option of equalizing their leg lengths, the complication rate remains high. The most common complica-

3: Malignant Primary Bone Tumors

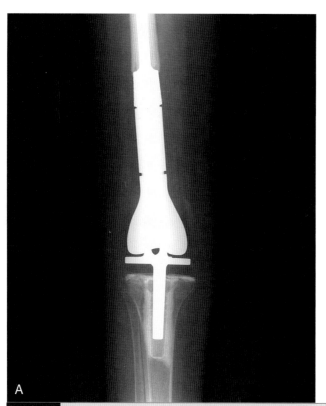
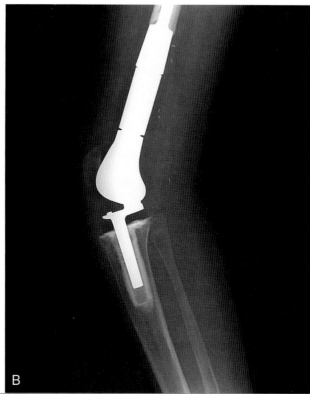

| **Figure 6** | Distal femur endoprosthesis. **A,** AP radiographic view. **B,** Lateral radiographic view. |

tions are related to a failure of the expansion mechanism, aseptic loosening, and infection. In addition, careful patient selection is important. An expandable prosthesis, no matter which component is used, is a large undertaking, not only for the surgeon but also for the patient and family. Diligent and close follow-up is necessary. Both the patient and her or his family have to be committed to the procedure and the long rehabilitation process. Failure to fully participate in rehabilitation can lead to fixed flexion contractures and poor functional results.[24-26]

Tibia

After the distal femur, the proximal tibia is the second most common site for primary tumors of bone. The reconstruction options include modular and expandable endoprosthesis, APC, osteoarticular graft, amputation, and rotationplasty. Soft-tissue considerations differ significantly between the proximal tibia and the distal femur. Wide excision of the proximal tibial tumors requires reconstruction of the extensor mechanism of the knee, as the insertion of the patella tendon on the tibial tubercle is usually resected with the tumor. In addition, the anterior-medial part of the tibia is subcutaneous, which can be problematic when the tibia is replaced with an endoprosthesis or an allograft. A gastrocnemius transposition flap can help obtain anterior-medial

soft tissue coverage and has been shown to decrease infection and wound complications.[27] Endoprosthetic reconstruction along with a muscle flap and reattachment of the patella tendon is an excellent reconstruction option after bone tumor resection at the proximal tibia. In the current literature, implant survivorships at 10 years and 20 years were 63% to 86% and 37% to 41%, respectively.[19]

APC reconstruction is also a viable option following resection of a tumor of the proximal tibia (**Figure 7**). It has the theoretical advantage of providing a biologic reattachment of the host's patella tendon to the allograft prosthetic composite, thus potentially improving the range of motion and decreasing the extensor lag. In addition, the allograft provides additional bone stock when the time comes for revision. A recent study reported good functional results with a low complication rate in 12 patients who had undergone resection of the proximal tibia and alloprosthetic reconstruction. However, APC reconstruction for the proximal tibia can be associated with fracture, nonunion, and infection as has been reported in earlier studies.[28]

The distal tibia is a rare site for malignant primary bone tumors. Despite current advances in biologic and prosthetic reconstructions, the distal tibia remains one of the few anatomic sites that have limited durable reconstruction options. Small case series have reported on allograft, autograft, and APC techniques.[29-31] Resection and allograft fusion offers a limb salvage option; however, it is fraught with the complications surround-

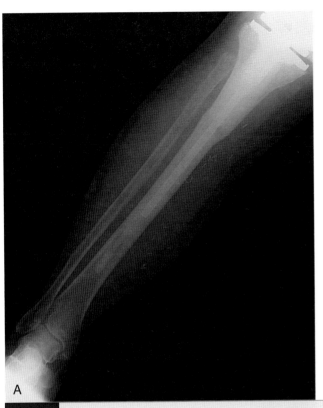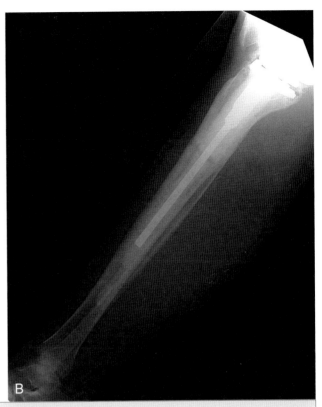

Figure 7   Tibia APC reconstruction. **A**, AP radiographic view. **B**, Lateral radiographic view.

ing the use of allograft: infection, fracture, delayed and nonhealing of the osteosynthesis site, and prolonged non–weight bearing. Range of motion is significantly reduced (fused), making high-impact activities quite difficult. Below-knee amputation is often the best oncologic and functional option for these patients, allowing the patient to return to high-impact activities.

Humerus

The proximal humerus is the third most common site for primary bone sarcomas. The limb salvage options include modular endoprosthesis, APC, osteoarticular graft, and fusion. As part of the wide excision of the proximal humerus, the rotator cuff is detached. Failure of functional reattachment of the cuff results in upward subluxation or dislocation of the endoprosthesis and severely limited shoulder function. Efforts have been made to develop new endoprosthesis or techniques to facilitate soft-tissue attachments. These include a constrained fixed-fulcrum endoprostheses and techniques using mesh that wraps around the endoprosthesis to provide mechanical constraint and anchor to the detached tendons.

APC reconstruction is a valuable reconstructive technique in the proximal humerus that provides the opportunity for soft-tissue reconstruction of the muscles of the shoulder girdle, which potentially improves stability

and function of the shoulder joint. Generally, a long-stemmed humeral component is cemented into the allograft and either press fit or cemented into the host bone. A compression plate can be added to the osteosynthesis site to provide further compression and rotational stability (**Figure 8**). Examples of APC reconstruction that have been reported include (1) anatomic (stemmed, nonreverse) hemiarthroplasty, (2) resurfacing hemiarthroplasty, and (3) reverse total shoulder arthroplasty. Anatomic hemiarthroplasty represents the standard APC reconstruction, in which a stemmed implant is inserted into the allograft-host bone component. Resurfacing hemiarthroplasty replaces only the surface of the allograft humeral head. Theoretical advantages of resurfacing hemiarthroplasty include preservation of bone stock, lower risk of periprosthetic fracture, and ease of conversion to a stemmed arthroplasty. Anatomic APC hemiarthroplasty and resurfacing APC hemiarthroplasty are indicated for reconstruction of intra-articular resection of the proximal humerus, where the detached host rotator cuff tendons are saved and can be repaired to the allograft tendons.[32,33] Reverse total shoulder arthroplasty are indicated for patients with severe cuff deficiency such as those undergoing extra-articular resection of the proximal humerus, because this procedure provides stability and active elevation without relying on the rotator cuff.[34]

Allograft and autograft arthrodesis is also a reconstructive option for tumors of the proximal humerus.

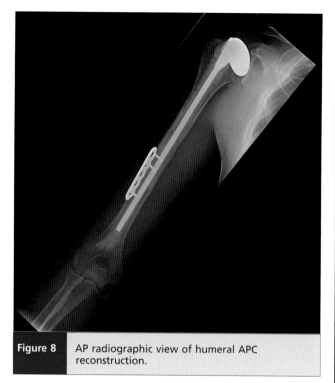

Figure 8 AP radiographic view of humeral APC reconstruction.

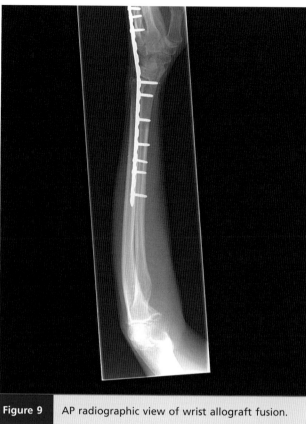

Figure 9 AP radiographic view of wrist allograft fusion.

This procedure offers a painless and stable shoulder girdle. However, shoulder arthrodesis is generally relegated to patients who have lost the function of both the deltoid muscle and the rotator cuff muscles, in addition to structure of the proximal humerus, or as a salvage of failed alloprosthesis or endoprosthesis reconstruction.

Intercalary spacer reconstruction is an option for lesions in the diaphysis of the humerus. Large segmental defects are amenable to resection and reconstruction with intercalary allografts, vascularized autografts, or intercalary metal spacers. As in the femur, intercalary bone grafts offer a biologic reconstruction option. Intercalary metal spacers offer a modular reconstruction option. This method of reconstruction has been shown to provide excellent and early return to function.[35,36]

Malignant tumors affecting the distal humerus or proximal ulna are rare. Large series of limb-salvage procedures in these areas are not available. Massive loss of bone and soft-tissue of the elbow following wide tumor excision of the distal humerus present a particular challenge in reconstructive surgery. As in other anatomic locations, reconstructive options include endoprosthesis, osteoarticular allograft, and APC. Recently, two studies with endoprosthetic reconstruction of the distal humerus (53 and 18 patients, respectively) reported a mean Musculoskeletal Tumor Society score of 76% and 78%, aseptic loosening rates of 8% and 17%, and infection in 15% and 11% of the patients, respectively. Total elbow reconstruction with an APC combined with musculocutaneous flap has also been shown to provide excellent functional and oncologic outcomes.[37,38]

Forearm

The forearm bones are rare sites for malignant primary bone tumors. Wide excision of the proximal radius or distal ulna can be performed without reconstruction or with the creation of a one-bone forearm. The main reconstruction options for the distal radius are allograft and autograft arthrodesis and osteoarticular allograft. Arthrodesis is recommended for patients who are manual laborers or who need a weight-bearing upper extremity. It provides a painless, stable, weight-bearing wrist (**Figure 9**). Osteoarticular allograft reconstruction is an option to restore the mobility of the wrist; however, it does not provide same stability and weight-bearing options as does wrist fusion. A recent study with 18 cases of osteoarticular allograft reconstruction of the distal radius following tumor excision demonstrated reconstruction of painless mobile wrist.[38]

Summary

The surgical management of malignant tumors of bone consists of two distinct objectives—adequate resection and functional, durable reconstruction. The goal of the surgery is to resect the entire tumor, with negative margins, and then reconstruct the limb in the best functional manner. Several reconstructive options for each surgical defect exist. However, the decision of which reconstructive option can be performed is multifactorial and should be based on the patient's comorbidities, prognosis and expectations, site of disease, size of the lesion, and resulting defect. Improvements in fixation techniques and prosthetic devices have allowed better and more durable fixation and hence improved patient outcomes. Amputation and rotationplasty remain good surgical options in selected patients.

Annotated References

1. Pisters PW, Leung DH, Woodruff J, Shi W, Brennan MF: Analysis of prognostic factors in 1,041 patients with localized soft tissue sarcomas of the extremities. *J Clin Oncol* 1996;14(5):1679-1689.

2. Simon MA, Springfield D, Conrad EU, et al: *Surgery for Bone and Soft-Tissue Tumors.* Philadelphia, PA, Lippincott-Raven, 1998.

3. Stojadinovic A, Leung DH, Hoos A, Jaques DP, Lewis JJ, Brennan MF: Analysis of the prognostic significance of microscopic margins in 2,084 localized primary adult soft tissue sarcomas. *Ann Surg* 2002; 235(3):424-434.

4. Enneking WF, Spanier SS, Goodman MA: A system for the surgical staging of musculoskeletal sarcoma: 1980. *Clin Orthop Relat Res* 2003;415:4-18.

5. King DM, Hackbarth DA, Kirkpatrick A: Extremity soft tissue sarcoma resections: How wide do you need to be? *Clin Orthop Relat Res* 2012;470(3):692-699.

   One hundred seventeen patients with soft-tissue sarcomas were resected with negative margins from 2001 to 2007. Gross specimens were inked and the closest macroscopic margins were sent for microscopic examination. Resection margins were categorized as smaller than 1 mm, 1 to 5 mm, or larger than 5 mm. The incidence of local recurrence was similar in patients with margins smaller than 1 mm and margins larger than 1 mm: 2 of 45 patients (4.4%) and 20 of 64 patients (3.1%), respectively. The power of the study was limited by the low number of local recurrences, but the authors concluded that relatively low local recurrence rates can be achieved even with close margins.

6. Avedian RS, Haydon RC, Peabody TD: Multiplanar osteotomy with limited wide margins: A tissue preserving surgical technique for high-grade bone sarcomas. *Clin Orthop Relat Res* 2010;468(10):2754-2764.

   In this retrospective review, six patients with sarcoma underwent resection and reconstruction with an intercalary allograft cut to fit the residual defect with multiplanar osteotomy. No patient experienced a local recurrence or metastasis, and all patients were alive and disease free at the most recent follow-up. All allografts healed during the study period. The authors concluded that with careful patient selection, the multiplanar osteotomy resection technique can be considered an option for treating patients with high-grade bone sarcomas, and can lead to improved healing and function of the involved extremity.

7. Li X, Moretti VM, Ashana AO, Lackman RD: Impact of close surgical margin on local recurrence and survival in osteosarcoma. *Int Orthop* 2012;36(1):131-137.

   In this retrospective review, 47 cases with conventional osteosarcoma underwent resection and reconstruction. Resection margins were classified. A close margin was defined as tumor present less than 5 mm from the closest resection margin. Positive margins had a greater risk of local recurrence (57.1%) than wide margins and close margins. There was no difference in local recurrence (8.3% versus 10.7%) between close margins and wide margins. Margin status was not correlated with osteosarcoma. In comparison with wide margins, close margins did not lead to increased local recurrence.

8. Enneking WF, Dunham WK: Resection and reconstruction for primary neoplasms involving the innominate bone. *J Bone Joint Surg Am* 1978;60(6):731-746.

9. Chang DW, Fortin AJ, Oates SD, Lewis VO: Reconstruction of the pelvic ring with vascularized double-strut fibular flap following internal hemipelvectomy. *Plast Reconstr Surg* 2008;121(6):1993-2000.

   In this retrospective review, six patients with sarcoma underwent internal hemipelvectomy and pelvic ring reconstruction with a vascularized double-strut fibular bone flap. The mean follow-up period was 18 months (range, 8 to 32 months). Radiographic evidence of bone bridging was seen at a mean of 2.5 months (range, 2 to 4 months). The mean time to ambulation without assistance was 8 months (range, 5 to 18 months). Five patients were ambulatory with a mild limp or no limp. Use of a vascularized double-strut fibular bone flap for pelvic ring reconstruction is effective in facilitating early ambulation and restoring normal to near-normal gait in patients undergoing internal hemipelvectomy.

10. Angelini A, Drago G, Trovarelli G, Calabrò T, Ruggieri P: Infection after surgical resection for pelvic bone tumors: An analysis of 270 patients from one institution. *Clin Orthop Relat Res* 2013. Epub ahead of print.

    Two hundred seventy patients with pelvic bone tumors were treated by surgical resection. The resection involved the periacetabular area in 166 patients. Reconstruction was performed in 137 patients. A deep infection developed in 20% of patients at a mean follow-up period of 8 months. Infection was more common in patients who underwent pelvic reconstruction after resection; no other risk factors were associated with an increased likelihood of infection. Despite surgical débridements and antibiotics, 46% underwent implant removal and 9% underwent external hemipelvectomy. The authors concluded that infection is a common complication of pelvic resection for bone tumors, and reconstruction after resection is associated with an increased risk of infection compared with resection alone. No significant difference between allograft and metallic prosthesis was noted.

11. Donati D, Di Bella C, Frisoni T, Cevolani L, DeGroot H: Alloprosthetic composite is a suitable reconstruc-

tion after periacetabular tumor resection. *Clin Orthop Relat Res* 2011;469(5):1450-1458.

Thirty-five patients underwent resection of the acetabulum and reconstruction with an allograft-prosthetic composite. Infection was a negative factor for allograft survival. More than 75% of the allografts were still in place at last follow-up, and the original prosthetic reconstruction was still in place in 56%. The average functional score was 72%. The authors concluded that allograft-prosthetic composite provides a valuable reconstructive option.

12. Ueda T, Kakunaga S, Takenaka S, Araki N, Yoshikawa H: Constrained total hip megaprosthesis for primary periacetabular tumors. *Clin Orthop Relat Res* 2013;471(3):741-749.

Twenty-five patients with primary periacetabular tumors treated using constrained total hip arthroplasty were retrospectively reviewed. The 10-year overall survival rate of all patients was 47%. Constrained total hip arthroplasty implants survived in 19 of 25 patients. Twenty-one patients acquired ambulatory activity, and there were seven local recurrences. Postoperative complications included deep infection in 8 of the 25 patients, dislocation in 4, and aseptic loosening in 2, necessitating 5 revision surgeries and 3 implant removals. The authors concluded that constrained total hip arthroplasty using an acetabular reconstruction cup is a useful reconstructive option after resection of periacetabular malignant tumors despite frequent postoperative complications.

13. Bell RS, Davis AM, Wunder JS, Buconjic T, McGoveran B, Gross AE: Allograft reconstruction of the acetabulum after resection of stage-IIB sarcoma: Intermediate-term results. *J Bone Joint Surg Am* 1997; 79(11):1663-1674.

14. Jansen JA, van de Sande MA, Dijkstra PD: Poor long-term clinical results of saddle prosthesis after resection of periacetabular tumors. *Clin Orthop Relat Res* 2013; 471(1):324-331.

Seventeen patients underwent periacetabular tumor resection and reconstruction with a saddle prosthesis in a retrospective review. Local complications were seen in 14 of the 17 patients. Thirteen of 17 patients used walking assistance for mobilization and the other 3 patients were not able to mobilize independently. The mean Musculoskeletal Tumor Society score at long-term follow-up was 47% (range, 20% to 77%), the mean Toronto Extremity Salvage Score was 53% (range, 41% to 67%), and the mean composite Short Form-36 physical and mental component summaries were 43.9 and 50.6, respectively. Reconstruction with saddle prostheses after periacetabular tumor surgery has a high risk of complications with poor long-term function.

15. Bernthal NM, Schwartz AJ, Oakes DA, Kabo JM, Eckardt JJ: How long do endoprosthetic reconstructions for proximal femoral tumors last? *Clin Orthop Relat Res* 2010;468(11):2867-2874.

Eighty-six proximal femoral replacements used for tumor reconstruction were retrospectively reviewed.

Five-, 10-, and 20-year implant survivorships were 93%, 84%, and 56%, respectively. Cemented bipolar proximal femoral replacement after tumor resection was a durable reconstruction technique. The implants outlived patients with metastatic disease and high-grade localized disease, but patients with low-grade disease outlived their implants.

16. Jeys LM, Kulkarni A, Grimer RJ, Carter SR, Tillman RM, Abudu A: Endoprosthetic reconstruction for the treatment of musculoskeletal tumors of the appendicular skeleton and pelvis. *J Bone Joint Surg Am* 2008; 90(6):1265-1271.

A consecutive series of 661 patients who had undergone endoprosthetic reconstruction following resection of a bone tumor with a minimum follow-up of 10 years was reviewed. Two hundred twenty-seven patients (34%) had revision surgery because of mechanical failure (116 patients), infection (75 patients), and locally recurrent disease (36 patients). Implant survival at 10 years was 75%.

17. Bergin PF, Noveau JB, Jelinek JS, Henshaw RM: Aseptic loosening rates in distal femoral endoprostheses: Does stem size matter? *Clin Orthop Relat Res* 2012; 470(3):743-750.

Ninety-three patients who underwent distal femoral replacements were retrospectively reviewed. Overall implant survival for 104 stems in 93 patients was 73.3% at 10 years, 62.8% at 15 years, and 46.1% at 20 years. Survival from aseptic loosening was 94.6% at 10 and 15 years and 86.5% at 20 years. Only the bone:stem ratio independently predicted aseptic failure. Patients with stable implants had larger stem sizes and lower bone stem ratios than those with loose implants, suggesting that durability is related to the size of stems that fill the canal.

18. Myers GJ, Abudu AT, Carter SR, Tillman RM, Grimer RJ: Endoprosthetic replacement of the distal femur for bone tumours: Long-term results. *J Bone Joint Surg Br* 2007;89(4):521-526.

Three hundred thirty-five patients with distal femoral replacement (162 with a fixed-hinge design and 173 with a rotating hinge) were retrospectively reviewed. The risk of revision for any reason was 17% at 5 years, 33% at 10 years, and 58% at 20 years. Aseptic loosening was the main reason for revision of the fixed-hinge knees, whereas infection and fracture of the stem were the most common for the rotating-hinge implant. The overall risk of revision for any reason decreased by 52% when the rotating-hinge implant was used. The rotating-hinge prosthesis with a hydroxyapatite collar offers the best chance for long-term survival of the prosthesis. Improvements in the design of distal femoral endoprostheses have substantially decreased the need for revision operations, but infection remains a serious problem.

19. Schwartz AJ, Kabo JM, Eilber FC, Eilber FR, Eckardt JJ: Cemented endoprosthetic reconstruction of the proximal tibia: How long do they last? *Clin Orthop Relat Res* 2010;468(11):2875-2884.

The authors retrospectively reviewed 52 patients with

proximal tibial endoprosthetic reconstructions for a tumor-related diagnosis. Overall prosthesis survival at 5, 10, 15, and 20 years was 94%, 86%, 66%, and 37%, respectively. The mean postoperative Musculoskeletal Tumor Society score at most recent follow-up was 82% of normal function (mean raw score, 24.6; range, 4–29).

20. Henderson ER, Groundland JS, Pala E, et al: Failure mode classification for tumor endoprostheses: Retrospective review of five institutions and a literature review. *J Bone Joint Surg Am* 2011;93(5):418-429.

    A multicenter review of the use of segmental endoprostheses is presented. A total of 2,174 skeletally mature patients were identified; among this group of patients, 534 failures were identified. Five modes of failure were identified and classified: soft-tissue failures (type 1), aseptic loosening (type 2), structural failures (type 3), infection (type 4), and tumor progression (type 5). The most common mode of failure in this series was infection. Modes of endoprosthetic failure and their incidences were significantly different and dependent on anatomic location. Mode of failure and time to failure also showed a significant dependence. Cumulative reporting of segmental failures should be avoided because anatomy-specific trends will be missed.

21. Farid Y, Lin PP, Lewis VO, Yasko AW: Endoprosthetic and allograft-prosthetic composite reconstruction of the proximal femur for bone neoplasms. *Clin Orthop Relat Res* 2006;442(442):223-229.

22. Aponte-Tinao L, Farfalli GL, Ritacco LE, Ayerza MA, Muscolo DL: Intercalary femur allografts are an acceptable alternative after tumor resection. *Clin Orthop Relat Res* 2012;470(3):728-734.

    Eighty-three patients who underwent reconstruction with femur segmental allograft after tumor resection were retrospectively reviewed. Survivorship was 85% (95% confidence interval: 93% to 77%) at 5 years and 76% (95% confidence interval: 89% to 63%) at 10 years. Nonunion rate was 19% for diaphyseal junctions and 3% for metaphyseal junctions. An increase in the diaphysis nonunion rate in patients who underwent nail fixations (28%) compared with those who underwent plate fixation (15%) was noted. The fracture rate was 17% and occurred in areas of the allograft not adequately protected with internal fixation. The authors concluded that the internal fixation should span the entire allograft to avoid the risk of fracture.

23. Raskin KA, Hornicek F: Allograft reconstruction in malignant bone tumors: Indications and limits. *Recent Results Cancer Res* 2009;179:51-58.

    The authors discussed the limitations, complications, survival rates, and indications for using bone allografts for reconstruction of skeletal defects after tumor resection.

24. Picardo NE, Blunn GW, Shekkeris AS, et al: The medium-term results of the Stanmore non-invasive extendible endoprosthesis in the treatment of paediatric

bone tumours. *J Bone Joint Surg Br* 2012;94(3):425-430.

    Forty-four patients with a mean age of 11.4 years who had undergone reconstruction with the Stanmore noninvasive extendible endoprosthesis were reviewed. The mean length gained per patient was 38.6 mm. Complications developed in 16 patients and 10 underwent revision.

25. Ruggieri P, Mavrogenis AF, Pala E, Romantini M, Manfrini M, Mercuri M: Outcome of expandable prostheses in children. *J Pediatr Orthop* 2013;33(3): 244-253.

    Thirty-two children with bone sarcomas of the femur who underwent reconstruction using expandable prostheses were evaluated in a retrospective review. The authors concluded that the growing prosthesis, although requiring an open lengthening procedure, was associated with a higher rate of survival when compared with the noninvasive prosthesis, which had low total lengthening and high complication rates.

26. Beebe K, Benevenia J, Kaushal N, Uglialoro A, Patel N, Patterson F: Evaluation of a noninvasive expandable prosthesis in musculoskeletal oncology patients for the upper and lower limb. *Orthopedics* 2010; 33(6):396.

    Twelve skeletally immature patients who underwent reconstruction with a noninvasive expandable prosthesis for the lower extremity and the upper extremity were retrospectively reviewed. The authors found that the noninvasive expandable prosthesis provided acceptable functional outcomes and had a potential advantage over conventional expandable prostheses, which required open procedures that potentially increase the risk of infection from repeated hardware exposure.

27. Grimer RJ, Carter SR, Tillman RM, et al: Endoprosthetic replacement of the proximal tibia. *J Bone Joint Surg Br* 1999;81(3):488-494.

28. Gilbert NF, Yasko AW, Oates SD, Lewis VO, Cannon CP, Lin PP: Allograft-prosthetic composite reconstruction of the proximal part of the tibia: An analysis of the early results. *J Bone Joint Surg Am* 2009;91(7): 1646-1656.

    Twelve patients who underwent allograft-prosthetic composite reconstruction of the proximal part of the tibia after tumor resection were evaluated. Nine patients had no extensor lag. Complete bone union occurred in nine patients, and partial union occurred in three patients. Technical aspects of the procedure that may favorably affect outcome include soft-tissue coverage with muscle flaps and rigid fixation with a long-stemmed implant.

29. Mavrogenis AF, Abati CN, Romagnoli C, Ruggieri P: Similar survival but better function for patients after limb salvage versus amputation for distal tibia osteosarcoma. *Clin Orthop Relat Res* 2012;470(6):1735-1748.

    The authors retrospectively evaluated 42 patients with

distal tibia osteosarcoma, 19 of whom had amputations and 23 who underwent limb salvage and allograft reconstructions. The minimum follow-up period was 8 months (median, 60 months; range, 8 to 288 months). The survival of patients who underwent limb salvage was similar to that of patients who underwent amputation, and the incidence of local recurrence and complications was similar. Better function is achievable for patients treated with limb salvage versus amputation.

30. Jamshidi K, Mazhar FN, Masdari Z: Reconstruction of distal fibula with osteoarticular allograft after tumor resection. *Foot Ankle Surg* 2013;19(1):31-35.

Four patients who underwent reconstruction of the distal fibula with an osteoarticular fibular allograft, after wide resection of a tumor, were retrospectively reviewed. The mean follow-up period was 3.2 years. There was no infection or wound healing problems, and union was achieved in all patients.

31. Shekkeris AS, Hanna SA, Sewell MD, et al: Endoprosthetic reconstruction of the distal tibia and ankle joint after resection of primary bone tumours. *J Bone Joint Surg Br* 2009;91(10):1378-1382.

The outcomes of six patients treated with endoprosthetic replacement of the distal tibia and ankle joint were reported. Two patients underwent a below-knee amputation for persistent infection after a mean 16 months (range: 1 to 31 months). Four patients retained their endoprosthesis and had a mean Musculoskeletal Tumor Society score of 70% and a mean Toronto Extremity Salvage score of 71%. Despite the risk of infection in these patients, the authors concluded that a custom-made endoprosthetic replacement of the distal tibia and ankle joint is a viable treatment option for carefully selected patients with a primary bone tumor.

32. Abdeen A, Hoang BH, Athanasian EA, Morris CD, Boland PJ, Healey JH: Allograft-prosthesis composite reconstruction of the proximal part of the humerus: Functional outcome and survivorship. *J Bone Joint Surg Am* 2009;91(10):2406-2415.

An allograft-prosthesis composite was used to reconstruct a proximal humeral defect following tumor resection in 36 consecutive patients. The overall estimated rate of survival of the construct was 88% at 10 years. There were three failures due to progressive prosthetic loosening. Four patients required an additional bone-grafting procedure to treat a delayed union.

33. Cannon CP, Paraliticci GU, Lin PP, Lewis VO, Yasko AW: Functional outcome following endoprosthetic reconstruction of the proximal humerus. *J Shoulder Elbow Surg* 2009;18(5):705-710.

The authors retrospectively reviewed 83 proximal humeral endoprosthetic reconstructions following an intra-articular, deltoid muscle, and axillary nerve-sparing resection. Mean active abduction was 41 degrees and mean active forward flexion was 42 degrees. The mean Musculoskeletal Tumor Society score was 63%. Implant-related complications included deep infections (2%) and proximal migration of the prosthesis (26%). Overall proximal humeral endoprosthesis provides a durable reconstruction with a relatively low complication rate and a stable platform for elbow and hand function, but limited shoulder function.

34. De Wilde L, Boileau P, Van der Bracht H: Does reverse shoulder arthroplasty for tumors of the proximal humerus reduce impairment? *Clin Orthop Relat Res* 2011;469(9):2489-2495.

The authors retrospectively reviewed 14 patients who had undergone reverse total shoulder arthroplasty for tumors of the proximal humerus. Four patients died, leaving nine patients for review. At last follow-up, mean active abduction was 157°. One patient had a deep infection and another developed a loose prosthesis. Radiographic graft resorption was seen in all except one patient.

35. Damron TA, Sim FH, Shives TC, An KN, Rock MG, Pritchard DJ: Intercalary spacers in the treatment of segmentally destructive diaphyseal humeral lesions in disseminated malignancies. *Clin Orthop Relat Res* 1996;324:233-243.

36. Damron TA, Leerapun T, Hugate RR, Shives TC, Sim FH: Does the second-generation intercalary humeral spacer improve on the first? *Clin Orthop Relat Res* 2008;466(6):1309-1317.

Thirty-two consecutive patients who underwent intercalary resection and reconstruction with an intercalary humeral spacer were retrospectively reviewed. The male-female taper implants were compared with the lap joint configuration. A lower complication rate was noted in the lap joint group, but aseptic loosening occurred more frequently in the lap joint group.

37. Funovics PT, Schuh R, Adams SB Jr, Sabeti-Aschraf M, Dominkus M, Kotz RI: Modular prosthetic reconstruction of major bone defects of the distal end of the humerus. *J Bone Joint Surg Am* 2011;93(11):1064-1074.

Fifty-three elbows in 52 patients underwent reconstruction with a modular prosthesis. The mean Musculoskeletal Tumor Society score was 78%. Eight patients had a deep periprosthetic infection. Four patients underwent implant revision for aseptic loosening.

38. Hanna SA, David LA, Aston WJ, et al: Endoprosthetic replacement of the distal humerus following resection of bone tumours. *J Bone Joint Surg Br* 2007;89(11):1498-1503.

Patients who underwent resection of the distal humerus with endoprosthetic reconstruction were evaluated. Complications occurred in nine patients and included aseptic loosening, local recurrence, infection, neurapraxia of the radial nerve, and a periprosthetic fracture. The mean Musculoskeletal Tumor Society score was 76% and mean Toronto Extremity Salvage score was 73%. Seventeen of 18 patients had substantial improvement in the degree of pain following surgery. The authors concluded that custom-made endoprosthetic reconstruction of the elbow for bone tumors is a viable treatment in carefully selected patients.

Section 4

Soft-Tissue Tumors

Section Editor:

Patrick P. Lin, MD

Chapter 21

The Evaluation and Diagnosis of Soft-Tissue Masses

Joel L. Mayerson, MD

4: Soft Tissue Tumors

Introduction

The true prevalence of soft-tissue masses is unknown. Many people have a mass that never causes pain and is clinically stable. Such a mass does not receive medical attention unless it changes significantly. By that point in the disease course, the mass may be large and, if malignant, the risk of metastatic disease may have increased.[1]

Benign soft-tissue masses appear to be common, although the exact prevalence is unknown, and are believed to occur at least 100 times more often than malignant soft-tissue lesions. Approximately 9,000 soft-tissue sarcomas are diagnosed in the United States each year. These malignant tumors can be extremely aggressive, and inappropriate evaluation, diagnosis, and management can lead to an adverse outcome.[2] It is important to properly evaluate and diagnose every soft-tissue mass.

Clinical Evaluation

History

Every clinician who treats musculoskeletal diseases must understand whether a patient's soft-tissue mass should be observed or requires further evaluation. A complete patient history and physical examination are the most important first steps. The clinician must have the answers to a number of questions: How long has the soft-tissue mass been present? Is the mass growing or has it been stable? Over what period has the mass been growing or stable? How large is the mass? Is the mass just under the skin, or is it deep in the muscle? Is there a history of trauma to the area? Has the patient had a recent infection elsewhere in the body? Does the patient have a personal history of malignancy? Is the

mass soft or firm? Is the mass painful? Are there any systemic symptoms such as fever, chills, or night sweats? Does the mass increase and decrease in size? Is the patient from an area of the world in which certain types of infection, such as tuberculosis, are prevalent? Is the patient taking a blood-thinning agent, or has the patient taken such an agent in the past? The answers to these questions allow the clinician to refine the list of possible diagnoses and follow an algorithm for treatment (**Figure 1**).

A soft-tissue mass that has been present for years and is stable in size, small, superficial, and soft is relatively unlikely to be malignant. A mass that is rapidly growing after a recent onset and is large, deep, and firm is more likely to be malignant. A history of trauma should lead the surgeon to consider etiologies such as hematoma and myositis ossificans. Current or past use of anticoagulants is a risk factor for hematoma. Systemic symptoms such as fever and chills suggest an infection. A mass that increases and decreases in size is almost never malignant and may be a cyst or a hemangioma–arteriovenous malformation.

Physical Examination

A complete, directed physical examination must always be performed. The area of the soft-tissue mass is inspected for any skin changes. The mass must be palpated, and its size, firmness, and depth must be determined. The mass also must be palpated for tenderness, increased warmth, erythema, purulent drainage, and fluctuance. A detailed motor and sensory examination determines whether the mass could be compressing a major nerve. A positive Tinel sign (paresthesias along a nerve dermatome with palpation) may be present over the mass. A regional lymph node evaluation must be performed. Gait should be analyzed for limping, pain, or any other type of weakness associated with ambulation.

Following the examination, a differential diagnosis is made. If a low level of concern exists for malignancy, the mass is followed clinically. Otherwise, imaging studies are used for further evaluation. In general, a small, soft, superficial mass that is stable in size can be observed. However, it should be recognized that a soft-

Dr. Mayerson or an immediate family member has received research or institutional support from Millennium Pharmaceuticals, and serves as a board member, owner, officer, or committee member of the American Academy of Orthopaedic Surgeons, the National Comprehensive Cancer Network, the Musculoskeletal Tumor Society, and the Ohio Orthopaedic Society.

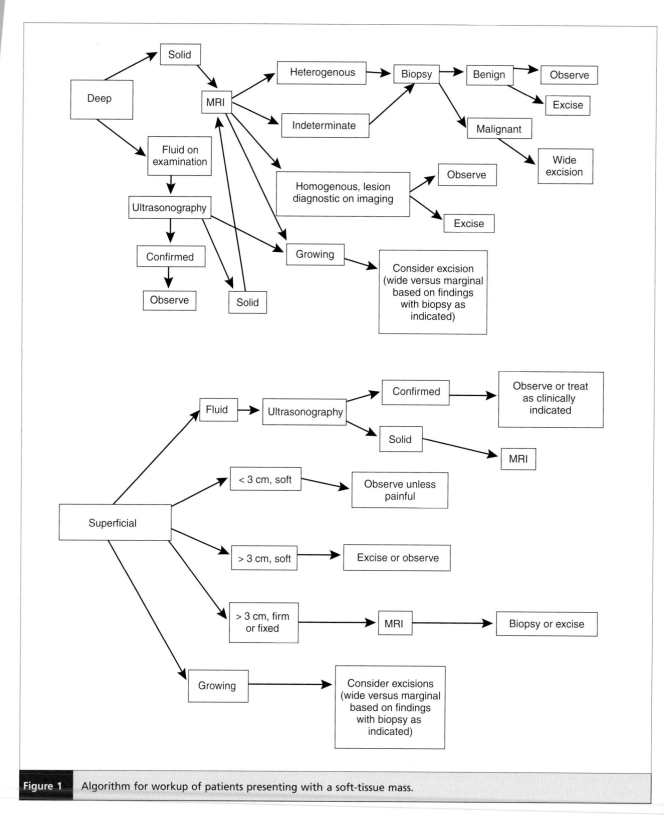

Figure 1 Algorithm for workup of patients presenting with a soft-tissue mass.

tissue sarcoma can appear as a small, superficial lesion. Early recognition of such a tumor is important because a small tumor has a relatively favorable prognosis. If any doubt exists regarding the diagnosis, it is always a good idea to schedule a follow-up examination. The patient must be informed of signs and symptoms that would necessitate further evaluation, such as pain or an increase in size. A soft-tissue mass that is larger than 3 cm, firm, deep to fascia, and/or painful typically is evaluated further using radiographic studies.

Imaging

Plain radiography is the first modality used to evaluate a soft-tissue mass in the pelvis or an extremity. An abnormal tissue plane or mineralization within the soft-tissue mass can be detected radiographically. Certain patterns of mineralization are useful in the differential diagnosis. It must first be determined whether ossification or calcification is present. Bone has a regular, ordered pattern of trabeculae, and calcification has a more random pattern. If bone is present centrally within the lesion, the possibility of maligancy such as soft-tissue osteosarcoma is cause for concern. When bone is present more peripherally, especially in the setting of trauma, myositis ossificans is a more likely diagnosis. Most calcifications are dystrophic and can occur around a venous valve such as a phlebolith or centrally within a lipoma. When calcifications occur with more aggressive-appearing soft-tissue masses, synovial sarcoma should be considered and biopsy performed for correct diagnosis of the lesion.

Ultrasonography frequently is used as an inexpensive screening tool for evaluating a soft-tissue mass.[3] Ultrasonography can reveal blood flow within the lesion and whether the lesion is cystic or solid (**Figure 2**). A fluid-filled cystic lesion with no blood flow most often is benign; a solid lesion or a lesion with significant blood flow often requires further evaluation with CT or MRI. CT is useful if a patient cannot undergo MRI because of the presence of a metallic implant, such as a cardiac stent or pacemaker. CT identifies the anatomic location of the mass as well as MRI but otherwise provides a lower level of information. MRI is the gold standard for evaluating almost every soft-tissue mass

that requires further investigation after completion of the history and physical examination.[4] MRI defines the lesion's size, depth, fluid content, signal intensity, and relation to other anatomic structures (**Figure 3**). The information is synthesized to determine whether additional investigation is warranted. Some entities, such as a lipoma or hemangioma, can be definitively diagnosed on MRI and do not require biopsy or further workup.[5] A mass with suspicious features must be biopsied by a specifically trained physician.

Positron emission tomography fused with CT (PET-CT) uses fluorodeoxyglucose, with the radioactive iso-

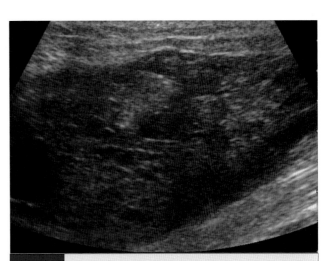

| **Figure 2** | Ultrasound of a large soft-tissue mass in the right buttock, showing areas of fluid and solid tissue that could represent a soft-tissue sarcoma. |

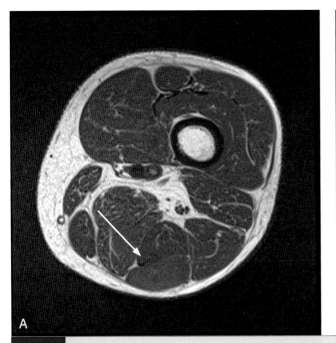

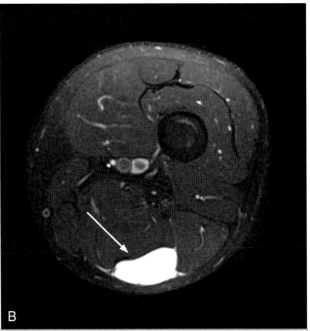

| **Figure 3** | MRI showing high fluid content in a soft-tissue sarcoma. The tumor (arrows) is isointense with muscle on a T1-weighted study (**A**) and bright on a T2-weighted study (**B**). |

4: Soft Tissue Tumors

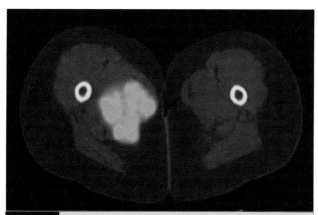

Figure 4 F18 fluorodeoxyglucose PET-CT showing a large soft-tissue mass in the medial thigh. The high standardized uptake value of 11.3 is consistent with a high-grade sarcoma.

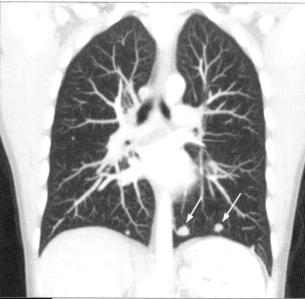

Figure 5 Chest CT showing multiple pulmonary nodules (arrows) that on biopsy proved to be metastatic sarcoma. A high-resolution coronal CT reconstruction is shown, rather than the traditional axial image.

tope fluorine-18 to determine the metabolic activity of a soft-tissue mass. The standardized uptake value, which is obtained from a nomogram for the individual machine, helps determine the probability that the lesion is malignant (**Figure 4**). A maximum standardized uptake value greater than 3 often suggests malignancy. PET-CT is also useful in staging malignant disease. For a high-grade soft-tissue sarcoma, PET-CT can be repeated after induction chemotherapy to help determine the response to treatment. Follow-up PET-CT generally is not warranted for a low-grade malignant lesion that does not require systemic therapy because the information obtained does not improve patient management.

Angiography can be performed if an exact roadmap of blood flow is vitally important to biopsy placement or surgical treatment. The test can be performed with fluoroscopic or CT guidance or in combination with MRI.

Because the lung is the most common organ site of metastasis in soft-tissue sarcomas, chest radiography and CT of the chest should be performed for any soft-tissue mass that is likely to be or is known to be a soft-tissue sarcoma. Plain chest radiographs are used as a screening tool and a baseline for comparison with future staging evaluations. Chest CT can evaluate for small (2 to 3 mm) lung nodules that may be metastatic disease (**Figure 5**).

Laboratory Studies

No specific blood tests exist for identifying a soft-tissue tumor. Basic laboratory studies, such as a complete blood count with differential, erythrocyte sedimentation rate, and C-reactive protein level, are important to assess for systemic issues such as bleeding or infection. Coagulation studies are useful before performing a biopsy or if hematoma is part of the differential diagnosis. Other studies may be appropriate.

Biopsy

Based on the history, physical examination, imaging studies, and laboratory tests, an improved differential diagnosis can be generated and a decision can be made as to whether a biopsy is necessary. The ideal biopsy minimizes the risk to the patient and expeditiously leads to an accurate diagnosis. A patient with a soft-tissue mass that may be malignant should be referred to a tertiary center specializing in musculoskeletal soft-tissue tumors. Expert biopsy planning can greatly affect the ability to provide proper care for a patient with a soft-tissue mass in an extremity or the pelvis. Patient outcomes improve as a result of subspecialty care.

Biopsy complications can be caused by inappropriate needle placement or failure to obtain hemostasis. Loss of function can result because a contaminated biopsy requires a larger resection field. Amputation occasionally is necessary as a result of a complication such as extensive postbiopsy bleeding.

Fine-Needle Aspiration

Fine-needle aspiration is less expensive than other biopsy methods and can be performed as an in-office procedure without the use of lidocaine. The results can be obtained quickly during the office visit. A palpable lesion can be biopsied without image guidance, but a biopsy of a nonpalpable lesion is best performed with image guidance, using ultrasonography, CT, or MRI. One study found sensitivity of 89.2% and specificity of 89.8% with fine-needle aspiration,[6] but another study found only 79.2% sensitivity and 72.7% specificity.[7]

These differences highlight the importance of the expertise of the cytopathologist in obtaining an accurate fine-needle aspiration. In the absence of a well-trained cytopathologist, fine-needle aspiration is not a good diagnostic option for a musculoskeletal tumor.

Core Needle Biopsy

Core needle biopsy is slightly more invasive than fine-needle aspiration but allows better analysis of the architecture, cell type, and histologic grade of the tumor. Core needle biopsy may require image guidance, typically with CT or ultrasonography, to ensure that the most representative portion of the mass is sampled. Lidocaine must be administered, and a small risk for complications exists from the use of this agent. Core needle biopsy is slightly more expensive than fine-needle aspiration because additional tissue handling is necessary. Core needle biopsy can be performed as an in-office procedure; according to one study, the sensitivity and specificity of this procedure are 79% and 82%, respectively.[7] This method requires a trained musculoskeletal pathologist, but because the evaluation is histologic rather than cytologic, more pathologists have the expertise required for this procedure than for fine-needle aspiration.

Open Surgical Biopsy

An open technique is the gold standard for biopsy. An open biopsy provides more tissue than fine-needle aspiration or core needle biopsy and therefore generally has greater sensitivity and specificity. However, an open biopsy carries a greater risk of infection or bleeding, which can contaminate normal tissue with malignant cells. The procedure must be performed in an operating room using strict aseptic technique; therefore, it is more expensive than needle biopsy.

The two types of open biopsy are excisional and incisional. The excisional type should be performed only if advanced imaging studies have definitively established the lesion as benign, as with a lipoma. A superficial lesion also is suitable for excisional biopsy if it is smaller than 3 cm and the surgeon can avoid violating the underlying deep fascia or compromising the principles of limb salvage surgery. It is important to keep in mind that a subsequent wide reexcision of the tumor bed will be necessary if a pathologic diagnosis of soft-tissue sarcoma is made.

The incisional type of open biopsy should be used to determine the diagnosis in most other instances. It is extremely important that the incision be performed in a longitudinal fashion to prevent contamination of other compartments. A frozen section should be obtained during every open biopsy to ensure that diagnostic tissue has been included. Tissue must be sent for culture if infection, rather than neoplasm, is a possibility. If a definitive diagnosis cannot be made with a frozen section, the procedure should be halted and the wound closed. Doing so ensures that the surgeon does not act on incomplete data. Modern pathology incorporates many immunostains and studies such as fluorescence in situ hybridization, and resection can be planned for a later date, when all results are available. Meticulous hemostasis always should be obtained before closure to prevent bleeding, which can cause widespread contamination of the surrounding soft tissues. Contamination leads to the need for a wider resection field and may result in an otherwise unnecessary amputation.

Summary

A proper algorithm must be followed for a patient with a soft-tissue mass. In addition, referral to a physician trained in the management of musculoskeletal tumors may be necessary for an optimal outcome. Benign lesions are far more common than malignant tumors, but it is vitally important to recognize signs of possible malignancy and not to assume that every soft-tissue mass is innocuous. Biopsy procedures must be performed with great care to avoid compromising any future limb salvage surgery.

Annotated References

1. Johnson GD, Smith G, Dramis A, Grimer RJ: Delays in referral of soft tissue sarcomas. *Sarcoma* 2008; 2008:378-574.

   The median times to disease appearance, evaluation by a medical professional, and referral to a tertiary center were studied for soft-tissue sarcomas. The greatest source of delay was in medical provider referral to a specialist. Published guidelines can be used to decrease this delay.

2. Qureshi YA, Huddy JR, Miller JD, Strauss DC, Thomas JM, Hayes AJ: Unplanned excision of soft tissue sarcoma results in increased rates of local recurrence despite full further oncological treatment. *Ann Surg Oncol* 2012;19(3):871-877.

   A study of 134 patients with an unplanned excision of soft-tissue sarcoma and 209 stage-matched control subjects found increased local recurrence in patients who underwent unplanned excision, especially in those with a stage III tumor. Metastasis-free and sarcoma-specific survival rates also were decreased after unplanned excision.

3. Newman B: Ultrasound body applications in children. *Pediatr Radiol* 2011;41(Suppl 2):555-561.

   The parameters for ultrasonography were defined in the initial evaluation of a clinically inconclusive mass in children. Ultrasonography was used to determine the anatomic origin of the mass and to distinguish between a cystic and a solid mass.

4. Chung WJ, Chung HW, Shin MJ, et al: MRI to differentiate benign from malignant soft-tissue tumours of the extremities: A simplified systematic imaging approach using depth, size and heterogeneity of signal in-

tensity. *Br J Radiol* 2012;85(1018):e831-e836.

The systematic combination of signal intensity, size, and depth was used to differentiate benign from malignant soft-tissue masses for nonexperts.

5. van Vliet M, Kliffen M, Krestin GP, van Dijke CF: Soft tissue sarcomas at a glance: Clinical, histological, and MR imaging features of malignant extremity soft tissue tumors. *Eur Radiol* 2009;19(6):1499-1511.

    The clinical, histologic, and MRI characteristics of soft-tissue sarcomas were classified by the World Health Organization. This overview is useful in creating a differential diagnosis for a soft-tissue mass.

6. Ng VY, Thomas K, Crist M, Wakely PE Jr, Mayerson J: Fine needle aspiration for clinical triage of extremity soft tissue masses. *Clin Orthop Relat Res* 2010;468(4):1120-1128.

    The institutional experience of fine-needle aspiration was described, as performed and analyzed in an office setting by an expert cytopathologist. With close clinical collaboration among the surgeon, pathologist, and radiologist, sensitivity and specificity of 89.2% and 89.8%, respectively, were found in 432 patients.

7. Kasraeian S, Allison DC, Ahlmann ER, Fedenko AN, Menendez LR: A comparison of fine-needle aspiration, core biopsy, and surgical biopsy in the diagnosis of extremity soft tissue masses. *Clin Orthop Relat Res* 2010;468(11):2992-3002.

    In 57 patients, open biopsy was found to be more accurate than core needle biopsy, which in turn was more accurate than fine needle aspiration in determining the presence of malignancy, reaching an accurate diagnosis, and guiding treatment of palpable musculoskeletal neoplasms.

Chapter 22

Benign Vascular Soft-Tissue Tumors

Yee-Cheen Doung, MD

Introduction

Vascular anomalies fall into two categories: vascular tumors, which are produced by neoplastic cell proliferation, and vascular malformations, which are characterized by abnormal vascular channels arising from aberrant development (**Table 1**). Historically, both tumors and malformations have been called hemangiomas, but some physicians think this usage is ambiguous and prefer to reserve the term hemangioma for certain true benign neoplasms of blood vessels.[1]

Vascular Malformations (Venous Malformations, Intramuscular Hemangiomas, and Arteriovenous Malformations)

Vascular malformations are grouped into low-flow lesions (venous, lymphatic, and capillary malformations) and high-flow lesions (arteriovenous malformations). They occur in approximately 0.3% to 0.5% of the population. Several notable syndromes are associated with vascular malformations (**Table 2**). The most common are Klippel-Trénaunay syndrome, Kasabach-Merritt syndrome, Parkes Weber syndrome, and Maffucci syndrome.

The most common vascular anomaly is the venous malformation.[1] When intramuscular, it is often referred to as an intramuscular hemangioma. Venous malformations occur more commonly in females than in males, in a 2:1 ratio. They are present at birth, but are often discovered during adolescence. The most common location is in the head and neck. In the limbs, the intramuscular venous malformation is more commonly seen in the lower extremity than in the upper extremity. They can also appear intra-articularly and can lead to hemarthrosis.

Etiology

Venous malformations are suspected to be formed by ectatic vessels morphologically similar to veins. They are hormonally modulated with estrogen receptors on endothelial cells. Symptoms are exacerbated during pregnancy or times of hormonal changes.[1]

Diagnosis

The patient often reports a history of painful symptoms. These symptoms vary from intermittent pain as-

Table 1

International Society for the Study of Vascular Anomalies: 1996 Adapted Classification of Vascular Anomalies

Category	Conditions
Vascular tumors Hemangiomas	Superficial hemangioma Deep hemangioma Combined hemangioma
Other tumors	Kaposiform hemangioendothelioma Spindle-cell hemangioendothelioma Tufted angioma Glomangioma Pyogenic granuloma Hemangiopericytoma Kaposi sarcoma Angiosarcoma
Vascular malformations Single	Capillary (port-wine stain or nevus flammeus) Venous Lymphatic Arterial
Combined	Arteriovenous fistula Arteriovenous malformation Capillary-lymphatic venous malformation Capillary venous malformation Lymphatic venous malformation Capillary arteriovenous malformation Capillary-lymphatic arteriovenous malformation

Table 2

Common Syndromes Associated With Vascular Malformations

Syndrome	Characteristics
Klippel-Trénaunay syndrome	Cutaneous nevus flammeus Varicose veins Venous and lymphatic malformation Skeletal hypertrophy
Kasabach-Merritt syndrome	Angiomatous lesions Bleeding diathesis resulting in thrombocytopenia and purpura
Parkes Weber syndrome	Cutaneous nevus flammeus Arteriovenous fistulae
Maffucci syndrome	Multiple cutaneous vascular malformations Multiple enchondromas Possible sarcomatous transformation

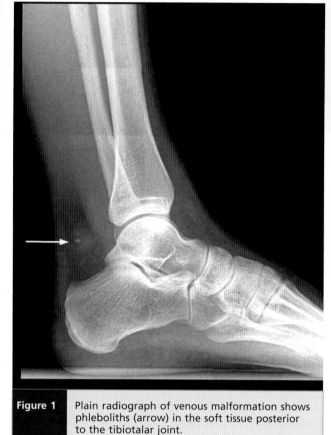

Figure 1 Plain radiograph of venous malformation shows phleboliths (arrow) in the soft tissue posterior to the tibiotalar joint.

sociated with swelling to mild persistent pain that worsens with activity. Placement of the extremity with the lesion in a dependent position usually leads to increasing size of the mass. The lesion can be cutaneous, subcutaneous, or intramuscular. Cutaneous lesions have skin changes and bluish discoloration and sometimes the presence of varicose veins. Subcutaneous and intramuscular lesions often do not have skin changes, but they feel boggy and have poorly defined borders. Often, the lesion is softer than the surrounding musculature. Arteriovenous malformations can sometimes be pulsatile. If the lesion is intra-articular, it can cause synovial irritation, and, if it bleeds, can cause hemarthrosis. The pain of hemangiomas is occasionally due to acute thrombophlebitis, which causes the lesions to be firm and exquisitely tender on palpation.

Imaging of the lesion on plain radiographs may sometimes show phleboliths (**Figure 1**), which probably represent calcified chronic thrombi within the vascular channels. MRI often shows a speckled, infiltrative pattern with multiple small focal areas that have high intensity on proton density, short tau inversion recovery, and T2-weighted images and are isointense to muscle on T1-weighted images (**Figure 2, A and B**). Small amounts of fat surrounding the vessels can cause scant areas surrounding the vessels to have bright signal on T1-weighted images. There is often some contrast enhancement around the vessel walls of the lesion (**Figure 2, C**). The pattern on these images can be described as serpiginous or as resembling grape clusters or a bag of worms. MRI can often distinguish venous malformation from arteriovenous malformation with a characteristic serpiginous flow void (**Figure 3, A through B**). Angiography can also be used to characterize arteriovenous malformation (**Figure 3, D**). Although ultrasonography is not often used for diagnosis, it is helpful in distinguishing between high-flow and low-flow malformations.

Histopathology of the lesion shows the characteristic abundance of vascular channels (**Figure 4, A**). Some hemorrhage is often visible within the channels. The endothelial cells do not show atypia or mitotic figures.

Treatment

Many vascular malformations can be treated with observation. Symptomatic lesions can be treated with compressive garments and aspirin. Because of hormonal modulation, cessation of oral contraceptive pills may also ease symptoms.[2]

Sclerotherapy may be effective for symptomatic lesions with well-defined vascular channels. Smaller lesions are often more successfully treated than larger ones. Sclerotherapy is often a series of treatments, separated by 2 to 3 months. The most common form of sclerotherapy is based on ethanol. It is often palliative but is not considered curative. Relative contraindications include lesions with multiple intralesional thrombosis, and preexisting neurologic impairment. A 2001 study with 30 patients showed complete or partial relief in 27 of 28 patients.[3] In 2004, a study with 21 patients showed complete or partial pain relief in 17 patients and no relief in 4 patients.[4]

Surgical excision can also be used either alone or in conjunction with sclerotherapy. Surgical excision can cause morbidity due to resection of surrounding tissue, especially for lesions that are intramuscular. Excision of

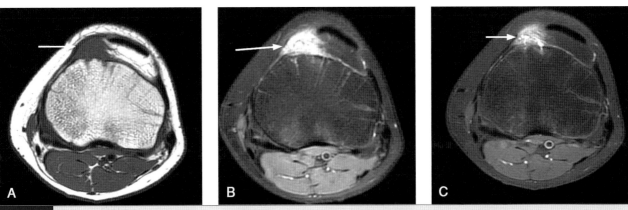

Figure 2 An intra-articular knee venous malformation is shown. **A,** T1-weighted MRI shows the lesion (arrow) as isointense with skeletal muscle adjacent to patellar tendon. **B,** Proton density-weighted MRI shows the lesion (arrow) as hyperintense within the joint. A vessel is present within the substance of the lesion. **C,** T1 and contrast-enhanced MRI shows contrast enhancement within the vessel in the substance of the lesion (arrow).

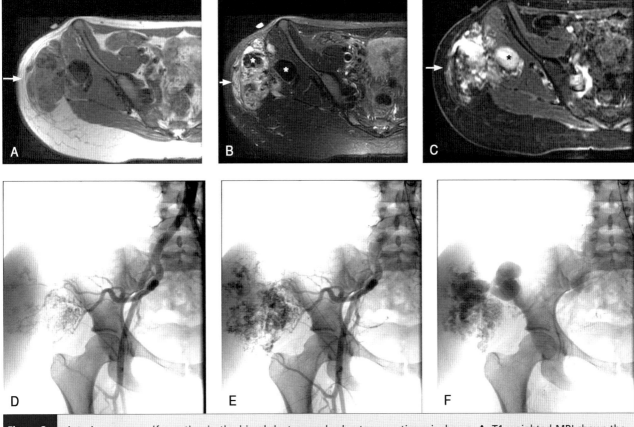

Figure 3 Arteriovenous malformation in the hip abductors and subcutaneous tissue is shown. **A,** T1-weighted MRI shows the lesion (arrow) as isointense both superficial to the fascia and deep within the gluteus medius. **B,** T2-weighted MRI shows the lesion (arrow) as hyperintense, again both superficial to fascia and deep within the gluteus medius. Note the presence of hypointense flow voids (starred). **C,** T1 and contrast–enhanced MRI shows the lesion (arrow) with serpiginous contrast enhancement. Flow voids on T2 are contrast enhancing in this lesion (starred). **D** through **F,** A rapid sequence of angiograms shows the multitude of vessels that comprise the lesion.

such lesions necessarily sacrifices muscle tissue because the vessels are intimately involved with the muscle fibers. A combination of embolization and surgical excision is often used for arteriovenous malformations. Embolization alone often fails as a result of neovascularization of the lesion. In a 2002 study of 89 patients, 74 patients (83%) showed excellent functional results at an average follow-up of 5 years.[5] There was an over-

4: Soft Tissue Tumors

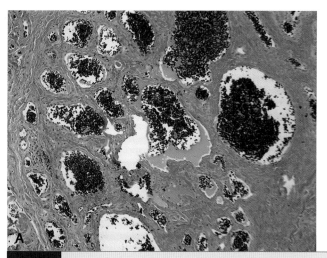
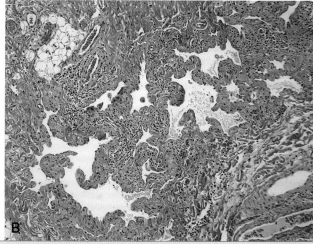

Figure 4 The histology of vascular malformations is shown. Large vascular spaces (filled with red blood cells) or lymphatic lumens (containing acellular proteinaceous material) are the most striking morphologic feature. **A,** Venous malformation is shown (hematoxylin and eosin stain, low power field). **B,** Lymphatic malformation is shown (hematoxylin and eosin stain, low power field).

all recurrence rate of 19%, with 13% of patients undergoing additional procedures. A 2012 study, which included patients with head and neck lesions, examined 48 patients who underwent excision. Thirty-six patients showed improvement, and 11 showed no improvement. There was a 10% recurrence rate at 4-year follow-up.[6] Another study, in 2002, discussed treatment of 176 patients, including patients with lesions in the head and neck. Forty-two patients (24%) were treated with observation, aspirin, and compressive garments. Fifty-four patients (31%) were treated with sclerotherapy, 35 patients (20%) were treated with surgical excision, and 48 patients (27%) were treated with both sclerotherapy and surgical excision. Full or partial relief of symptoms was reported by 39 of 54 patients treated with sclerotherapy, 23 of 35 patients treated with surgical excision, and 44 of 48 patients treated with combined therapy.[7]

Lymphatic Malformation/Lymphangioma

Lymphatic malformations are most often seen at birth, and 90% are detected by 2 years of age. They are thought to be developmental defects. During intrauterine fetal development, primordial lymphatic cell buds fail to reestablish a connection with the remaining venous system.[1]

Lymphangioma has three clinical forms: cystic hygroma, which most often occurs in the neck, axilla, and retroperitoneum; cavernous lymphangioma, which occurs in the subcutaneous tissue, salivary gland, tongue, and lips; and capillary lymphangioma, which is uncommon and can be seen as a wart or a cluster of small vesicles. Seventy-five percent of lymphangiomas occur in the head and neck.

The lesion is often associated with pain, warmth, swelling, and occasionally fever. Skeletal hypertrophy is often related to lymphangioma. The appearance of these lesions depends on size, depth, and location. Often, they appear vesicular and have normal surrounding skin. Deeper lesions feel softer than the surrounding musculature and have poorly defined borders.

On MRI scans, the lesions appear isointense to muscle on T1-weighted images and hyperintense on T2-weighted images. Gadolinium contrast enhancement can be seen along vessel walls. Fluid-fluid levels can be present in cavernous vessels. Histologically, the lesion has lymph channels with interstitial lymphoid tissue (**Figure 4, B**).

The lesion is treated with sclerotherapy, surgery, or a combination of the two. Bleomycin and OK-432 are the sclerosing agents of choice. A study in 2011 showed intralesional bleomycin to have partial or complete resolution in 19 of 24 patients.[8] There were 2 recurrences. In a 2006 study, surgical excision was performed in 23 of 27 patients with cystic hygroma; 6 of the surgical patients developed recurrences. Head and neck lesions have a high complication rate, with five deaths reported in one series.[9]

Vascular Tumors

Hemangioma

The true cutaneous hemangioma is characterized by cellular proliferation with expression of glucose transporter protein (GLUT1). This protein is not expressed in vascular malformations. These lesions are found in the head and neck in about 40% of patients, and they are usually seen in infancy. Hemangiomas have a pro-

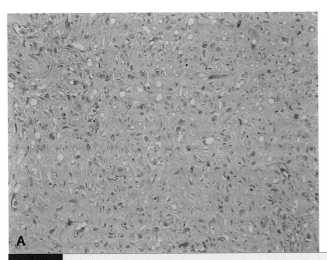
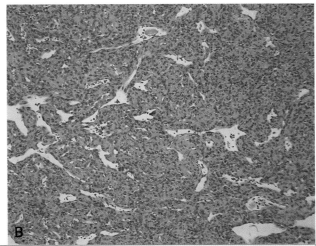

Figure 5	The histology of vascular tumors is shown. In contrast to vascular malformations, the lesions are much more cellular. **A,** Epithelioid hemangioendothelioma is shown. Note the sheets of cells with nonspindle, epithelioid appearance and minute vascular spaces (hematoxylin and eosin stain, high-power field). **B,** Hemangiopericytoma is shown. Prominent vascular channels resembling branching "antlers" are visible (hematoxylin and eosin stain, low-power field).

liferating phase and an involuting phase: a biphasic process not seen in vascular malformations. During the proliferating phase, the lesion increases cell proliferation, vessel diameter, and lumen formation. During the involuting phase, these vessels mature and organize into lobules and slowly recede. Remaining tissue may result in telangiectasia.[10]

Because hemangiomas spontaneously involute, they may be observed. However, between 20% and 40% of involutions either take more than 6 years or produce aesthetically unacceptable results, especially on the face. Other treatments include laser therapy, systemic steroids, propranolol, and sometimes systemic interferon. Surgery is rarely performed. It is reserved for lesions that cause functional deficits, and should be done during the involuting stage.[10]

Hemangioendothelioma

Hemangioendothelioma comes in four forms, of which epithelioid hemangioendothelioma is the most common. It occurs as excessive endothelial proliferation within lumens of medium-sized vessels. It is thought to arise from unusual thrombus organization and may be stimulated by an autocrine loop involving endothelial growth factor. Endothelial growth factor secretion that is triggered by macrophages may also play a role in the pathogenesis.

Hemangioendothelioma occurs slightly more often in females than in males. The average lesion is smaller than 2 cm and often occurs in the head and neck, fingers, or trunk. It is often solitary and cutaneous. It can appear reddish in nature and well circumscribed. Microscopically, endothelial cell hyperplasia is visible in the intravascular spaces without atypia (**Figure 5, A**). However, hemangioendothelioma can be confused with angiosarcoma at times, and roughly 15% to 25% of

hemangioendotheliomas exhibit malignant or aggressive behavior. As a result, treatment is usually with wide resection. Radiation therapy can be considered for positive margins. Chemotherapy is reserved for patients with metastatic disease.[11]

Hemangiopericytoma and Solitary Fibrous Tumor

Historically, hemangiopericytoma and solitary fibrous tumor were considered two different entities, with many similar histologic features. Solitary fibrous tumor represents a spectrum of mesenchymal tumors. Hemangiopericytoma is now considered a cellular variant of solitary fibrous tumor.

Solitary fibrous tumor is a soft-tissue tumor with variable malignant potential. This tumor is composed of variably pleomorphic spindle cells arranged haphazardly or in short fascicles. It is CD34 reactive and has a staghorn-like vascular network. The chief characteristic of hemangiopericytoma, or the cellular variant of solitary fibrous tumor, is the presence of mesenchymal cells that have pericytic differentiation. It occurs in both infantile and adult forms. Infantile hemangiopericytoma is congenital and occurs mostly in the head and neck. It responds well to chemotherapy, and cases of spontaneous regression have been observed. Prognosis is usually favorable.

Adult solitary fibrous tumor often occurs in the sixth and seventh decades of life but can occur as early as the third decade of life. It can form in an intramuscular compartment of the lower extremities, pelvis, head, or neck. The mass is typically painless but can cause discomfort from distension of the muscles. It is also commonly seen in the abdomen and the pleura. Imaging shows a soft-tissue mass that can be either hyperintense or heterogeneous on T2-weighted MRI, isointense on

T1-weighted MRI, and bright with contrast enhancement. Histologically, there is a perivascular pattern of cell proliferation with multiple prominent vascular channels (**Figure 5, B**). Because 15% to 20% of solitary fibrous tumors exhibit malignant behavior, there is controversy regarding whether solitary fibrous tumor should be classified as a benign or malignant tumor. A study in 2012 showed that the 5-year metastasis-free rate was 73% and disease-specific survival was 89%.[12] Risk factors included patient age, tumor size, and mitotic index. The mainstay of treatment of solitary fibrous tumor is wide resection. Because of its ability to metastasize, it is often treated as a malignancy. Like other soft-tissue sarcomas, it can be treated with adjuvant radiation therapy for better local control of disease. Chemotherapy can also be considered for patients with metastatic and overtly malignant disease, but the response to traditional cytotoxic chemotherapy has been disappointing. Because of the vascularity of the tumor, newer treatment strategies with antiangiogenic agents may offer hope for these patients, but results are still preliminary.[13]

Summary

Vascular malformations are common and present often during adolescence. They can be treated with observation, sclerotherapy, or surgical excision. Vascular tumors include hemangioma, hemangioendothelioma, and solitary fibrous tumor. Hemangiomas are benign and most will involute. Hemangioendothelioma and solitary fibrous tumor exhibit a wide spectrum of disease, from benign to malignant. Because of their potential for malignancy, they are treated with wide excision.

Annotated References

1. Redondo P, Aguado L, Martínez-Cuesta A: Diagnosis and management of extensive vascular malformations of the lower limb: Part I. Clinical diagnosis. *J Am Acad Dermatol* 2011;65(5):893-906, quiz 907-908.

   This article is the first part of a review of the definition, etiology, description, and diagnosis of vascular malformations and associated syndromes.

2. Redondo P, Aguado L, Martínez-Cuesta A: Diagnosis and management of extensive vascular malformations of the lower limb: Part II. Systemic repercussions [corrected], diagnosis, and treatment. *J Am Acad Dermatol* 2011;65(5):909-923, quiz 924.

   This article is the second part of a review of vascular malformations and focuses on diagnosis, natural history, and treatment.

3. Lee BB, Kim DI, Huh S, et al: New experiences with absolute ethanol sclerotherapy in the management of a complex form of congenital venous malformation. *J Vasc Surg* 2001;33(4):764-772.

4. Rimon U, Garniek A, Galili Y, Golan G, Bensaid P, Morag B: Ethanol sclerotherapy of peripheral venous malformations. *Eur J Radiol* 2004;52(3):283-287.

5. Tang P, Hornicek FJ, Gebhardt MC, Cates J, Mankin HJ: Surgical treatment of hemangiomas of soft tissue. *Clin Orthop Relat Res* 2002;399:205-210.

6. Roh YN, Do YS, Park KB, et al: The results of surgical treatment for patients with venous malformations. *Ann Vasc Surg* 2012;26(5):665-673.

   This study reviewed 48 patients who underwent surgical excision of venous malformations with minimum 1 year follow-up. The lesions were in the head and neck in 17 patients (35%), in the upper extremities in 12 patients (25%), in the lower extremities in 15 patients (31%), in the abdomen and pelvis in 1 patient (2%), and in the perineum and genitalia in 3 patients (6%). Twenty-five patients (52%) had remission, 11 (23%) had improvement, and 12 (25%) had no change. Recurrence after wide excision occurred in 3 patients of 31 (10%), and size increase after debulking occurred in 4 patients of 17 (25%). Complications including arteriovenous fistula with bleeding, peripheral nerve palsy, skin necrosis, and wound dehiscence occurred in four patients (8%). Level of evidence: IV.

7. Hein KD, Mulliken JB, Kozakewich HP, Upton J, Burrows PE: Venous malformations of skeletal muscle. *Plast Reconstr Surg* 2002;110(7):1625-1635.

8. Rozman Z, Thambidorai RR, Zaleha AM, Zakaria Z, Zulfiqar MA: Lymphangioma: Is intralesional bleomycin sclerotherapy effective? *Biomed Imaging Interv J* 2011;7(3):e18.

   This study reviewed the effectiveness of intralesional bleomycin in 24 patients. Fifteen patients (63%) had complete response, 5 patients (21%) had good response, and 4 patients (16%) had poor response. Two patients had tumor recurrence. Two patients had a complication consisting of abscess formation at the site of injection. Level of evidence: IV.

9. Uba AF, Chirdan LB: Management of cystic lymphangioma in children: Experience in Jos, Nigeria. *Pediatr Surg Int* 2006;22(4):353-356.

10. Hochman M, Adams DM, Reeves TD: Current knowledge and management of vascular anomalies: I. Hemangiomas. *Arch Facial Plast Surg* 2011;13(3):145-151.

    This study is a review of the diagnosis, pathogenesis, history, and treatment of cutaneous hemangiomas.

11. Deyrup AT, Tighiouart M, Montag AG, Weiss SW: Epithelioid hemangioendothelioma of soft tissue: A proposal for risk stratification based on 49 cases. *Am J Surg Pathol* 2008;32(6):924-927.

    This study reviewed the pathology and natural history of epithelioid hemangioendothelioma and a risk stratification was proposed. Among the 49 patients reviewed, 32 tumors were in the extremities. The 5-year disease-specific survival was 81%. Eleven patients

(22%) had metastatic disease: 6 metastases were to the lungs, 4 were to the lymph nodes, and 2 were to the liver. Mitotic activity and size were associated with greater mortality. High-risk tumors demonstrated 59% disease-specific survival at 5 years, compared to 100% in low-risk tumors. Level of evidence: IV.

12. Demicco EG, Park MS, Araujo DM, et al: Solitary fibrous tumor: A clinicopathological study of 110 cases and proposed risk assessment model. *Mod Pathol* 2012;25(9):1298-1306.

   This study reviews 103 cases of solitary fibrous tumor. Hemangiopericytoma is a part of the spectrum of solitary fibrous tumor, a cellular variant. These tumors were most commonly found in the abdomen and pleura. Five-year and 10-year metastasis-free rate was

74% and 55%, respectively. Five-year and 10-year disease-specific survival was 89% and 73%, respectively. Patient age, tumor size, and mitotic index predicted time to metastasis as well as disease-specific survival. Poor outcomes were seen in patients ≥ 55 years with tumors ≥ 15 cm and mitotic rates ≥ 4/10 per high-power field. Level of evidence: IV.

13. Park MS, Araujo DM: New insights into the hemangiopericytoma/solitary fibrous tumor spectrum of tumors. *Curr Opin Oncol* 2009;21(4):327-331.

   This article is a review of the etiology, pathology, and current treatment of hemangiopericytoma and solitary fibrous tumor.

Chapter 23

Benign Cystic Soft-Tissue Lesions

Jeffrey E. Krygier, MD

Introduction

Benign cystic soft-tissue tumors are a heterogeneous group including all soft-tissue lesions with a true cyst or pseudocyst lining and fluid or proteinaceous content. Hamartomatous, reactive, degenerative, and neoplastic processes all are capable of producing cystic masses.

Synovial Cysts

A synovial epithelial lining distinguishes true synovial cysts from other periarticular cystic structures. Despite the synovial lining, not all synovial cysts have identifiable contiguity with their presumed joint of origin. All synovial cysts have a layer of synovial epithelium as well as fluid content of variable viscosity. Varying quantities of inflammatory tissue may be present secondary to attempted aspiration or trauma.

Popliteal Cysts

Popliteal (Baker) cysts represent a distension of the gastrocnemius-semimembranosus bursa. The cyst contents likely originate from within the knee joint and traverse a relatively weak portion of the posteromedial knee capsule.[1] Most extend superficially, intermuscularly, and inferiorly, but variants may progress laterally (toward or into the popliteal fossa), proximally, or intramuscularly. Affected patients have a wide age range, but the incidence rises significantly in individuals older than 50 years.

As with most other synovial cysts, varying theories exist as to the origin of popliteal cysts. Synovial outpouching through a capsular defect, fluid extension through a valvular conduit into the gastrocnemius-semimembranosus bursa, and encapsulation of extravasated synovial fluid are often-described mechanisms. Most popliteal cysts in adults are secondary to an underlying intra-articular joint condition, frequently a degenerative condition. The high incidence of popliteal cysts in patients with an injury of the posterior horn of the medial meniscus suggests that the tear further weakens the posterior capsule and decreases resistance to fluid egress.[2]

The patient may have a variety of symptoms. Usually, all symptoms are consistent with the underlying knee pathology, but the patient may attribute the symptoms to the visible, palpable mass. A patient with a true symptomatic or isolated popliteal cyst describes pain, swelling, or loss of flexion. The symptoms may mimic those of a deep vein thrombosis.

The most common neurovascular insults secondary to a popliteal cyst are entrapment neuropathy, vascular compression, pseudothrombophlebitis, and compartment syndrome, but few patients experience such sequelae.[3] Patients with a ruptured cyst have distant swelling, bruising, ecchymosis, and sometimes severe pain simulating acute venous thrombophlebitis. Patients often can recall the cyst before it ruptured. Compartment syndrome has been described after cyst rupture. Because symptoms of a popliteal cyst can mimic those of deep vein thrombosis, many such lesions are identified through an ultrasound meant to evaluate for a clot. Ultrasound has diagnostic accuracy comparable to that of MRI.

On MRI the cyst origin often can be seen between the semimembranosus and the medial head of gastrocnemius tendons. Low signal T1-weighted, high signal T2-weighted, and short tau inversion recovery studies characterize synovial cysts (**Figure 1**). Areas of increased T1 signal may represent intracystic hemorrhage or protein-rich synovial fluid. The cyst wall and internal septae can be enhanced with contrast administration. Simple, loculated, and septated variants have been reported. Loculated variants may represent the two distinct components of the gastrocnemius-semimembranosus bursa.[4] Loose bodies and calcifications can be seen within the cyst (**Figure 2**). Ruptured cysts show significant edema and fluid tracking along the posterior calf.

The presence of an arthritic knee may incorrectly lead the provider to conclude that a soft-tissue mass behind the knee is a benign cyst. Patients in the age group in which a popliteal cyst is most likely to develop also are in an age group in which soft-tissue sarcoma most often occurs. The presence of a deep, firm, and proximal soft-tissue mass must raise suspicion that the mass is not a cyst, but a lesion requiring further evaluation (**Figure 3**).

Neither Dr. Krygier nor any immediate family member has received anything of value from or has stock or stock options held in a commercial company or institution related directly or indirectly to the subject of this chapter.

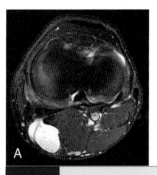
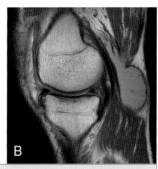

Figure 1 Proton density MRIs of a popliteal cyst in a 55-year-old man. **A,** Fat-saturated axial study showing the stalk traversing the interval between the semimembranosus tendon and medial head of the gastrocnemius. The bilobar appearance may represent the engorged bursa of the respective tendons. **B,** Sagittal study showing the superficial location of the cyst.

Treatment of the cyst itself often is not warranted. Instead, the treatment focuses on the underlying pathology. Intra-articular injection of corticosteroid can result in diminution of cyst volume. Reassurance and patient education are integral to the management of a popliteal cyst. In the rare instances in which the cyst is responsible for neurovascular compromise, excision with dissection of the compromised structure is indicated. Compartment syndrome secondary to a cyst or a cyst rupture is treated immediately to diminish the associated morbidity. The likelihood of recurrence is high unless the primary knee pathology is treated. Arthroscopic techniques can be used if the cyst itself remains symptomatic, with posterior knee pain and flexion difficulty. Reported recurrence rates are low if arthroscopy is combined with treatment of the underlying pathology. An intracystic dye injection can be useful for visualizing the stalk arthroscopically.[5]

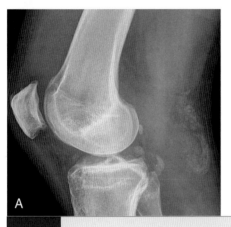
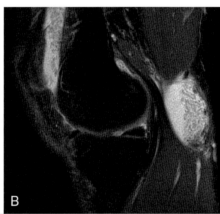
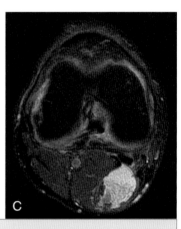

Figure 2 **A,** Lateral radiograph of the knee of a 50-year-old man showing calcification within the popliteal space. Proton density fat-saturated MRI (**B,** sagittal; **C,** axial) showing heterogeneous signal of the popliteal cyst originating between the medial head of the gastrocnemius and semimembranosus, consistent with the calcification in **A.** Similar debris can be seen intra-articularly.

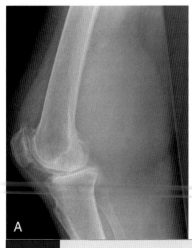
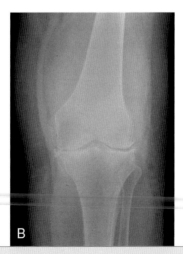
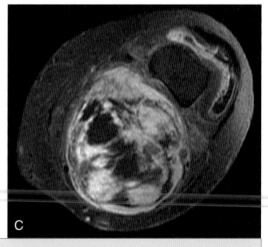

Figure 3 Lateral (**A**) and AP (**B**) radiographs of the knee of an 80-year-old woman with advanced osteoarthrosis. A posterior thigh mass can be seen immediately adjacent to the femur and extending proximal to the knee joint. T1-weighted fat-suppressed axial MRI with gadolinium contrast (**C**) shows a heterogenous mass with central cystic degeneration. Biopsy revealed a high-grade soft-tissue sarcoma.

Popliteal cysts occur in pediatric patients much less frequently than in adult patients (**Figure 4**). In a review of 80 consecutive pediatric patients with a clinically suspected popliteal cyst, ultrasound confirmed a cyst in 55 of 147 knees (37%) evaluated. In the 17 patients with a confirmed arthritis, the incidence increased to 57% (16 of 28 knees evaluated by ultrasound). The incidence of an underlying arthritis prompted the authors to conclude that pediatric patients presenting with a popliteal cyst and no previously diagnosed arthritis should undergo a diagnostic workup. Most pediatric cysts communicated with the knee joint. Spontaneous regression or induced regression was common after treatment of the underlying condition.[6]

Acromioclavicular Cysts

Acromioclavicular cysts are fluid collections over the acromioclavicular joint and superior shoulder. These cysts can be striking in size and are indicative of underlying degenerative shoulder girdle pathology. Two types of acromioclavicular cysts have been identified, based on etiology. A type 1 cyst originates from the acromioclavicular joint proper and communicates with the underlying subacromial bursa. The more common type 2 cyst is the result of fluid extravasation from a degenerative glenohumeral joint through an incompetent rotator cuff.[7]

On examination, the patient has a large supraclavicular, transilluminating mass without a thrill or bruit. The physical examination often elucidates signs of underlying rotator cuff disease or degenerative arthritis. In evaluating the MRI of a shoulder with a cyst, it is important to look for the presence and extent of rotator cuff injury. The pathognomonic geyser sign represents the conduit of glenohumeral synovial fluid through the acromioclavicular joint into the cephalad cyst.

As with all secondary findings, treatment of the pathology underlying these synovial cysts provides the best chance of definitive resolution. Observation and reassurance are an acceptable treatment because the cyst is not dangerous to the patient. Physical therapy, medication, and injections may safely be used to manage the underlying condition. Aspiration may provide transient resolution of the cyst, but a recurrence is likely without management of the underlying condition. Open excision often is performed with a reconstructive or salvage procedure for the underlying pathology. With a type 1 cyst, distal clavicle excision, bursectomy, and cyst removal may be indicated after unsuccessful nonsurgical treatment. Management of a type 2 cyst may involve surgical reconstruction to treat an irreparable rotator cuff tear or advanced glenohumeral degenerative arthropathy.

Other Synovial Cysts

Synovial cysts have been described in myriad locations. Many small cysts are identified incidentally. Digital lesions (digital mucous cysts) often are located over ar-

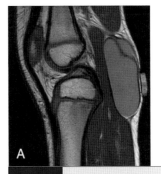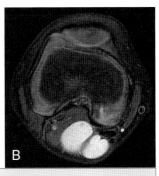

Figure 4 Proton density sagittal (**A**) and fat-saturated T2-weighted axial (**B**) MRIs of the knee of a 4-year-old patient showing a popliteal cyst with characteristics similar to those of adult variants. The mass spontaneously resolved. The only other MRI finding of concern was medial femoral condyle subchondral edema suggestive of recent trauma.

thritic interphalangeal joints. Pedal lesions can affect shoe wear and irritate adjacent nerves.

Ganglion Cysts

Ganglia are firm periarticular or pretendinous pseudocysts with mucinous contents. The viscosity may be thin, comparable to synovial fluid, or thick as in mucin, rich in high molecular weight proteins and glycosaminoglycans. They may be unilocular or multilocular. Because they are lined with dense fibrous tissue and lack a synovial lining, ganglia are pseudocysts.

The etiology of ganglia is unclear. The observed unilateral flow of material from the joint space to the ganglion cavity supports a one-way valve theory of synovial fluid extravasation. Other theories include mucinous degeneration of ligament or capsule and metaplasia of fibroblasts or synovial cells into mucin-producing cells.[8]

Wrist Ganglia

Despite the high incidence of wrist ganglia, controversies remain as to their etiology, ability to cause wrist pain, and management.[9] Wrist ganglia can be dorsal or volar (palmar). Volar ganglia are most commonly identified over the scapholunate interval but also may be at the interval between the radial artery and the flexor carpi radialis tendon, adjacent to the scaphoid tubercle, within the anatomic snuffbox, or more distally over the hand. Ulnar-sided lesions have been reported.

The patient's history and physical examination are important for accurate diagnosis of wrist ganglia. A host of lesions can mimic a ganglion, most notably small neoplasms, vascular malformations, osteophytes, and even sarcoma.

An MRI study identified ganglia in more than half of a group of asymptomatic volunteers.[10] Extraosseous wrist ganglia have been identified in 67% of asymp-

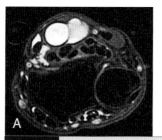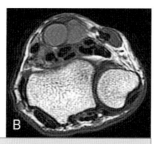

Figure 5 Axial MRIs showing a multilobular volar ganglion in a 42-year-old woman. **A,** T2-weighted fat-suppressed study showing uniform high signal intensity. **B,** T1-weighted study showing an intermediate signal. The mass appears to closely adhere to the flexor carpi radialis tendon. Post-contrast sequences showed trace peripheral uptake.

tomatic computer users and 75% of symptomatic computer users; ganglia were the most common MRI finding in this cohort.[11] The prevalence of wrist ganglia and the relative rarity of symptomatic ganglia leads to questions about the role of the ganglion itself as a pain generator.

Arthroscopy has allowed better identification of intra-articular pathology associated with ganglia as well as the presence of altered wrist mechanics in patients with a ganglion. The symptomatology of ganglia still remains unclear. Small, occult ganglia and intraosseous lesions most likely cause symptoms from pressure within the scapholunate ligament or on the posterior interosseous nerve.[11]

The patient may describe unsightliness, pain, fear of malignancy, and dysesthesias and often the patient cannot recall an inciting trauma. Left or right handedness has not been shown to affect incidence. A small lesion may be detectable only with wrist extension (for a volar lesion) or flexion (for a dorsal lesion). The lesion often can be transilluminated, and lacks a thrill or bruit.

A recent prospective study found that patients were concerned about pain or functional impairment less often than cosmesis or fear of malignancy (34% and 76%, respectively).[12] In contrast, other reports describe pain and dysesthesias as a substantial percentage of presenting patient concerns.[13-15]

The occult ganglion can be challenging to diagnose clinically. Scapholunate tenderness and painful wrist extension without a palpable nodule are the hallmarks of an occult ganglion. A loss of extension may be present.[16] Plain radiography may demonstrate a soft-tissue density in the area of the ganglion. A 2007 retrospective review of 103 radiographic studies found a 13% incidence of radiographic abnormalities on a three-view series of wrist radiographs of patients being evaluated for wrist ganglia, but treatment was altered only for one patient.[17] The role of routine radiography for a clinically suspected ganglion is being questioned in the current era of attention to health care spending.

MRI will reveal a discrete mass with homogenous signal. T1-weighted studies show low to intermediate signal, and T2-weighted studies show high signal (**Figure 5**). High sensitivity has been reported for MRI in the evaluation of occult ganglia.[18] A small sarcoma or tumor can have a similar appearance, but administration of gadolinium contrast should allow the lesions to be distinguished. Ganglia have low enhancement with contrast. The cost-efffectiveness of MRI in diagnosing overt ganglia has not been reported. Given the generally high accuracy with which wrist ganglia can be diagnosed on history and physical examination, MRI should be reserved for incidences in which the diagnosis is in question or an otherwise unidentifiable process may be responsible for symptoms.

The role of routine histologic evaluation of most ganglia has also come into question based on cost considerations. A recent Massachusetts General Hospital study of 429 patients found no treatment-changing disagreements between clinical and histologic diagnoses.[19] In the five discrepancies between the clinical and histologic diagnoses, no fluid ganglion contents could be expressed during surgery. State law may obligate the surgeon to provide all excised samples for histologic examination.

Accounts of nonsurgical treatment have provided insight into the natural history of wrist ganglia. In a large UK study, 42% of dorsal lesions resolved with observation, and a similar persistence-recurrence rate was reported in volar ganglia.[20,21] Observation and patient education can lead to satisfying results, particularly if the patient's primary concern is the malignant potential of the lesion. The absence of documented malignant degeneration indicates there is no need for routine surveillance of a clinically diagnosed ganglion. Although significantly lower patient satisfaction has been reported after reassurance alone when compared to aspiration and excision, no specific posttreatment finding was correlated with patient satisfaction.[20]

Aspiration of the mucinous cyst contents can provide an immediate cosmetic improvement and possibly relief of pressure. Injection of steroid has not been found to decrease the recurrence rate in adults. Open excision is an option for a symptomatic lesion after unsuccessful nonsurgical care. Excessive ligament resection must be avoided to prevent iatrogenic carpal instability. Reported recurrence rates have greatly varied.[21-24] Advances in arthroscopic techniques have made arthroscopic débridement of wrist ganglia an attractive option. In addition to smaller incisions, arthroscopy allows dynamic evaluation of the wrist and anatomic evaluation of ligamentocapsular structures. Recurrence rates were found to be comparable to those of open surgery.[25]

Wrist ganglia can occur in children, although they are less common than in adults. A study of 48 patients younger than 12 years who had a wrist ganglion found a greater prevalence of tendon sheath origin than is found in adult patients.[26] Observation with splinting and reassurance was found to be effective in several studies.[12,20,21] Tendon sheath ganglia often are difficult to treat and have relatively high recurrence rates after aspiration and/or excision.

Meniscal Ganglia

Meniscal cysts are uncommon and may arise from the lateral or medial meniscus. Though meniscal cysts are grouped with ganglion cysts, histologic evaluation of meniscal cysts has identified both synovial lining and dense fibrous tissue in the cyst wall, components defining both synovial cysts and ganglia. Most meniscal cysts are identified incidentally in association with a horizontal meniscal tear and probably represent a synovial cyst formed by excursion of intra-articular fluid through the tear.

Isolated symptomatic meniscal cysts are uncommon. If a cyst extends to the meniscal periphery, it can appear as a tender, palpable joint line mass. The patient may experience a sense of tightness in the affected knee even while retaining a normal range of motion. MRI is sensitive and specific for identifying meniscal cysts. Many of these cysts are multilocular and have a low-intensity signal with T1 weighting and a high-intensity signal with T2 weighting (**Figure 6**). Hemorrhage into a cyst, with subsequent deposition of proteinaceous material and hemoglobin, can result in a heterogeneous appearance. Fluid-fluid levels, a nonspecific finding, can be seen if bleeding into the cyst occurs. A heterogeneous cyst in the absence of a meniscal tear can mimic both a benign and a malignant tumor.[27]

Asymptomatic and symptomatic lesions can safely be observed. However, lesions with a heterogeneous MRI appearance and without an associated meniscal tear should be followed closely, and biopsy may be necessary to rule out an intra-articular neoplasm.

Decompression can be done during meniscal surgery for a patient with an associated tear. An isolated, symptomatic lesion can be excised arthroscopically, but an open approach may be warranted for a large lesion. Little is known about the recurrence rate of meniscal cysts, but recurrence is less likely when the underlying pathology is treated.

Intraneural Ganglia

Intraneural ganglia are most commonly identified in the tibial nerve and likely represent an intraneural advancement of a degenerative cyst of the proximal tibiafibula joint; this is the articular or synovial theory of pathogenesis.[28] The patient may have symptoms of nerve compression.

Periosteal Ganglia

Knowledge of periosteal ganglia (originally called periostitis albuminosa) largely has been garnered from case reports and small studies. These lesions often are identified in adults adjacent to tubular bones of the lower extremity, with an apparent proclivity for the proximal tibia and fibula near the pes anserinus attach-

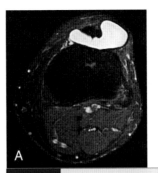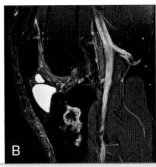

Figure 6	Axial (A) and sagittal (B) T2-weighted fat-suppressed MRIs showing a lateral parapatellar mass in a 36-year-old man with knee pain. A lateral meniscal cyst can be seen, with extrusion through the capsule, as well as a horizontal lateral meniscal tear and incidental tibia bone infarct.

ments. Two reports of periosteal ganglia in children have been published.[29]

The mass is atraumatic and can be painful or pain free. A palpable lesion is firm and immobile. Plain radiographs may be unremarkable or show cortical scalloping with reactive bone formation underlying the ganglion. CT demonstrates a soft-tissue mass adjacent to the cortical surface and may also show cortical erosion and periosteal new bone formation. On MRI, a homogenous, well-defined mass is seen with signal isointense to muscle on T1-weighted studies and high signal on T2-weighted studies. Unlike soft-tissue ganglia, periosteal lesions do not have internal septae.

Excision is the treatment for a symptomatic lesion. Although some lesions recur locally, the cause may be further mucoid degeneration rather than inadequate excision.

Other Ganglia

Like synovial cysts, ganglia can appear in seemingly any joint or tendon sheath. The treatment is based on symptoms and often includes excision (**Figure 7**).

Myxomas

The myxoid soft-tissue tumors are a clinically, histologically, and genetically diverse group of tumors with the commonality of an extracellular matrix rich in polysaccharide (glycosaminoglycans) and fibrous structural proteins. Myxoid tumors can be benign or malignant.

Intramuscular Myxomas

Intramuscular myxomas are benign and believed to be true mesenchymal neoplasms consisting of undifferentiated stellate cells. The architecture resulting from the elaborate arrangement of cellular and extracellular components gives myxoid lesions their gel-like consistency. Intramuscular myxomas often are identified in

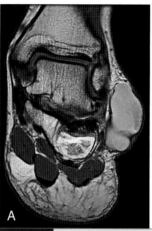
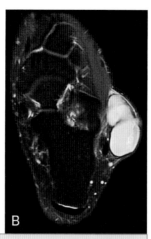

Figure 7 Proton density coronal **(A)** and T2-weighted fat-suppressed axial **(B)** MRIs showing a foot mass in a 47-year-old patient. A lobular mass with internal fluid signal can be seen adjacent to the peroneal tendons, without communication with the ankle, subtalar, or midfoot joints. An incidental intraosseous lipoma can be seen in **A**. This painless cystic mass interfered with shoe wear. Histologic examination of the excised specimen confirmed the diagnosis of a ganglion.

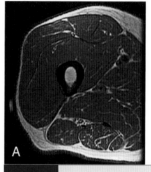
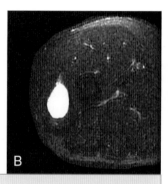

Figure 8 Axial MRIs showing an asymptomatic thigh mass in a 61-year-old man demonstrate an intramuscular mass isointense to muscle on a T1-weighted axial image **(A)** and very bright on a T2-weighted fat-suppressed axial image **(B)**. Biopsy confirmed an intramuscular myxoma.

older adults, with a slightly higher incidence among women.[30]

Physical findings often do not differentiate an intramuscular myxoma from other benign or malignant soft-tissue tumors. These nontender, soft, mobile tumors are most commonly identified in proximal large muscles. Their location and the lack of pain mean that these lesions may become quite large. MRI shows a low signal intensity with T1-weighted imaging and a high signal intensity with T2-weighted imaging because of the lesion's high water content. Often low signal areas of bridging septae can be seen inside the lesion with T2-weighted sequences (**Figure 8**).

The tumor is soft and lobular with a gelatinous, whitish gray appearance. Histologically, there is an abundance of mucinous extracellular matrix. The tumors are hypovascular and paucicellular. The cells are stellate or spindle shaped, with hyperchromatic nuclei without mitoses. The more vascular variants are more cellular, and differentiating them from a low-grade myxoid malignancy is a diagnostic challenge.

Genetic methods have been used experimentally to establish the diagnosis and pathogenesis of these tumors. Coamplification at lower denaturation temperature polymerase chain reaction was used to reveal an increased prevalence of guanine nucleotide-binding protein alpha-stimulating activity 1 (*GNAS1*) mutation (seen in fibrous dysplasia) in both the classic tumor and cellular variants. No *GNAS1* mutations were identified in myxoid sarcomas.[31]

Although asymptomatic lesions can be treated with observation, the differentiation of benign intramuscular myxomas from low-grade malignant myxoid neoplasms can be challenging. Surveillance of a confirmed intramuscular myxoma should be performed if the patient chooses observation. Marginal excision is an acceptable surgical treatment with a low rate of local recurrence.

A periarticular (or juxta-articular) myxoma most typically occurs around large joints. Though histologically similar to its intramuscular counterparts, this lesion has a significantly higher rate of local recurrence after excision.

Mazabraud Syndrome

Mazabraud syndrome is defined by the presence of intramuscular myxomas in association with fibrous dysplasia. The most common type of this rare disease is polyostotic fibrous dysplasia with multiple myxomas, although there have been incidences of monostotic disease with a solitary soft-tissue lesion. The extent of the disease varies as the causative *GNAS1* mutation occurs as a postzygotic event, creating a mosaic of affected and unaffected cell populations. Theoretically, the earlier in development the mutation occurs, the more affected the individual will be.

Nerve Sheath Myxoma

A nerve sheath myxoma (neurothekeoma) presents as a small, often asymptomatic mass. If the lesion is sufficiently large or is in a confined space, it may cause a compressive neuropathy. Head and neck sites predominate, though approximately 25% occur in an upper extremity. These lesions are most commonly identified in patients younger than 30 years and are rare in the pediatric population. The anatomic depth of the lesions ranges from superficial dermal to deep along a peripheral nerve. The etiology of nerve sheath myxoma remains unresolved, but the architecture and nodularity suggest a relationship to neurofibroma.

Histologically, nerve sheath myxomas are classified as cellular, mixed, or myxoid. Fibrous bands compartmentalize areas of varying myxoid and cellular content. A cellular variant may be confused with a sarcoma because cellular atypia and extension into adjacent tissues are common. A superficial lesion may mimic a dermatologic malignancy. The cellular and mixed variants may represent a heterogeneous group of lesions not properly classified as nerve sheath myxomas. Marginal excision is curative, and the local recurrence rates are low.

Aneurysmal Soft-Tissue Cysts

The aneurysmal soft-tissue cyst is a rarely occurring counterpart to the aneurysmal bone cyst and is most often described in case reports and small studies. The lesion can occur in both axial and appendicular sites.[32] Like aneurysmal bone cysts, the soft-tissue lesions have been identified adjacent to other processes, suggesting the existence of secondary aneurysmal cysts. Soft-tissue seeding and secondary aneurysmal cyst formation were described after intralesional excision of an aneurysmal bone cyst.[33]

A soft-tissue aneurysmal cyst presents as a firm, growing, mobile, painful or pain-free mass. The lesion may have calcification on radiographs but no contiguity with adjacent bone; it can mimic myositis ossificans. CT shows a septated lesion with peripheral calcification. Histological examination reveals a giant, cell-rich lesion with numerous blood-filled cavities. Reactive bone often is identified on the lesion's periphery.

Marginal excision is the treatment of choice; otherwise lesions will continue to grow. There are no reports of malignant degeneration or metastasis.

Epidermoid Cysts

Epidermoid cysts are not commonly seen by orthopaedic surgeons. Large lesions, though, can mimic any of several soft-tissue tumors. The etiology is unclear, but traumatic implantation of epidermis, human papillomavirus, and hair follicle occlusion have been proposed. The lesion often is painless and very slow growing. On MRI, the features include a nonenhancing, homogenous intermediate high signal with T1 weighting and high proton density. The lesions are not aggressive and do not invade adjacent structures (Figure 9).

Histologically, the lesion is lined with epithelium, and therefore it is a true cyst. Treatment is excision of a symptomatic lesion. In rare instances, squamous cell carcinoma has arisen in an epidermoid cyst.

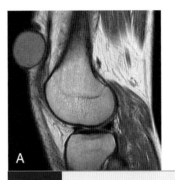
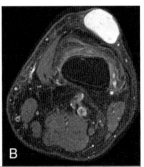

Figure 9 Proton density MRIs showing a well-encapsulated mass in a 66-year-old man with no history of significant trauma. The lesion had slowly grown over more than 20 years, mimicking a bursitis. The homogenous intermediate high signal intensity on the T1-weighted sagittal study **(A)** and high signal intensity on the fat-suppressed axial study **(B)** were not enhanced by contrast administration. Biopsy confirmed an epidermoid inclusion cyst.

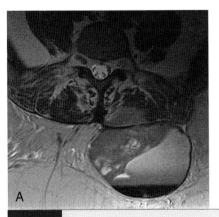
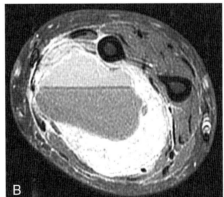
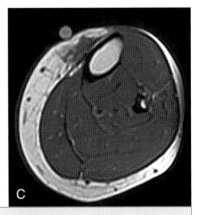

Figure 10 Axial MRIs showing large fluid-fluid levels within two soft-tissue masses, both of which had a significant solid portion adjacent to the cyst. Synovial sarcoma **(A)** and leiomyosarcoma **(B)** are among the many soft-tissue neoplasms that may show fluid-fluid levels on MRI. **C,** Axial T1 MRI showing a small homogenous area adjacent to the tibia in an active 51-year-old woman diagnosed with a stress reaction of the tibia and a periosteal ganglion. Excisional biopsy revealed a poorly differentiated sarcoma.

4: Soft Tissue Tumors

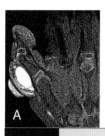
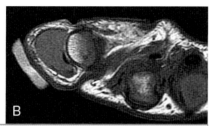

Figure 11 Proton density fat-suppressed coronal **(A)** and T1-weighted axial **(B)** MRIs showing a painless thumb mass in a 2-year-old girl. A unilocular fluid-filled mass is adjacent to the metacarpophalangeal joint. Despite the cystic appearance, histologic and immunohistochemical findings were consistent with a hemangioma.

Lesions Masquerading as Cysts

Sarcomas

Mismanagement of a soft-tissue sarcoma is a rational fear among physicians. Though the typical soft-tissue sarcoma appears as a painless, deep, proximal mass in an adult, an atypical sarcoma can mimic a cyst. MRI findings can contribute to the confusion because the fluid-fluid levels in several sarcomas can be similar to those of a benign cyst and may create a false sense of security (**Figure 10**). A pericystic solid component likely represents the primary pathology and is the most appropriate area for biopsy.[34]

Vascular Malformations

A vascular malformation can appear as a large vascular dilation resembling a cyst. Gross and histologic examination may be necessary for identification (**Figure 11**).

Summary

The benign soft-tissue cystic masses are a heterogeneous collection. Though these tumors are often concerning to the patient, most pose no serious threat to life or limb and some merely serve as an indicator that underlying pathology is present. Observation with an emphasis on treatment of the underlying condition often is the most prudent course of management, but it is important to be vigilant for symptoms or signs that are inconsistent with a benign cystic process.

Annotated References

1. Baker WM: On the formation of synovial cysts in the leg in connection with disease of the knee-joint: 1877. *Clin Orthop Relat Res* 1994;299(299):2-10.

2. Labropoulos N, Shifrin DA, Paxinos O: New insights into the development of popliteal cysts. *Br J Surg* 2004;91(10):1313-1318.

3. Sanchez JE, Conkling N, Labropoulos N: Compression syndromes of the popliteal neurovascular bundle due to Baker cyst. *J Vasc Surg* 2011;54(6):1821-1829.

   This 2011 literature review identified 16 published cases of entrapment neuropathy, 46 of popliteal vein compression, and 5 of popliteal artery compression secondary to a popliteal cyst.

4. Beaman FD, Peterson JJ: MR imaging of cysts, ganglia, and bursae about the knee. *Radiol Clin North Am* 2007;45(6):969-982, vi.

   This 2007 pictorial review highlighted MRI findings of common cystic knee and periarticular pathology with an emphasis on cystic lesions and diseases of bursae.

5. Satyajit S, Paode V, Campbell AC: Popliteal cysts: A technique of methylene blue dye-assisted arthroscopic decompression. *Eur J Orthop Surg Traumatol* 2009;19(5):373-375.

   This 2009 technique paper described the use of methylene blue as a safe adjunct to the identification of the stalk of a popliteal cyst during arthroscopic surgery.

6. Neubauer H, Morbach H, Schwarz T, Wirth C, Girschick H, Beer M: Popliteal cysts in paediatric patients: Clinical characteristics and imaging features on ultrasound and MRI. *Arthritis* 2011;2011:751-593.

   In 80 consecutive patients with a clinically suspected popliteal cyst, 55 popliteal cysts were confirmed by ultrasound. An increased incidence of popliteal cysts was observed in patients with associated knee pathology such as arthritis and hypermobility.

7. Hiller AD, Miller JD, Zeller JL: Acromioclavicular joint cyst formation. *Clin Anat* 2010;23(2):145-152.

   In this 2010 review article, the authors summarized two mechanisms by which acromioclavicular cysts arise. Type 1 cysts originate at the acromioclavicular joint overlying an intact rotator cuff. Type 2 cysts orginate in the glenohumeral joint with synovial fluid traversing a torn rotator cuff (creating the MRI "Geyser sign") and acromioclavicular joint to the subcutaneous surface.

8. Watson HK, Rogers WD, Ashmead D IV : Reevaluation of the cause of the wrist ganglion. *J Hand Surg Am* 1989;14(5):812-817.

9. Gant J, Ruff M, Janz BA: Wrist ganglions. *J Hand Surg Am* 2011;36(3):510-512.

   This concise 2011 review article summarized the best available evidence in counseling a patient on the most prudent course for management of a ganglion cyst. This report also reviewed utility of diagnostic data as pertains to establishing a diagnosis and guiding therapy.

10. Lowden CM, Attiah M, Garvin G, Macdermid JC, Osman S, Faber KJ: The prevalence of wrist ganglia in an asymptomatic population: Magnetic resonance evaluation. *J Hand Surg Br* 2005;30(3):302-306.

11. Burgess RA, Pavlosky WF, Thompson RT: MRI-identified abnormalities and wrist range of motion in asymptomatic versus symptomatic computer users. *BMC Musculoskelet Disord* 2010;11:273.

    An MRI study of 24 computer users identified a 66.6% prevalence of extraosseous wrist ganglia in the 10 without symptoms and a 75% prevalence in the 14 with symptoms. Of the multiple pathologic findings, only intraosseous ganglia were significantly more common in symptomatic volunteers.

12. Westbrook AP, Stephen AB, Oni J, Davis TR: Ganglia: The patient's perception. *J Hand Surg Br* 2000;25(6): 566-567.

13. Rizzo M, Berger RA, Steinmann SP, Bishop AT: Arthroscopic resection in the management of dorsal wrist ganglions: Results with a minimum 2-year follow-up period. *J Hand Surg Am* 2004;29(1):59-62.

14. Luchetti R, Badia A, Alfarano M, Orbay J, Indriago I, Mustapha B: Arthroscopic resection of dorsal wrist ganglia and treatment of recurrences. *J Hand Surg Br* 2000;25(1):38-40.

15. Varley GW, Needoff M, Davis TR, Clay NR: Conservative management of wrist ganglia: Aspiration versus steroid infiltration. *J Hand Surg Br* 1997;22(5):636-637.

16. Osterwalder JJ, Widrig R, Stober R, Gächter A: Diagnostic validity of ultrasound in patients with persistent wrist pain and suspected occult ganglion. *J Hand Surg Am* 1997;22(6):1034-1040.

17. Wong AS, Jebson PJ, Murray PM, Trigg SD: The use of routine wrist radiography is not useful in the evaluation of patients with a ganglion cyst of the wrist. *Hand (N Y)* 2007;2(3):117-119.

    Of 103 consecutive patients with wrist ganglia, 13 had radiographically identified abnormalities and 1 had a treatment change secondary to imaging findings. Radiography was found not cost-effective in this clinical setting.

18. Goldsmith S, Yang SS: Magnetic resonance imaging in the diagnosis of occult dorsal wrist ganglions. *J Hand Surg Eur Vol* 2008;33(5):595-599.

    This is a retrospective review of 20 wrists in 20 patients who underwent MRI and surgery for a suspected occult dorsal wrist ganglion. Sixteen of the 20 wrists demonstrated a ganglion on MRI. Eighteen of the 20 had gross findings of a ganglion. Sixteen of the 20 had histological evidence of a ganglion. Overall sensitivity and specificity of MRI to identify an occult ganglion were 80% and 20% when using histology to determine disease.

19. Guitton TG, van Leerdam RH, Ring D: Necessity of routine pathological examination after surgical excision of wrist ganglions. *J Hand Surg Am* 2010;35(6): 905-908.

    In 429 consecutive ganglion excisions, there was a 98.6% concordance between clinical and histologic diagnosis, with no treatment change indicated in the incidences of discrepancy. Abandoning the practice of pathologic examination of wrist ganglia was found not to compromise patient care.

20. Dias JJ, Dhukaram V, Kumar P: The natural history of untreated dorsal wrist ganglia and patient reported outcome 6 years after intervention. *J Hand Surg Eur Vol* 2007;32(5):502-508.

    Thirty-two (58%) of 55 patients were successfully treated nonsurgically for a dorsal wrist ganglion. No significant benefit was observed in patients treated with aspiration or excision compared with reassurance.

21. Dias J, Buch K: Palmar wrist ganglion: Does intervention improve outcome? A prospective study of the natural history and patient-reported treatment outcomes. *J Hand Surg Br* 2003;28(2):172-176.

22. Wright TW, Cooney WP, Ilstrup DM: Anterior wrist ganglion. *J Hand Surg Am* 1994;19(6):954-958.

23. Kang L, Akelman E, Weiss AP: Arthroscopic versus open dorsal ganglion excision: A prospective, randomized comparison of rates of recurrence and of residual pain. *J Hand Surg Am* 2008;33(4):471-475.

    This randomized study from 2008 compared open versus arthroscopic dorsal wrist ganglion excision, and no significant difference in recurrence or residual pain could be identified.

24. Craik JD, Walsh SP: Patient outcomes following wrist ganglion excision surgery. *J Hand Surg Eur Vol* 2012; 37(7):673-677.

    This 2012 study reported an 8% recurrence rate and 98% patient satisfaction in 48 patients responding to a questionnaire at least 21 months following open wrist ganglion excision.

25. Gallego S, Mathoulin C: Arthroscopic resection of dorsal wrist ganglia: 114 cases with minimum follow-up of 2 years. *Arthroscopy* 2010;26(12):1675-1682.

    This South American study described 114 patients treated with arthroscopic ganglion excision. The recurrence rate was 12.3%, with high patient satisfaction and early return of function as measured by grip strength and range of motion.

26. Coffey MJ, Rahman MF, Thirkannad SM: Pediatric ganglion cysts of the hand and wrist: An epidemiologic analysis. *Hand (N Y)* 2008;3(4):359-362.

    A retrospective study of 48 patients younger than 12 years with hand and wrist ganglia found that tendon sheath-associated cysts and spontaneous regression were more commonly identified than in studies of adult patients.

27. Roidis N, Zachos V, Basdekis G, Hantes M, Khaldi L, Malizos K: Tumor-like meniscal cyst. *Arthroscopy* 2007;23(1):e1-e6.

    A case report described an atypical meniscal cyst mimicking a neoplastic process. An excellent literature review was included.

28. Spinner RJ, Scheithauer BW, Amrami KK: The unifying articular (synovial) origin of intraneural ganglia: Evolution-revelation-revolution. *Neurosurgery* 2009; 65(suppl 4)A115-A124.

29. Abdelwahab IF, Kenan S, Hermann G, Klein MJ, Lewis MM: Periosteal ganglia: CT and MR imaging features. *Radiology* 1993;188(1):245-248.

30. Graadt van Roggen JF, Hogendoorn PC, Fletcher CD: Myxoid tumours of soft tissue. *Histopathology* 1999; 35(4):291-312.

31. Delaney D, Diss TC, Presneau N, et al: GNAS1 mutations occur more commonly than previously thought in intramuscular myxoma. *Mod Pathol* 2009;22(5): 718-724.

   Coamplification at lower denaturation temperature polymerase chain reaction was used to maximize yield from relatively hypocellular intramuscular myxoma tissue. An increased prevalence was identified of the GNAS1 mutation seen in fibrous dysplasia. The lack of mutation in sarcomatous tissue suggests a role in diagnosis of histologically unclear tissue.

32. Sahu A, Gujral SS, Gaur S: Extraosseous aneurysmal cyst in hand: A case report. *Cases J* 2008;1(1):268.

   This case was the first reported soft-tissue aneurysmal bone cyst of the hand. At 2 years follow-up from excisional biopsy, the patient was without signs of recurrence.

33. Karkuzhali P, Bhattacharyya M, Sumitha P: Multiple soft tissue aneurysmal cysts: An occurrence after resection of primary aneurysmal bone cyst of fibula. *Indian J Orthop* 2007;41(3):246-249.

   This case report was the first description of an iatrogenic secondary aneurysmal bone cyst of soft tissue. Seeding of the excision bed during treatment of a fibular aneurysmal bone cyst led to development of multiple soft tissue masses histologically consistent with the primary osseous lesion.

34. Van Dyck P, Vanhoenacker FM, Vogel J, et al: Prevalence, extension and characteristics of fluid-fluid levels in bone and soft tissue tumors. *Eur Radiol* 2006; 16(12):2644-2651.

Chapter 24

Lipoma and Other Benign Lipomatous Tumors

Sean V. McGarry, MD

4: Soft Tissue Tumors

Introduction

A lipoma is a benign tumor consisting of mature adipose tissue. Lipomas are the most commonly reported mesenchymal tumor (benign or malignant) in humans. However, there is a relative paucity of literature on their treatment and outcomes. Most recent studies report on the use of molecular and cytogenetic markers to classify and diagnose the histologic variants of lipoma. Little has changed in the actual treatment of lipoma.

A lipoma can be classified as superficial or deep in relation to the fascia, and it can be a discrete mass or a diffuse infiltration of adipose tissue. Several histologic subtypes have subtle pathologic and prognostic differences. A borderline malignancy is called atypical lipomatous tumor or well-differentiated liposarcoma (ATL/WDL).

Incidence and Anatomic Location

Considering the indolent behavior of most lipomas, it can be assumed that most such tumors are not reported. In addition, many surgically excised lipomas are never confirmed by pathology. The true incidence therefore is difficult to assess. Lipomas appears to occur slightly more often among men than women. Lipomas are extremely rare in children and uncommon in young adults. Most lipomas occur in middle-aged adults, and they may be more common in sedentary or obese individuals. There is no racial variation in the incidence.

Superficial lipomas occur significantly more frequently than deep lipomas and are the most common type of soft-tissue tumor. The common anatomic locations include the back, shoulder, posterior neck, and abdomen. These locations are those of the highest density of subcutaneous fat in the body. Lipomas occur much more commonly in the trunk than in the extremities, and they are more common proximally than distally in the extremity.

Clinical Evaluation

Superficial and deep lipomas have a bimodal presentation. In the subcutaneous tissue, lipoma is a small (less than 5 cm), slowly enlarging, nonpainful mass just below the skin. The tumor has a rubbery consistency and is freely mobile. A deep lipoma is found incidentally on imaging or as a fullness in the involved area. The tumor usually is much larger (10 to 15 cm) and not discretely palpable. Often a patient who is obese describes an increase in size of the lesion in proportion to weight gain. The lesion typically is not painful unless it is encroaching on an adjacent anatomic structure, such as a nerve. Frequently the first symptom is a cosmetic asymmetry.

Imaging

Plain radiographs are not specific but may show a soft-tissue shadow suggesting the presence of a mass. CT shows a homogenous soft-tissue mass with the same radiodensity of subcutaneous fat. MRI often is diagnostic. In all sequences, MRI typically shows a homogenous mass with signal intensity isointense to that of subcutaneous fat. Specifically, a lipoma has high signal intensity with T1 weighting and intermediate signal intensity with T2 weighting (**Figure 1**). Occasionally a lipoma has a heterogeneous signal intensity, either centrally as a result of central necrosis or calcification, or more diffusely secondary to prominent vascular septa. This factor increases the difficulty of a radiographic diagnosis.[1]

Pathology

A subcutaneous lipoma is a beige to yellowish, roughly spherical mass ranging in diameter from 1 to 2 cm to 6 to 8 cm. The tumor usually is well circumscribed by a thin capsule, which when opened reveals a lobular, irregularly shaped lesion. A deep lesion usually is larger;

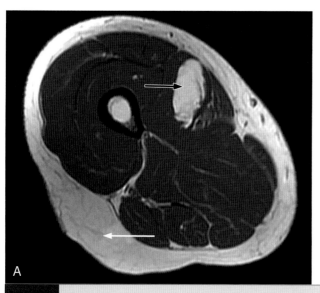

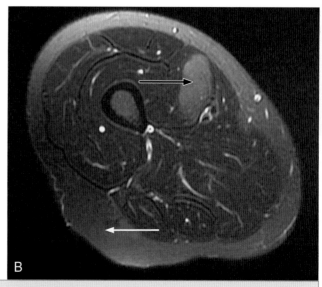

Figure 1 Axial MRI studies showing a lipoma (black arrow) isointense to subcutaneous fat (white arrow) with T1 (**A**) and T2 (**B**) weighting.

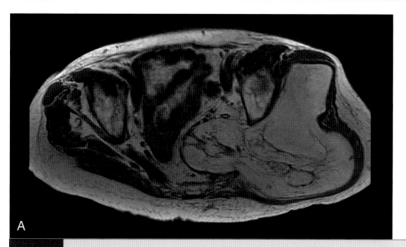

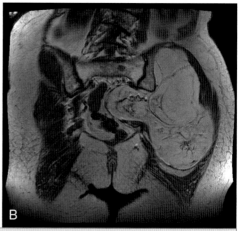

Figure 2 T1-weighted axial (**A**) and coronal (**B**) MRI showing both centripetal and longitudinal lipoma growth.

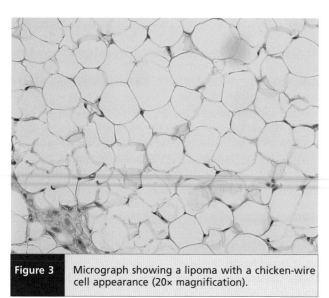

Figure 3 Micrograph showing a lipoma with a chicken-wire cell appearance (20× magnification).

in the thigh, it can be larger than 15 to 20 cm. A deep lipoma is yellowish to orange on gross inspection and is irregularly shaped; the size is dictated by the space in which it was growing. The growth pattern is centripetal in the axial plane, and growth in a more longitudinal plane occurs when the tumor meets resistance, filling the available space in the compartment (**Figure 2**).

Lipoma cells are histologically indistinguishable from mature adipocytes. The cells are oval in appearance, with a central lipid droplet composing most of the cell and the remainder of the cytoplasm and bland basophilic nuclei pushed to a more peripheral location (the appearance resembles that of a engagement ring). In a large microscopic field, the cells are seen to form an interlocking pattern similar to that of chicken wire (**Figure 3**). Lobules of these cells are separated by fibrous septa through which the blood vessels course. A thin capsule usually surrounds the tumor. Occasionally muscle fibers are present at the periphery of a deep lipoma where the lipoma is infiltrating into the adjacent muscle. The subtypes of lipomas are distinguished by an admixture of cells and matrix of other types, such as spindle cells, blood vessels, and chondroid matrix.

Chromosomal abnormality is found in most lipomas, frequently as a balanced translocation involving the chromosomal segments 12q13-15 and 3q27-28. The high-mobility group AT-hook 2 *(HMGA2)* and lipoma-preferred partner *(LPP)* genes form a fusion gene. The expression of *HGMA2-LPP* or *LPP-HGMA2* is found in almost 25% of all lipomas.[2] Most other cytogenetic abnormalities in lipoma involve a combination of the *HGMA2* gene and one of the following: the nuclear factor I/B *(NFIB)*, chemokine (C-X-C motif) receptor 7 *(CXCR7)*, early B-cell factor 1 *(EBF1)*, or lipoma HMGIC fusion partner *(LHFP)* gene. The translocation partner chromosome segments for those genes are t(9; 12)(p22;q13-15), t(2;12)(q37;q13-15), t(5;12)(q32-33; q13-15), and t(12;13)(q13-15;q12), respectively.[3]

Treatment and Prognosis

Lipomas have an indolent growth pattern. After the initial growth, most tumors become stable and further growth is not significant. Many lipomas that are in a subcutaneous location and smaller than 5 cm can be treated nonsurgically with observation. Many patients find such a tumor to be cosmetically unacceptable, and this factor can be an indication for surgery. Other surgical indications include relatively large size or continuing lesion growth. If the diagnosis remains questionable after appropriate imaging, the patient should be referred to an orthopaedic oncologist. A deep lesion usually appears as a relatively large lesion and can be challenging to diagnose. Referral may be warranted to an orthopaedic oncologist in a center with multidisciplinary specialists including a musculoskeletal radiologist and a soft-tissue pathologist.

For a true lipoma, surgical excision usually is curative. Recurrence rate is reportedly less than 5%.[4] A poorly encapsulated or infiltrative tumor is more difficult to completely excise and therefore more likely to recur. With the exception of an ATL/WDL, malignant degeneration of a lipoma into a liposarcoma is extremely rare. In some reported incidences of malignant degeneration, questions arose as to whether the tumor originally was misdiagnosed secondary to sampling error.[4]

Histologic Variants

Lipomatosis

Lipomatosis is a diffuse overgrowth of normal adipose tissue that can affect the trunk or extremities. Histologically, lipomatosis is identical to lipoma. Its rapid growth pattern and infiltrative nature can cause concern. Lipomatosis is impossible to completely excise, and the treatment is debulking when necessary for cosmetic or functional reasons. Debulking has a high incidence of recurrence and may provide only temporary cosmesis or relief of symptoms.

Familial Lipomatosis

Familial lipomatosis occurs in several different clinical presentations and syndromes depending where in the body the disease manifests. A cohort of patients with lipomatosis have a family history suggesting autosomal dominant inheritance.[5] There is some evidence to suggest that a mitochondrial DNA mutation is associated with familial lipomatosis.[6]

Lipoma Arborescens

Lipoma arborescens is a fatty infiltration of the synovium of a joint. The most commonly affected joint is the knee, and the most common location within the knee is the suprapatellar pouch. There is some question as to whether lipoma arborescens is a reactive process, because it almost always occurs in association with other intra-articular pathology. The treatment is synovectomy of the involved joint.

Lipoblastoma

Lipoma is rare in patients younger than 20 years. The equivalent tumor in infants and young children is a lipoblastoma. Like lipoma, lipoblastoma also occurs in a diffuse form, known as diffuse lipoblastomatosis. The radiographic and clinical appearance is similar to that of adult lipoma and is characterized by abundant fat. MRI shows nonenhancing cystic change, representing necrosis and myxoid stroma; and enhancing areas containing soft-tissue nodules, representing the relatively vascular and cellular nodules of lipoblasts.[7] Histologically, lipoblastoma consists of lobules of lipoblasts (immature adipocytes) in various stages of differentiation and separated by vascular fibrous stroma with an underlying myxoid stroma. Fluorescence in-situ hybridization and cytogenetic studies can be used to search for the pleomorphic adenoma gene 1 *(PLAG1)* gene rearrangement (8q11-13) and confirm a diagnosis of lipoblastoma.[8] The treatment is marginal surgical resection. Lipoblastoma may mimic liposarcoma radiographically, but the clinical setting generally clearly sets it apart.

Spindle Cell and Pleomorphic Lipomas

Spindle cell and pleomorphic lipomas occur during the fifth or sixth decade of life and are more common in men than in women. As a subcutaneous mass of the posterior shoulder or the back, the clinical appearance is similar to that of lipoma. Histologically, the lesion is well circumscribed and consists of a mixture of benign spindle cells and adipocytes (in spindle cell lipoma) or floretlike giant cells, adipocytes, and a myxoid stroma (in pleomorphic lipoma). Cytogenetic studies have found deletions on 13q in almost all spindle cell lipomas.[9] Pleomorphic lipoma shows 13q and/or 16q deletions.[3] Marginal excision is curative for spindle cell and pleomorphic lipomas.

Hibernoma

Hibernoma is a benign lipoma of brown fat, most commonly occurring in young adults. The common locations include the thigh, shoulders, back, neck, and chest. The clinical appearance is similar to that of lipoma. MRI findings for hibernoma are similar to other lipomatous tumors and not reliably diagnostic. Histologically hibernoma is clearly different, with the cells ranging from a granular eosinophilic appearance to multivacuolated. Cytogenetic abnormalities on 11q13, deleting the tumor suppressor genes multiple endocrine neoplasia 1 (MEN1) and aryl hydrocarbon receptor-interacting protein (AIP), have been found in hibernoma.[10] The treatment is marginal surgical excision.

Neural Fibrolipoma

Neural fibrolipoma (also called lipofibromatous hamartoma of nerve, fibrolipomatous hamartoma of nerve, or neurolipomatosis) is a lipomatous infiltration of peripheral nerves. It occurs most commonly on the volar surface of the upper extremity. The clinical appearance is that of a slow-growing, diffuse lipomatous mass in the distribution of the involved peripheral nerve. Neural fibrolipoma often is associated with bone overgrowth or macrodactyly. Patients are in the first three decades of life, and they experience a slowly enlarging mass or a compressive neuropathy, such as carpal tunnel syndrome. The treatment (in the case of median nerve involvement) usually is a carpal tunnel release to preserve nerve function.

Myolipoma

Myolipoma is a benign tumor consisting of an admixture of mature adipose tissue and mature smooth muscle tissue. Like lipoma, myolipoma appears in a middle-aged adult as a painless superficial or deep mass. In the subcutis, a myolipoma usually is small (3 to 5 cm). In a subfascial location, a myolipoma can be much larger (10 to 15 cm or more) and often is found incidentally. Histologically, the tumor appears as a mixture of eosinophilic smooth muscle cells interspersed with typical adipocytes. The treatment is marginal resection.

Angiolipoma

Angiolipoma is a benign tumor composed of mature adipose tissue with an abundant interspersed vascular component. Typically an angiolipoma is a subcutaneous nodule smaller than 2 cm that is painful or tender to the touch. Often these tumors are multiple, and the most common location is the forearm. Histologically, the appearance is that of mature adipocytes divided by a branching vascular network. Angiolipomas are distinguished from lipomas with a prominent vasculature by the presence of fibrin thrombi in the vascular channels. The treatment is marginal surgical resection.

Chondroid Lipoma

Chondroid lipoma is a benign variant of lipoma that consists of mature adipose tissue admixed with a chondroid matrix. A firm, painless mass is found in the subcutis or the deeper tissues of a proximal extremity. Most commonly, chondroid lipoma occurs in middle-aged adults, but the age range is wide. Significantly more women than men are affected. The microscopic architecture is lobular, with nests of vacuolated cells resembling adipocytes and small round cells with a granular cytoplasm, within a chondroid matrix. Marginal surgical resection is curative.

Atypical Lipomatous Tumor/ Well-Differentiated Liposarcoma

ALT/WDL is a lesion of late adult life. The most common locations are a deep muscle compartment and the retroperitoneum. The gross and imaging appearance is similar to that of a typical lipoma, although there may be more fibrous stranding. On resection, these lesions are found to have less distinct margins and tend to be more infiltrative than lipoma. Histologically, the cells appear as mature fat, with fibrous septa containing spindle cells with occasional atypia. The tumor sometimes is indistinguishable from lipoma on light microscopy. Fluorescence in-situ hybridization and cytogenetic findings include ring and giant marker chromosomes with amplification of the HMGA2 and mouse double-minute 2 homolog (MDM2) genes.[11]

Historically, such a lesion was called an atypical lipomatous tumor when found in an extremity. In the retroperitoneum, the lesion was called a well-differentiated liposarcoma. Both lesions have a high recurrence rate and the potential for dedifferentiation into a fully malignant sarcoma with an ability to metastasize. Cytogenetic and molecular testing has revealed that the two types of tumor are closely related, and the two terminologies now are used interchangeably. In one study, MDM2 amplification (which does occur in many other cancers) was found to be 100% sensitive and specific for ALT/WDL compared with simple lipoma.[12] One large group of patients with a primary ATL/WDL lesion had a recurrence rate of 11%, and patients with a recurrent ATL/WDL lesion had a 52% re-recurrence rate.[13] The rate of dedifferentiation in the recurrent tumors was 4%. Marginal surgical excision of ALT/WDL is the appropriate treatment because of the lesion's benign nature. With dedifferentiation, the tumor is fully malignant and capable of metastasizing. The area of dedifferentiation requires wide surgical excision.

Summary

Lipoma, the most common soft-tissue tumor in humans, often goes unnoticed or undiagnosed. Usually it appears as a painless, superficial mass with a rubbery consistency, and often it can be managed nonsurgically. The lesion can be removed if it is symptomatic, growing, or cosmetically unacceptable. Marginal surgical resection usually is curative. A lesion found deep to the fascia usually is larger and of more concern than a superficial lesion, and in general should be removed to rule out a malignant or borderline malignant lesion (ALT/WDL). ATL/WDL can be difficult to distinguish from lipoma radiologically or histologically. Molecular genetics is useful for distinguishing between ALT/WDL and benign lipoma. ATL/WDL is characterized by a higher local recurrence rate and potential for dedifferentiation relative to benign lipoma.

Annotated References

1. Toirkens J, De Schepper AM, Vanhoenacker F, et al: A comparison between histopathology and findings on magnetic resonance imaging of subcutaneous lipomatous soft-tissue tumors. *Insights Imaging* 2011;2(5): 599-607.

   A diagnostic protocol was described for the treatment of lipomatous tumors.

2. Kubo T, Matsui Y, Naka N, et al: Specificity of fusion genes in adipocytic tumors. *Anticancer Res* 2010; 30(2):661-664.

   A retrospective review of a large study of lipomatous tumors established the specificity of fusion gene expression in benign and malignant fatty tumors.

3. Nishio J: Contributions of cytogenetics and molecular cytogenetics to the diagnosis of adipocytic tumors. *J Biomed Biotechnol* 2011;2011:524067.

   The contributions of cytogenetics to the diagnosis of adipocytic tumors over the last 15 years were described.

4. Weiss SW, Goldblum JR: *Enzinger and Weiss's Soft-Tissue Tumors*, ed 5. St. Louis, MO, Mosby-Elsevier, 2007.

   This comprehensive text discusses tumors of muscle, fat, and connective tissue and latest developments in the field.

5. Keskin D, Ezirmik N, Celik H: Familial multiple lipomatosis. *Isr Med Assoc J* 2002;4(12):1121-1123.

6. Gámez J, Playán A, Andreu AL, et al: Familial multiple symmetric lipomatosis associated with the A8344G mutation of mitochondrial DNA. *Neurology* 1998; 51(1):258-260.

7. Chen C-W, Chang W-C, Lee H-S, Ko K-H, Chang C-C, Huang G-S: MRI features of lipoblastoma: Differentiating from other palpable lipomatous tumor in pediatric patients. *Clin Imaging* 2010;34(6):453-457.

   This review and summary of MRI findings in lipoblastoma can aid in the differentiation of lipomatous tumors in children.

8. Bartuma H, Domanski HA, Von Steyern FV, Kullendorff C-M, Mandahl N, Mertens F: Cytogenetic and molecular cytogenetic findings in lipoblastoma. *Cancer Genet Cytogenet* 2008;183(1):60-63.

   The incidence of chromosomal aberrations in the region of the *PLAG1* gene was reviewed in seven incidences of lipoblastoma, which represented almost 20% of the reported incidences.

9. Bartuma H, Nord KH, Macchia G, et al: Gene expression and single nucleotide polymorphism array analyses of spindle cell lipomas and conventional lipomas with 13q14 deletion. *Genes Chromosomes Cancer* 2011;50(8):619-632.

   Molecular cytogenetics was used to localize the specific genetic alterations that occur in spindle cell lipomas as an aid in diagnosis.

10. Nord KH, Magnusson L, Isaksson M, et al: Concomitant deletions of tumor suppressor genes MEN1 and AIP are essential for the pathogenesis of the brown fat tumor hibernoma. *Proc Natl Acad Sci U S A* 2010; 107(49):21122-21127.

    Molecular cytogenetics was used to map the sequence of genetic events preceding the development of a hibernoma. The information gained can help in the diagnosis of this subtype of lipomatous tumor.

11. Mandahl N, Bartuma H, Magnusson L, Isaksson M, Macchia G, Mertens F: HMGA2 and MDM2 expression in lipomatous tumors with partial, low-level amplification of sequences from the long arm of chromosome 12. *Cancer Genet* 2011;204(10):550-556.

    The differential expression of two specific genes found in lipomatous tumor aided the differential diagnosis of benign, borderline, and malignant fatty tumors.

12. Weaver J, Downs-Kelly E, Goldblum JR, et al: Fluorescence in situ hybridization for MDM2 gene amplification as a diagnostic tool in lipomatous neoplasms. *Mod Pathol* 2008;21(8):943-949.

    Molecular cytogenetic findings for a single gene were useful for differentiation of purely benign and borderline malignant fatty tumors.

13. Mavrogenis AF, Lesensky J, Romagnoli C, Alberghini M, Letson GD, Ruggieri P: Atypical lipomatous tumors/well-differentiated liposarcomas: Clinical outcome of 67 patients. *Orthopedics* 2011;34(12):e893-e898.

    In a retrospective review of a large group of patients with ALT/WDL with good long-term follow-up, the outcome parameters of recurrence rates and dedifferentiation rates in the recurrent tumors were analyzed.

Chapter 25

Benign Neural Tumors

Shahram Bozorgnia, MD

4: Soft Tissue Tumors

Introduction

The neural tumors and associated tumorlike lesions originate from the nerve sheath of a peripheral nerve and include schwannomas, neurofibromas, perineuromas, nerve sheath myxoma, traumatic neuroma, and Morton neuroma. These tumors, especially schwannomas and neurofibromas, are among the most common benign soft-tissue tumors. Although usually they are benign, some of these tumors have potential for malignant degeneration.

Schwannomas

Schwannomas, also known as neurilemomas, represent approximately 5% of all benign soft-tissue tumors.[1] Schwannomas can affect patients in any age group but are most common in adults age 20 to 40 years, with no predilection for women or men. A schwannoma can occur anywhere that nerve fibers exist. The most common locations include the head and neck, flexor surfaces of extremities, spinal nerve roots (the paraspinal region), and nerves in the mediastinum or retroperitoneum. The etiology may be related to the neurofibromatosis type 2 (*NF2*) gene.

In 95% of patients, the tumor is an isolated mass characterized by a noninfiltrating pattern of growth.[1,2] Often the tumor is found incidentally as a painless mass, but it may cause neurologic symptoms by compressing surrounding nerves. The Tinel sign may be present on physical examination. Two types of multiple schwannomas exist. NF2 is characterized by germline mutation of the *NF2* gene and by bilateral schwannomas of the eighth cranial (auditory) nerve. The less common type is schwannomatosis, in which multiple schwannomas are associated with a somatic mutation of the *NF2* gene.[3] In addition, schwannomas infrequently are associated with neurofibromatosis type 1 (NF1, formerly known as von Recklinghausen disease), in which large plexiform tumors are formed and multiple tumors may be present.

Neither Dr. Bozorgnia nor any immediate family member has received anything of value from or has stock or stock options held in a commercial company or institution related directly or indirectly to the subject of this chapter.

Imaging

Schwannomas do not have specific imaging characteristics and share some features with neurofibromas. Often the two lesions cannot be distinguished. MRI is particularly useful for depicting the tumor; a fusiform, ovoid, or dumbbell-shaped tumor located on a large peripheral nerve often can be seen with a low- to intermediate-intensity T1 signal or a high-intensity T2 signal (**Figure 1**). Sometimes the nerve of origin can be detected next to the tumor. T2-weighted studies may reveal the nonspecific target sign, which consists of a central, relatively low signal intensity with a peripheral rim of high signal intensity. The target sign corresponds pathologically to central fibrocollagenous tissue and predominantly myxoid peripheral tissue.[1] T1-weighted studies may show the nonspecific split-fat sign, in which there is a high signal rim of fat surrounding the tumor. This sign can occur if the tumor originated in an intermuscular location, where there is adipose tissue in the adventitia between muscles[4] (**Figure 2**). A so-called dumbbell lesion may be seen in an enlarging tumor lo-

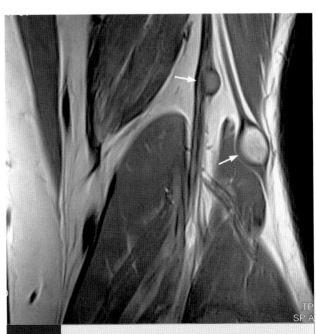

| **Figure 1** | T1-weighted MRI showing two schwannomas (arrows). The nerves of origin (the tibial nerve and common peroneal nerve) can be seen next to the tumors. |

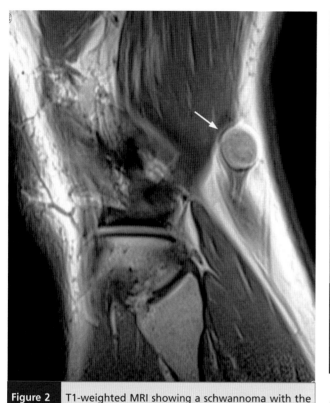

Figure 2 T1-weighted MRI showing a schwannoma with the nonspecific split-fat sign (arrow), in which there is a high signal rim of fat surrounding the tumor.

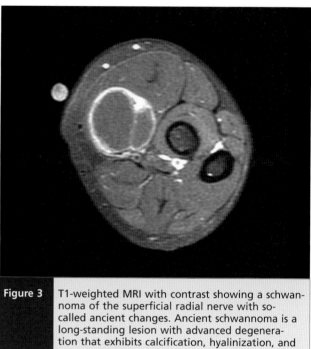

Figure 3 T1-weighted MRI with contrast showing a schwannoma of the superficial radial nerve with so-called ancient changes. Ancient schwannoma is a long-standing lesion with advanced degeneration that exhibits calcification, hyalinization, and cystic cavitation.

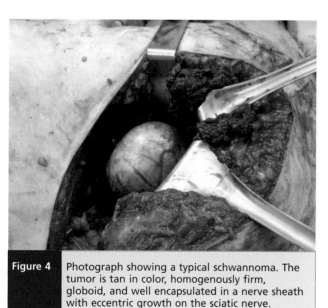

Figure 4 Photograph showing a typical schwannoma. The tumor is tan in color, homogenously firm, globoid, and well encapsulated in a nerve sheath with eccentric growth on the sciatic nerve.

that exhibits calcification, hyalinization, and cystic cavitation; these features can be identified to a varying extent on all imaging modalities[5] (**Figure 3**). A heterogeneous appearance with degeneration and cystic cavitation is more likely in schwannoma than neurofibroma.[5]

Pathology

A schwannoma usually is tan in color, homogenously firm, globoid, and well encapsulated in a nerve sheath, with eccentric growth on the parent nerve (**Figure 4**). Cut sections show a mixture of gray or white fibrous tissue and bright yellow lipid-rich foci. The schwannoma may have cysts or calcifications. Tumor size varies greatly and usually depends on anatomic location.

The schwannoma is composed of Schwann cells, which are spindle shaped with poorly defined eosinophilic cytoplasm and a basophilic nucleus. The cells often assume a teardrop shape. These tumors have two distinct histologic regions. The Antoni A regions are highly ordered and compact collections of Schwann cells arranged in short, intersecting bundles, linear arrays, or sheets. Nuclei tend to palisade around eosinophilic anuclear areas containing cell processes. These stacked arrangements of elongated palisading nuclei are called Verocay bodies (**Figure 5**). The Antoni B regions are loosely arranged and less cellular because of accumulation of extracellular mucin, which gives the region a myxoid appearance (**Figure 6**).

The capsule of a schwannoma consists of spindle cells with associated collagen from perineurial and epineurial connective tissue. Common vascular changes are thick-walled, hyalinized vessels with perivascular

cated in the neural foramen or in the internal acoustic meatus, where the tumor has eroded or compressed the adjacent bone.

On ultrasound, a schwannoma appears as a well-defined hypoechoic mass. On CT the mass is well defined and hypodense. A so-called ancient schwannoma is a long-standing lesion with advanced degeneration

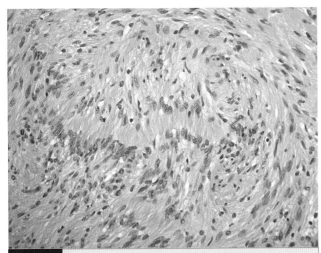

Figure 5 High-power photomicrograph (×200) of Verocay bodies of schwannomas with standard hematoxylin-eosin stain. These are composed of palisaded arrays of nuclei separated by vaguely fibrillary collections of cell processes.

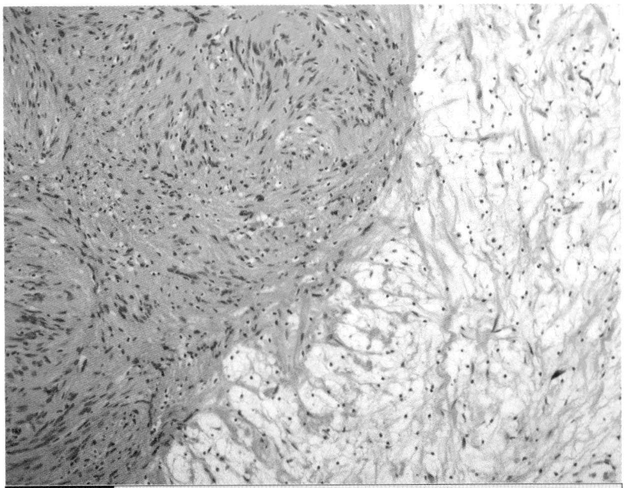

Figure 6 Low-power photomicrograph (×100) of Schwannomas with standard hematoxylin-eosin stain, are characterized by alternating compact Antoni type A tissues (left side) and loose Antoni type B tissues (right side).

deposits of hemosiderin. In Antoni B areas, thin-walled vessels surrounded by edematous stroma is common as well. Infiltrates of lymphocytes and plasma cells as well as collections of lipid-laden foamy macrophages are common. Special studies are not required for a typical schwannoma; all variants uniformly stain positive for S100 protein.

Variants
Although a conventional schwannoma or neurilemoma is most common, several other types of schwannoma exist. Cellular schwannoma is characterized by Antoni A architecture, high cellularity, and proliferative activity. The cells are mostly spindle shaped. Histologically, a cellular schwannoma can simulate a malignant peripheral nerve sheath tumor, with its high mitotic rate; however, it is benign and does not transform into a malignant peripheral nerve sheath tumor. Usually a cellular schwannoma occurs in the posterior mediastinum or pelvis.[6] The recurrence rate after incomplete excision can be as high as 40%.[7]

A plexiform schwannoma is characterized by multinodular or wormlike cutaneous tumors. Visceral types can occur but are rare. Histologically, a plexiform schwannoma has typical Schwann cells with more Antoni A areas than Antoni B areas, and lacks a thick capsule, especially in the cutaneous type. Recurrence can result from incomplete excision, irregular fingerlike growth, or lack of thick encapsulation. There is no association with NF1.[3] The tumors are benign, and, as with cellular schwannomas, a high mitotic index is not prognostically important.

Melanotic schwannoma, often mistaken for melanoma, are rare, tarlike tumors that lack a grossly defined capsule. Plump, spindle-shaped to epithelioid cells are arranged in sheets, lobules, and fascicles and often

are accompanied by densely pigmented histiocytes. These tumors tend to arise from spinal nerves and paraspinal ganglia.[8] About 10% are malignant, and the presence of macronucleoli or necrosis suggests malignancy. Psammomatous melanotic schwannomas often are associated with the Carney complex, a rare autosomal dominant heritable syndrome that includes cutaneous lentigines, cardiac myxomas, and endocrine neoplasms. Psammoma bodies and cells resembling adipocytes typify these tumors. The diagnosis of this variant is important because of the morbidity associated with cardiac myxoma and the potential for metastasis.

Schwannomatosis
Schwannomatosis is a syndrome characterized by the presence of multiple schwannomas in the absence of the diagnostic criteria for NF2 (that is, no evidence of vestibular tumor). The criteria for definite schwannomatosis are fulfilled if the patient has two or more nonintradermal schwannomas, is older than 30 years, has no evidence of vestibular schwannomas on high-quality MRI, and does not have a known constitutional NF2 mutation.[9] Alternatively, definite schwannomatosis can be diagnosed if the patient has a first-degree relative with definite schwannomatosis and has one or more pathologically confirmed nonvestibular schwannomas, without reference to patient age, MRI findings, or results of NF2 mutation testing. Possible schwannomatosis can be diagnosed without MRI if the patient does not have symptoms of eighth nerve dysfunction, is older than 45 years, has two or more nonintradermal schwannomas, and does not have a known constitutional NF2 mutation. The schwannomatosis diagnostic criteria have been modified to state that patients with definite or possible schwannomatosis must not possess

any of the existing diagnostic criteria for NF2, including evidence of vestibular schwannomas on high-quality MRI, a first-degree relative with NF2, and a constitutional *NF2* mutation.[10]

In the absence of classic NF2, schwannomatosis occurs in 2% to 4% of patients with schwannomas.[9] Schwannomatosis affects men and women equally and becomes symptomatic when the patient is age 20 to 50 years.[11] The patients tend to be younger than patients with a solitary schwannoma. The physician therefore should suspect schwannomatosis in a relatively young patient with multiple schwannomas who does not meet the criteria for NF2.[11] The first-appearing symptom is pain from the mass or spinal cord compression.[11] In most patients, schwannomatosis is sporadic; familial schwannomatosis accounts for fewer than 20% of incidences.[10,12] Because the spine is affected in most patients, MRI of the spine should be part of the routine evaluation. Routine whole-spine MRI imaging is recommended regardless of the location of the symptomatic tumor, because schwannomatosis-related schwannomas tend to enlarge and grow into previously healthy nerves.[11]

Genetics

Mutations in the *NF2* gene at position 22q12.2 are the basis of schwannoma formation in both sporadic schwannomas and NF2.[13] This tumor-suppressor gene codes for moesin-ezrin-radixin-like protein (MERLIN, also called schwannomin), a cell membrane–associated protein that links the cell membrane and the cytoskeleton and functions in intracellular signaling pathways.[14] The mutations decrease the synthesis of MERLIN. The *NF2* gene follows the two-hit hypothesis: the mutation must affect both alleles that code for MERLIN protein to reduce its expression sufficiently to cause tumor formation.[15]

The molecular basis of schwannomatosis is being actively investigated. A mosaic alteration of the *NF2* gene mutation was found in 1997, but a non-*NF2* locus was suggested in some patients.[16] The calcineurin-binding protein 1 (*CABIN1*) gene, adjacent to the *NF2* gene on chromosome 22, has been implicated in the pathogenesis of both NF2 and schwannomatosis.[17] The SW1/SNF–related, matrix-associated, actin-dependent regulator of chromatin B1 (*SMARCB1*) tumor-suppressor gene and its product, the integrase interactor 1 (INI1) protein, are involved in 50% of incidences of familial schwannomatosis and 10% of sporadic incidences. The familial and sporadic forms of schwannomatosis also differ in their patterns of INI1 staining.[12,18-20]

Treatment

Marginal excision of a schwannoma usually can spare the parent nerve because the tumor is separable from the underlying nerve fibers. The excision usually is over the nerve parallel to the fascicles so that the mass can be almost extruded. The encapsulation of the tumor facilitates the excision. Occasionally, partial resection is performed to spare the nerve; despite the incomplete removal, recurrence or progression is unusual.[1] Treatment of schwannomatosis follows the same principles. Many experts surgically treat only symptomatic tumors or those that are enlarged at follow-up.[11]

Prognosis

The prognosis of a solitary schwannoma is excellent if the tumor was completely excised. Recurrences are uncommon and vary by location and completeness of tumor excision. Malignant transformation is very rare.

Schwannomatosis has a less certain outcome. The disease ranges from indolent to malignant variations. This broad spectrum of behavior must be taken into account during family counseling. In the future, prenatal *INI1-SMARCB1* testing may become available for the familial forms of schwannomatosis.[11]

Neurofibromas

Neurofibromas can occur at any age but are most common in adults age 20 to 30 years, with no sex-based predilection. Neurofibromas represent slightly more than 5% of all benign soft-tissue tumors.[1] These tumors can occur in any peripheral nerve as well as soft tissue, skin, and bone. The etiology is only partially understood but appears to be related to the *NF1* gene. Superficial neurofibromas typically are small, painless masses, whereas deeper neurofibromas are commonly associated with neurologic symptoms. Pain and tenderness may be present with a positive Tinel sign on physical examination.[21]

Neurofibromas can grow as solitary or multiple tumors. Most lesions are solitary, but as many as 10% are associated with NF1. In the setting of neurofibromatosis, tumors tend to be larger, multiple, and deep, and they have a higher incidence of malignant transformation.[21]

Solitary and multiple tumors are categorized into four types. Localized intraneural neurofibroma, the most common form of neurofibroma, is an intraneural nodule involving a peripheral nerve. Localized cutaneous neurofibroma is a cutaneous nodule that rarely exceeds 3 cm in diameter. The lesion appears at puberty and can enlarge with age or pregnancy.[22] Cutaneous neurofibromas may develop from the multipotent cells present in hair follicles rather than from the cutaneous small nerve twigs.[3] Diffuse neurofibroma is an infiltrative lesion involving skin or soft tissue, typically restricted to the subcutaneous tissues and most commonly occurring in children and young adults.[1,4] Plexiform neurofibroma originates in multiple fascicles of a peripheral nerve and infiltrates the surrounding tissues to form a large, disfiguring mass with a bag-of-worms appearance. The tumor expands during early childhood and is pathognomonic for NF1.[23] Its clinical importance stems from an increased risk of malignant transformation.

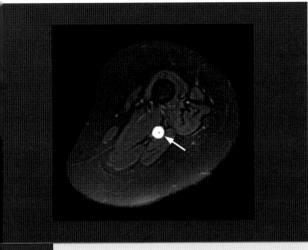

Figure 7 | T2-weighted MRI of a neurofibroma showing the target sign (arrow), in which there is a central low signal intensity and a peripheral high signal intensity.

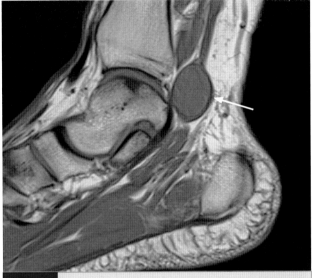

Figure 8 | T1-weighted MRI showing a neurofibroma (arrow) originating from the tibial nerve.

Imaging

The imaging characteristics of neurofibromas are not specific. Some characteristics on MRI are shared with schwannomas, including the split-fat sign, the dumbbell lesion in an enlarging tumor located in the neural foramen, and the target sign. The target sign is considered to be more typical of neurofibromas than schwannomas (**Figure 7**). MRI is particularly useful in showing extension of the lesion as well as the parent nerve as it enters and exits the tumor. Another typical feature is a fusiform shape that is oriented longitudinally in a nerve distribution, often with tapered ends that blend into the parent nerve (**Figure 8**). When the nerve of origin is identified, a lesion that is eccentrically positioned in relation to the nerve suggests a schwannoma, whereas a centrally located mass suggests a neurofibroma[21] (**Figure 9**).

A neurofibroma typically has low T1 signal intensity, high T2 signal intensity, and avid gadolinium contrast enhancement. Ultrasound shows the neurofibroma as a well-defined hypoechoic mass. CT shows hypodensity relative to muscle; the lesion is enhanced after contrast administration. A tumor adjacent to a bone can compress and erode the cortex. Sometimes the tumor can appear as an intraosseous lytic lesion or even simulate a cyst. Large, nonossifying fibromas can be associated with NF1.

The diffuse form of neurofibroma is ill defined and extensively reticulates through the subcutaneous tissue.[4] Its imaging characteristics can be markedly different from those of the other forms of neurofibroma.

Pathology

A neurofibroma typically is a firm, gray-white, rubbery mass that appears homogenous and translucent. There is an intimate association with the parent nerve; the tumor grows in a longitudinal fusiform manner with the

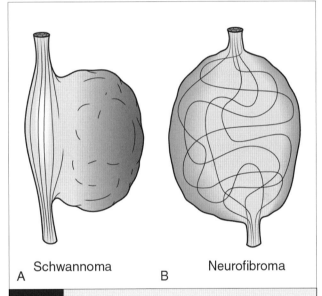

Figure 9 | Schematic drawing showing the eccentric position of a schwannoma (A) in relation to the parent nerve and the central location of a neurofibroma (B).

nerve. Unlike a schwannoma, the tumor is not encapsulated.[21] Most neurofibromas range in size from a few millimeters to 5 cm. Plexiform neurofibromas are a tangle of expanded nerve fascicles that can reach a larger size. In diffuse neurofibroma, severe thickening of the subcutaneous tissues can result in marked enlargement of the affected extremity. The exact size often is difficult to appreciate.

Neurofibromas contain bundles of spindle cells (Schwann cells and fibroblasts), often with wavy nuclei that are embedded in myxoid stroma and wavy colla-

© 2014 American Academy of Orthopaedic Surgeons

4: Soft Tissue Tumors

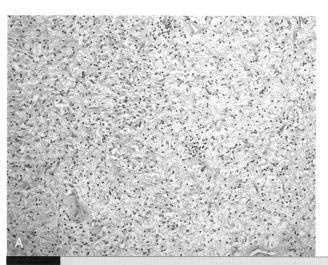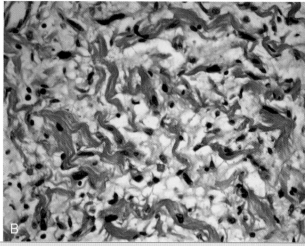

Figure 10 **A,** Low-power photomicrograph (×100) of a neurofibroma with standard hematoxylin-eosin stain showing the characteristic low cellularity and bands of collagen. **B,** High-power photomicrograph (×400) of a neurofibroma with standard hematoxylin-eosin stain showing the waviness of collagen (sometimes described as the shredded carrot appearance) and tumor cell nuclei.

gen bundles (similar in appearance to shredded carrots) (**Figure 10, B**). The cellularity and the amount of stroma differ from lesion to lesion, but in general, neurofibromas are less cellular than schwannomas.[24] Nerve fibers are commonly found among the tumor cells as the tumor expands inside a nerve. Mitoses, a rare finding, should alert the clinician to the possibility of malignant transformation. Neurofibromas have variable S100 protein expression.

Neurofibromatosis

Neurofibromatosis is a phakomatosis (neurocutaneous syndrome) with a wide spectrum of clinical expression that can include neurocutaneous abnormalities and involvement of multiple organ systems. The two forms, NF1 and NF2, are clinically and genetically distinct. NF1 is commonly associated with peripheral nerve sheath tumors and is caused by a mutation in the neurofibromin 1 (*NF1*) gene, whereas NF2 primarily affects the central nervous system and is largely attributed to mutation in the neurofibromin 2 (*NF2*) gene. NF1 affects approximately 1 in 3,500 persons worldwide.[25] The clinical findings and severity of the disease are highly variable. The hallmarks of NF1 include café-au-lait macules and multiple cutaneous neurofibromas. The clinical diagnosis is based on the presence of at least two of the following findings: six or more café-au-lait macules with a diameter of more than 5 mm in a prepubertal patient or 15 mm in an adult; two or more neurofibromas of any type or one plexiform neurofibroma; freckling of axillary or inguinal areas; two or more Lisch nodules of the iris; optic glioma; a distinctive osseous lesion such as sphenoid wing dysplasia, congenital tibial pseudarthrosis, or severe scoliosis; and a first-degree relative in whom a diagnosis of NF1 has been made. It has been suggested that the pathognomonic mutation in the *NF1* gene should be added to

the list of diagnostic criteria. The lifetime risk of malignant tumors arising from peripheral nerves is estimated to be 10% to 13%.[26] All patients with NF1 have cutaneous neurofibromas, but clinically detectable plexiform neurofibromas develop only in approximately one third of these patients.

Genetics

NF1 results from an autosomal dominant trait caused by germline mutation in the *NF1* gene, which is located on chromosome 17q.[27] Approximately 50% of incidences of NF1 are caused by a new sporadic germline mutation in the *NF1* gene. More than 80% of new sporadic germline *NF1* gene mutations are of paternal origin.[28] The penetrance of NF1 is 100%, which means that all patients with an *NF1* mutation have NF1, but the extent of penetrance varies considerably.

The *NF1* gene is translated into a protein called neurofibromin.[29] All patients with NF1 are heterozygous for an *NF1* mutation that causes haploinsufficiency; the single functional copy of the gene does not produce enough neurofibromin to ensure normal development and regulation of cell growth, thereby leading to a disease state. Neurofibromin function is not clear, and none of the known interactions alone can explain all symptoms related to NF1. One of the functional domains of neurofibromin, the RasGAP-related domain (Ras-GRD), accelerates the conversion of active Ras–guanosine triphosphate (Ras-GTP) to inactive Ras–guanosine diphosphate (Ras-GDP) in various cell types and acts as a negative regulator of P21Ras. The Ras guanosine triphosphatases interact with multiple pathways, including the Raf-MEK-ERK mitogen-activated protein kinase cascade, which regulates cellular growth and differentiation.[30]

Like the tumor-suppressor gene *NF2* that underlies schwannoma formation, the *NF1* gene fulfills the two-

4: Soft Tissue Tumors

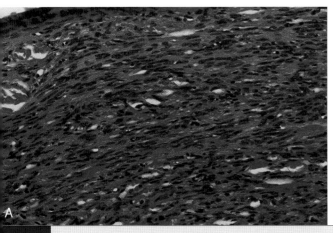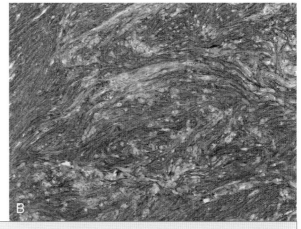

Figure 11 Histologic findings in perineurioma. **A,** High-power photomicrograph (×200) with standard hematoxylin-eosin stain of the longitudinal section of the affected nerve shows parallel, ill-defined perineurial cells around nearly indistinguishable nerve fibers. **B,** Immunohistochemical study ×100. Perineurial cells stain positive for epithelial membrane antigen encircling negative nerve fibers and their accompanying Schwann sheaths.

it hypothesis: the mutation must inactivate both alleles that code for neurofibromin protein to result in marked reduction of neurofibromin levels and formation of tumors such as neurofibroma, café-au-lait macules, and glomus tumors.[31] Solitary neurofibromas also are characterized by biallelic inactivation of the *NF1* gene in a subpopulation of Schwann cells.[32]

Approximately 5% of patients with NF1 develop a malignant peripheral nerve sheath tumor in a large or plexiform neurofibroma. Biallelic inactivation of the *NF1* gene appears to be a first step in the development of a malignant peripheral nerve sheath tumor but certainly is not sufficient by itself. Other mutations appear to be necessary for full malignant transformation.

Treatment

Surgical resection requires sacrificing the parent nerve because neurofibroma expands inside the nerve without any capsule and cannot be separated from the nerve fibers. If a large nerve is involved, excision of the tumor may result in a major neurologic deficit. Unless the pain is intolerable, it may be preferable to leave a lesion in an important large nerve rather than to risk major functional disability. Meticulous dissection of the tumor from stretched-out nerve fascicles may be possible. The diffuse type generally is treated nonsurgically, with surgical resection reserved for intolerable lesions. A patient with a single plexiform neurofibroma or multiple neurofibromas should be evaluated for NF1.

Prognosis

Although the prognosis usually is excellent after complete excision of a solitary lesion, recurrences do occur. The risk of malignant degeneration is approximately 5% in plexiform and large neurofibromas. The presence of a rapidly enlarging or painful lesion should alert the clinician to the possibility of malignant transformation and lead to a biopsy. If malignancy occurs,

only approximately 16% of patients survive for 5 years or longer.[33]

Perineuriomas

Perineurioma is a rare, benign, soft-tissue tumor composed exclusively of perineurial cells. The most common location is the dermis and subcutis of the limbs or trunk. This tumor should be considered in the differential diagnosis of spindle cell lesions in any location, because it has been reported in many unusual sites, such as the intestinal tract.[34] Perineurioma tends to occur in patients from age 10 to 80 years (mean age, 46 years) and is slightly more common among women than men.[35] The two distinct subtypes are soft-tissue perineurioma and intraneural perineurioma. The clonal nature of both subtypes can be confirmed by a lack of all or a portion of chromosome 22, but this cytogenic change is not always present.[36] Soft-tissue perineurioma, formerly known as storiform perineurial fibroma, is not associated with a nerve and appears as a painless, often superficial mass on the trunk or an extremity. The size of the tumor can range from 0.3 to 20 cm.[35] Intraneural perineurioma, formerly known as localized hypertrophic neuropathy, usually is limited to a segment of nerve in an extremity and often results in loss of sensorimotor function.[36] Hybrid tumors composed of perineurioma and either schwannoma or neurofibroma have been reported.[37]

Pathology

Perineurioma typically is an unencapsulated mass with proliferation of spindle cells, exclusively of perineurial cells, arranged in a storiform pattern within a variably collagenized stroma (**Figure 11,** *A*).[35] Pseudo-onion bulbs can form, composed of perineurial neoplastic cells surrounding one or more nerve fibers and

4: Soft Tissue Tumors

Schwann sheaths. Immunohistochemistry is important for the diagnosis and accurate classification of perineurioma. Most perineuriomas express epithelial membrane antigen (EMA) (**Figure 11,** *B*), CD34, smooth muscle actin, and Glut-1, which is a human red blood cell glucose transporter.[38] Some tumors also express claudin-1, but they do not express S100 protein or glial fibrillary acidic protein. Schwannoma, neurofibroma, and cutaneous meningioma do not stain for Glut-1. Claudin-1 reactivity is not found in dermatofibrosarcoma protuberans, low-grade fibromyxoid sarcoma, or fibromatosis. Claudin-1 therefore is useful in distinguishing perineurioma from its mimicking lesions.[39]

Soft-tissue perineurioma has three variants. Sclerosing soft-tissue perineurioma occurs in young adults and involves the digits or palms of the hands.[40] Its unique epithelioid perineurial cells are arranged in a trabecular or storiform pattern in a heavily collagenized stroma. The appearance of soft-tissue perineurioma can be similar to that of sclerotic fibroma of tendon sheath, except that there is no association with tendons, and soft-tissue perineurioma expresses EMA. The reticular soft-tissue perineurioma has a prominent lacelike reticular arrangement of lesional cells within a variably myxoid stroma. The plexiform soft-tissue perineurioma is rare and must be distinguished from multiple neoplasms having a plexiform pattern of growth, such as plexiform neurofibroma, plexiform schwannoma, and plexiform circumscribed neuroma. In contrast to perineurioma, the other lesions typically are S100 positive and EMA negative. Intraneural perineurioma is characterized by the wrapping of neoplastic perineurial cells around endoneurial structures. Involvement of multiple nerve fascicles produces a ropelike thickening of the nerve.[36]

Treatment

Excision is usually curative, and recurrence is rare. Malignant transformation has not been reported.[41]

Nerve Sheath Myxoma

Nerve sheath myxoma is a rare, histologically distinctive benign neural tumor of the dermis. It occurs in patients with a wide age range, beginning in childhood, with a peak incidence in the fourth decade of life. There is no sex-based predilection. Eighty-five percent of incidences occur in an extremity, particularly in the fingers or in the vicinity of the knee (especially the infrapatellar pretibial region). This tumor characteristically forms superficial, highly myxoid, multilobular masses with a dense peripheral fibrous border. The lesions contain spindled, stellate-shaped, ring-shaped, and epithelioid Schwann cells.[42] The tumor is immunoreactive for S100 protein and glial fibrillary acidic protein and typically has very limited reactivity for EMA and CD34. Axons are only rarely identifiable within these tumors, and when present they are typically organized into

small, compact clusters. Wide excision and follow-up are recommended because of the relatively high recurrence rate after incomplete excision.[42]

Traumatic Neuroma

Traumatic neuroma is a nonneoplastic, nonencapsulated lesion that can occur wherever a nerve is divided or injured. Although most commonly the lesion is found in a laceration or an amputation stump (amputation neuroma) or postoperatively at the site of sensory nerve transection, it also can occur after a minor trauma, even with a blunt nonpenetrating injury. Typically there is a painful or tender nodule with a positive Tinel sign. Histologically, the lesion is characterized by a disorganized outgrowth of all normal components of a nerve fascicle on the proximal side of the injured nerve. The regenerative nerve twigs, which consist of axons and Schwann cells surrounded by perineurial cells, are located in a dense collagenous matrix with surrounding fibroblasts. The Schwann cells are S100 positive, and the perineurial cells are EMA and Glut-1 positive.[43] Excision followed by recession of the nerve end into deep muscle or soft tissue that is not easily stimulated by pressure on the skin can be curative, but the neuroma sometimes re-forms.

Morton Neuroma

Morton neuroma is a compression neuropathy of the common digital nerve. It most often occurs in the third intermetatarsal space but can occur in other intermetatarsal spaces. Morton neuromas are most common in the third decade of life and among women rather than men.[44] The diagnosis primarily is clinical and is reached after other etiologies of symptoms have been ruled out by examination and diagnostic testing. The patient may report burning pain or numbness and tingling and has a lump at the plantar aspect of the intermetatarsal space. Typically the pain can be reproduced with palpation of the intermetatarsal space. Ultrasound can confirm the neuroma, which appears as a ovoid mass with hypoechoic signal. The symptoms can be exacerbated by wearing closed-toe shoes, especially if they are tight fitting. The lesion is characterized by endoneurial, perineurial, and epineurial fibrosis and hyalinization associated with loss of axons and mural thickening in nearby blood vessels. Adjacent blood vessels have fibrosis and thickening of the walls.

The initial treatment is nonsurgical. Pressure on the neuroma can be alleviated by wearing shoes with a wide toe box, using metatarsal pads in the shoe, and avoiding high-heeled shoes. Injection with corticosteroids or alcohol agents has had variable success.[45,46] Cryogenic neuroablation of the neuroma has been reported, but the results are not permanent and are relatively ineffective on larger neuromas.[47] The most commonly used surgical option is excision of the affected portion of the nerve. The second option is decompression of the nerve by releasing the deep transverse intermetatarsal ligament and external neurolysis.[44]

Summary

The neural tumors are common and usually benign. Physical examination and imaging characteristics are generally nonspecific, but findings on MRI scans may suggest a neural tumor. It is important to be aware of the potential for malignant degeneration associated with certain neural tumors as well as the genetic syndromes with which they are associated.

Annotated References

1. Murphey MD, Smith WS, Smith SE, Kransdorf MJ, Temple HT: Imaging of musculoskeletal neurogenic tumors: Radiologic-pathologic correlation. *Radiographics* 1999;19(5):1253-1280.

2. Kang HJ, Shin SJ, Kang ES: Schwannomas of the upper extremity. *J Hand Surg Br* 2000;25(6):604-607.

3. Kurtkaya-Yapicier O, Scheithauer B, Woodruff JM: The pathobiologic spectrum of Schwannomas. *Histol Histopathol* 2003;18(3):925-934.

4. Peh WC, Shek TW, Yip DK: Magnetic resonance imaging of subcutaneous diffuse neurofibroma. *Br J Radiol* 1997;70(839):1180-1183.

5. Schultz E, Sapan MR, McHeffey-Atkinson B, Naidich JB, Arlen M: Case report 872. "Ancient" schwannoma (degenerated neurilemoma). *Skeletal Radiol* 1994; 23(7):593-595.

6. White W, Shiu MH, Rosenblum MK, Erlandson RA, Woodruff JM: Cellular schwannoma: A clinicopathologic study of 57 patients and 58 tumors. *Cancer* 1990;66(6):1266-1275.

7. Casadei GP, Scheithauer BW, Hirose T, Manfrini M, Van Houton C, Wood MB: Cellular schwannoma: A clinicopathologic, DNA flow cytometric, and proliferation marker study of 70 patients. *Cancer* 1995;75(5): 1109-1119.

8. Font RL, Truong LD: Melanotic schwannoma of soft tissues: Electron-microscopic observations and review of literature. *Am J Surg Pathol* 1984;8(2):129-138.

9. MacCollin M, Chiocca EA, Evans DG, et al: Diagnostic criteria for schwannomatosis. *Neurology* 2005; 64(11):1838-1845.

10. Baser ME, Friedman JM, Evans DG: Increasing the specificity of diagnostic criteria for schwannomatosis. *Neurology* 2006;66(5):730-732.

11. Gonzalvo A, Fowler A, Cook RJ, et al: Schwannomatosis, sporadic schwannomatosis, and familial schwannomatosis: A surgical series with long-term follow-up. *J Neurosurg* 2011;114(3):756-762.

   The aim of this study was to provide disease-specific information about schwannomatosis in its different forms. Of the 158 patients, 142 had a solitary schwannoma, 2 had familial schwannomatosis (an inherited *NF2* mutation), and 14 had sporadic schwannomatosis.

12. Boyd C, Smith MJ, Kluwe L, Balogh A, Maccollin M, Plotkin SR: Alterations in the SMARCB1 (INI1) tumor suppressor gene in familial schwannomatosis. *Clin Genet* 2008;74(4):358-366.

   This study supported the hypothesis that *SMARCB1* is a tumor suppressor for schwannomas in the context of familial disease. The coding region of *SMARCB1* was studied by direct sequencing of DNA from 19 schwannomatosis kindreds.

13. Wolff RK, Frazer KA, Jackler RK, Lanser MJ, Pitts LH, Cox DR: Analysis of chromosome 22 deletions in neurofibromatosis type 2-related tumors. *Am J Hum Genet* 1992;51(3):478-485.

14. Rouleau GA, Merel P, Lutchman M, et al: Alteration in a new gene encoding a putative membrane-organizing protein causes neuro-fibromatosis type 2. *Nature* 1993;363(6429):515-521.

15. Louis DN, Ramesh V, Gusella JF: Neuropathology and molecular genetics of neurofibromatosis 2 and related tumors. *Brain Pathol* 1995;5(2):163-172.

16. Jacoby LB, Jones D, Davis K, et al: Molecular analysis of the NF2 tumor-suppressor gene in schwannomatosis. *Am J Hum Genet* 1997;61(6):1293-1302.

17. Buckley PG, Mantripragada KK, Díaz de Ståhl T, et al: Identification of genetic aberrations on chromosome 22 outside the NF2 locus in schwannomatosis and neurofibromatosis type 2. *Hum Mutat* 2005;26(6): 540-549.

18. Hadfield KD, Newman WG, Bowers NL, et al: Molecular characterisation of SMARCB1 and NF2 in familial and sporadic schwannomatosis. *J Med Genet* 2008; 45(6):332-339.

   DNA sequencing and dosage analysis of *SMARCB1* and *NF2* were performed for 28 sporadic and 15 familial incidences of schwannomatosis. A four-hit model with mutations in both *SMARCB1* and *NF2* defined a subset of patients with schwannomatosis.

19. Hulsebos TJ, Kenter SB, Jakobs ME, Baas F, Chong B, Delatycki MB: SMARCB1/INI1 maternal germ line mosaicism in schwannomatosis. *Clin Genet* 2010; 77(1):86-91.

   Germline mosaicism, a condition in which the precursor cells to ova and spermatazoa are a mixture (mosaic) of two or more genetically different cell lines, may occur in schwannomatosis. This finding has implications for genetic counseling. Although schwanno-matosis is not typically a heritable trait, germline mosaicism in these genes might occasionally lead to inheritance.

20. Patil S, Perry A, Maccollin M, et al: Immunohisto-chemical analysis supports a role for INI1/SMARCB1 in hereditary forms of schwannomas, but not in solitary, sporadic schwannomas. *Brain Pathol* 2008;18(4):517-519.

    This study confirmed a role for INI1/SMARCB1 in multiple schwannoma syndromes and suggested that a different pathway of tumorigenesis occurs in solitary, sporadic tumors.

21. Lin J, Martel W: Cross-sectional imaging of peripheral nerve sheath tumors: Characteristic signs on CT, MR imaging, and sonography. *AJR Am J Roentgenol* 2001;176(1):75-82.

22. Jouhilahti EM, Peltonen S, Callens T, et al: The development of cutaneous neurofibromas. *Am J Pathol* 2011;178(2):500-505.

    The multiple manifestations of NF1 and the wide spectrum of different clinical phenotypes were evaluated. The biallelic inactivation of the *NF1* gene through a second hit seems to be crucial to the development of certain manifestations.

23. Ferner RE: The neurofibromatoses. *Pract Neurol* 2010;10(2):82-93.

    The current NF1 and NF2 nomenclature is awkward because these are clinically and genetically separate disorders. The goal was to provide cohesive standards of care with neurofibromatosis and to devise standardized protocols for assessment and management within a multidisciplinary setting.

24. Peltonen J, Jaakkola S, Lebwohl M, et al: Cellular differentiation and expression of matrix genes in type 1 neurofibromatosis. *Lab Invest* 1988;59(6):760-771.

25. Lammert M, Friedman JM, Kluwe L, Mautner VF: Prevalence of neurofibromatosis 1 in German children at elementary school enrollment. *Arch Dermatol* 2005;141(1):71-74.

26. Evans DG, Baser ME, McGaughran J, Sharif S, Howard E, Moran A: Malignant peripheral nerve sheath tumours in neurofibromatosis 1. *J Med Genet* 2002;39(5):311-314.

27. Legius E, Marchuk DA, Collins FS, Glover TW: Somatic deletion of the neurofibromatosis type 1 gene in a neurofibrosarcoma supports a tumour suppressor gene hypothesis. *Nat Genet* 1993;3(2):122-126.

28. Jadayel D, Fain P, Upadhyaya M, et al: Paternal origin of new mutations in von Recklinghausen neurofibromatosis. *Nature* 1990;343(6258):558-559.

29. Hermonen J, Hirvonen O, Ylä-Outinen H, et al: Neurofibromin: Expression by normal human keratino-cytes in vivo and in vitro and in epidermal malignancies. *Lab Invest* 1995;73(2):221-228.

30. Le LQ, Parada LF: Tumor microenvironment and neurofibromatosis type I: Connecting the GAPs. *Oncogene* 2007;26(32):4609-4616.

    There appears to be a role for the microenvironment in plexiform neurofibroma genesis. The emerging evidence points to mast cells as crucial contributors to neurofibroma tumorigenesis.

31. Jouhilahti EM, Peltonen S, Heape AM, Peltonen J: The pathoetiology of neurofibromatosis 1. *Am J Pathol* 2011;178(5):1932-1939.

    Although a mutation in the *NF1* gene is the only factor required to initiate the NF1, the wide spectrum of different clinical phenotypes and their development, severity, and prognosis seem to result from the cross-talk between numerous cell types, cell signaling networks, and cell-extracellular matrix interactions.

32. Serra E, Rosenbaum T, Winner U, et al: Schwann cells harbor the somatic NF1 mutation in neurofibromas: Evidence of two different Schwann cell subpopulations. *Hum Mol Genet* 2000;9(20):3055-3064.

33. Ducatman BS, Scheithauer BW, Piepgras DG, Reiman HM, Ilstrup DM: Malignant peripheral nerve sheath tumors: A clinicopathologic study of 120 cases. *Cancer* 1986;57(10):2006-2021.

34. Hornick JL, Fletcher CD: Intestinal perineuriomas: Clinicopathologic definition of a new anatomic subset in a series of 10 cases. *Am J Surg Pathol* 2005;29(7):859-865.

35. Hornick JL, Fletcher CD: Soft tissue perineurioma: Clinicopathologic analysis of 81 cases including those with atypical histologic features. *Am J Surg Pathol* 2005;29(7):845-858.

36. Giannini C, Scheithauer BW, Jenkins RB, et al: Soft-tissue perineurioma: Evidence for an abnormality of chromosome 22, criteria for diagnosis, and review of the literature. *Am J Surg Pathol* 1997;21(2):164-173.

37. Kazakov DV, Pitha J, Sima R, et al: Hybrid peripheral nerve sheath tumors: Schwannoma-perineurioma and neurofibroma-perineurioma. A report of three cases in extradigital locations. *Ann Diagn Pathol* 2005;9(1):16-23.

38. Yamaguchi U, Hasegawa T, Hirose T, et al: Sclerosing perineurioma: A clinicopathological study of five cases and diagnostic utility of immunohistochemical staining for GLUT1. *Virchows Arch* 2003;443(2):159-163.

39. Folpe AL, Billings SD, McKenney JK, Walsh SV, Nusrat A, Weiss SW: Expression of claudin-1, a recently described tight junction-associated protein, distinguishes soft tissue perineurioma from potential mimics. *Am J Surg Pathol* 2002;26(12):1620-1626.

40. Fetsch JF, Miettinen M: Sclerosing perineurioma: A clinicopathologic study of 19 cases of a distinctive soft tissue lesion with a predilection for the fingers and palms of young adults. *Am J Surg Pathol* 1997;21(12): 1433-1442.

41. Duncan L, Tharp DR, Branca P, Lyons J: Endobronchial perineurioma: An unusual soft tissue lesion in an unreported location. *Patholog Res Int* 2010;2010:613-824.

    The first case of an endobronchial perineurioma, a rare, benign neoplasm typically occurring in soft tissue, is reported.

42. Fetsch JF, Laskin WB, Miettinen M: Nerve sheath myxoma: A clinicopathologic and immunohistochemical analysis of 57 morphologically distinctive, S-100 protein- and GFAP-positive, myxoid peripheral nerve sheath tumors with a predilection for the extremities and a high local recurrence rate. *Am J Surg Pathol* 2005;29(12):1615-1624.

43. Argenyi ZB, Santa Cruz D, Bromley C: Comparative light-microscopic and immunohistochemical study of traumatic and palisaded encapsulated neuromas of the skin. *Am J Dermatopathol* 1992;14(6):504-510.

44. Keh RA, Ballew KK, Higgins KR, Odom R, Harkless LB: Long-term follow-up of Morton's neuroma. *J Foot Surg* 1992;31(1):93-95.

45. Greenfield J, Rea J Jr, Ilfeld FW: Morton's interdigital neuroma: Indications for treatment by local injections versus surgery. *Clin Orthop Relat Res* 1984;185:142-144.

46. Hyer CF, Mehl LR, Block AJ, Vancourt RB: Treatment of recalcitrant intermetatarsal neuroma with 4% sclerosing alcohol injection: A pilot study. *J Foot Ankle Surg* 2005;44(4):287-291.

47. Caporusso EF, Fallat LM, Savoy-Moore R: Cryogenic neuroablation for the treatment of lower extremity neuromas. *J Foot Ankle Surg* 2002;41(5):286-290.

4: Soft Tissue Tumors

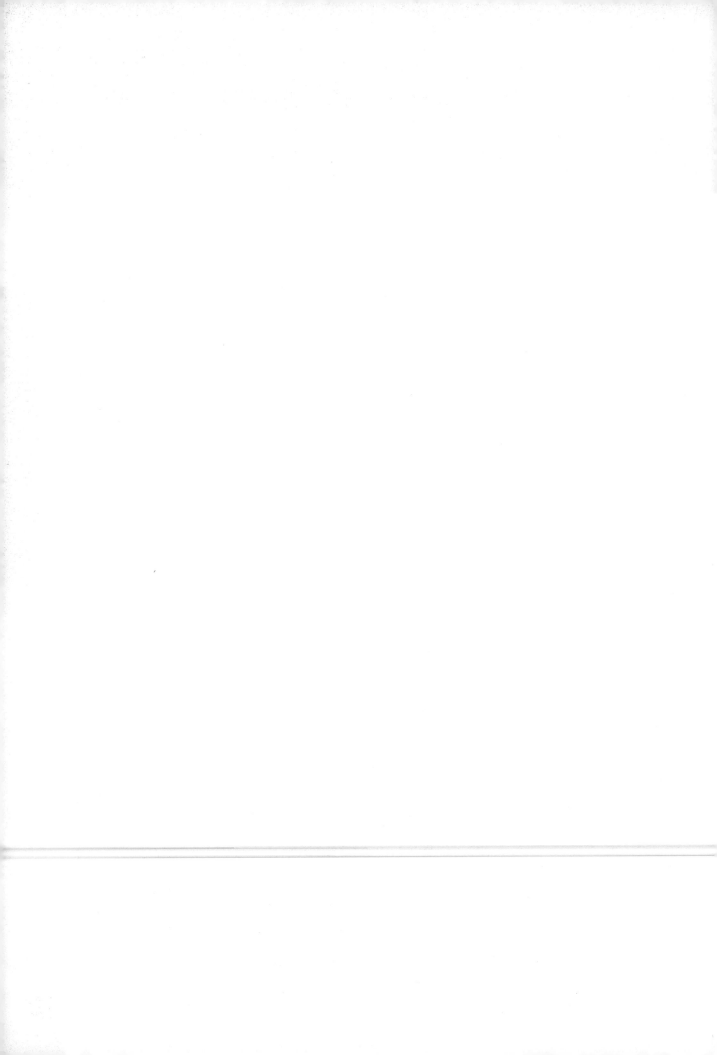

Chapter 26

Benign Fibrous Tumors

Robert L. Satcher Jr, MD, PhD

Desmoid Tumors/Fibromatosis

Desmoid tumors are locally aggressive neoplasms that most commonly occur in men in proximal areas about the shoulder and buttock, followed by the posterior thigh (**Figure 1**), popliteal space, arm, and forearm. They are benign, enlarging tumors without metastatic potential. Despite their benign nature, they can infiltrate and/or engulf surrounding vessels and nerves, causing dysfunction. Desmoid tumor is also referred to as extra-abdominal desmoid tumor, aggressive fibromatosis, or simple desmoid tumor. These tumors are distinct from abdominal desmoid tumors, which are usually seen in young women following pregnancy. Desmoid tumors most commonly occur in older children or young adults. In most patients, a solitary tumor is present. Multicentric involvement can occur in association with the familial adenomatous polyposis (FAP) variant known as Gardner syndrome. Gardner syndrome is now considered a phenotypic variant of FAP and is characterized by polyposis of the large bowel and craniofacial osteomas. It is caused by a mutation in the adenomatous polyposis coli gene (*APC*) located at chromosome band 5q21, and is inherited in an autosomal dominant manner. Intra-abdominal (rather than extra-abdominal or abdominal) desmoid tumors are the most common in patients with FAP.[1,2]

Desmoid tumors originate from muscle fascial planes and can also occur in tendon sheaths, in joint capsules, and inside bone. Clinically and histologically, they resemble low-grade fibrosarcomas, but they are locally aggressive and tend to recur even after complete resection. Compared with sarcomas, desmoids are poorly encapsulated, making them difficult to resect with negative margins.[1,3]

Clinically, desmoid tumors are firm to palpation, and frequently cause pain. They tend to grow along muscle planes and often reach considerable size, leading to restricted joint motion about the shoulder, hip, or knee. Diagnosis requires a biopsy, and microscopically the tumor is heavily collagenized but has a low mitotic index, with an appearance similar to plantar fibromatosis. Longitudinally oriented sheaths of fibro-

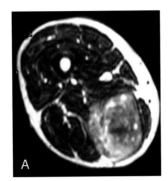
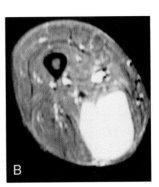
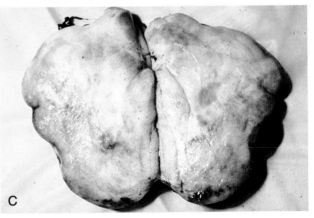
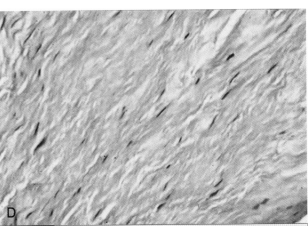

Figure 1 Desmoid tumor of the posterior thigh is shown. **A,** Axial T1-weighted MRI. **B,** Axial T2-weighted MRI. **C,** Resected specimen. **D,** Histologic section of specimen at low power showing fibroblasts with low mitotic index surrounded by collagenous background.

Dr. Satcher or an immediate family member serves as a board member, owner, officer, or committee member of the American Academy of Orthopaedic Surgeons.

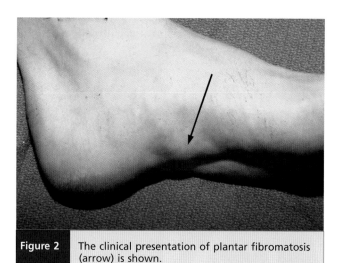

Figure 2 | The clinical presentation of plantar fibromatosis (arrow) is shown.

blasts and myofibroblasts are surrounded by a collagenous background. For desmoid tumors that do not calcify, imaging is best achieved with MRI, where the tumor will be low signal on T1-weighted images, and intermediate to high signal on T2 (**Figure 1**).

In some patients, particularly when the tumor is asymptomatic and found incidentally, observation may be a reasonable form of management. Published data suggest that the disease may stabilize in some patients over time.[4] However, many patients report pain and an enlarging mass. In these patients, the preferred treatment is surgical resection with negative margins. Without additional treatment, recurrences are reported in the range of 25% to 50%.[3] Radiation therapy is an effective adjuvant, usually starting 2 weeks postoperatively, to the extent of 50 Gy to the surgical site. Radiation therapy reduces the chance of local recurrence to 0% to 40%. In patients for whom surgery would be significantly disfiguring or result in increased morbidity, irradiation can be used as the sole treatment. Irradiation doses of 60 to 65 Gy for gross residual disease and 50 to 60 Gy for microscopic residual disease are recommended. Amputation may be necessary in rare cases, usually when the patient has multiple recurrences following radiation therapy. Spontaneous involution of desmoid tumors is rare, but has been reported in patients older than 40 years.

Estrogen may play a role in the development of desmoid tumors. Antiestrogenic agents such as tamoxifen are being used in some centers with some reported clinical benefit. Other adjuvant therapies include NSAIDs. In selected patients with progressive disease, chemotherapeutic agents including low-dose vinblastine and methotrexate also can be used.[2]

Palmar/Plantar Fibromatosis

Fibromatoses are benign, fibrous, clinically aggressive, proliferative processes that occur in the palmar fascia (Dupuytren disease), plantar fascia (Ledderhose syndrome), and penile fascia (Peyronie disease). Palmar fibromatosis is typically seen in older patients and can result in contracture of a finger. Plantar fibromatosis is more common in children and young adults, and usually occurs on the medial portion of the arch of the foot (**Figure 2**). There can be a familial association (in Scandinavians), with a greater incidence in males.[5,6] The etiology is a nodular proliferation of fibrous tissue. On histology, both palmar and plantar fibromas are typically cellular, and can be misdiagnosed as a malignant sarcoma. If the lesions are asymptomatic, observation is warranted. However, if pain results, a simple surgical resection can be performed and can be curative. In the most severe cases, complete fasciectomy may be indicated; partial or subtotal fasciectomy frequently results in local recurrence. Most recently, clinical trials have shown that injections of collagenase clostridium histolyticum are an effective, minimally invasive option for treatment of Dupuytren contracture. In a prospective randomized trial, collagenase clostridium histolyticum injection followed by joint manipulation improved outcomes compared with placebo.[7]

Benign Fibrous Histiocytoma

Benign fibrous histiocytoma (BFH) is typically a cutaneous, solitary, slowly growing nodule that occurs in patients aged 20 to 40 years, most commonly in the extremities. About one third occur as multiple tumors, often in the setting of immunosuppression, but not associated with human herpesvirus 8 as has been demonstrated with Kaposi sarcoma. BFH is a benign tumor composed of a mixture of fibroblastic and histiocytic cells that are often arranged in a cartwheel or storiform pattern. The tumor also occurs, although infrequently, in deep soft tissue and more rarely in parenchymal organs. Tumors in deep tissues tend to be larger than cutaneous tumors. Grossly, they are yellow or white masses that can have focal areas of hemorrhage. BFH is distinguished from the low-grade malignant variant dermatofibrosarcoma protuberans by the presence of foamy and hemosiderin-laden macrophages and multinucleated giant cells.[8,9]

The benign nature of BFH is usually apparent histologically. Deep fibrous histiocytomas usually have a more prominent storiform pattern and fewer secondary elements such as foamy macrophages, compared with cutaneous lesions. BFH is most frequently confused with the benign lesions of nodular fasciitis, neurofibroma, and leiomyoma. The differential diagnosis for aggressive forms of the fibrohistiocytic tumors includes dermatofibrosarcoma protuberans and malignant fibrous histiocytoma. Distinguishing BFH from these tumors is based on immunostaining in addition to histologic features.

Treatment of BFH is wide surgical excision, with no defined role for adjuvant chemotherapy or radiation therapy. Local recurrence rates of 5% to 10% have been reported, with more frequent recurrences for deeper and larger lesions. It is sometimes difficult to predict biologic behavior on the basis of cellular features. Correspondingly, rare metastases have been reported with large (greater than 6 cm), deep tumors that were histologically identical to nonmetastasizing lesions. For this reason, extended follow-up is recommended after surgical removal.[8]

Infantile Digital Fibromatosis

Infantile digital fibromatoses are fibrous proliferations that occur in infancy and childhood, and are most often diagnosed in the first 3 years of life, although confirmed cases have been reported in adolescents and young adults. Compared with the adult analogue, they are characterized by abundant cellularity and the presence of necrosis. Infantile digital fibromas are rare benign neoplasms that are usually confined to the digits. Most lesions are found between toes and fingers, in the exact location where programmed cell death leads to separation of the fetal digits. The usual appearance of the tumor is a flesh-colored or slightly red nodule on the lateral side of the digits. However, histologically identical tumors have been reported in the breast, mouth, hand, upper arm, thigh, and foot. Biopsy is often required to confirm the diagnosis because the lesions are similar in appearance to several benign and malignant lesions.[10,11] On histology the tumor consists of myofibroblasts that contain pathognomonic eosinophilic actin-positive intracellular inclusion bodies. The surrounding stroma is collagenous and dense. The histologic features are relatively aggressive, with proliferation and cellularity. As the tumor ages and degenerates, the number and density of the inclusion bodies decrease. Management of these lesions remains controversial. Excision is recommended rather than amputation, but recurrences are frequent. Spontaneous regression of both solitary and multicentric lesions has been observed, and has led to the advocacy of nonsurgical management by some.

Nodular Fasciitis

Nodular fasciitis is a self-limiting, reactive process that is the most common type of benign fibrous proliferation. It usually occurs in patients age 20 to 40 years, equally affecting men and women. The etiology is a reactive process rather than a neoplastic one. It typically arises spontaneously and rapidly (within a few weeks), and is tender and painful. In addition to its dramatic clinical presentation, tumors can have high cellularity, a high mitotic index, and infiltrative borders, which can lead to erroneous diagnosis as a malignancy. Lesions most commonly occur in the upper extremity, trunk, chest wall, and back, but can occur in almost any connective tissues. Most lesions are less than 2 cm in size but larger lesions do occur. Histologically, larger lesions can be difficult to distinguish from fibrosarcoma. Grossly, the lesions have a grayish-white appearance and can have myxoid changes. The histology is characterized by variable amounts of collagen, fibroblasts, infiltrating lymphocytes, and mucoid material. Marginal excision is usually curative, with a local recurrence rate of 1% to 2%. Spontaneous resolution has also been observed, and no adjuvant therapy is indicated.[5,12]

Solitary Fibrous Tumor

Solitary fibrous tumors principally occur in patients age 40 to 70 years, and most often are located in the thoracic cavity, where they are usually asymptomatic and are discovered incidentally on routine chest imaging. They can exhibit unpredictable behavior, and therefore in some systems are classified as intermediate grade rather than benign. Extrathoracic sites are much less common and include the liver, meninges, skin, respiratory tract, thyroid, orbit nasal passages, and soft tissues of the limbs. The tumor was originally described as a pleural lesion of mesothelial origin. Subsequently, it was shown to lack mesothelial cells, and currently it is defined as a ubiquitous mesenchymal tumor, most likely of fibroblastic origin, containing myxoid changes and containing branching vascular channels that are indistinguishable from those of hemangiopericytoma.[13,14]

Extrapleural solitary fibrous tumors are usually slow growing and asymptomatic (**Figure 3**). Grossly, the lesions are nodular, firm, partially encapsulated, gray-white masses measuring 1 to 25 cm, with occasional myxoid areas, hemorrhage, and necrosis. Larger tumors are associated with hypoglycemia in about 5% of patients because of the secretion of insulin-like growth factors (IGFs) by the tumor. When IGF secretion by the tumor occurs, typical symptoms can include profuse sweating, headaches, restlessness, and, in the most severe cases, disorientation, convulsion, and coma. In contrast to typical hemangiopericytomas, the solitary fibrous tumor is composed of spindle cells, rather than round or fusiform cells, characterized by zones of cells organized in short fascicles, alternating with areas of random arrangement (the "patternless pattern"). There are also usually areas of hyalinization with cells interspersed with dense collagen.[13]

Although the typical solitary fibrous tumor is benign, aggressive behavior and/or malignancy is reported in 10% to 20% of patients. The features correlated with malignancy include increased cellularity, pleomorphism, increased mitotic activity (> 4 mitoses per 10 high-power fields), necrosis, and hemorrhage. Metastases are rare but can develop in lungs, liver, and bone. The recommended treatment of benign extrapleural solitary fibrous tumors is complete marginal excision, followed by close surveillance. For malignant tumors, complete wide excision (with or without adjuvant radi-

4: Soft Tissue Tumors

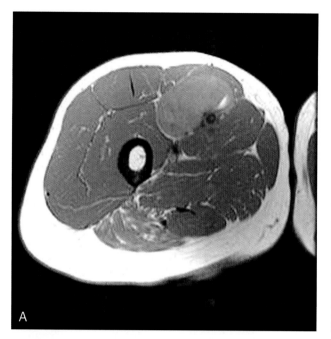

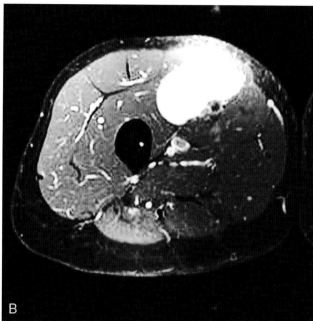

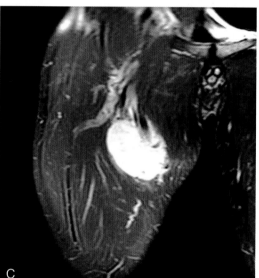

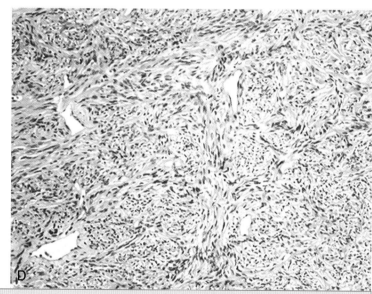

Figure 3 Solitary fibrous tumor of the anterior thigh is shown. **A,** Axial T1-weighted MRI scan. **B,** Axial T2-weighted MRI scan. **C,** Coronal T2-weighted MRI scan. **D,** Low-power magnification shows spindle cells, characterized by zones of cells organized in short fascicles, alternating with areas of random arrangement (the "patternless pattern"). There are also areas of hyalinization with cells interspersed with dense collagen.

ation therapy) is recommended. Preoperative radiation therapy is occasionally used for large tumors regardless of whether the tumor is determined to be benign or malignant from biopsy, on the suspicion that there may be aggressive or malignant areas of the tumor.

cal presentation, natural history, diagnosis, and current treatment options for desmoid tumors, fibromatoses, benign fibrous histiocytosis, infantile digital fibromatosis, nodular fasciitis, and solitary fibrous tumors. Areas of ongoing research and future treatment approaches have been identified.

Summary

It is important for the orthopaedic surgeon to be able to recognize the main features of benign tumors of fibrous origin, and to be knowledgeable about the clini-

Annotated References

1. Gronchi A, Casali PG, Mariani L, et al: Quality of surgery and outcome in extra-abdominal aggressive fibro-

matosis: A series of patients surgically treated at a single institution. *J Clin Oncol* 2003;21(7):1390-1397.

2. Merchant NB, Lewis JJ, Woodruff JM, Leung DH, Brennan MF: Extremity and trunk desmoid tumors: A multifactorial analysis of outcome. *Cancer* 1999; 86(10):2045-2052.

3. Murphey MD, Ruble CM, Tyszko SM, Zbojniewicz AM, Potter BK, Miettinen M: From the archives of the AFIP: Musculoskeletal fibromatoses. Radiologic-pathologic correlation. *Radiographics* 2009;29(7): 2143-2173.

   The authors describe pathologic and clinical features of musculoskeletal fibromatoses. Pathologic features are correlated with radiologic features; treatment options and outcomes are described. Most patients fared well, but cure is difficult because of the infiltrative growth pattern of these tumors. Level of evidence: IV.

4. Nakayama T, Tsuboyama T, Toguchida J, Hosaka T, Nakamura T: Natural course of desmoid-type fibromatosis. *J Orthop Sci* 2008;13(1):51-55.

   A retrospective review of 11 patients with extremity and trunk desmoid fibromatoses who were observed without treatment following diagnosis is presented. Ten tumors eventually stopped growing spontaneously; and three of these tumors also regressed. In one patient, the tumor enlarged and caused a substantial functional deficit. It was concluded that observation can be done in some patients with desmoid tumors, rather than treating. Level of evidence: IV.

5. Konwaler BE, Keasbey L, Kaplan L: Subcutaneous pseudosarcomatous fibromatosis (fasciitis). *Am J Clin Pathol* 1955;25(3):241-252.

6. Rayan GM: Dupuytren disease: Anatomy, pathology, presentation, and treatment. *J Bone Joint Surg Am* 2007;89(1):189-198.

   Anatomy, pathophysiology, clinical features, diagnosis, and treatment options for Dupuytren disease are reviewed. A comprehensive summary of more than 100 articles is provided, with a thorough review of complications from surgical treatments. Level of evidence: V.

7. Hurst LC, Badalamente MA, Hentz VR, et al; CORD I Study Group: Injectable collagenase clostridium histolyticum for Dupuytren's contracture. *N Engl J Med* 2009;361(10):968-979.

   The primary metacarpophalangeal or proximal interphalangeal joints of 308 patients were randomly assigned to receive up to three injections of collagenase clostridium histolyticum (at a dose of 0.58 mg per injection) or placebo in the contracted collagen cord at 30-day intervals. Twenty-six secondary end points were evaluated, and data on adverse events were collected. Collagenase treatment significantly improved outcomes. Three treatment-related serious adverse events were reported: two tendon ruptures and one

case of complex regional pain syndrome. No significant changes in flexion or grip strength, no systemic allergic reactions, and no nerve injuries were observed. Level of evidence: I.

8. Gleason BC, Fletcher CD: Deep "benign" fibrous histiocytoma: Clinicopathologic analysis of 69 cases of a rare tumor indicating occasional metastatic potential. *Am J Surg Pathol* 2008;32(3):354-362.

   The authors describe pathologic details and present a retrospective study of 69 patients with BFH arising from nonvisceral soft tissues. Marginal or incomplete excision was associated with local recurrence. Metastasizing tumors were large but otherwise histologically identical to nonmetastasizing lesions. Level of evidence: III.

9. Fletcher CD: Benign fibrous histiocytoma of subcutaneous and deep soft tissue: A clinicopathologic analysis of 21 cases. *Am J Surg Pathol* 1990;14(9):801-809.

10. Taylor HO, Gellis SE, Schmidt BA, Upton J, Rogers GF: Infantile digital fibromatosis. *Ann Plast Surg* 2008;61(4):472-476.

    The authors provide a review of current knowledge about infantile digital fibromas. The clinical, histologic, and etiologic features of these tumors are discussed. The clinical course following surgery is generally unpredictable, and treatment recommendations remain controversial. Level of evidence: V.

11. Reye RD: Recurring digital fibrous tumors of childhood. *Arch Pathol* 1965;80:228-231.

12. Tomita S, Thompson K, Carver T, Vazquez WD: Nodular fasciitis: A sarcomatous impersonator. *J Pediatr Surg* 2009;44(5):e17-e19.

    The authors present cases of nodular fasciitis that illustrate typical features. The clinical presentation is consistently aggressive. Diagnosis is consequently challenging, and must be made by histology to avoid mistaking this condition for malignancy. Most patients fared well after surgical resection. Level of evidence: IV.

13. Musyoki FN, Nahal A, Powell TI: Solitary fibrous tumor: An update on the spectrum of extrapleural manifestations. *Skeletal Radiol* 2012;41(1):5-13.

    A review of solitary fibrous tumors is presented. Clinical, radiologic, and histologic features are summarized. Treatment is generally surgical, augmented with irradiation. The rate of malignancy is reported to range from 11% to 22%, and malignancy is predictive of poorer outcome. Level of evidence: V.

14. Briselli M, Mark EJ, Dickersin GR: Solitary fibrous tumors of the pleura: Eight new cases and review of 360 cases in the literature. *Cancer* 1981;47(11):2678-2689.

4: Soft Tissue Tumors

Chapter 27

Synovial Chondromatosis and Pigmented Villonodular Synovitis

Bryan S. Moon, MD

Synovial Chondromatosis

Synovial chondromatosis is a rare metaplastic process that occurs in synovium-lined joints. Cells of the synovium produce loose bodies composed of hyaline cartilage. Once formed, these loose bodies remain in the joint cavity and receive nourishment from the synovial fluid. Symptoms eventually occur as a result of mechanical damage and the action of inflammatory mediators.

Etiology

The exact etiology of synovial chondromatosis is unknown. Although karyotype abnormalities and malignant progression have been identified, the process is considered metaplastic rather than neoplastic. The involvement of transforming growth factor–β, fibroblast growth factor, and bone morphogenetic protein has been suggested. Interleukin-6 and vascular endothelial growth factor-A have been suggested as inflammatory mediators.[1,2] In some instances of osteoarthritis, formation of scattered chondroid bodies may be secondary to degenerative changes within the joint.

Clinical Evaluation

Synovial chondromatosis affects more men than women and typically occurs in adults age 30 to 50 years. The knee joint is most commonly affected, followed by the hip, shoulder, elbow, and ankle. Although synovial chondromatosis has a predilection for large joints, it has been reported in smaller joints, such as the temporomandibular joint. The typical symptoms include pain, swelling, loss of motion, popping, catching, and crepitus. These symptoms are similar to those of osteoarthritis. Synovial chondromatosis is not evident on plain radiographs until calcification of the loose body occurs. For these reasons, the diagnosis typically is delayed, and the patient may already have degenera-

tive changes at the first appointment. Although the clinical course typically is benign, there have been rare instances of malignant progression.

Imaging

Findings on plain radiographs are varied. If calcification is minimal, the cartilaginous nodules may be difficult to identify. The nodules are easily seen as they enlarge and calcify (**Figure 1**). The calcification typically is densest at the periphery of the nodule. In advanced disease, joint erosion and advanced degenerative changes can be identified. The differential diagnosis based on plain radiographs includes myositis ossificans and synovial chondrosarcoma. Degenerative changes can produce loose bodies reminiscent of synovial chondromatosis, sometimes called secondary synovial chonodromatosis; however, in this instance there are generally far fewer of the nodules and moderate to advanced degenerative joint disease. Secondary synovial chonodromatosis is treated in accordance with the underlying arthritis.

MRI can lead to an earlier diagnosis because the cartilaginous nodules can easily be identified before calci-

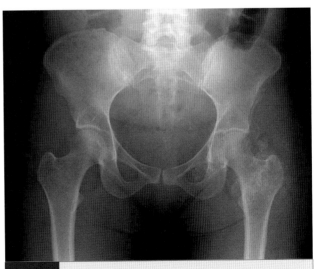

Figure 1 AP radiograph of the pelvis of a patient with synovial chondromatosis of the left hip, in which intra-articular and extra-articular calcified lobules of cartilage can be seen.

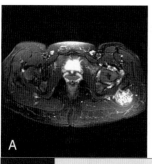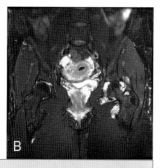

Figure 2 T2-weighted axial (A) and coronal (B) MRI showing synovial chondromatosis of the pelvis and left hip, respectively. Lobules of cartilage with increased signal can be seen centrally, with the low-signal rim indicating peripheral calcification.

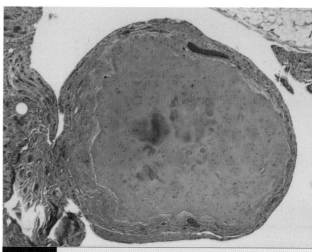

Figure 3 Low-power micrograph (×40) showing synovial chondromatosis. A nodule of cartilage can be seen within the synovial tissue.

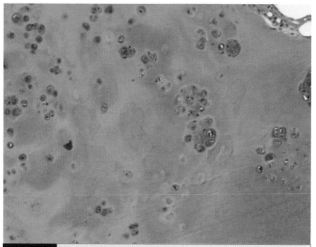

Figure 4 Medium-power micrograph (×100) showing synovial chondromatosis. Foci of increased cellularity can be seen, with clustering of chondrocytes and nuclear enlargement.

fication (**Figure 2**). The nodules are hypointense with T1 weighting and hyperintense with T2 weighting. Any calcifications are seen as signal voids. Joint effusions also can be readily identified. CT is the most precise modality for identifying the mineralization of the nodules and is useful in identifying the extent of joint erosion or degenerative change.

Pathology

Synovial chondromatosis is seen as multiple glistening white loose bodies that typically are small and can number into the hundreds. Occasionally the nodules are large and confluent. Although the nodules typically are loose and free floating in the joint, they also can be found embedded in the synovial lining. Histologically, well-circumscribed nodules of hyaline cartilage are identified with clusters of chondrocytes (**Figures 3** and **4**).

Treatment

The mainstay treatment of synovial chondromatosis is surgical removal of the loose bodies and synovectomy of the joint through an open or arthroscopic approach. Although arthroscopy is a less invasive procedure, the risk of recurrence may be higher than after an open procedure. The synovectomy is more limited with an arthroscopic rather than an open approach, and it may be difficult to arthroscopically remove large loose bodies. The rate of local recurrence has not been clearly defined. In the hip, open treatment may require a dual anterior-posterior approach or dislocation of the femoral head, which can lead to osteonecrosis. An arthroscopic approach therefore may be preferable.[3] If degenerative changes of the involved joint are advanced, the treatment includes joint arthroplasty at the time of synovectomy.

Pigmented Villonodular Synovitis

Pigmented villonodular synovitis (PVNS) is a proliferative disease of the intra-articular and periarticular synovium. It occurs in both nodular (localized) and diffuse forms and typically appears with pain or swelling. The presence of hemosiderin leads to the classic gross and radiographic appearance. Advanced PVNS can cause significant joint destruction.

Etiology

The pathogenesis of PVNS is controversial. Although it has been suggested that PVNS is a reactive process, there is recent evidence that the disease is at least in part neoplastic.[4] A recurrent translocation of t(1p13; 2q35) has been identified that leads to overexpression of the colony-stimulating factor–1 *(CSF1)* gene. *CSF1* recruits reactive macrophages that bear a *CSF1* receptor. These reactive macrophages account for most of

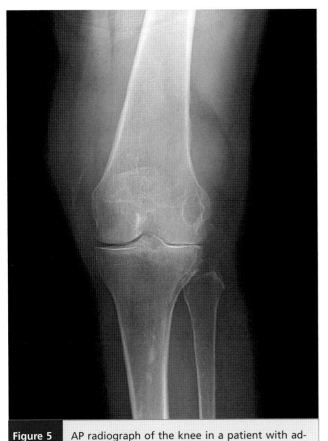

Figure 5 AP radiograph of the knee in a patient with advanced degenerative changes from recurrent PVNS, showing significant bone destruction.

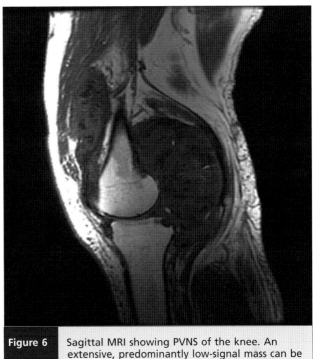

Figure 6 Sagittal MRI showing PVNS of the knee. An extensive, predominantly low-signal mass can be seen in the anterior and posterior joint, with bony erosion.

the cells in PVNS. It has also been postulated that apoptosis resistance may be a critical event that contributes to the progressive nature of the disease.[5]

Clinical Evaluation

PVNS has a slightly higher incidence in women than in men and most commonly occurs in adults age 30 to 50 years. The knee is the most common location, followed by the hip, but any joint can be affected. PVNS usually is monoarticular, but polyarticular disease has been described. PVNS is relatively rare, with an annual incidence of approximately 600 patients per year in the United States. Most PVNS occurs in the diffuse or generalized form of the disease, with abnormal tissue appearing diffusely throughout the joint. A localized form of the disease, presenting with one large mass and sparing the remainder of the joint, has been described and unsurprisingly is associated with a lower relapse rate after surgical treatment.

The clinical course and natural history of PVNS tend to be insidious, with intermittent bouts of joint swelling and discomfort that progress over time. The localized form may appear with only mechanical symptoms, such as popping, catching, and locking, and may be confused with meniscal pathology. The diagnosis may

be made incidentally during arthroscopy, with no preoperative imaging.

In advanced disease, significant joint destruction and bone erosion can lead to pain and dysfunction. The nodules may proliferate so that a soft-tissue mass is palpable, and soft-tissue sarcoma may be suspected. Malignant PVNS is rare.

Joint aspiration can be helpful in diagnosis and alleviation of symptoms until the time of definitive treatment. Although a hemarthrosis is typical, it is not present in all patients. The presence of fluid that is clear or only blood tinged does not rule out the diagnosis of PVNS.

Imaging

Other than showing a joint effusion, plain radiographs may be completely normal. In the more advanced stages of PVNS, severe arthritis, periarticular erosions, and substantial bone invasion may be present (**Figure 5**). MRI is excellent for diagnosing PVNS because it readily shows a synovial mass from villous or nodular synovial proliferation, along with a joint effusion (**Figure 6**). As a result of ferromagnetic hemosiderin deposition, PVNS has the classic diagnostic low signal intensity on all pulse sequences and blooming artifact with gradient echo sequences. The radiographic differential diagnosis includes hemophilic arthropathy, hemorrhagic synovitis, and inflammatory arthropathies.

Pathology

The gross appearance of PVNS classically includes a villous proliferation of synovium that is stained deep

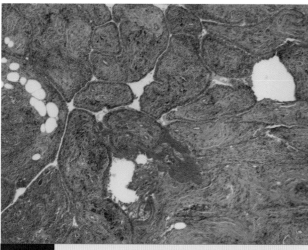

Figure 7 Low-power micrograph (×40) showing PVNS. Villous hyperplasia of the synovium can be seen, with villi containing prominent hemosiderin pigment.

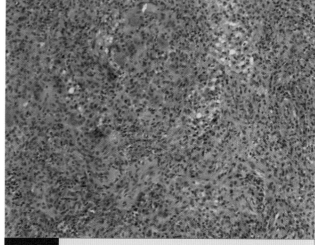

Figure 8 Medium-power micrograph (×100) showing PVNS. The proliferation includes mononuclear fibrohistiocytic cells with foamy and pigment-laden macrophages, as well as giant cells.

brown. The joint is typically laden with this tissue and associated xanthochromic fluid, and in long-standing disease it may have extruded out of the joint capsule into adjacent soft tissues or bursae. On low-power magnification, highly vascularized villous synovium is readily identifiable, and the hemosiderin deposition is easily seen (**Figure 7**). Higher power magnification reveals the presence of pigment-laden macrophages and multinucleated giant cells (**Figure 8**).

Treatment

The mainstay of treatment is surgical resection through complete synovectomy. Open synovectomy is the gold standard for the diffuse villous form, but arthroscopy may be adequate for resection of isolated nodules. In a patient with advanced disease with bone erosion, adequate curettage and bone grafting or cementation of the involved bone also should be performed. Joint arthroplasty at the time of synovectomy is indicated if the degenerative changes are significant.

The recurrence rate after surgical resection is approximately 20% to 30%, although the reported rates vary widely and in part depend on the type of management.[6,7] As a result of concern about the risk of recurrence, other modalities have been used as adjuvant treatments. The primary adjuvants include the use of intra-articular radioisotopes and external beam radiation therapy.[8,9] Although both modalities have reported recurrence rates lower than those of surgery alone, they have not yet gained widespread acceptance because of the limited availability of radioisotopes and the risk of radiation-induced malignancy.

Because of the evidence of a malignant component or uncontrolled aggressive growth in PVNS, chemotherapy may be considered in rare instances. The relative indications for chemotherapy include disease for which resection would result in significant morbidity,

unresectable disease that would require amputation, or multiple recurrences. Tyrosine kinase inhibitors that target CSF1 receptor are occasionally used, generally in recurrent or unresectable disease.

Summary

Synovial chondromatosis and PVNS usually are benign diseases of the synovium. Synovial chondromatosis may be a metaplastic condition, and there is evidence that PVNS has a neoplastic component. Both diseases cause significant local destruction, can locally recur, and have rare malignant counterparts. Surgical resection is the treatment of choice, but adjuvant treatment may be considered for some patients with PVNS.

Annotated References

1. Wake M, Hamada Y, Kumagai K, et al: Up-regulation of interleukin-6 and vascular endothelial growth factor-A in the synovial fluid of temporomandibular joints affected by synovial chondromatosis. *Br J Oral Maxillofac Surg* 2013;51(2):164-169.

   Synovial fluid was analyzed in 10 patients with synovial chondromatosis, and the important role of IL-6 and VEGF-A was described.

2. Nakanishi S, Sakamoto K, Yoshitake H, Kino K, Amagasa T, Yamaguchi A: Bone morphogenetic proteins are involved in the pathobiology of synovial chondromatosis. *Biochem Biophys Res Commun* 2009;379(4):914-919.

   Loose bodies from patients with synovial chondromatosis were analyzed with reverse transcription polymerase chain reaction and immunohistochemistry. The authors proposed that BMPs promote cartilaginous and osteogenic metaplasia.

3. Boyer T, Dorfmann H: Arthroscopy in primary synovial chondromatosis of the hip: Description and outcome of treatment. *J Bone Joint Surg Br* 2008;90(3): 314-318.

    In a study of 120 patients with synovial chondromatosis of the hip, 45 (38%) required open surgery, and 24 (20%) eventually required total hip arthroplasty.

4. Ravi V, Wang W-L, Lewis VO: Treatment of tenosynovial giant cell tumor and pigmented villonodular synovitis. *Curr Opin Oncol* 2011;23(4):361-366.

    The treatment options and molecular biology of PVNS were described, and the neoplastic role in PVNS was supported.

5. Berger I, Aulmann S, Ehemann V, Helmchen B, Weckauf H: Apoptosis resistance in pigmented villonodular synovitis. *Histol Histopathol* 2005;20(1):11-17.

    Immunohistochemistry and flow cytometry were used to analyze the role of apoptosis resistance for sustained cell proliferation in PVNS.

6. Mankin H, Trahan C, Hornicek F: Pigmented villonodular synovitis of joints. *J Surg Oncol* 2011; 103(5):386-389.

    In 215 patients with PVNS treated primarily with surgery, the rate of local recurrence was 1.4%.

7. Ottaviani S, Ayral X, Dougados M, Gossec L: Pigmented villonodular synovitis: A retrospective single-center study of 122 cases and review of the literature. *Semin Arthritis Rheum* 2011;40(6):539-546.

    In 122 patients, there was a 30% rate of recurrence for PVNS of the knee and a 9% rate for PVNS at other sites. Most patients were treated with synovectomy and radioisotopes. The researchers were unable to confirm the usefulness of radioisotopes.

8. Zook JE, Wurtz DL, Cummings JE, Cárdenes HR: Intra-articular chromic phosphate (^{32}P) in the treatment of diffuse pigmented villonodular synovitis. *Brachytherapy* 2011;10(3):190-194.

    The outcomes of nine patients treated for diffuse PVNS with ^{32}P were described. Patients without bulky diffuse PVNS at the time of injection had a better outcome.

9. Park G, Kim YS, Kim JH, et al: Low-dose external beam radiotherapy as a postoperative treatment for patients with diffuse pigmented villonodular synovitis of the knee: 4 recurrences in 23 patients followed for mean 9 years. *Acta Orthop* 2012;83(3):256-260.

    In 23 patients with diffuse PVNS who underwent postoperative radiation therapy, a relatively low dosage (20 Gy) appeared to be as effective as a moderate dosage (35 Gy).

4: Soft Tissue Tumors

Chapter 28

Miscellaneous Benign Soft-Tissue Tumors

Spencer J. Frink, MD   Robert L. Satcher Jr, MD, PhD

4: Soft Tissue Tumors

Introduction

Many of the miscellaneous benign soft-tissue tumors discussed in this chapter are brought to clinical attention because of a palpable mass. Pain is a symptom of some of these tumors. Most are true neoplasms, but others are considered reactive.

Elastofibroma

The elastofibroma is a reactive pseudotumor with an excellent prognosis. It has a peak incidence in the sixth and seventh decades of life, and occurs more commonly in women than men. Most patients have a history of involvement in heavy manual labor or sports that require extensive use of the upper extremities. Autopsy studies have shown that elastofibromas occur in up to 17% of elderly patients. The tumor is an ill-defined mass that almost always occurs between the inferior angle of the scapula and the chest wall (between the latissimus/rhomboid muscles and the chest wall), and is firmly attached to the chest wall in the area of the seventh and eighth ribs posteriorly. They often present with unilateral disease, but up to 60% are bilateral.[1] Clinically, elastofibromas are rarely painful, and patients most often report the symptom of a snapping sensation in the lower portion of the scapula. Occurrence of this tumor is considered secondary to repeated trauma, but a genetic predisposition is suspected in those with a high familial incidence and the rare occasion when it occurs in the gastrointestinal tract.[2,3]

Grossly, the tumor has an appearance similar to a desmoid tumor, and can contain mature fat (**Figure 1**). Histologically, elastofibromas are composed of intertwining eosinophilic collagen fibers and thick elastic fi-

bers. The elastin fibers have a degenerated, beaded appearance, or are fragmented into small globules or droplets that are visualized with antibodies or Verhoeff stain (specific for elastin fiber). CT reveals an inhomogeneous soft-tissue mass with densities approximating muscle, and with poorly defined margins. MRI demonstrates a fairly well-circumscribed mass with intermediate signal intensive on T1-weighted and T2-weighted images with interlaced areas of fat. There is heterogeneous enhancement with gadolinium. Ultrasound can also demonstrate these masses.[4] Simple excision is curative with an extremely low recurrence rate. There are also reports of curative treatment with radiation therapy alone without surgery.[2] There are no reports of malignant transformation.

Giant Cell Tumor of Tendon Sheath

Giant cell tumor of tendon sheath (GCTTS) (also known as nodular tenosynovitis or localized pigmented villonodular synovitis) is a slow-growing, benign soft-tissue tumor that typically occurs as a solitary lesion in the hand. It is the second most common tumor of the hand (after ganglions) and also can occur in other areas, such as the foot, knee, elbow, and wrist.[5] These tumors are more common in adults (30 to 50 years of age).[6] The lesion is rare in children, but when it is found in children, its presentation and treatment are similar to those in adults.[7] Lesions typically appear as a painless mass that has existed for several years. Pain can be a sign of neurovascular bundle involvement.[8]

Histologically, GCTTS is composed of multinucleated giant cells, round to polygonal mononuclear cells, and collagen fibers. Mitotic figures, which occur in more than 50% of patients, can lead to a misdiagnosis of malignancy.[6]

GCTTS has a reported recurrence rate of 9% to 45%.[3] Risk factors for recurrence have included the presence of adjacent degenerative joint disease, location at the distal interphalangeal joint of the finger or interphalangeal joint of the thumb, and the presence of osseous pressure erosions or indentation.[9]

MRI of GCTTS is distinctive and sometimes diagnostic, showing the characteristic low signal intensity

Dr. Satcher or an immediate family member serves as a board member, owner, officer, or committee member of the American Academy of Orthopaedic Surgeons. Neither Dr. Frink nor any immediate family member has received anything of value from or has stock or stock options held in a commercial company or institution related directly or indirectly to the subject of this chapter.

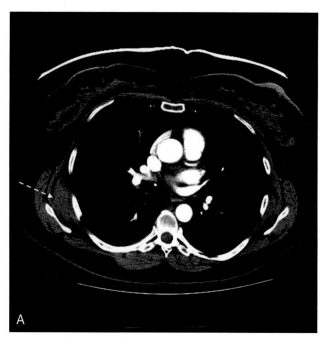

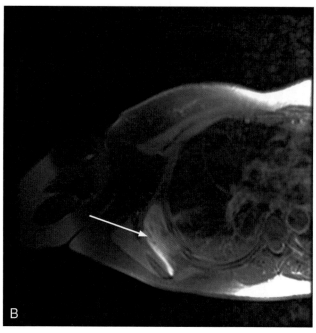

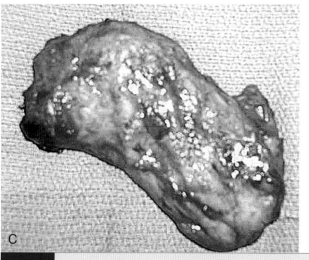

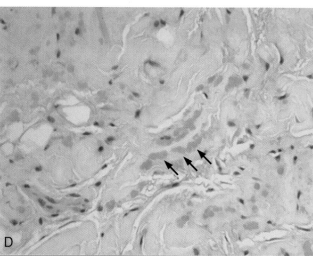

Figure 1   Elastofibroma. **A,** Axial CT scan. **B,** Axial MRI with contrast. **C,** Resected specimen. **D,** Histological section of specimen at low power showing thick elastin fibers with a beaded appearance (arrows).

on both T1-weighted and T2-weighted images (**Figure 2**). Treatment of GCTTS is complete surgical excision under loupe magnification to reduce local recurrence. Recurrent or infiltrative tumors can be treated with radiation therapy with acceptable results.[10] Locally advanced or metastatic GCCTS has recently been treated with imatinib (Gleevec), with 19% of patients having a partial or complete response and 74% having the disease stabilize. Mechanism of action of imatinib is inhibition of the colony stimulating factor 1 (CSF-1) receptor. CSF-1 is overexpressed by tumor cells in GCTTS in a paracrine fashion.[11]

Glomus Tumor

Glomus tumor is a benign neoplastic process named for the identification of cells that resemble the modified smooth muscle cells of the normal glomus body under light microscopy.[6] The normal glomus body is a specialized arteriovenous anastomosis (Sucquet-Hoyer canal) that provides a thermoregulatory function and is likely unrelated to these tumors. These uncommon tumors represent less than 2% of soft-tissue tumors and 1% to 5% of tumors of the upper extremity.[12] They occur in the third through fifth decades with no sex predilection.[13] They appear as small, blue-red nodules in the deep dermis or subcutaneous area of the upper or lower extremity. The most common site is the subun-

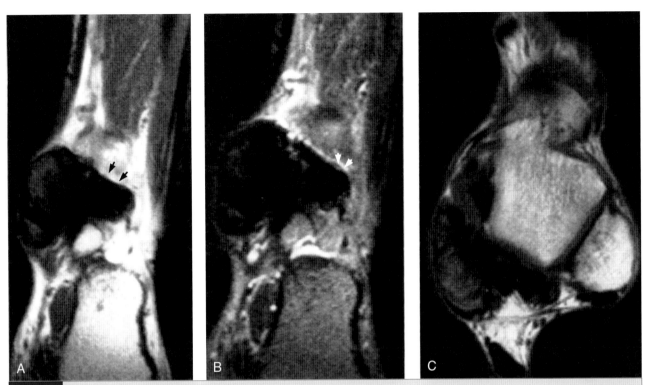

Figure 2   Giant cell tumor of tendon sheath is shown in T1-weighted (**A**), T2-weighted (**B**), and gadolinium postcontrast (**C**) images. The lesion (arrowheads) often appears dark on MRI sequences as a result of high hemosiderin (iron) content.

gual region of the finger, where the tumor occurs more frequently in females (3:1 ratio). Other common locations include the palm, wrist, forearm, and foot.[6] However, glomus tumors can occur in less common locations such as the gastrointestinal tract, the female reproductive tract, mesentery, the trachea, and bone.[14] The lesions are usually solitary, but multiple lesions have been reported in 10% of patients. In the multifocal form, they occur more frequently in children, are usually not in a subungual location, and are less likely to be painful. Multiple glomus tumors are typically associated with a mutation in the glomulin gene, located at chromosome band 1p21-22, which codes for synthesis of the glomulin protein. This mutation is inherited in an autosomal dominant pattern.[15] Multiple glomus tumors have also been associated with neurofibromatosis type 1 due to biallelic loss in the *NF-1* gene.

Glomus tumors produce the characteristic symptom of paroxysms of lancinating pain that is out of proportion to the size of the lesion. The pain is usually elicited by changes in temperature or touch/pressure to the area of the lesion.[16] Subungual glomus tumors can cause nail changes and pressure erosion into the underlying distal phalanx. The mechanism of pain is thought to be mediated by the release of substance P from nerve fibers contained in glomus tumors.

Histologically, glomus tumors can have varying proportions of glomus cells, vascular structures, and smooth muscle tissue. They are categorized into three groups on the basis of these proportions and include glomus tumor proper (75%), glomangioma (20%), and glomangiomyomas. Treatment of glomus tumors involves simple excision.[17] There is a 15% recurrence rate.

Granuloma Annulare

Granuloma annulare represents a group of benign dermatoses of unknown etiology. These include cutaneous (localized, disseminated, and perforating) and subcutaneous types. They typically appear as grouped papules in an enlarging annular shape. They can occur anywhere on the body but occur most often on the lateral or dorsal sides of the hands and feet. When granuloma annulare occurs in the subcutaneous region, it is known as a pseudorheumatoid nodule. This is the form that is most commonly encountered by orthopaedic surgeons and can be mistaken for a possible malignancy (pseudotumorous condition). Subcutaneous granuloma annulare is most common in children 2 to 5 years of age but can occur from infancy to adolescence.[18] It occurs as painless, immobile, usually solitary or clustered masses on the lower extremities. Biopsy is rarely indicated, but histology reveals palisading granulomas with a small area of central necrosis.[19] Imaging studies are not specific, but MRI typically reveals an ill-defined lesion in the subcutaneous fat that does not extend to the

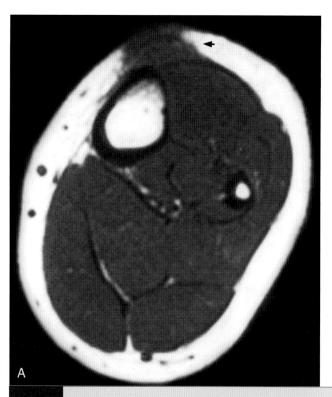
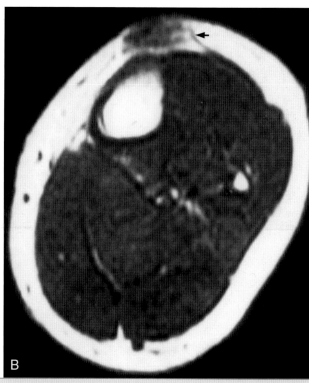

Figure 3 **A,** Subcutaneous granuloma annulare (arrow) is shown in a T1-weighted image. **B,** Subcutaneous granuloma annulare (arrow) is shown in a T2-weighted image.

deep tissue or fascia. The lesions are isointense to muscle on T1-weighted images, are heterogeneously hyperintense on T2-weighted images, and have a variable degree of enhancement.[20]

The cause of granuloma annulare is unknown, but it has been reported to occur following trauma and insect bites as well as in association with chronic disease related to immune dysfunction (viral infections, autoimmune disease, Rosai-Dorfman disease).[21] It is thought to be due to a delayed hypersensitivity and cell-mediated immune response. Granuloma annulare has occurred in association with malignancies, most commonly with lymphoma.[22]

Because granuloma annulare, including the subcutaneous type (**Figure 3**), is a self-limiting condition that resolves spontaneously over several months to 2 years, most patients with granuloma annulare do not require treatment.

Leiomyoma

Leiomyomas are benign smooth muscle tumors that are categorized by location and depth. They include cutaneous leiomyomas, angiomyomas (also called angioleiomyomas or vascular leiomyomas), and leiomyomas of the deep soft tissue.

Cutaneous leiomyomas include those that arise from the arrector pili muscle of the skin and genital leiomyomas, which occur in scrotal, labial, and nipple areas.

Pilar leiomyomas are usually multiple red-brown nodules that coalesce into a linear pattern that follows a dermatomal distribution. They occur in adolescents and young adults. Pain is usually associated with exposure to cold.[6] Treatment of large lesions is surgical, but 50% of patients develop recurrences or new lesions in the same area. Genital leiomyomas are twice as common as pilar leiomyomas. They are small nodules (less than 2 cm) that are not painful. Treatment is observation unless the lesions are symptomatic.[23]

Angiomyomas are thought to originate in the tunica media of veins, and they occur in cutaneous, subcutaneous, and superficial fascial locations. They usually occur as subcutaneous masses in middle-aged women and are painful in 67% of patients. They are found most often in the lower extremity but can occur elsewhere.[24] A unique feature of angiomyomas is an increase in size or swelling of the lesion with physical activity. This increase is often noted when angiomyomas occur in the hand.[25] They have also been reported to cause nerve compression syndromes such as tarsal tunnel syndrome.[26] MRI is nonspecific but shows isointense signal to muscle on T1-weighted images and heterogeneous linear or branching increased signal on T2-weighted images with heterogeneous enhancement. There are usually adjacent tortuous vascular structures.[27] Treatment of angiomyomas is marginal excision.

Leiomyomas of the deep soft tissue are rare tumors that occur either in deep somatic soft tissue with no sex predilection or in the retroperitoneum in women. They

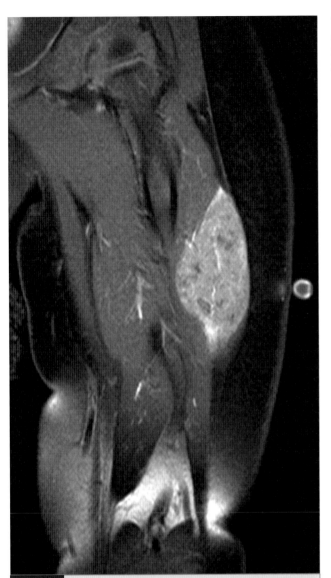

Figure 4 Leiomyoma of deep somatic soft tissue is shown in a T2-weighted fat-suppressed image of the thigh. Benign leiomyomas can occasionally attain large size, as in this example. This makes histologic differentiation from leiomyosarcoma critically important.

test positive for hormone receptors (estrogen receptor and progesterone receptor).[29] Long-term follow-up is necessary to ensure that the tumor is not a low-grade malignancy (**Figure 4**).

Summary

The benign soft-tissue lesions discussed in this chapter are classified on the basis of clinical, radiologic, and histologic characteristics. They include elastofibroma, GCTTS, glomus tumor, granuloma annulare, and leiomyoma. Most require only observation for treatment. Simple excision of symptomatic lesions is usually curative. Exceptions include cutaneous leiomyomas, in which recurrence is common; GCTTS, in which complete excision is necessary to prevent recurrence; and deep-seated leiomyomas, which can be difficult to distinguish from leiomyosarcomas.

Annotated References

1. Nagamine N, Nohara Y, Ito E: Elastofibroma in Okinawa: A clinicopathologic study of 170 cases. *Cancer* 1982;50(9):1794-1805.

2. Järvi OH, Länsimies PH: Subclinical elastofibromas in the scapular region in an autopsy series. *Acta Pathol Microbiol Scand A* 1975;83(1):87-108.

3. Suresh SS, Zaki H: Giant cell tumor of tendon sheath: Case series and review of literature. *J Hand Microsurg* 2010;2(2):67-71.

   The authors retrospectively reviewed 14 patients with GCTTS treated at their institution. There was a predilection for the thumb, and bony changes were noted in two patients. Meticulous excision of all tumor including satellite lesions kept the recurrence rate low (8.3%). The use of loupe magnification or operating microscope is recommended. Level of evidence: II.

4. Ochsner JE, Sewall SA, Brooks GN, Agni R: Best cases from the AFIP: Elastofibroma dorsi. *Radiographics* 2006;26(6):1873-1876.

5. Darwish FM, Haddad WH: Giant cell tumour of tendon sheath: Experience with 52 cases. *Singapore Med J* 2008;49(11):879-882.

   The authors retrospectively reviewed 52 patients with GCTTS treated over a 7-year period. These tumors appeared as painless swelling in the hand and wrist. There was a female predilection. The recurrence rate was 24%. Wide local excision was recommended. Level of evidence: II.

6. Weiss SW, Goldblum JR (eds): *Enzinger and Weiss's Soft Tissue Tumors*, ed 4. St Louis, MO, Mosby, 2001.

   Three retrospective reviews of tenosynovial giant cell tumors and pigmented villonodular synovitis were used for clinical data cited. Level of evidence: II.

occur as large masses and are often diagnosed late because they cause few symptoms. Histologically, they are similar to cutaneous leiomyomas but usually have degenerative or regressive changes such as fibrosis, calcification, or even ossification, which can be seen on radiographs.[6] Surgical treatment is excision with a surrounding margin of normal tissue. Differentiating deep soft-tissue leiomyomas from leiomyosarcomas can be difficult histologically. Some authors suggest that only very low mitotic rates (< 1 mitosis per 50 high-power fields) are acceptable for deep somatic soft-tissue leiomyomas.[28] Retroperitoneal leiomyomas in females should have low mitotic rates (< 10 mitoses per 50 high-power fields), resemble uterine leiomyomas, and

4: Soft Tissue Tumors

7. Gholve PA, Hosalkar HS, Kreiger PA, Dormans JP: Giant cell tumor of tendon sheath: Largest single series in children. *J Pediatr Orthop* 2007;27(1):67-74.

   The authors retrospectively reviewed 29 children with GCTTS. Clinical and radiographic presentation was similar to presentation in adults. Treatment was meticulous dissection and excision using loupe magnification. There were no recurrences after more than 2-year follow-up. Level of evidence: II.

8. Garg B, Kotwal PP: Giant cell tumour of the tendon sheath of the hand. *J Orthop Surg (Hong Kong)* 2011; 19(2):218-220.

   The authors retrospectively reviewed 106 patients with GCTTS. Pain often indicated neurovascular involvement. Patients at high risk for recurrence were treated with radiation therapy with acceptable morbidity. Level of evidence: II.

9. Reilly KE, Stern PJ, Dale JA: Recurrent giant cell tumors of the tendon sheath. *J Hand Surg Am* 1999; 24(6):1298-1302.

10. Coroneos CJ, O'Sullivan B, Ferguson PC, Chung PW, Anastakis DJ: Radiation therapy for infiltrative giant cell tumor of the tendon sheath. *J Hand Surg Am* 2012;37(4):775-782.

    This study was a retrospective review of 58 patients treated at a single center. Fourteen patients had infiltrative tumors and were treated with postoperative radiation therapy. There were no recurrences in patients treated with radiation therapy at 3-year follow-up. Hand function was not adversely affected. Level of evidence: II.

11. Cassier PA, Gelderblom H, Stacchiotti S, et al: Efficacy of imatinib mesylate for the treatment of locally advanced and/or metastatic tenosynovial giant cell tumor/pigmented villonodular synovitis. *Cancer* 2012; 118(6):1649-1655.

    A multi-institutional retrospective study was conducted to examine imatinib mesylate activity in patients with locally advanced and/or metastatic tenosynovial giant cell tumor/pigmented villonodular synovitis. It was shown that the benefits of alleviating morbidity in these patients must be balanced with the likelihood of toxicity of chronic drug therapy.

12. Paliogiannis P, Trignano E, Trignano M: Surgical management of the glomus tumors of the fingers: A single center experience. *Ann Ital Chir* 2011;82(6):465-468.

    The authors reported a single-center experience of four patients with digital glomus tumors. Duplex ultrasound was employed for diagnosis and during surgery to ensure complete excision. Classic symptoms of intense pain and sensitivity to cold were noted preoperatively. Surgical excision was curative with no recurrences.

13. Ozdemir O, Coşkunol E, Ozalp T, Ozaksar K: Glomus tumors of the finger: A report on 60 cases [in Turkish]. *Acta Orthop Traumatol Turc* 2003;37(3):244-248.

14. Schiefer TK, Parker WL, Anakwenze OA, Amadio PC, Inwards CY, Spinner RJ: Extradigital glomus tumors: A 20-year experience. *Mayo Clin Proc* 2006;81(10): 1337-1344.

15. Boon LM, Brouillard P, Irrthum A, et al: A gene for inherited cutaneous venous anomalies ("glomangiomas") localizes to chromosome 1p21-22. *Am J Hum Genet* 1999;65(1):125-133.

16. Heys SD, Brittenden J, Atkinson P, Eremin O: Glomus tumour: An analysis of 43 patients and review of the literature. *Br J Surg* 1992;79(4):345-347.

17. McDermott EM, Weiss AP: Glomus tumors. *J Hand Surg Am* 2006;31(8):1397-1400.

18. Takeyama J, Sanada T, Watanabe M, Hatori M, Kunikata N, Aiba S: Subcutaneous granuloma annulare in a child's palm: A case report. *J Hand Surg Am* 2006;31(1):103-106.

19. Cyr PR: Diagnosis and management of granuloma annulare. *Am Fam Physician* 2006;74(10):1729-1734.

20. Van Hul E, Vanhoenacker F, Van Dyck P, De Schepper A, Parizel PM: Pseudotumoural soft tissue lesions of the foot and ankle: A pictorial review. *Insights Imaging* 2011;2(4):439-452.

    The imaging features of the most common pseudotumors of the soft tissues in the foot and ankle were reviewed. A specific diagnosis was suggested in most cases, when imaging characteristics were combined with lesion location and clinical features.

21. Marie I, Verdier E, Courville P, et al: Rosai-Dorfman disease and granuloma annulare. *Acta Derm Venereol* 2007;87(4):375-377.

    The authors reported on a patient with granuloma annulare associated with Rosai-Dorfman disease (sinus histiocytosis with massive lymphadenopathy). Level of evidence: III.

22. Li A, Hogan DJ, Sanusi ID, Smoller BR: Granuloma annulare and malignant neoplasms. *Am J Dermatopathol* 2003;25(2):113-116.

23. Holst VA, Junkins-Hopkins JM, Elenitsas R: Cutaneous smooth muscle neoplasms: Clinical features, histologic findings, and treatment options. *J Am Acad Dermatol* 2002;46(4):477-490, quiz, 491-494.

24. Freedman AM, Meland NB: Angioleiomyomas of the extremities: Report of a case and review of the Mayo Clinic experience. *Plast Reconstr Surg* 1989;83(2):328-331.

25. Ramesh P, Annapureddy SR, Khan F, Sutaria PD: Angioleiomyoma: A clinical, pathological and radiological review. *Int J Clin Pract* 2004;58(6):587-591.

26. Hamoui M, Largey A, Ali M, et al: Angioleiomyoma in the ankle mimicking tarsal tunnel syndrome: A case report and review of the literature. *J Foot Ankle Surg* 2010;49(4):e9-e15.

    The authors discussed the case of a 64-year-old woman with tarsal tunnel syndrome symptoms due to a subcutaneous angioleiomyoma. Level of evidence: III.

27. Yoo HJ, Choi JA, Chung JH, et al: Angioleiomyoma in soft tissue of extremities: MRI findings. *AJR Am J Roentgenol* 2009;192(6):W291-W294.

    The authors retrospectively reviewed the MRI characteristics of eight patients with angioleiomyomas of the soft tissue. These soft-tissue tumors appeared as a well-demarcated subcutaneous mass of isointense signal on T1-weighted images, heterogeneous high signal intensity on T2-weighted images with homogeneous strong enhancement, and an adjacent tortuous vascular structure in the extremities. Level of evidence: II.

28. Kilpatrick SE, Mentzel T, Fletcher CD: Leiomyoma of deep soft tissue: Clinicopathologic analysis of a series. *Am J Surg Pathol* 1994;18(6):576-582.

29. Paal E, Miettinen M: Retroperitoneal leiomyomas: A clinicopathologic and immunohistochemical study of 56 cases with a comparison to retroperitoneal leiomyosarcomas. *Am J Surg Pathol* 2001;25(11):1355-1363.

4: Soft Tissue Tumors

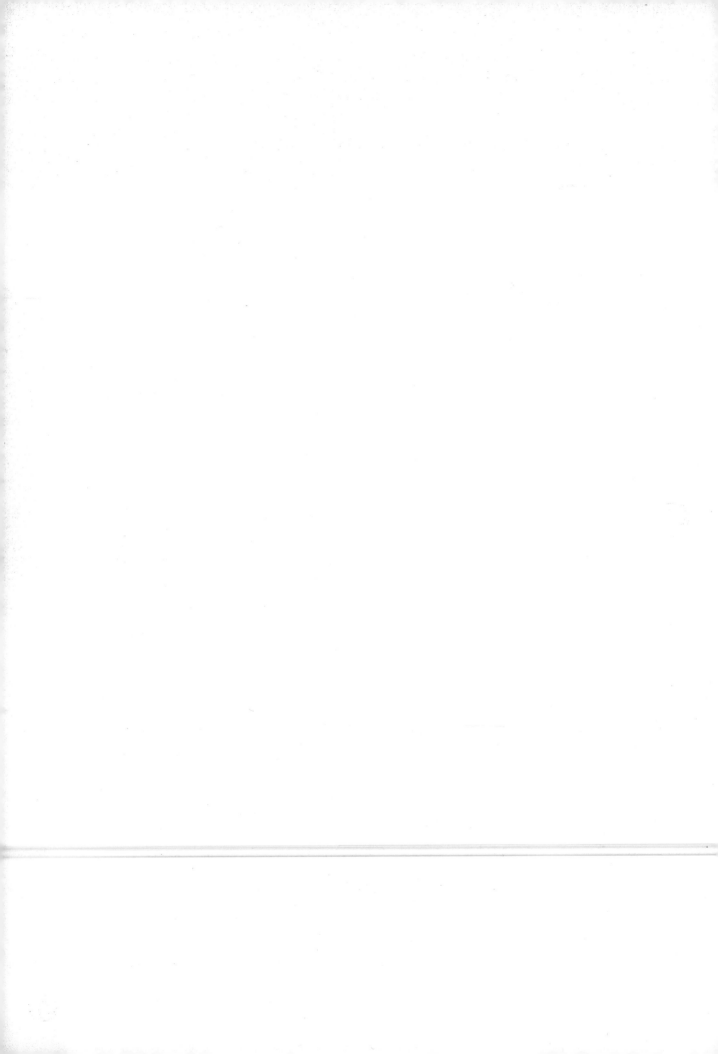

Chapter 29

Soft-Tissue Sarcomas

Robert J. Esther, MD

Introduction

Soft-tissue sarcomas are a relatively rare, heterogeneous group of malignancies. Although research continues into the molecular and cytogenetic pathogenesis of these tumors, their infrequent occurrence and variable clinical outcomes pose ongoing challenges.

Soft-tissue sarcomas arise from mesenchymal tissue. Aside from this presumed common tissue of origin, these types of tumors display an exceedingly wide range of clinical behavior, anatomic location, and histologic findings.

Some of the challenges of treating soft-tissue sarcoma arise from this wide degree of variability. For most patients and clinicians, the notion of cancer brings to mind a painful, rapidly growing mass. Some soft-tissue sarcomas, however, can display indolent clinical characteristics that contrast with their histology and potential for metastasis. This counterintuitive behavior can lead to a delay in seeking medical attention and to unplanned, inadequate initial surgical resections. Soft-tissue sarcomas often cause few local symptoms and many patients have no pain. For this reason, proximal lesions, especially around the thigh and pelvis, can reach significant size before patients seek medical attention (**Figure 1**). Although osseous sarcomas frequently spread into adjacent soft tissues, soft-tissue sarcomas rarely invade bone.[1] Although 25% to 30% of soft-tissue sarcomas occur superficially, most occur deep to investing fascia. The relationship between duration of symptoms and survival is not clearly defined.[2] Despite their malignant nature, sarcomas often respect fascial boundaries. Evidence exists that fascial invasion can portend worse prognosis.[3] Superficial fungating masses can also have a worse outcome.[4]

Incidence and Epidemiology

Approximately 11,000 new cases of soft-tissue sarcoma occur in the United States each year. Compared to other malignancies, these tumors are exceedingly un-common, comprising less than 1% of all cancers in the United States.

Commensurate with the wide array of histologic subtypes, soft-tissue sarcoma affects patients throughout life. Most soft-tissue sarcomas develop during adulthood, but 15% to 20% of tumors develop in patients younger than 15 years. Some types of sarcoma occur more commonly in different age groups. Synovial sarcoma is more commonly seen in younger patients; angiosarcomas and pleomorphic undifferentiated sarcomas are more commonly seen in older adults. Recent data suggest that older patients may develop more clinically aggressive tumors.

Despite improved molecular characterization of soft-tissue sarcomas, their pathogenesis is largely unknown. Although some data correlate the risk of soft-tissue sarcoma with genetic conditions, much remains unknown.[5,6] Definitive tissue diagnosis is possible through open or percutaneous techniques.[7,8]

As with any tumor, treatment involves coordinated multidisciplinary care to manage local and systemic issues. Local treatment of soft-tissue sarcoma is largely successful, with a recurrence rate of 10% to 15%. Local recurrence is multifactorial, with recent data suggesting that margin status, tumor size, and primary versus recurrent status all play a role.[9] Evidence also suggests that older patients may be more likely to experience a recurrence.[10] For instances in which the tumor is large and deep, neoadjuvant or adjuvant radiation therapy should be strongly considered. Systemic therapy is usually reserved for large, deep, high-grade extremity sarcomas, for which meta-analysis has shown an improvement in survival.[11,12] No established role exists for stem cell transplants.[13] Because of the intensity of the doxorubicin-based regimens, greater consideration for chemotherapy is given in younger patients with high-grade tumors. Local recurrence is a challenging clinical problem that can affect prognosis;[14] the relationship between recurrence and survival is uncertain.[15]

Soft-tissue sarcomas typically spread hematogenously to the lungs. Although visceral and skeletal metastases do occur, these events are considerably less common than pulmonary involvement.[16] Nodal disease is also rare and occurs most commonly with certain histologic subtypes: epithelioid sarcoma, synovial sarcoma, clear cell sarcoma, and rhabdomyosarcoma. Staging evaluations typically include local imaging of

Neither Dr. Esther nor any immediate family member has received anything of value from or has stock or stock options held in a commercial company or institution related directly or indirectly to the subject of this chapter.

4: Soft Tissue Tumors

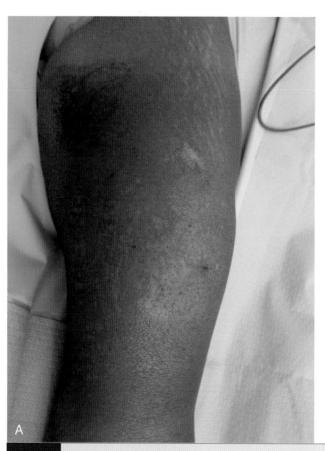 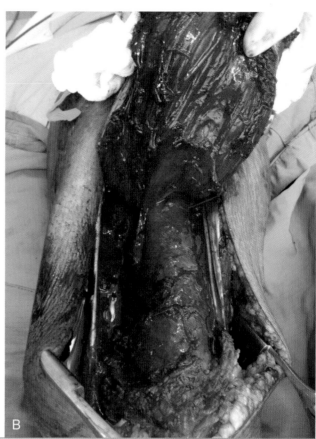

Figure 1 Intraoperative photographs of a high-grade pleomorphic sarcoma in the thigh of a 65-year-old woman. Despite the high grade of the tumor and large size, the mass was painless.

the tumor (plain radiographs, MRI) as well as cross-sectional chest imaging (CT). Given the relatively low incidence of nodal and other nonpulmonary metastases, the role of positron emission tomography (PET) scans in systemic evaluation is not yet fully defined for sarcoma care. Often, sarcomas are more aggressive when they originate from preexisting tumors or other conditions. Malignant peripheral nerve sheath tumors (MPNSTs), for example, can be high grade even though they occur in neurofibromas. Similarly, postradiation sarcomas have a poor prognosis.[17-19]

Staging

American Joint Committee on Cancer Staging System

The staging system used by the American Joint Committee on Cancer (AJCC, **Table 1**) is based on three main characteristics: tumor size, lymph node involvement, and metastatic disease. The system is a modification of the tumor-node-metastasis system. The AJCC system, therefore, is a modification of a staging schema developed for carcinomas.

The most recent modifications of the system included the addition of tumor depth (superficial or deep

to fascia) and transition from three to four histologic grades. Tumor grading is assessed by mitotic figures, cytologic atypia, and extent of necrosis. Grades 1 and 2 are low-grade tumors; grades 3 and 4 are considered high grade. The AJCC system uses nodal involvement as a separate category. As with all staging systems, the AJCC system is useful for classifying tumors, database management at large cancer centers, and communication between providers. As with all staging systems, however, limitations exist regarding the implications of prognosis between different AJCC grades. Also, despite its widespread use, the system also has not been rigorously validated in multi-institutional studies.

Enneking System

The Enneking staging system of the Musculoskeletal Tumor Society (MSTS), developed in 1980,[20] relies on three elements: tumor grade (high or low), anatomic location and extent, and presence of metastatic disease. The system has a more surgical perspective in that the tumor's anatomic site is characterized as intracompartmental or extracompartmental. In contrast with the AJCC system, the MSTS system does not distinguish between nodal and distant metastatic disease, with both entities characterized as stage III disease. Compared to the AJCC system, the Enneking system is not as widely used and is primarily of historic interest, because of its failure to incorporate subsequently discovered prognostic variables, most notably size.

Table 1

American Joint Committee on Cancer Staging System for Soft-Tissue Sarcoma (2010)

Stage IA	Low grade sarcoma, less than or equal to 5 cm without spread to lymph nodes or more distant sites
Stage IB	Low grade sarcoma, larger than 5 cm without spread to lymph nodes or more distant sites
Stage IIA	Intermediate or high grade sarcoma, less than or equal to 5 cm, without spread to lymph nodes or more distant sites
Stage IIB	Intermediate grade sarcoma, larger than 5 cm, without spread to lymph nodes or more distant sites
Stage III	Either high grade sarcoma larger than 5 cm without spread to lymph nodes or more distant sites OR Any grade or size sarcoma that has spread to nearby lymph nodes but not spread to distant sites
Stage IV	Any grade or size sarcoma that has spread to distant sites

Modified from American Joint Committee on Cancer: Soft tissue sarcoma, in Edge SB, Byrd DR, Compton CC, et al, eds: AJCC Cancer Staging Manual, ed 7. New York, NY, Springer, 2010, pp 291-298.

Undifferentiated Pleomorphic Sarcoma

Malignant fibrous histiocytoma (MFH) was a widely used term to describe many high-grade, pleomorphic sarcomas in adults. Over time, the histiocytic origin of these tumors was called into question. Therfore, the current preferred term is undifferentiated pleomorphic sarcoma. Despite the change in terminology and classification of these tumors, use of the term MFH largely persists in clinical practice. The molecular characteristics of these tumors can vary.[21,22] Some of these tumors also display lipogenic markers.[23]

With a slight male predominance, these tumors tend to occur in patients older than 50 years. These tumors usually occur in a subfascial location in the proximal extremities, with a preponderance in the lower extremities. Imaging findings show nonspecific, heterogeneous signal on MRI (**Figure 2**).

Histologically, these tumors show significant pleomorphism and aggressive mitotic activity (**Figure 3**). Pleomorphic sarcomas do not show distinctive characteristics on immunostaining or karyotype analysis, and their negative histochemical staining patterns can help differentiate them from other histologic subtypes.

Lipomatous Sarcomas

Liposarcomas represent a wide range of soft-tissue sarcomas and are the second most common histologic subtype following undifferentiated pleomorphic sarcoma.

Well-differentiated liposarcomas, also known as atypical lipomatous tumors, are slow-growing tumors that usually do not present any significant risk for metastatic

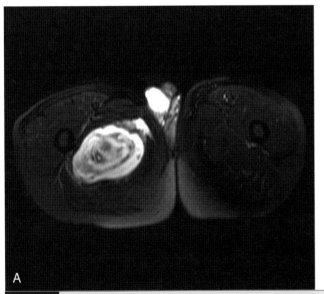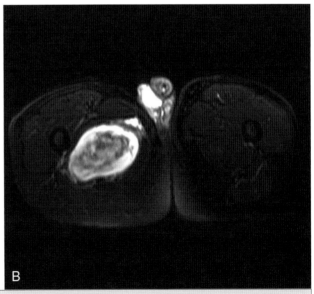

Figure 2 Axial T2 fat-suppressed (**A**) and postcontrast images (**B**) showing an undifferentiated pleomorphic sarcoma of the posteromedial thigh in a 46-year-old man. Note the heterogenous signal and areas without enhancement suggestive of possible necrosis.

spread when located in the extremities (**Figure 4**). Many pathologists use the term atypical lipoma to describe extremity lesions that clinically and histologically are identical to retroperitoneal tumors classified as well-differentiated liposarcoma. Often, classification of this entity as either a well-differentiated liposarcoma or an atypical lipoma is center dependent. In the extremities, these tumors are essentially a local problem with a 5-year local recurrence rate of up to 50%. Treatment involves local resection—usually a marginal or a conservative wide resection—with no role for adjuvant radiation or chemotherapy.

These tumors display very little cellularity and show lipomatous differentiation (**Figure 5**). Karyotype analysis can demonstrate supernumerary ring chromosomes. Amplification of the protein MDM2 and the enzyme CDK4 can also aid in diagnosis.

Dedifferentiated Liposarcoma

A dedifferentiated component occurring in a preexisting, low-grade lipomatous tumor is a rare event (accounting for less than 10% of cases). These dedifferentiated liposarcomas have a heterogenous appearance with areas of nonlipomatous signal on MRI (**Figure 6**) and microscopically show high-grade characteristics juxatoposed with lower-grade lipomatous areas.

Myxoid Liposarcoma

Myxoid liposarcoma tends to occur in adults age 30 to 60 years. As with other sarcomas, patients with myxoid liposarcoma will have few symptoms and the masses can reach significant size, especially in the thigh. The tumors have a myxoid background (**Figure 7**) and display a typical t(12;16)(q13;p11) translocation on karyotype analysis. Prognosis is thought to be worse if the tumor has a significant component of round cell differentiation. Myxoid liposarcoma can metastasize to unconventional, nonpulmonary sites. It is one of the few sarcomas that may benefit from wider surveillance, such as CT scans of the abdomen and pelvis, in addition to chest imaging. Myxoid liposarcoma is also notable for being relatively more responsive to chemotherapy and radiation.

Pleomorphic Liposarcoma

As with dedifferentiated liposarcomas, pleomorphic liposarcomas are rare and account for 5% or less of liposarcomas. Clinically, these tumors occur in patients older than 60 years. These tumors are usually painless and can become large when located in areas such as the thigh or pelvis.

The histologic diagnosis can be challenging because areas of at least focal lipoblastic differentiation must be noted. Documenting such differentiation can be difficult in a large mass. The distinction between a pleo-

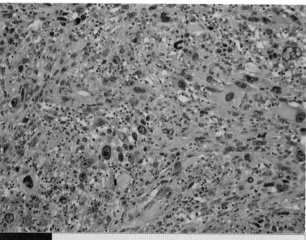

| Figure 3 | High-power photomicrograph of a high-grade pleomorphic sarcoma in a man with Li Fraumeni Syndrome. Note the considerable atypia and frequent number of bizarre-appearing cells arranged in a haphazard fashion. |

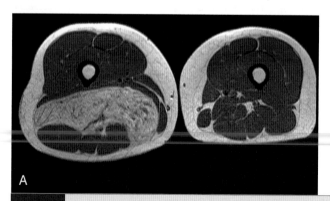
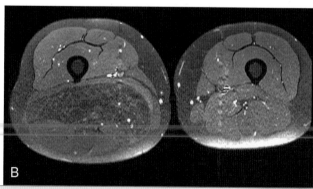

| Figure 4 | Axial T1 (**A**) and postcontrast (**B**) images of an atypical lipomatous tumor/well-differentiated liposarcoma in the posterior thigh of a 48-year-old woman. Note the stranding intermixed between the lipomatous areas of the mass. No significant areas of focal enhancement are seen on the postcontrast images. |

4: Soft Tissue Tumors

morphic liposarcoma and other high-grade soft-tissue sarcomas may be less critical, however, for treatment is largely determined by grade, size, and depth. These tumors have no distinctive immunohistochemical or chromosomal findings.

Synovial Sarcoma

Although the term synovial sarcoma originated because of the tumor's microscopic resemblance to mature synovium, the actual cell of origin is not known. Although these tumors are frequently juxta-articular, they, like other soft-tissue sarcomas, occur within joint spaces extremely rarely. Synovial sarcomas display a wide range of clinical presentations. Considered by convention to be high-grade tumors, some synovial sarcomas occur as large, rapidly-growing masses deep in the extremities. Synovial sarcomas can also be small, clinically indolent neoplasms (**Figure 8, A**). Some tumors can be present for years with little apparent change in size. Synovial sarcomas have also been described as a cause of joint contractures in pediatric patients. This type of tumor can be very challenging for clinicians because of its variable behavior.

Histologically, synovial sarcoma usually demonstrates either monophasic or biphasic architecture (**Figure 8, B**), with epithelioid and spindle-cell areas present. The tumor also has some staining characteristics similar to epithelial tumors. Some pathologists have suggested that the tumor be renamed a carcinosarcoma.[7,24] In some cases, the histology and immunohis-

tochemistry of synovial sarcoma can closely mimic those of an MPNST.

The cytogenetic profile of synovial sarcoma can aid in diagnosis. A characteristic translocation t(X; 18)(p11.2;11.2) is present in most instances. Two transcription products of this chromosomal rearrangement have been characterized: SYT-SSX1 and SYT-SSX2. These findings help confirm a diagnosis of synovial sar-

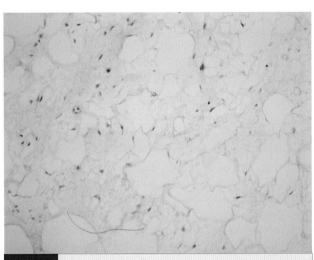

| **Figure 5** | Photomicrograph of atypical lipomatous/well-differentiated liposarcoma. These lesions are bland, hypocellular tumors with occasional lipoblasts. |

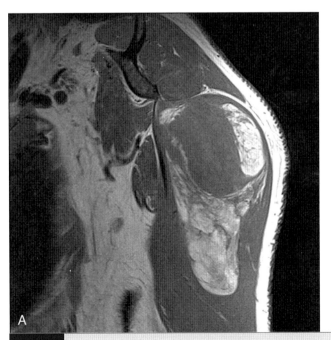
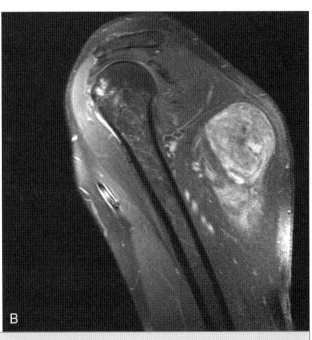

| **Figure 6** | **A,** Sagittal proton density MRI of a dedifferentiated liposarcoma arising in the triceps of a 60-year-old man. Although the tumor has some regions where signal appears fatty, there is a large area of nonlipomatous signal. **B,** Gadolinium-enhanced MRI shows markedly different amounts of enhancement between the low- and high-grade areas of the tumor. |

coma for cases in which the histology and immunohistochemistry may be nonspecific. Moreover, some data suggest that synovial sarcomas with different transcription products can have different clinical outcomes. Poorly differentiated synovial sarcoma is a rare subset of synovial sarcoma with newly recognized molecular attributes.[25]

Synovial sarcoma is considered to be one of the more chemosensitive soft-tissue sarcomas. Because most patients with synovial sarcoma tend to be younger than the average patient with soft-tissue sarcoma, chemotherapy is often discussed with the patient. Despite this fact, adjuvant systemic treatment is largely center dependent and also must account for other variables such as size, depth, grade, patient age, presence of metastatic disease, and comorbidities.

Clear Cell Sarcoma

Clear cell sarcoma is also known as malignant melanoma of soft parts. As with melanoma, clear cell sarcomas have a characteristic immunohistochemistry staining pattern (including positivity for HMB-45, a melanoma marker). A characteristic cytogenetic translocation—t(11;22)(p13;q12)—is also seen in almost all cases. These tumors have also been found to express antiapoptotic protein Bcl-2.[24]

Among soft-tissue sarcomas, clear cell sarcomas have a somewhat distinctive capacity for nodal spread. These tumors most commonly occur in the distal extremities and can be associated with tendon sheaths. As with other soft-tissue sarcomas, clear cell sarcomas can be present for years without substantial change in size. As with some synovial sarcomas, this indolent clinical behavior can lead to errors in diagnosis or delays in

treatment. Given the anatomic constraints in the distal extremities, local management can be very challenging after unplanned resections of these tumors.

Angiosarcoma

Angiosarcomas tend to develp in patients older than 60 years. These lesions are often superficial and, as opposed to other soft-tissue sarcomas, commonly arise in the skin.

Angiosarcomas have a wide degree of histologic variability, although most are high-grade tumors. As commonly seen in mesenchymal tumors, these sarcomas display vimentin positivity on immunohistochemistry. Many display positivity for vascular-specific mark-

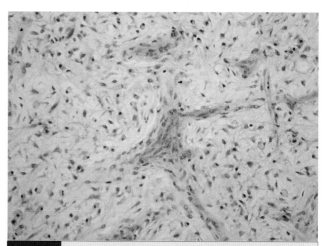

Figure 7   Intermediate-power photomicrograph of myxoid liposarcoma. Note the myxoid stroma, moderate cellularity, and occasional lipoblast.

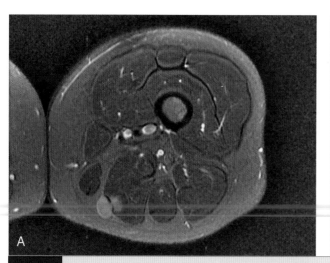

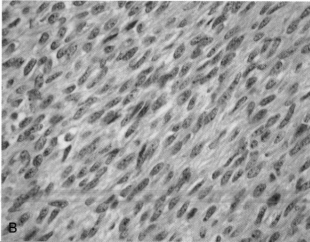

A

B

Figure 8   **A,** T2-weighted axial MRI of a 35-year-old woman with a small, painless posteromedial thigh mass. A portion of the mass is in the substance of the semimembranosus. **B,** High-power photomicrograph of the biopsy specimen of the tumor in **A** demonstrating monophasic synovial sarcoma. Karyotype analysis demonstrated the characteristic t(X; 18)(p11.2;11.2) translocation.

ers. They have no reproducible cytogenetic findings.

Angiosarcomas tend to display aggressive clinical behavior, with local recurrence and pulmonary metastasis as common occurrences. Chemotherapy plays a limited role for these tumors. Moreover, given the increased patient age, toxicity from systemic agents is often not well tolerated. Surgery and radiation therapy can provide good local control, but the possibility for extensive skin involvement can lead to considerable morbidity. Plastic surgery involvement is often required for soft-tissue coverage.

Kaposi Sarcoma

Kaposi sarcoma (KS) is a vascular-based endothelial sarcoma that has a wide range of clinical presentations. There are four forms of KS (**Table 2**). Some forms of KS are associated with immunosuppression from HIV infection or from iatrogenic causes after solid organ transplant. Spontaneous KS can be indolent or aggressive depending on the age of presentation and other clinical variables. The treatment of KS depends on the stage and local extent of disease and involves a combination of resection, chemotherapy, and radiation therapy.

Epithelioid Sarcoma

Epithelioid sarcoma is the most common soft-tissue sarcoma of the hand. As is the case with synovial sarcomas, epithelioid sarcomas can display very slow growth and are easily mistaken clinically for benign lesions such as fibromatosis. Epithelioid sarcomas tend to occur in patients younger than 40 years. Despite their occasional slow growth, these tumors have a high likelihood of local recurrence and pulmonary metastasis.

Epithelioid sarcomas have the capacity to spread to local and regional lymph nodes. The benefit of sentinel node dissection remains unclear for many soft-tissue sarcomas, but may be a reasonable consideration in patients with epithelioid sarcoma.

Grossly, these tumors have a firm consistency. Microscopically, plump, epithelioid-type cells as well as areas of possible central caseation are seen that can mimic benign granulomatous conditions.

Dermatofibrosarcoma Protuberans

Dermatofibrosarcoma protuberans is a typically low-grade, superficial sarcoma that occurs in young adults. A superficial, painless mass develops that can be present for months or years before presentation. These tumors involve the skin and subcutaneous fat (**Figure 9, A**). These tumors are usually nonaggressive and respond well to wide local resection. Given the occasionally extensive superficial location, soft-tissue reconstruction with skin grafting is sometimes required.

These tumors can develop fibrosarcomatous changes (**Figure 9, B**).

Ewing Sarcoma

Extraskeletal Ewing sarcoma and primitive neuroectodermal tumors are considerably more rare than their skeletal counterparts. The local principles of treatment are the same as for other soft-tissue sarcomas, including wide surgical resection and consideration of adjuvant external beam radiation therapy. Unlike many other types of soft-tissue sarcomas, however, these tumors are considered to be relatively chemosensitive and are generally treated with high-dose chemotherapy regardless of tumor size.

Extraskeletal Osteosarcoma

Extraskeletal osteosarcoma tends to occur in older adults. These tumors are very rare and comprise only 1% to 2% of all soft-tissue sarcomas. Most extraskeletal osteosarcomas arise in the deep tissue of the proximal lower extremity. They can display mineralization patterns suggestive of osteoid on plain radiographs.

Histologically, these tumors display findings similar to those seen in their osseous counterparts, with malignant cells producing osteoid. These tumors have no characteristic immunohistochemistry or cytogenetic findings.

The prognosis for extraskeletal osteosarcoma tends to be poor, perhaps related to the fact that these neoplasms are usually high grade in elderly patients. Unlike extraskeletal Ewing sarcoma, not all patients receive chemotherapy because the value of chemotherapy for extraskeletal osteosarcoma is not well established.

Extraskeletal Myxoid Chondrosarcoma

Extraskeletal myxoid chondrosarcoma is a rare soft-tissue sarcoma. These tumors more commonly occur in an older patient population. These tumors can occasionally display calcification suggestive of chondroid tumors on plain radiographs. The designation of these tumors as chondrosarcoma is a misnomer because there no true cartilage is present in the tumors.

Extraskeletal myxoid chondrosarcomas tend to develop in the deep tissues of the lower extremity. They occasionally demonstrate very slow growth, and in some patients may have been present for a considerable time before a health care provider is consulted.

Microscopically, these types of tumors display lobular architecture. Cytogenetic evaluation demonstrates two characteristic translocations: t(9;22)(q22;q12) and t(9;17)(q22;q11). Systemic chemotherapy is not helpful in most cases. Although overall survival is relatively good at 5 years, the disease tends to exhibit slow pro-

Table 2

Vascular Sarcomas

Sarcoma	Clinical	Histopathology	IHC/Genetics	Prognosis
Retiform hemangioendothelioma	Dermis, subcutaneous red/blue plaque Located in distal extremity Locally aggressive Rarely metastasizes Males = Females	Arborizing vascular channels Simulate rete testis No pleomorphism Rare mitoses	IHC: *CD31, CD34, VWF*	Local recurrence up to 60% No distant metastases or death from disease
Composite hemangioendothelioma	Dermis, subcutaneous tissue red/purple mass Swelling Located in distal extremties Males = Females 25% associated with lymphedema	Complex admixture of benign, malignant characteristics	IHC: *CD31, CD34, VWF*	Local recurrence up to 50%
Epithelioid hemangioendothelioma	Higher metastatic potential than RH and CH Affects patients of all ages except young children Males = Females Deep or superficial soft tissue of extremities involving a small vessel Pain is not uncommon Thrombophlebitis Ossification may be present	Fusiform intravascular mass Epithelioid or histiocytoid eosinophilic rounded spindle cells with endothelial differentiation Bland with little mitotic activity Metaplastic bone One third of patients with higher grade characteristics	IHC: *CD31, CD34, FLI1, VWF* 25% to 30% cytokeratin t(1;3)(p36.3;q25)	Local recurrence: 10% to 15%; Metastatic rate: 20% to 30% Mortality: 10% to 20%; High-grade tumors are more aggressive
Kaposi sarcoma	Four subtypes: (1) Classic indolent (2) Endemic African (3) Iatrogenic (4) AIDS-related Location: skin, subcutaneous, distal lower extremity Purple, nodular Affects adults Males > Females	Aggressive vascular pattern with rare mitosis Tumor may progress into angiosarcoma or fibrosarcoma	IHC: *CD31, CD34,* HHV-8, *FLI1* VEGF and FGF implicated in pathogenesis	Function of clinical subtype
Angiosarcoma	1% of all sarcomas Cutaneous > deep Upper extremity Peak occurance in seventh decade of life Males > Females Associated with lymphedema, coagulopathy, anemia, neurofibromatosis, Klippel-Trénauny	Multinodular hemorrhagic masses Anaplastic spindle and epithelial cells Rudimentary vascular channels Reticulum fiber Epithelioid variant	IHC: *CD31, CD34,* and *VWF* Up to one third will express cytokeratin Laminin and type IV collagen occur in the vascular channels Complex karyotypic abnormalities	Risk factors for progression include local recurrence, older age, retroperitoneal location, large size, and high *Ki-67* values

IHC = immunohistochemistry; RH = retiform hemangioendothelioma; CH = composite hemangioendothelioma; VEGF = vascular endothelial growth factor; FGF = fibroblast growth factor
(Reproduced from Randall RL: Malignant soft-tissue tumors, in Schwartz HS, ed: *Orthopaedic Knowledge Update: Musculoskeletal Tumors 2.* Rosemont, IL, American Academy of Orthopaedic Surgeons, 2007, pp277-287.)

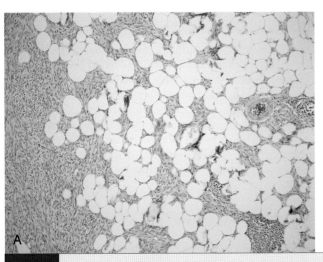 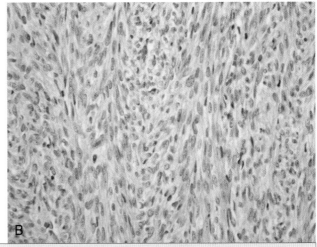

Figure 9 **A,** Low-power photomicrograph of a 42-year-old man with fibrosarcoma arising in the setting of dermatofibrosarcoma protuberans of the skin overlying the deltoid. Note the presence of adipocytes within the section. **B,** High-power photomicrograph showing histopathologic findings of fibrosarcoma seen in other areas of the patient's tumor. Note the nuclear atypia, frequent mitotic figures, and overall cytoarchitecture suggestive of a fibrosarcoma.

gression that can take 10 to 20 years. Up to 50% of patients can develop late pulmonary metastases and local recurrence.

Alevolar Soft-Part Sarcoma

Alveolar soft-part sarcoma usually occurs in patients younger than 30 years. The tumor is more commonly seen in the deep tissues of the proximal lower extremity (thigh and buttock), and is more likely to develop in females. As seen in **Figure 10**, these tumors can have a rich vascular supply and, like other soft-tissue sarcomas, can reach a large size before diagnosis.

Alveolar soft-part sarcoma has an alveolar architectural pattern on histologic examination. A misdiagnosis of alveolar rhabdomyosarcoma is a possibility. Although this type of tumor has aggressive clinical behavior, frequent mitotic figures and nuclear pleomorphism are not characteristically seen. These tumors have no specific immunohistochemical staining patterns. The most commonly seen cytogenetic finding is t (X;17)(p11;q25).

Prognosis is relatively poor for this type of sarcoma. Pulmonary metastases, often appearing early in tumor development, are common. Treatment involves a combination of wide surgical resection with chemotherapy and radiation therapy.

Leiomyosarcoma

Leiomyosarcoma is a relatively uncommon soft-tissue sarcoma. As the name implies, the cell of origin is smooth muscle. These types of tumors occur in an older population, more often affecting women. These tumors can display aggressive local characteristics (**Figure 11**).

Leiomyosarcomas tend to occur more commonly in

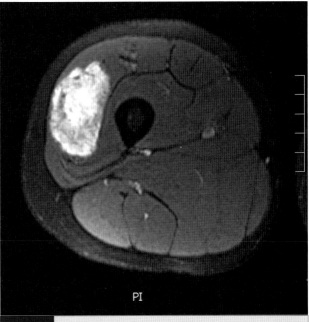

Figure 10 Axial T2 fat-suppressed MRI showing an alveolar soft part sarcoma of the vastus lateralis. The mass, as do most soft-tissue sarcomas, has nonspecific signal characteristics. Its large size and location deep to investing fascia are concerning for possible malignancy.

the retroperiteum and abdomen than in the extremities. These tumors can occasionally be very superficial and associated with veins. Prognosis is thought to be worse for tumors that originate from the venous wall.

Histologic classification of these tumors can be facilitated by immunohistochemistry because leimyosarcomas have strong actin positivity. This type of subclassification does not have a significant bearing on clinical

4: Soft Tissue Tumors

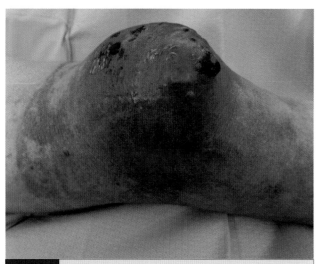

Figure 11   Photograph of a leiomyosarcoma arising from the distal vastus medialis in a 75-year-old woman. She noted rapid growth of the mass and was first evaluated after developing necrotic skin from the fungating tumor.

treatment, however, because tumors are treated locally with the customary combination of wide resection and radiation therapy. Some evidence exists that leiomyosarcomas are not especially sensitive to chemotherapy.[26]

Nerve-Associated Sarcomas

MPNST, once more commonly referred to as neurofibrosarcoma, typically arises secondarily in the setting of multiple neurofibromas. Patients with type 1 neurofibromatosis are at a particularly increased risk for developing MPNST. Typical hallmarks of clinical concern include increasing size and pain in a preexisting asymptomatic neurofibroma. Interest is increasing regarding the use of PET scanning to evaluate neurofibromas for possible malignant change.

Although MPNST usually originates in a longstanding neurofibroma, it tends to exhibit very aggressive clinical behavior. These tumors are typically fast growing and most are high grade. Survival is poor, with reported 5-year survival rates of 30% to 40%. Although these tumors often involve major peripheral nerves, they can also develop in small, unnamed superficial or deep nerves.

MPNST does not have specific histologic findings. Most commonly, fascicles of malignant spindle cells with frequent mitotic figures are seen. Occasionally, epithelioid morphology can make definitive histologic diagnosis more challenging. Tumors are usually positive for S-100 protein and display no characteristic cytogenetic abnormalities.

Summary

Soft-tissue sarcoma remains a broad category that includes a neoplasms with a wide array of histologic and clinical characteristics. Aside from sharing a presumed mesenchymal lineage, these tumors show markedly different histologic and clinical characteristics. For many of these tumors, the actual cell of origin remains unknown. As increasing interest is directed toward the molecular and cytogenetic basis of sarcomas, classification and treatment will continue to be refined.

Annotated References

1. Ferguson PC, Griffin AM, O'Sullivan B, et al: Bone invasion in extremity soft-tissue sarcoma: Impact on disease outcomes. *Cancer* 2006;106(12):2692-2700.

   Soft-tissue sarcomas rarely spread into the adjacent bone. The authors of this study reviewed 874 patients with soft-tissue sarcoma and found that 5.5% had evidence of bone invasion. Bone invasion was associated with a more aggressive clinical course of the tumors and found to be prognostic of lower overall survival. Level of evidence: III.

2. Rougraff BT, Lawrence J, Davis K: Length of symptoms before referral: Prognostic variable for high-grade soft tissue sarcoma? *Clin Orthop Relat Res* 2012;470(3):706-711.

   In a review of 381 patients treated with high-grade soft-tissue sarcoma, the authors did not find that longer symptom length before diagnosis was predictive of overall or disease-free survival.

3. Tsukushi S, Nishida Y, Shido Y, Wasa J, Ishiguro N: Clinicopathological prognostic factors of superficial non-small round cell soft tissue sarcomas. *J Surg Oncol* 2012;105(7):668-672.

   A review of 105 patients with superficial soft-tissue sarcomas showed fascial invasion to be a significant adverse prognostic factor. The authors suggested that this histologic finding could be used to assess benefit of adjuvant treatments. Level of evidence: IV.

4. Potter BK, Adams SC, Qadir R, Pitcher JD, Temple HT: Fungating soft-tissue sarcomas: Treatment implications and prognostic importance of malignant ulceration. *J Bone Joint Surg Am* 2009;91(3):567-574.

   The authors reviewed 24 patients with a high-grade soft-tissue mass with associated skin ulceration and compared results to a cohort without skin breakdown. Ulceration portended a significant difference in outcome this study. Patients with malignant ulceration had a higher rate of metastatic disease and amputation than the control group. Five-year survival of the patients with ulceration was 20% compared with 63% in the control group. Level of evidence: II.

5. Ognjanovic S, Olivier M, Bergemann TL, Hainaut P: Sarcomas in TP53 germline mutation carriers: A

review of the IARC TP53 database. *Cancer* 2012; 118(5):1387-1396.

A review of data in the International Agency for Research on Cancer (IARC) database found that 95.6% of sarcomas occurred in patients younger than 50 years compared with 38.3% in a database reflective of the general population. Level of evidence: III.

6. Mastrangelo G, Coindre J-M, Ducimetière F, et al: Incidence of soft tissue sarcoma and beyond: A population-based prospective study in 3 European regions. *Cancer* 2012;118(21):5339-5348.

    In this population-based study, the authors reviewed findings associated with soft-tissue sarcomas including extremity, retroperitoneum, and viscera. The authors indicated the findings suggest that of a role for sex hormones in the pathogenesis of adult soft-tissue sarcoma should be considered. Level of evidence: III.

7. Adams SC, Potter BK, Pitcher DJ, Temple HT: Office-based core needle biopsy of bone and soft tissue malignancies: An accurate alternative to open biopsy with infrequent complications. *Clin Orthop Relat Res* 2010;468(10):2774-2780.

    The preferred type of biopsy, whether open, image-guided percutaneous, or office-based percutaneous, can vary between centers. The authors reviewed 234 patients who underwent 252 core needle biopsies of musculoskeletal tumors in an outpatient office setting and found a low rate (6%) of nondiagnostic specimens. No biopsy-related complication were reported. The authors noted a minor error rate of 10%, a major error rate of 3%, but no resulting errors in selection of appropriate surgical treatment. Level of evidence: IV.

8. Strauss DC, Qureshi YA, Hayes AJ, Thway K, Fisher C, Thomas JM: The role of core needle biopsy in the diagnosis of suspected soft tissue tumours. *J Surg Oncol* 2010;102(5):523-529.

    The authors reviewed 426 patients with soft-tissue tumors. Outpatient core biopsy without imaging guidance demonstrated the capability to differentiate benign from malignant soft-tissue tumors (97.6% success) with very few complications. Level of evidence: IV.

9. Biau DJ, Ferguson PC, Chung P, et al: Local recurrence of localized soft tissue sarcoma: A new look at old predictors. *Cancer* 2012;118(23):5867-5877.

    The authors reviewed possible contributors to local recurrence in 1,668 patients with localized soft-tissue sarcomas. Using a statistical technique known as a competing risk scenario, the study found that surgical margins, histologic grade, and presentation status (recurrent or primary) were the most significant influences on local recurrence. The authors also suggested that consideration of adjuvant radiation be based on presentation status and margins. Level of evidence: III.

10. Biau DJ, Ferguson PC, Turcotte RE, et al: Adverse effect of older age on the recurrence of soft tissue sarcoma of the extremities and trunk. *J Clin Oncol* 2011; 29(30):4029-4035.

    The authors reviewed 2,385 patients with soft-tissue sarcoma at several institutions. The authors found that increasing age at presentation was associated with an increased risk for metastasis and local recurrence that could not be accounted for by tumor histology or treatment type. Level of evidence: III.

11. von Mehren M, Benjamin RS, Bui MM, et al: Soft tissue sarcoma, version 2.2012: Featured updates to the NCCN guidelines. *J Natl Compr Canc Netw* 2012; 10(8):951-960.

    The authors updated the 2011 guidelines for staging, treatment, and follow-up care for soft-tissue sarcoma.

12. Sarcoma Meta-analysis Collaboration (SMAC): Adjuvant chemotherapy for localised resectable soft tissue sarcoma in adults. *Cochrane Database Syst Rev* 2000; 2:CD001419.

13. Peinemann F, Smith LA, Kromp M, Bartel C, Kröger N, Kulig M: Autologous hematopoietic stem cell transplantation following high-dose chemotherapy for non-rhabdomyosarcoma soft tissue sarcomas. *Cochrane Database Syst Rev* 2011;2:CD008216.

    The authors reviewed 54 studies that reported results from 177 patients who underwent autologous stem cell transplantation and 69 patients who did not. The data were not sufficient to indicate a survival benefit from stem cell transplantation in this patient population. Level of evidence: III.

14. Toulmonde M, Bellera C, Mathoulin-Pelissier S, Debled M, Bui B, Italiano A: Quality of randomized controlled trials reporting in the treatment of sarcomas. *J Clin Oncol* 2011;29(9):1204-1209.

    The authors reviewed 72 randomized clinical sarcoma trials published between 1988 and 2008. Quality of studies was measured using a 15-item instrument from the revised Consolidated Standards of Reporting Trials (CONSORT) statement. Although they found a trend toward improved study quality over time, the authors found that, overall, methodology reporting in sarcoma randomized controlled trials was inadequate. Level of evidence: II.

15. Sawamura C, Springfield DS, Marcus KJ, Perez-Atayde AR, Gebhardt MC: Factors predicting local recurrence, metastasis, and survival in pediatric soft tissue sarcoma in extremities. *Clin Orthop Relat Res* 2010; 468(11):3019-3027.

    The authors reviewed 98 pediatric patients with soft-tissue sarcomas of the extremities treated over an 18-year period. The authors found that local recurrence did not influence the risk for developing metastatic disease. Radiation therapy reduced the risk of local recurrence; chemotherapy did not affect the risk of developing metastatic disease. Level of evidence: II.

16. King DM, Hackbarth DA, Kilian CM, Carrera GF: Soft-tissue sarcoma metastases identified on abdomen and pelvis CT imaging. *Clin Orthop Relat Res* 2009; 467(11):2838-2844.

    The authors reviewed 124 patients with soft-tissue sarcoma and found 16% either presented with or devel-

© 2014 American Academy of Orthopaedic Surgeons

oped abdominal or pelvic metastases. Five percent of patients developed such metastases without pulmonary disease. These results suggest that there may be a role for inclusion of the abdomen and pelvis in staging CT scans. Level of evidence: III.

17. Gladdy RA, Qin LX, Moraco N, et al: Do radiation-associated soft tissue sarcomas have the same prognosis as sporadic soft tissue sarcomas? *J Clin Oncol* 2010;28(12):2064-2069.

The authors reviewed 130 radiation-associated sarcomas treated over a 25-year period at the same institution. They compared findings to a cohort of more than 7,000 soft tissue sarcomas. Disease-free survival was significantly worse in the radiation sarcoma group. Level of evidence: III.

18. Mavrogenis AF, Pala E, Guerra G, Ruggieri P: Post-radiation sarcomas: Clinical outcome of 52 patients. *J Surg Oncol* 2012;105(6):570-576.

The authors reviewed 52 patients with postradiation sarcoma treated over a 26-year period and found the mean latency period of 15 years between radiation and tumor diagnosis. All of the tumors were high grade. Five-year survival was 45%. Level of evidence: IV.

19. Keel SB, Jaffe KA, Petur Nielsen G, Rosenberg AE: Orthopaedic implant-related sarcoma: A study of twelve cases. *Mod Pathol* 2001;14(10):969-977.

20. Enneking WF, Spanier SS, Goodman MA: A system for the surgical staging of musculoskeletal sarcoma. *Clin Orthop Relat Res* 1980;153:106-120.

21. Matsuo T, Shay JW, Wright WE, et al: Telomere-maintenance mechanisms in soft-tissue malignant fibrous histiocytomas. *J Bone Joint Surg Am* 2009;91(4):928-937.

The authors reviewed 43 soft-tissue sarcomas classified as MFH to assess the activity of telomerase, a chromosomal maintenance enzyme. The authors did not find telomerase to be a significant prognostic variable across all patients with MFH. Level of evidence: II.

22. Dei Tos AP: Classification of pleomorphic sarcomas: Where are we now? *Histopathology* 2006;48(1):51-62.

23. Chung L, Lau SK, Jiang Z, et al: Overlapping features between dedifferentiated liposarcoma and undifferentiated high-grade pleomorphic sarcoma. *Am J Surg Pathol* 2009;33(11):1594-1600.

The authors reviewed 15 cases of dedifferentiated liposarcoma and 45 cases of high-grade pleomorphic sarcoma. The authors found that MDM2 and CDK4 markers were present in approximately one fourth of pleomorphic sarcomas, suggesting that some undifferentiated sarcomas may be dedifferentiated liposarcomas. Level of evidence: III.

24. Hisaoka M, Ishida T, Kuo TT, et al: Clear cell sarcoma of soft tissue: A clinicopathologic, immunohistochemical, and molecular analysis of 33 cases. *Am J Surg Pathol* 2008;32(3):452-460.

In a review of 33 cases of clear cell sarcoma, the authors found a mortality rate of 43%, varying histologic patterns, and expression of two fusion proteins: EWSR1-ATF1 and EWSR1-CREB1. The authors also noted diffuse expression of antiapoptotic mitochondrial protein bcl-2. Level of evidence: IV.

25. Nakayama R, Mitani S, Nakagawa T, et al: Gene expression profiling of synovial sarcoma: Distinct signature of poorly differentiated type. *Am J Surg Pathol* 2010;34(11):1599-1607.

Although most synovial sarcomas are either monophasic or biphasic, rare instances of poorly differentiated tumors occur. The authors reviewed 34 cases of synovial sarcoma to better define the genetic basis of poorly differentiated synovial sarcoma. The authors noted a downregulation of neuronal and skeletal genes, and upregulation of genes on locus 8q21.11. These results may give further insight into the pathogenesis of poorly differentiated synovial sarcoma. Level of evidence: IV.

26. Stacchiotti S, Verderio P, Messina A, et al: Tumor response assessment by modified Choi criteria in localized high-risk soft tissue sarcoma treated with chemotherapy. *Cancer* 2012;118(23):5857-5866.

The authors evaluated RECIST and Choi criteria for assessment of response to neoadjuvant chemotherapy (epirubicin and ifosfamide) in soft-tissue sarcoma. The authors found that response to chemotherapy was predictive of better outcome. Leimyosarcoma was the least responsive histologic subtype. Level of evidence: III.

Chapter 30

Surgical Management of Soft-Tissue Sarcomas

Justin E. Bird, MD

Introduction

Soft-tissue sarcomas are rare limb- and life-threatening malignancies that occur at a rate of approximately 11,000 new patients per year in the United States.[1] They arise within tissues of mesenchymal origin such as muscle, ligament, tendon, and nerve. Any suspicious extremity mass should be managed as a sarcoma until proven otherwise. Treatment is recommended on the basis of the histologic grade, anatomic location, the presence and degree of metastatic disease, and both physical and social factors related to the patient. Surgery remains the cornerstone of multimodal treatment; however, current strategies include various combinations of radiation therapy, chemotherapy, and surgery. Although surgery alone can be curative in select patients, adjuvant treatments are indicated in most patients. Despite sophisticated surgical advances over the past few decades, significant variability in patient outcomes exists. Outcomes vary significantly for several reasons; perhaps the most frustrating, however, is treating physicians' poor adherence to surgical principles and recommendations that have been well documented to improve outcomes. Unfortunately, improper referrals, poor adherence to biopsy and surgical recommendations, and ignorance still exist. These factors are modifiable and should be persistently addressed within the larger medical community, wherein many of the management errors occur. One should also remember, however, that sarcomas are a heterogeneous group of malignancies with a great degree of biologic variability, and despite physicians' best efforts, tumor biology plays an important role and cannot be altered by even the sharpest blade, the keenest eye, and the most dutiful set of surgical hands.

Neither Dr. Bird nor any immediate family member has received anything of value from or has stock or stock options held in a commercial company or institution related directly or indirectly to the subject of this chapter.

Imaging

Any patient with a suspected soft-tissue sarcoma should be referred to a specialized center for a comprehensive evaluation that includes a thorough history, physical examination, review of appropriate imaging, and biopsy.[2] The general approach is illustrated in Figure 1.[3] Any mass greater than 5 cm or deep to fascia should be considered suspicious and evaluated appropriately. The preferred method of imaging soft-tissue tumors is MRI, with and without contrast. MRI should include the entire region of interest and provide thin slices with maximum detail in axial, coronal, and sagittal planes. Contrast studies are critical in evaluating sarcomas and should be routinely included. The imaging should be reviewed by the surgical specialist and the radiologist, and when feasible, both parties should review the imaging together so that the radiographic characteristics, involved structures, and overall extent of disease are clearly defined. Ultrasound can be a useful screening tool to determine depth and size of the mass and helpful in demonstrating the internal characteristics of the mass, particularly if there is a cystic component.[4] Ultrasound is also a useful tool in image-guided biopsy techniques and for localizing small tumors intraoperatively. Plain radiographs should be reviewed to evaluate the local bony anatomy to determine if the mass has caused any collateral damage to the bone. Calcifications within the soft-tissue mass can also be visualized on plain radiographs. CT may be used in patients in whom MRI is contraindicated, and is the imaging modality of choice to evaluate the chest for metastatic disease. Whole-body bone scanning is not recommended as a routine staging study. CT scans of the abdomen and pelvis can be useful in certain types of soft-tissue sarcomas, such as myxoid liposarcomas, which may be associated with concomitant visceral or retroperitoneal disease. Certain sarcoma subtypes that spread to lymph nodes with higher frequency are synovial sarcoma, epithelioid sarcoma, angiosarcoma, rhabdomyosarcoma, and clear cell sarcoma. Lymph node evaluation should be performed in these subtypes with available imaging. Positron emission tomography (PET) is still investigational and not part of the routine staging; however, its utility has been shown in monitoring

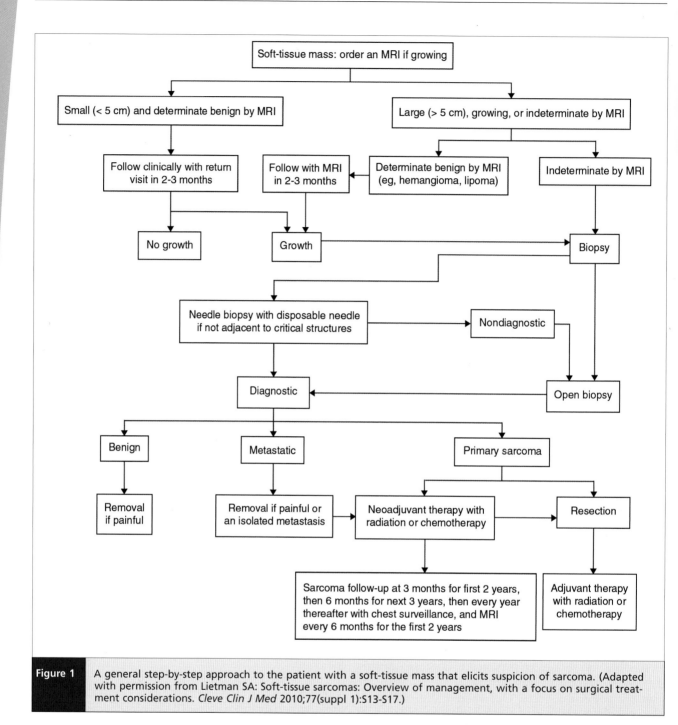

Figure 1 A general step-by-step approach to the patient with a soft-tissue mass that elicits suspicion of sarcoma. (Adapted with permission from Lietman SA: Soft-tissue sarcomas: Overview of management, with a focus on surgical treatment considerations. *Cleve Clin J Med* 2010;77(suppl 1):S13-S17.)

treatment response and evaluating metastatic disease. PET could also be useful in the future for determining safe surgical margins by measuring standardized uptake values (SUVs) in the tissues surrounding the tumor.[5]

Biopsy

The biopsy is a critical aspect in the workup of a patient with a suspected sarcoma and should be managed in a multidisciplinary manner by radiologists and surgeons with specific expertise in this field. Sarcomas are fundamentally dissimilar from their more common epithelially derived counterparts in that en bloc resections are indicated because intraoperative contamination with tumor frequently leads to seeding and local recurrence. As a result, the manner in which the biopsy is performed becomes critically important in determining patient outcomes. Surprisingly, biopsies are performed before resection less than 50% of the time when management is initiated in community-based practices (low volume settings).[6] Unplanned excisions are performed despite the fact that biopsies have been shown to decrease the number of operations that patients with soft-tissue sarcomas undergo to clear their local disease.[5] Core biopsy is currently the standard approach. Core biopsies are performed increasingly by interventional radiologists and less often by surgeons; therefore, clear communication among the members of the team is critical to ensure that surgical options are not compromised. The imaging should be carefully reviewed, and particular areas of concern should be targeted. Multiple cores should be taken through the same tract to maximize diagnostic yield. When feasible, the surgeon should communicate the surgical approach being considered to the person performing the biopsy so that it is performed such that the tract can easily be excised at the time of surgery. This communication can be achieved by marking potential surgical approaches on the patient with permanent marker before the patient's visit with the interventionalist performing the biopsy. The interventionalist can use the marks to plan placement of the needle and its trajectory. To avoid contamination, it is important that adjacent compartments are not crossed during the biopsy.

Incisional biopsy may be necessary if the core biopsy is nondiagnostic. Transverse incisions should routinely be avoided because they lead to contamination of adjacent compartments and may necessitate much wider excision and/or amputation. Maintaining meticulous hemostasis and placing the drain in line with the incision during the biopsy are also critical to prevent contamination.

Fine-needle aspiration (FNA) biopsy is not generally recommended as a primary diagnostic modality because of the limited retrievable tissue volume; however, it may be useful in confirming disease recurrence. Cytologic analysis of fine-needle aspirate can sometimes help establish a diagnosis when performed in conjunction with core biopsy.

Diagnosis

A diagnosis should always be pursued before treatment. This remains true even when a patient with a known primary malignancy has a new soft-tissue mass. Numerous documented cases have clearly demonstrated the serious limb-threatening and life-ending complications that occur when treatments are performed without a clear diagnosis. The pretreatment diagnosis is based on key factors drawn from the comprehensive workup. These factors include elements of the history, constitutional symptoms, physical examination, imaging, and biopsy. Biopsy should not be performed without appreciating the key factors of the comprehensive evaluation, because doing so can lead to improper conclusions. The pathologic diagnosis relies on careful inspection of the morphologic characteristics of the sample. Tissue sampling is therefore extremely important and should be based upon the imaging findings. Morphologic analysis may be complemented by immunohistochemical and molecular analyses if necessary to reach a firm diagnosis.

Staging

Appropriate staging should be performed according to the American Joint Committee on Cancer staging system before surgical treatment. Lymph node evaluation via ultrasound should be considered in the subtypes that have higher incidence of lymph node metastasis (synovial sarcoma, epithelioid sarcoma, angiosarcoma, rhabdomyosarcoma, and clear cell sarcoma). Selected patients with these malignancies may be considered for sentinel node biopsy. Because of the paucity of patients, sentinel node biopsy has not been studied in a randomized fashion to determine its effect on outcome.

Adjuvant Therapy

Radiation Therapy

The goal of radiation therapy is to destroy any microscopic tumor cells that may reside beyond the surgical margin while minimizing damage to important nearby structures. The most common type of radiation therapy is external-beam photon therapy. Newer modalities such as intensity-modulated radiation therapy are designed to decrease the irradiation of important normal structures adjacent to the tumor. Radiation therapy can be performed either preoperatively, intraoperatively, or postoperatively for local control. Preoperative and postoperative radiation strategies have been shown to be equally effective in terms of local control. Preoperative radiation therapy has been shown to be associated with increased postoperative wound complications compared to the standard postoperative treatment (35% versus 17%);[7] however, preoperative radiation therapy has less late toxicity, because less volume is targeted and dosing is less (50 Gy preoperatively compared with 66 Gy postoperatively). Surgery is performed approximately 4 to 6 weeks after completion of radiation therapy for patients undergoing preoperative radiation therapy. Additional radiation therapy can also be done postoperatively if tumor margins are positive. Postoperative radiation therapy can generally be initiated 2 to 3 weeks after surgery, once the incision has healed. Alternatively, brachytherapy can be used postoperatively, although superiority of this technique compared to external-beam photon therapy has not been demonstrated. Brachytherapy requires close cooperation between the surgeon and the radiation oncologist, and is subject to anatomic constraints in the sarcoma tumor bed.

Chemotherapy

Chemotherapy is usually considered either preoperatively or postoperatively in the setting of large, deep, high-grade soft-tissue sarcoma. Chemotherapy regimens are generally based on doxorubicin and ifosfamide; however, individualized therapy based on the patient's particular tumor genomics may provide the

Table 1

Chemosensitivities of Soft-Tissue Sarcomas

Relative Chemosensitivity	Examples of Soft-Tissue Sarcomas
Chemotherapy integral to management	Ewing sarcoma family tumors Embryonal and alveolar rhabdomyosarcoma
Chemosensitive	Synovial sarcoma Myxoid/round cell liposarcoma Uterine leiomyosarcoma
Moderately chemosensitive	Pleomorphic liposarcoma Myxofibrosarcoma Epithelioid sarcoma Pleomorphic rhabdomyosarcoma Leiomyosarcoma Malignant peripheral nerve sheath tumor Angiosarcoma Desmoplastic small round cell tumor Scalp and face angiosarcoma
Relatively chemoinsensitive	Dedifferentiated liposarcoma Clear cell sarcoma Endometrial stromal sarcoma
Chemoinsensitive	Alveolar soft part sarcoma Extraskeletal myxoid chondrosarcoma

(Reproduced with permission from Grimer R, Judson I, Peake D, Seddon B: Guidelines for the management of soft tissue sarcomas. *Sarcoma* 2010;2010:506182.)

best hope for survival in the future. For relatively sensitive sarcomas, therapeutic response not only facilitates surgery but also has valuable prognostic implications. Neoadjuvant treatment has been shown to alter the tumor periphery and promote the formation of a fibrous capsule surrounding the tumor.[8] This finding may improve the ability to achieve local control of disease. Care should be taken to assess the preoperative patient who has undergone neoadjuvant chemotherapy to ensure restoration of sufficient counts of neutrophils and platelets before surgery. Isolated limb perfusion with melphalan and other agents are investigational techniques for delivering high-dose regional chemotherapy and have limited utility.

Small sarcomas and low-grade sarcomas are most commonly considered for surgical treatment alone following biopsy. However, in the case of several sarcomas that are refractory to currently identified chemotherapies, the surgeon may be called upon to perform resection even in the setting of high-grade bulky disease. Relative chemosensitivities are listed in **Table 1**.[2]

Principles of Surgical Management

Surgery is the standard treatment of all patients with localized soft-tissue sarcomas, and should be performed by an appropriately trained surgeon, ideally at a center that specializes in sarcoma management. The goal of surgery is to completely eradicate the primary tumor via excision of the tumor with a cuff of normal tissue.

Goals of Surgical Treatment

The primary goal of sarcoma surgery is to remove all local disease. Secondary goals are to minimize morbidity and maximize postoperative function. Surgery is also important for diagnostic purposes, and surgical biopsy is necessary in certain patients. At times, with massive recurrence, surgery may be necessary for palliation. Sarcomas, more so than carcinomas, create difficult problems in the extremities when they recur.

Surgical Margins

The four categories in the Enneking classification of surgical margins are often based on the histologic analysis of the specimen. The categories are intralesional, marginal, wide, and radical. Limb-sparing surgery with a wide margin is generally preferred, because it can achieve a low rate of recurrence with an acceptable level of morbidity.

Intralesional

The surgical plane runs through tumor. Intralesional procedures are often incomplete resections that leave microscopic and possibly gross tumor behind and are seldom if ever indicated in the treatment of soft-tissue sarcomas.

Marginal

The surgical plane runs extremely close to the tumor, through the pseudocapsule, also known as the reactive zone. The local recurrence rate is high because of tumor satellites in the reactive tissue.

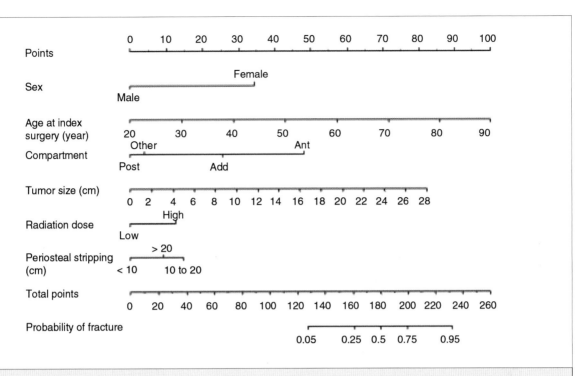

Figure 2 A nomogram to predict an irradiation-associated fracture of the femur after combined modality treatment of a soft-tissue sarcoma of the thigh is shown. A patient's probability of fracture can be calculated by finding the number of points on the top axis (which corresponds to each variable's value for that individual), summing these points, and then drawing a vertical line from the resulting total points axis to the probability of fracture axis. (Reproduced with permission from Gortzak Y, Lockwood GA, Mahendra A, et al: Prediction of pathologic fracture risk of the femur after combined modality treatment of soft tissue sarcoma of the thigh. *Cancer* 2010;116(6):1553-1559.)

Wide
The surgical plane runs through normal tissue surrounding the tumor but within the same anatomic compartment as the tumor. The recurrence rate is low and is presumed to be related to skip lesions in the affected compartment.

Radical
All affected compartments are excised in their entirety. There is a minimal risk of local recurrence.

Neurovascular and Periosteal Considerations
The resectability of the tumor depends, in part, on the relative proximity and involvement of neurovascular structures. Therefore, careful and meticulous study of the preoperative imaging is critical. If the tumor encases vital vasculature, resection can proceed if bypass grafting is feasible; however, complication rates can be high.[9] Careful coordination with a vascular surgeon is important in these cases. Nerve resections are considered if the expected deficit will leave an acceptable degree of meaningful function agreed upon by the surgeon and the patient. As a rule of thumb, one can expect an acceptable degree of function after resection of one major motor nerve. Resection of certain nerves, such as the femoral nerve, result in significant morbidity; therefore, careful preoperative counseling is extremely impor-

tant.[10] Function can be improved with the use of braces, and, in certain patients, nerve grafts and muscle transfers. Soft-tissue sarcomas can abut long bones and require stripping of the periosteum to obtain an adequate margin. Stripping the periosteum more than 10 cm is thought to put the bone at risk for fracture. The risk of fracture increases with radiation therapy, and the nonunion rate of irradiation-associated pathologic fractures after surgical resection of soft-tissue sarcomas is extremely high. Prophylactic intramedullary fixation should be considered on the basis of a combination of high-risk factors. Risk assessment can be performed using the nomogram in **Figure 2**.[11]

Careful and meticulous surgical technique should ensure that a cuff of normal tissue is maintained around the tumor at all times. If the tumor is inadvertently exposed during excision, the defect should be promptly closed. After resection of the tumor, samples of the surgical bed can be sent for frozen analysis, particularly if there is an area of suspicion, or if the resection was marginal because of the presence of neurovascular structures. The surgical bed should be marked with surgical clips to identify areas from which margins were selected. The specimen should be tagged with marking sutures that help the pathologist orient it so that the location of close or positive margins can be communicated to the multidisciplinary team.

Table 2

Factors to Be Considered When Deciding Between Limb Salvage and Amputation

Limb Salvage	Amputation
Low grade	Neurovascular structures encased (no bypass options)
Neurovascular structures free of disease	No adequate soft-tissue coverage options
Adequate margin achievable on imaging	Fungating tumor
Expected residual postoperative function acceptable	Multiple compartments involved (ie, previous surgery, transverse incisions)
Good response to systemic therapy	Palliation in the setting of metastatic disease

---

Limb Salvage Versus Amputation

Limb salvage is appropriate when resection can be performed with a reasonable degree of certainty that negative margins are achievable without causing unacceptable disability (**Table 2**). Soft-tissue sarcomas that involve critical structures that cannot be sacrificed without causing major dysfunction are best managed with amputation. Soft-tissue sarcomas involving the brachial plexus, hand, groin, popliteal fossa, or foot are particularly challenging and often require amputative procedures to achieve negative margins. Although amputation confers a lower local recurrence rate than does limb salvage, similar survival rates can be expected when comparing limb salvage performed with negative margins and amputation.

Wound Management

Resection of large soft-tissue sarcomas results in sizable defects. Meticulous hemostasis should be maintained. Soft-tissue defects may require muscle transfers to fill the void and/or cover vital structures. Wound closure should be performed in layers when possible. Surgical drains should be placed close to and, when possible, in line with the incision to facilitate excision of the tract if a recurrence occurs. Consultation with a plastic surgeon should be done preoperatively whenever feasible,[12] specifically if the surgical defect is expected to be large or if the patient has significant comorbidities that could affect healing. The plastic surgeon may perform muscle flap procedures or transfers either immediately or after a delay (staged) to improve local healing rates. Compressive dressings should be applied after closure to prevent hematoma and seroma formation. Vacuum therapy can be particularly beneficial in large defects. Incisional vacuum therapy (placement of the vacuum sponge over the closed surgical incision; **Figure 3**) has recently been employed and may decrease seroma formation and improve healing rates.[13] Perioperative nutrition should be maximized, and a consultation with a nutritionist should be considered to determine the appropriateness of supplementation.

Surgical Treatment of Local Control Failures

Although local recurrences can occur even in the most experienced hands, the local recurrence rate is higher when treatment is provided by individuals without expertise in the surgical management of soft-tissue sarcomas. Improper surgical treatment generally occurs because the tumor was not worked up appropriately, an unplanned excision without diagnosis was performed, and the basic principles of sarcoma surgery were not followed. Outcomes are generally poor for patients who have undergone improper surgical treatment even when subsequent treatment is performed by experienced sarcoma surgeons.[14] A multimodal treatment strategy should be used for patients who have either positive margins or local recurrence. Restaging should be completed to evaluate the patient for metastatic disease. In the absence of widely metastatic disease, re-excision should be performed when possible to gain local control. Positive margins occur in approximately 15% of re-excisions even when performed by specialized sarcoma surgeons. Amputation may be considered when local treatment options including radiation therapy and surgery are exhausted.

Metastatic Disease

The decision to surgically treat patients with metastatic disease is based on the disease-free period following primary surgery, the location and total number of metastases, observed tumor growth, and overall performance status of the patient. The most common site of metastasis is the lung, and a chest CT scan should be repeated in 3 months to determine if any new lesions have appeared before metastasectomy. In general, metastasectomy for cure can be attempted if all sites of metastasis are amenable to resection.

Surgery may also be indicated for palliation in patients with metastatic disease. Occasionally, major limb amputations can provide improved pain control and function for disease not controllable by other means, even when amputation is not intended to be curative.[15,16]

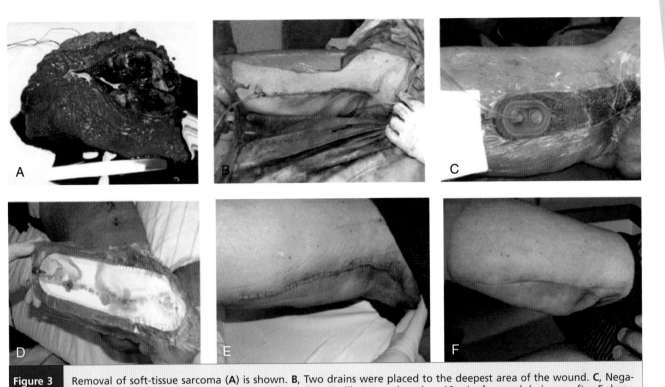

Figure 3 Removal of soft-tissue sarcoma (**A**) is shown. **B**, Two drains were placed to the deepest area of the wound. **C**, Negative pressure wound therapy was applied for 5 days. **D**, There was less than 10 mL of wound drainage after 5 days of negative pressure wound therapy. **E**, Primary healing of incision 14 days after surgery. **F**, Healed incision at 4 months postoperatively. (Reproduced with permission from Stannard JP, Gabriel A, Lehner B: Use of negative pressure wound therapy over clean, closed surgical incisions. *Int Wound J* 2012;9:32-39.)

Complications in Surgical Treatment

Common complications encountered in the surgical treatment of soft-tissue sarcomas include postoperative bleeding, infection, seroma formation, stiffness, chronic lymphedema, pain, fracture, deep vein thrombosis, wound dehiscence, and tumor recurrence. These potential complications should be clearly discussed with the patient before treatment. Complications should be managed early and aggressively to limit the degree of immediate and future morbidity. In large or anatomically unfavorable tumors, some complications including chronic lymphedema and stiffness may be unavoidable. Thorough preoperative counseling can help ameliorate a mismatch between surgeon and patient expectations.

Follow-up

Immediate postoperative follow-up is planned to monitor wound healing and manage the patient's rehabilitation to maximize function. Follow-up thereafter is focused on disease surveillance and generally performed every 3 to 4 months for the first 2 to 3 years, then twice a year for up to 5 years, and then annually.[17] Follow-up visits should include physical examination of the surgical site, inspection for palpable lymph nodes, and appropriate imaging of the surgical site and the chest.

Summary

Tumors that are greater than 5 cm or deep to fascia are considered soft-tissue sarcomas until proven otherwise and are ideally evaluated by a sarcoma specialist, preferably at a multidisciplinary sarcoma center. MRI, appropriate staging studies, and core biopsy should always be performed before definitive surgery. Surgery is the standard treatment of patients with localized soft-tissue sarcoma, in conjunction with adjuvant radiation therapy and/or chemotherapy as appropriate. A wide surgical margin is the goal of resection. Re-resection and radiation therapy are recommended for positive margins and/or unplanned excisions. Patients should have regular posttreatment surveillance with physical examination and imaging of the surgical site, chest, and other anatomic sites at risk for metastasis on the basis of histologic subtypes.

Annotated References

1. American Cancer Society: *Cancer Facts and Figures 2013*. Atlanta, GA, American Cancer Society, 2013.

2. Grimer R, Judson I, Peake D, Seddon B: Guidelines for the management of soft tissue sarcomas. *Sarcoma* 2010;2010:506182.

4: Soft Tissue Tumors

The authors present guidelines drawn from a consensus meeting of UK sarcoma specialists intended to provide a framework for the multidisciplinary care of patients with soft-tissue sarcomas. Level of evidence: V.

3. Lietman SA: Soft-tissue sarcomas: Overview of management, with a focus on surgical treatment considerations. *Cleve Clin J Med* 2010;77(suppl 1):S13-S17.

The author provides a succinct overview of the surgical management of soft-tissue sarcomas and a step-by-step algorithm for the management of suspicious soft-tissue masses. Level of evidence: V.

4. Widmann G, Riedl A, Schoepf D, Glodny B, Peer S, Gruber H: State-of-the-art HR-US imaging findings of the most frequent musculoskeletal soft-tissue tumors. *Skeletal Radiol* 2009;38(7):637-649.

The authors reviewed high-resolution ultrasounds performed between 2000 and 2007 and present common findings in both benign and malignant soft-tissue tumors. They concluded that high-resolution ultrasound is a quick, inexpensive, reliable first-line examination and a useful modality for image-guided core biopsies. Level of evidence: IV.

5. Yokouchi M, Terahara M, Nagano S, et al: Clinical implications of determination of safe surgical margins by using a combination of CT and 18FDG-positron emission tomography in soft tissue sarcoma. *BMC Musculoskelet Disord* 2011;12:166.

The authors compared SUV levels measured on PET to postoperative histopathology. On the basis of the study of 7 patients, they concluded that a safe surgical margin free of viable tumor cells can be ensured if the SUV cutoff level is set at 1.0. FDG PET-CT or PET-CT may be a useful diagnostic imaging technique to determine safe minimal margins for surgical resection of soft-tissue sarcoma. Level of evidence: IV.

6. Guadagnolo BA, Xu Y, Zagars GK, et al: A population-based study of the quality of care in the diagnosis of large (≥5 cm) soft tissue sarcomas. *Am J Clin Oncol* 2012;35(5):455-461.

Using the Surveillance, Epidemiology, and End Results (SEER)–Medicare database, the authors determined that only 40.6% of patients with tumors of 5 cm or larger underwent biopsy as the initial step in the management of their soft-tissue sarcoma. Biopsy was the only significant factor that decreased the likelihood of multiple soft-tissue sarcoma operations. They concluded that biopsies are underutilized and should always be performed for a suspicious mass that is 5 cm or larger, or deep to the fascia. Level of evidence: IV.

7. O'Sullivan B, Davis AM, Turcotte R, et al: Preoperative versus postoperative radiotherapy in soft-tissue sarcoma of the limbs: A randomised trial. *Lancet* 2002;359(9325):2235-2241.

8. Grabellus F, Podleska LE, Sheu SY, et al: Neoadjuvant treatment improves capsular integrity and the width of the fibrous capsule of high-grade soft-tissue sarcomas. *Eur J Surg Oncol* 2013;39(1):61-67.

This histopathologic study compared extremity soft-tissue sarcomas treated with neoadjuvant chemotherapy versus soft-tissue sarcomas treated without neoadjuvant therapy. The authors concluded that neoadjuvant treatment stabilized the tumor periphery and may improve resectability of soft-tissue sarcoma with negative margins. Level of evidence: III.

9. Muramatsu K, Ihara K, Miyoshi T, Yoshida K, Taguchi T: Clinical outcome of limb-salvage surgery after wide resection of sarcoma and femoral vessel reconstruction. *Ann Vasc Surg* 2011;25(8):1070-1077.

The authors present their experience of 15 patients with soft-tissue sarcomas involving vascular structures that were treated with resection and vascular reconstruction. In 12 patients, femoropopliteal reconstruction was performed with a contralateral great saphenous vein graft. In two patients with femoroinguinal reconstruction, expanded polytetrafluoroethylene grafts were used because of unacceptable size discrepancy between the artery and vein graft diameter. Level of evidence: IV.

10. Jones KB, Ferguson PC, Deheshi B, et al: Complete femoral nerve resection with soft tissue sarcoma: Functional outcomes. *Ann Surg Oncol* 2010;17(2):401-406.

The authors present their experience and functional outcomes after complete femoral nerve resection for the treatment of soft-tissue sarcomas in 10 women between 47 and 78 years of age. Six patients sustained fractures from falls related to absent knee extensors. The authors concluded that femoral nerve resections are more morbid than previously anticipated, and nerve-specific functional implications should be considered when counseling patients in preparation for possible resection of the femoral nerve when it is directly involved in a soft-tissue sarcoma. Level of evidence: IV.

11. Gortzak Y, Lockwood GA, Mahendra A, et al: Prediction of pathologic fracture risk of the femur after combined modality treatment of soft tissue sarcoma of the thigh. *Cancer* 2010;116(6):1553-1559.

The authors developed a logistic regression model to assess fracture risk after combined therapy for soft-tissue sarcoma with radiation therapy and surgery. The model was found to have 91% sensitivity and 81% specificity. A nomogram was created for risk assessment. Level of evidence: IV.

12. Marré D, Buendía J, Hontanilla B: Complications following reconstruction of soft-tissue sarcoma: Importance of early participation of the plastic surgeon. *Ann Plast Surg* 2012;69(1):73-78.

A retrospective analysis of 30 patients referred for reconstruction following soft-tissue sarcoma resection demonstrated that early reconstruction decreased the risk of complications. The authors concluded that early involvement of plastic surgeons in the management of soft-tissue sarcoma should be routine. Level of evidence: IV.

13. Stannard JP, Gabriel A, Lehner B: Use of negative pressure wound therapy over clean, closed surgical incisions. *Int Wound J* 2012;9(suppl 1):32-39.

The authors illustrate the clinical use of negative pressure wound therapy on closed surgical wounds. Level of evidence: IV.

14. Venkatesan M, Richards CJ, McCulloch TA, Perks AG, Raurell A, Ashford RU; East Midlands Sarcoma Service: Inadvertent surgical resection of soft tissue sarcomas. *Eur J Surg Oncol* 2012;38(4):346-351.

    The authors reported on 42 patients over a 3-year period who were seen in a sarcoma specialist center after unplanned excision. Limb salvage surgery was not possible in five patients. Level of evidence: IV.

15. Puhaindran ME, Chou J, Forsberg JA, Athanasian EA: Major upper-limb amputations for malignant tumors. *J Hand Surg Am* 2012;37(6):1235-1241.

    A retrospective review of the current indications and patient outcomes after major upper-limb amputations for malignant tumors is presented. Survival after major upper-limb amputation is poor, especially because amputations are reserved for patients with advanced tumors. However, amputation remains an option for local tumor control and can palliate symptoms in selected patients. Improvement of survival requires more effective systemic treatment strategies. Level of evidence: IV.

16. Parsons CM, Pimiento JM, Cheong D, et al: The role of radical amputations for extremity tumors: A single institution experience and review of the literature. *J Surg Oncol* 2012;105(2):149-155.

    Forty patients who underwent forequarter or hindquarter amputations were reviewed. Despite a 91% negative margin rate, 79% of patients had recurrent tumors either locally or distantly. In the absence of nonsurgical options, major amputations are indicated for the management of advanced tumors. These procedures can be performed safely, resulting in effective palliation of debilitating symptoms. Although recurrence rates remain high, some patients can achieve prolonged survival.

17. von Mehren M, Benjamin RS, Bui MM, et al: Soft tissue sarcoma, version 2.2012: Featured updates to the NCCN guidelines. *J Natl Compr Canc Netw* 2012; 10(8):951-960.

    The major changes to the 2012 and 2011 NCCN Guidelines for Soft Tissue Sarcoma pertain to the management of patients with gastrointestinal stromal tumors and desmoid tumors (aggressive fibromatosis). Observation was included as an option for patients with resectable desmoid tumors that are small and asymptomatic, and not causing morbidity, pain, or functional limitation. Sorafenib is included as an option for systemic therapy for patients with desmoid tumors. Level of evidence: V.

4: Soft Tissue Tumors

Metastatic Disease to Bone

SECTION EDITOR:

Joseph Benevenia, MD

Chapter 31

The Pathophysiology of Bone Metastasis

Valerie A. Fitzhugh, MD

Introduction

Tumor metastasis involves growth and arrest in different microenvironments. The process of tumor metastasis involves multiple stages during which malignant tumor cells spread from a primary site to other parts of the body. The behavior of a tumor may be benign or malignant; malignant tumors have the capacity to metastasize. A benign tumor often is well encapsulated, slow growing, noninvasive, and histologically similar to the cell of origin. In contrast, a malignant tumor tends to be poorly encapsulated, invasive, and rapid growing; the cell of origin may be difficult to postulate.[1] Metastasis is unpredictable in many cancers, and many patients are first seen with metastatic disease.

The skeletal system has long been known to be the target of metastasis in many malignant tumors, and bone is one of the organs most commonly invaded by metastatic malignancies. Certain malignancies are believed to be osteotropic; the most common of these in clinical practice are prostate carcinoma and breast carcinoma.[2] In a postmortem study, 70% of patients with one of these two malignancies had evidence of metastatic bone disease.[2] Carcinomas of the lung, thyroid, and kidney also account for a significant percentage of bone metastases. Gastrointestinal carcinomas are responsible for less than 10% of bone metastases; of these, colon carcinomas contribute a significant proportion.[2] Hematologic malignancies also are well known to involve bone.

It has been more than 100 years since Stephen Paget described metastatic disease from his analysis of autopsy reports on 735 women who had died of metastatic breast cancer.[2,3] The result of Paget's research was the classic seed-and-soil hypothesis of metastasis, in which metastasis is likened to the growth of vegetation: the seeds (cancer cells) are able to colonize and grow only in receptive soil (particular environments in the body). Researchers have confirmed and expanded this hypothesis, which forms the basis of many of the general principles of the biology of bone metastasis.

The Biology of Metastasis

Bone is a highly mineralized tissue that contributes both metabolic function and mechanical support to the skeleton.[2] Embryologically, bone is formed by endochondral or intramembranous ossification. At the ends of the long bones, bone formation occurs from a cartilaginous scaffold. In flat bones, such as those of the skull, bone can form from intramembranous ossification, which occurs when mesenchymal precursor cells differentiate into osteoblasts that stimulate bone production.

Bone cells are the basis of production in this metabolically active environment. Recent research and innovation into tumor metastasis to bone has focused on the products of these cells. Osteoclasts are derived from the same precursor as monocytes. Once activated, osteoclasts are responsible for the degradation of bone matrix. Macrophage colony-stimulating factor (M-CSF) and receptor activator of nuclear factor κB ligand (RANKL) are essential to the production of osteoclasts. M-CSF is produced by stromal cells within the bone marrow and is important in the beginning of osteoclast formation, whereas RANKL is involved in the maturation, differentiation, and activation of the osteoclast (**Figure 1**). Matrix metalloproteinases (MMPs) control the bioavailability and function of RANKL, and this function may make them key players in the process of bone metastasis.[4]

Osteoblasts are the producers of bone. Differentiation of the osteoblast is fine tuned by the parathyroid hormone-related protein (PTHrP), an important product that is a focus of current research into bone metastasis. As osteoblasts are embedded into the bone matrix, they undergo terminal differentiation into osteocytes, which further modulate changes in the bone microenvironment.[2]

Bone is composed of an organic matrix that is strengthened by calcium; most of the matrix is composed of type I collagen.[2] Bone is a dynamic substance that turns over 20% of its mass each year through the

Neither Dr. Fitzhugh nor any immediate family member has received anything of value from or has stock or stock options held in a commercial company or institution related directly or indirectly to the subject of this chapter.

5: Metastatic Disease to Bone

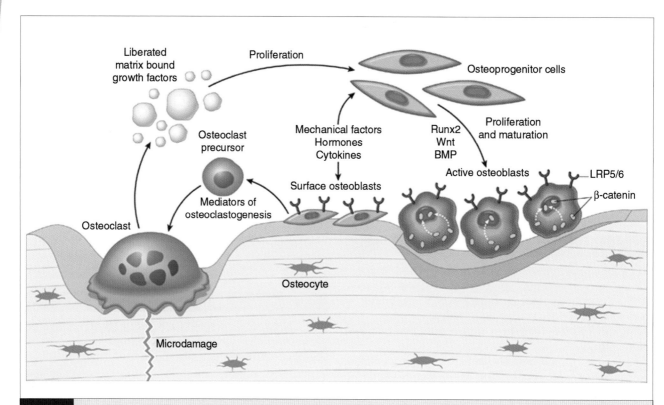

Figure 1 The RANK (receptor activator of nuclear factor-kappa B)-RANK ligand (RANKL) pathway of osteoclastogenesis. RANKL binds to RANK on the osteoclast precursor. Concurrently, interactions with macrophage colony-stimulating factor drive the early stages of osteoclast formation. RANKL is a key molecule in the maturation, differentiation, and activation of the osteoclast. (Adapted with permission from Rosenberg AB: Bones, joints, and soft tissue tumors, in Kumar V, Abbas AK, Fausto N, Aster JC, eds: *Robbins and Cotran Pathologic Basis of Disease*, ed 8. Philadelphia, PA, Saunders Elsevier, 2010, p 1208.)

process of remodeling. Because bone continuously remodels, bone-stored growth factors are continuously released by resorption of bone by osteoclasts.[2] The release of growth factors provides a fertile soil for metastatic tumor cells to reproduce within the bone.

The Physiology of Metastasis

Tumor cells must survive to metastasize. The tumor cells that develop the appropriate genetic changes to survive are transported through the blood to the bone marrow. Within the bone marrow, the tumor cells must adapt to the new environment for continued survival. Tumor cells, and in particular, epithelial tumor cells, are well known to develop a mesenchymal phenotype. In essence, the relatively low cohesion that is characteristic of the mesenchymal phenotype allows cancer cells to migrate away from the main neoplasm to other areas of the body[2,5] (**Figure 2**). Bone is a site in which cancer cells can reproduce exceptionally well.

The first site of interaction between the metastatic tumor cell and the bone marrow is the endothelial cell.[2] The combination of adhesion and chemoattractive molecules within the bone marrow endothelium makes it especially favorable for attracting circulating cancer cells. Stromal-derived factor–1 (SDF-1) induces hematopoietic stem cells of the bone marrow to undergo transmembrane migration mediated by P- and E-selectins. Some carcinoma cells use the same mechanism.[2]

Osteopontin is a major component of bone that mediates motility, survival, local adhesion, and growth by integrins. Cancer cell adhesion to osteopontin is integrin dependent. Therefore, integrins are critical not only in the movement of hematopoietic stem cells to hematopoietic sites but also in bone marrow colonization by cancer cells. Particularly, the integrins $\alpha IIb\beta 3$ and $\alpha v\beta 3$ play a role in bone marrow colonization in several cancers.[2,5]

For malignant cells to enter the bone marrow, they must be able to penetrate the basement membrane and traverse the extracellular matrix. This movement can occur only if the normal balance between proteases and their inhibitors is disturbed.[4,5] The family of MMPs is central to the process of invasion. MMPs play a critical role in the process of bone remodeling, which is necessary for bone metastasis to occur. It is not surprising, then, that MMPs are upregulated in sites in which bone metastasis has occurred.[4] MMPs can be derived from several types of cells within the bone microenvironment, in addition to osteoclasts, osteoblasts, and tumor

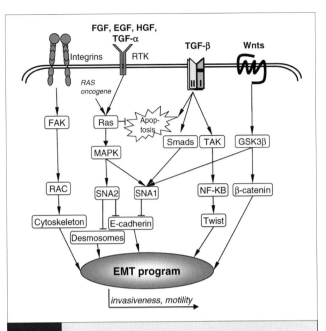

Figure 2 The necessary molecular networks in the epithelial-to-mesenchymal transition (EMT). Epithelial tumor cells are thought to develop from an epithelial phenotype into a mesenchymal phenotype with the involvement of many factors. Transforming growth factor (TGF)–β is thought to be one of the most important molecules in EMT. EGF = epidermal growth factor, FGF = fibroblast growth factor, FAK = focal adhesion kinase, HGF = hepatocyte growth factor, GSK3β = glycogen synthase kinase-3β, MAPK = mitogen-activated protein kinase, NF-KB = nuclear factor–kappa B, RTK = receptor tyrosine kinase, TAK = TGF-β–activated kinase-1. (Adapted with permission from Buijs JT, van der Pluijm G: Osteotropic cancers: From primary tumor to bone. *Cancer Lett* 2009;273[2]:177-193.)

cells.[4] Metastatic tumor cells produce MMPs that are specific to individual tumor types; for example, metastatic breast cancer cells produce MMP-2 and MMP-13. Osteoblasts produce MMPs that are thought to be integral to skeletogenesis. The function of osteoclast MMPs is still unclear.[4]

Although these molecules are important in providing the conditions for metastatic lesions, an event must occur to allow metastasis.[2] Vascular endothelial growth factor–1 (VEGFR1)–positive, bone marrow–derived, hematopoietic progenitor cells were found to be mobilized by factors secreted by tumor cells to create niches in target organs. Remarkably, this premetastatic niche hypothesis assumes that long-range communication exists between the primary malignant cell and the future site of metastasis.[2]

Once cancer cells are in bone, they are required to undergo genetic changes that allow them to establish residence.[5] During this process, called osteomimicry, metastatic tumor cells acquire genetic changes that allow them to produce bone matrix proteins. For example, bone sialoprotein is produced by metastatic breast cancer cells and assists in bone metastasis. Osteopontin is related to bone sialoprotein and also is important in the process of osteomimicry.[5]

Osteolytic bone resorption is key to the establishment of residence in bone. Active osteoclasts are associated with bone metastasis deposits and often are adjacent to these deposits. The ability of the cancer cells to promote the formation of active osteoclasts is a special property of tumors that produce bone metastases and is required for initiating and sustaining tumor expansion. Cancer cells promote the formation of osteoclasts by acting on host bone cells to induce the changes needed for osteoclast generation.[5] Several cancers also directly produce RANKL, an important molecule in osteoclastogenesis.

The hypothesis of the vicious cycle of bone metastasis summarizes the steps in the process of bone metastasis (**Figure 3**). Much of the research into bone metastasis is based on the vicious cycle hypothesis.[4] In the first step of the cycle, bone-lining osteoblasts proliferate and/or differentiate through metastasis-derived signals. PTHrP is a mediator of this process. Bone morphogenetic proteins; fibroblast growth factors (FGFs) such as FGF-9; endothelins; interleukins (ILs) such as IL-1, IL-6, and IL-8; wingless-type (Wnt) signaling pathways; and epidermal growth factor receptor (EGFR) ligands such as transforming growth factor (TGF)–α also have been implicated in the formation of metastatic bone lesions.[4] In the second step, the metastatic cancer cells produce factors that stimulate osteoblasts. The osteoblasts express factors that result in the activation of osteoclasts such as RANKL.[4] The presence of membrane-bound RANKL is an important step in the activation of osteoclast precursors. In the third step, RANKL promotes maturation of the osteoclast precursors into active multinucleated osteoclasts. Mature osteoclasts subsequently form a seal on the mineralized bone matrix surface, and, through acidification and the secretion of acidophilic proteases, mediate the process of bone resorption.[4] Osteoclasts are major mediators of angiogenesis in the bone microenvironment via the regulation of the bioavailability of vascular endothelial growth factor–A (VEGF-A). In addition, bone destruction results in the release of TGF-β, which causes further production of PTHrP, completing the vicious cycle.[4]

Disease-Specific Pathophysiology of Bone Metastasis

Prostate Cancer

Prostate cancer is the second most common cause of deaths from cancer among men in the United States. Androgen-refractory prostate cancer can lead to bone metastasis. More than 80% of all men who die of prostate cancer have some evidence of bone metastasis at autopsy.[6]

Prostate cancers are unusual in that they tend to produce osteoblastic metastases.[7] This process is less well

5: Metastatic Disease to Bone

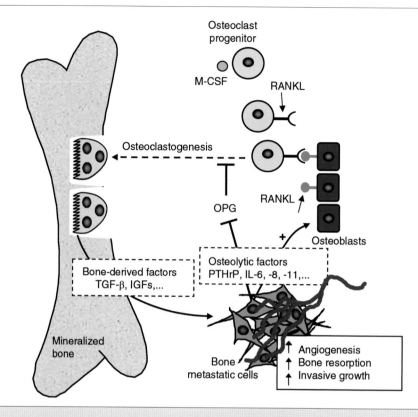

Figure 3	The vicious cycle of bone metastasis. Bone-lining osteoblasts differentiate in response to metastasis-derived signals mediated by parathyroid hormone-related protein (PTHrP). The osteoblasts are stimulated and release M-CSF and RANKL, leading to increased osteoclast production and maturation. Mature osteoclasts secrete acidophilic proteases that mediate bone resorption. The release of TGF-β stimulates the production of PTHrP, thus completing the cycle. IGF = insulin-like growth factor, IL = interleukin, OPG = osteoprotegerin; M-CSF = macrophage colony stimulating factor; RANKL = receptor activator or nuclear factor-kappa B ligand. (Adapted with permission from Buijs JT, van der Pluijm G: Osteotropic cancers: From primary tumor to bone. *Cancer Lett* 2009;273[2]:177-193.)

understood than the processes involving metastasis in osteolytic malignancies such as breast and lung cancers.[7] Endothelin-1 (ET-1) is produced by prostate cancer cells and appears to be a major determinant of osteoblastic bone metastasis, although the mechanism of action has not been fully explained.[7] ET-1 is produced as Big ET-1 and is converted to its active 21 amino acid form by endothelin-converting enzymes.[4] MMP-2 also generates ET-1 from Big ET-1. Therefore, the expression of MMP-2 by metastatic prostate cancer cells might result in the generation of active ET-1, which would lead to osteoblastic bone metastasis.[4]

High-level expression of PTHrP also is seen in prostate cancer metastases. This fact is important because prostate-specific antigen, which has extremely high concentration in prostate cancer metastasis, deactivates the osteolytic effects of PTHrP, thereby stimulating bone formation.[7] This factor may be important in the formation of osteoblastic bone metastasis. Additional growth factors implicated in osteoblastic bone metastasis of prostate cancer include TGF-β, bone morphogenetic proteins, platelet-derived growth factor, FGF, and insulinlike growth factor.[7]

Recently, microRNAs 143 and 145 were implicated

in the epithelial-to-mesenchymal transition in prostate carcinoma, and they have been shown to be upregulated in prostate cancer with bone metastases.[8] These markers may be useful as predictive biomarkers for bone metastasis, and they may serve as a therapeutic target.[8] Another recent study found upregulation of katanin p60 in prostate cancer progression.[6] Katanin p60 is a microtubule-severing protein that is involved in microtubule cytoskeleton organization in nonmitotic and mitotic processes. Although its role in cancer metastasis is unknown, it is aberrantly expressed during prostate cancer progression. Elevation of katanin p60 may contribute to prostate cancer metastasis through a stimulatory effect on cell motility.[6] These research findings may have a future role in the development of a therapeutic target.

Breast Cancer
Breast cancer is the second most common cause of deaths from cancer among women in the United States. Approximately 70% of patients with advanced breast cancer have bone metastasis.[9] The proximal long bones, pelvis, spine, and ribs are most commonly involved.

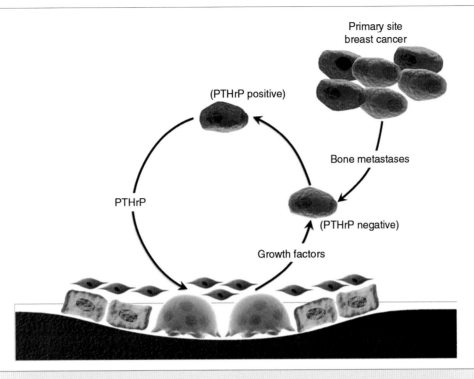

Figure 4 The phenotype of breast cancer cells can be PTHrP negative (purple) or PTHrP positive (green). PTHrP-negative cells have a higher rate of bone metastasis. When these cells reach bone, they convert to a PTHrP-positive phenotype, and the change facilitates the vicious cycle of osteolytic bone metastasis. Blue = stroma, gray = bone, green square = osteoblasts, pink = osteoclasts. (Adapted with permission from Sterling JA, Edwards JR, Martin TJ, Mundy GR: Advances in the biology of bone metastasis: How the skeleton affects tumor behavior. *Bone* 2011;48[1]:6-15.)

PTHrP is believed to have a role in the normal processes of breast development and lactation. Although PTHrP cannot be detected by plasma assay in most adults, it is readily identified in lactating women.[5] Studies of PTHrP expression in mice models have yielded important results. If the *PTHrP* gene lacks function, mice die shortly after birth because of skeletal abnormalities. If the *PTHrP* gene is rescued by shifting of production to cartilage, mice experience failure of breast development.[5] These studies indicate a very important role for PTHrP in breast development.

A small clinical study found that patients who had PTHrP production in their breast carcinomas were significantly more likely to experience later osseous metastasis.[5] One group of researchers has proposed that PTHrP is a bone-resorbing factor.[5] Such resorption may be a property of breast cancer that favors its growth in bone. PTHrP production may provide a niche for the growth of tumor within bone, as it appears to enhance the ability of tumor cells to grow within bone.[5]

A study of 526 patients found that patients with a PTHrP-positive primary breast cancer had better survival and fewer bone metastases when compared to patients with PTRrP-negative primary breast cancers.[5] A smaller study subsequently found that six of seven women whose primary and metastatic breast cancers were concurrently resected had a PTHrP-negative primary tumor but PTHrP-positive metastatic tumors.[5]

These two studies showed that changes in PTHrP status in bone may allow metastatic cells to take hold and grow[5] (**Figure 4**). These study results may lead to a clinical model for the identification of patients at high risk of bone metastasis.

An indirect function of PTHrP is to promote the production of TGF-β, which is released from bone matrix by osteoclasts.[10] PTHrP is produced by metastatic tumor cells in the bone microenvironment. In metastases, PTHrP leads to the production of RANKL, which, when bound to RANK, has a proliferative effect on osteoclasts. The osteoclasts drive production of TGF-β, which leads to the production of more tumor cells, creating a vicious cycle. If TGF-β is blocked, less PTHrP is produced, and fewer osseous metastases develop.[10] TGF-β is a possible therapeutic target for osseous metastases of breast cancer.

Other genes have been implicated in the metastasis of breast cancer. In a recent study, A disintegrin and metalloproteinase with thrombospondin motifs–1 *(ADAMTS-1)*, connective tissue growth factor *(CTGF)*, and *IL-11* each were found to be overexpressed in primary human cancers of the breast with bone metastasis.[9] *MMP-1*, chemokine (C-X-C motif) receptor–4 *(CXCR-4)*, *CTGF*, and *FGF-5* were found to be overexpressed in bone metastases compared with normal human epithelial cells. A strong correlation was found between the expression of *IL-11, CTGF, CXCR-4,*

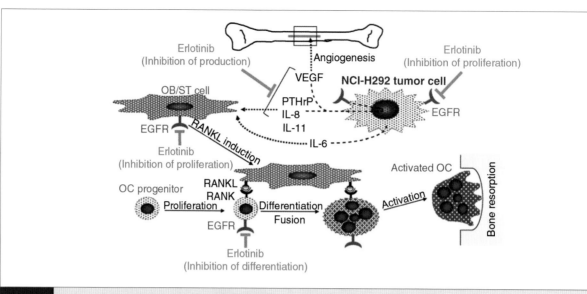

Figure 5 The mechanism of erlotinib in a human osteolytic metastasis model, in which erlotinib decreased osteolytic lesions by the suppression of RANKL activity. OB/ST = osteoblast/stromal, EGFR = epidural growth factor receptor, OC = osteoclast, VEGF = vascular endothelial growth factor. (Reproduced with permission from Furugaki K, Moriya Y, Iwai T, et al: Erlotinib inhibits osteolytic bone invasion of human non-small-cell lung cancer cell line NCI-H292. *Clin Exp Metastasis* 2011;28[7]:649-659.)

ADAMTS-1, and *MMP-1* in different combinations.[9] Like *PTHrP,* these genes are overexpressed in metastases, but they are not overexpressed in primary cancers. The overexpression may represent a late event in tumor progression.[9] To date, these genes do not appear to have predictive potential.

The vicious cycle of bone metastasis applies to breast cancer, but an intricate balance exists between the cell types and factors required to stimulate the bone microenvironment to become susceptible to metastasis. Interactions between osteoclasts and tumor cells are thought to be important, and interactions among immune cells, tumor cells, and stroma also may be important.[5] TGF-β, RANKL, and PTHrP are important in the development of bone metastasis from breast cancer, and other genes and proteins are also likely to be important. Further research is needed to continue to understand the intricate pathways that lead to osseous metastasis of breast cancer.

Lung Cancer

Lung cancer is the most important cancer in terms of disease incidence as well as mortality. Lung cancer is categorized on a histologic basis as small cell neuroendocrine carcinomas and non–small cell lung carcinomas (NSCLCs), which include adenocarcinoma, squamous cell carcinoma, and large cell neuroendocrine carcinoma. Bone metastases are more common in NSCLCs, occurring in 30% to 40% of patients.[11] The incidence of osseous metastasis is lower in patients with lung cancer than in those with breast or prostate cancer, and less research is being conducted on osseous metastasis in lung cancers.

Epidermal growth factor is well known to be a stimulator of osteoclast activity by binding to EGFR, which is overexpressed in many lung carcinomas and may have some effect on the presence of osseous metastasis.[12] Erlotinib, an EGFR tyrosine kinase inhibitor, is used as a standard therapy in previously treated advanced NSCLC.[11] Erlotinib reversibly binds to the intracellular tyrosine kinase domain of EGFR. This mechanism of action is important because the EGFR signaling network, which is disregulated in many carcinomas, affects inhibition of apoptosis, cell proliferation, angiogenesis, and metastasis.[11]

Recently, an osteolytic bone invasion model was studied using the human NSCLC cell line NCI-H292 implanted into the tibiae of mice. The human NSCLC cell line induced the production of RANKL in the tibiae of the transfected mice.[11] Upregulation of RANKL resulted in increased osteoclast activity, leading to osteolytic bone lesions. In mice that subsequently received doses of erlotinib, the number of osteolytic lesions decreased.[11] Furthermore, the mice that received erlotinib had complete suppression of RANKL expression[11] (Figure 5). Erlotinib may prove clinically useful for the inhibition of osteoclast-induced bone destruction by inhibiting activated osteoclast accumulation. Research is needed to determine whether the effects in mice will also occur in humans.

Multiple Myeloma

Multiple myeloma is a fatal hematologic malignancy that develops in multiple bones. It is the second most common hematologic malignancy. The clinical hallmark is multiple osteolytic lesions, which are unique to this disease.[13] Histologically, the lesion is characterized

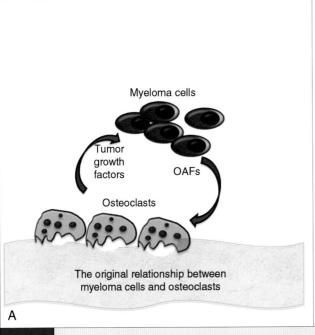

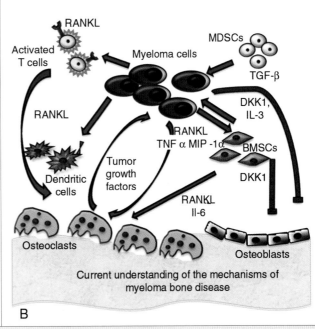

Figure 6 **A,** Monoclonal plasma cells formerly were thought to express an osteoclast-activating factor (OAF) responsible for osteolytic bone disease in multiple myeloma. **B,** It now is understood that many factors, including RANKL, are responsible for destructive bone disease in patients with multiple myeloma. BMSC = bone marrow stromal cell, DKK1 = dickkopf-related protein 1, MDSC = myeloid-derived suppressor cell. (Adapted with permission from Fowler JA, Edwards CM, Croucher PI: Tumor-host cell interactions in the bone disease of myeloma. *Bone* 2011;48[1]:121-128.)

by a proliferation of monoclonal plasma cells in various stages of maturity. For many years, plasma cells have been known to produce an elusive osteoclast-activating factor (**Figure 6, *A***). In the past decade, several pathways have been found to have a crucial role in the genesis of osteolytic bone lesions.[13]

RANKL plays a critical role in the pathogenesis of multiple myeloma. RANKL has been found in increased levels in the bone marrow of patients with multiple myeloma.[13-15] More recently, monoclonal plasma cells have been shown to express RANKL, thereby having the ability to directly induce osteoclastogenesis (**Figure 6, *B***).[13] Myeloma cells induce the production of RANKL in other cells of the bone microenvironment, including T lymphocytes.[13] RANKL may represent an opportunity for targeted therapy in patients with multiple myeloma.

IL-6 is a potent stimulator of osteoclastogenesis.[14] IL-6 is important in disease progression because it inhibits the apoptosis of monoclonal plasma cells and induces their proliferation.[14] When monoclonal plasma cells adhere to bone marrow stem cells, IL-6 production is increased by the bone marrow stem cells, resulting in another vicious cycle. Although levels of IL-6 are not correlated with the extent of bone disease in patients with multiple myeloma, a higher IL-6 level is correlated with a poorer prognosis.[14]

The osteolytic features of multiple myeloma are well known, and osteoblasts were found to be inhibited by the disease process.[13,14] Patients whose multiple my-

eloma is in remission have persistent lytic bone lesions. Osteoblasts derived from patients with multiple myeloma are more susceptible to tumor necrosis factor–induced apoptosis.[14] A more recently studied factor, dickkopf-related protein–1 (DKK-1), is a member of the Wnt signaling pathway, which contributes to the development, growth, and functioning of osteoblasts.[13] DKK-1 is a Wnt signaling antagonist. Not only do patients with multiple myeloma have significantly increased concentrations of DKK-1, but levels of DKK-1 are correlated with the extent of osteolytic bone disease.[13] Furthermore, DKK-1 levels are reduced in many patients after treatment for multiple myeloma. DKK-1 may represent an important therapeutic target for patients with multiple myeloma.

Levels of IL-3 and IL-7 are elevated in the bone marrow and serum of patients with multiple myeloma.[14] It has been determined that these interleukins both stimulate osteoclast formation and act as a myeloma growth factor.[14] IL-3 inhibits osteoblast differentiation, thus mediating the disease.[14]

Recently, a crucial molecule, macrophage inflammatory protein–1α (MIP-1α), has been identified in the pathogenesis of multiple myeloma.[13,15] MIP-1α levels are elevated in the serum of patients with multiple myeloma and is associated with the development of bone disease. MIP-1α is a member of the Regulated on Activation Normal T cell Expressed and Secreted (RANTES) family of chemokines. It is an important activator and chemoattractant of phagocytes.[14] Some studies assert that

5: Metastatic Disease to Bone

RANKL is required for the function of MIP-1α, but other studies have refuted this claim.[13] MIP-1α is thought to be produced by monoclonal plasma cells in most patients with multiple myeloma.[14,15] Therefore, MIP-1α, like DKK-1, may have potential as a target in the treatment of multiple myeloma.

Kidney Cancer

Each year 200,000 cases of renal cancer are diagnosed worldwide, and the mortality rate approaches 50%. Renal cell carcinoma is the most common renal cancer, representing 80% to 90% of the incidence.[16,17] The incidence in North America has increased to 2% of cancers diagnosed per year. Recognized histologic variants of renal cell carcinoma include translocation associated, sarcomatoid, papillary, chromophobe, and clear cell, of which the clear cell variant is by far the most common. The highest cure rates are achieved with early nephrectomy, but 20% to 50% of patients are first seen with advanced disease.[16,17] The lungs are the most common site of renal cell carcinoma metastasis. However, 20% to 35% of patients will have a skeleton-related event caused by the disease, the most common of which is skeletal metastasis.[16,18] Fewer than 10% of patients survive 5 years after the onset of metastatic renal cell carcinoma.[19]

EGFR is known to have a role in renal cell carcinoma metastasis.[19] EGFR is increased in patients with renal cell carcinoma. When the epidermal growth factor binds to EGFR, angiogenesis and tumor proliferation result. Some of the first targeted therapies for renal cell carcinoma metastasis involved EGFR blockade.[19] More recent research found that TGF-β is an important molecule in renal cell carcinoma metastasis to bone. TGF-β is a cytokine with effects on both tumor and normal cells. Advanced tumors become resistant to the inhibitory effects of TGF-β, resulting in a microenvironment ripe to receive metastatic cancer cells.[20] Bone is the most abundant source of TGF-β in the human body. Bone is therefore a prime site for metastasis in renal cell carcinoma because TGF-β is expressed in renal cell carcinoma bone metastasis tissue. TGF-β is released during osteoclast-mediated osteolysis, and is believed to play a central role in the signaling of renal cell carcinoma cells to the bone microenvironment.[20]

Research has revealed that RANKL, an important molecule that causes the osteoclast-mediated bone destruction necessary to release TGF-β, is expressed in 60% to 85% of renal cell carcinomas, with the clear cell subtype having the highest rate of expression.[21] The protein is expressed in both the primary carcinoma and the bone metastasis. Some patients, particularly patients with clear cell renal cell carcinoma, have very high levels of RANKL, but other patients have low levels. In at least one study, this distinction was specified as a prognostic factor: the patients with a low RANKL level had a longer interval to metastasis than those with a high RANKL level.[21] The survival of patients with a low RANKL level also was better than that of the pa-tients with a high RANKL level.[21] The vicious cycle concept can now be applied to renal cell carcinoma. Increased RANKL leads to osteoclastogenesis, and the increase in osteoclasts leads to bone destruction, which releases TGF-β, allowing for homing of renal cell carcinoma cells to the bone microenvironment.

Thyroid Cancer

Most thyroid carcinomas are well differentiated. In the absence of metastasis, the rate of survival associated with these carcinomas is as high as 80%. Most patient deaths are secondary to metastatic disease.[22,23] Follicular carcinoma is the most common of the differentiated thyroid carcinomas to metastasize by hematogenous means. The lung and bone are the most common sites of disease spread.[22]

Integrins, which are transmembrane proteins involved in signal transduction pathways, may have a role in the binding of follicular carcinoma cells to bone.[22] EGFR and VEGF also have been shown to exist in increased levels in the cells of follicular thyroid carcinomas and therefore have increased metastatic potential.[22]

More recent data suggest the production of osteoprotegerin, RANK, and RANKL by malignant follicular cells.[24,25] All three molecules are increased in carcinomas of follicular cell origin, but the effect of this increased production on bone metastasis has not been established.[24,25] Given the importance of these three molecules in the bone microenvironment, their production may be directly linked to bone metastasis, but research is needed to confirm this theory.

Lymphoma

Lymphoma is most often identified as bone disease if it is part of a systemic disease or is a primary localized disease of bone. Primary lymphoma of bone accounts for only 1% to 2% of all bone tumors and fewer than 1% of all non-Hodgkin lymphomas.[26] Secondary involvement of bone by lymphoma occurs in as many as 15% of patients with systemic lymphoma.[26] Adults are most commonly affected, but primary lymphomas of bone have been documented in children.[26]

The most common histologic subtypes in adults are diffuse large B-cell lymphoma and its variants. Approximately 60% of incidences are of the germinal center type, and the others are of the activated B-cell type.[26] The activated B-cell type of diffuse large B-cell lymphoma has a poorer prognosis than the germinal center type.[26] Primary bone lymphomas are more variable in the pediatric population and include lymphoblastic lymphoma, Burkitt lymphoma, and diffuse large B-cell lymphoma.[26]

Possibly because of the low incidence of the disease as a primary bone tumor, little research has been conducted on the pathophysiology of lymphoma in bone. Lymphomas, particularly B-cell lymphomas of bone, were shown to produce RANKL.[27] Lymphomas of bone, like many other malignant neoplasms that involve bone, produces osteolysis. Many malignant B cells also were shown to produce VEGF, which has important roles in both angiogenesis and osteoclastogenesis. Thus, the vicious cycle of bone destruction and tumor expansion was shown to occur in lymphoma of bone.[27]

Research has further indicated the importance of the RANK-OPG-RANKL pathway in the regulation of bone disease in patients with lymphoma. When the RANK-OPG-RANKL pathway is disrupted, B cells cannot form.[28] This disruption suggests that the pathway must be upregulated for B-cell lymphomas to survive in the bone microenvironment, thus contributing to the vicious cycle. Research is needed to understand some of the other players in the pathophysiology of bone disease as it relates to lymphoma.

Summary

Most current research into the pathophysiology of bone metastasis involves lung, breast, and prostate carcinomas, which are the three most common cancers in the United States. Multiple myeloma also is being researched because of the great involvement of bone pathology and subsequent skeleton-related events. The RANK-OPG-RANKL pathway has potential as a therapeutic target against bone disease because it is implicated in many metastatic diseases of bone. Targeting this and other pathways may lead to a new era in personalized medicine.

Annotated References

1. Talmadge JE, Fidler IJ: AACR centennial series: The biology of cancer metastasis: Historical perspective. *Cancer Res* 2010;70(14):5649-5669.

   The authors reviewed the history of observations on the biology of bone metastasis, with current research controversies in the biology and pathophysiology of bone metastases. Level of evidence: V.

2. Buijs JT, van der Pluijm G: Osteotropic cancers: From primary tumor to bone. *Cancer Lett* 2009;273(2): 177-193.

   The seed-and-soil hypothesis, which states that cancer cells circulate in all directions but can metastasize only to organs that permit their proliferation, was applied to bone metastasis research. Level of evidence: V.

3. Coghlin C, Murray GI: Current and emerging concepts in tumour metastasis. *J Pathol* 2010;222(1):1-15.

   The authors reviewed tumor metastasis with recognition of host factors outside the primary site that lead to the development of metastatic disease. The premetastatic niche hypothesis is evolving and being defined. Level of evidence: V.

4. Lynch CC: Matrix metalloproteinases as master regu-

lators of the vicious cycle of bone metastasis. *Bone* 2011;48(1):44-53.

   The authors reviewed the role of MMPs in the vicious cycle of bone metastasis. MMPs are intimately involved with the bioavailability and bioactivity of RANKL and TGF-β, two factors known to have major roles in bone metastasis. Level of evidence: V.

5. Sterling JA, Edwards JR, Martin TJ, Mundy GR: Advances in the biology of bone metastasis: How the skeleton affects tumor behavior. *Bone* 2011;48(1):6-15.

   The authors reviewed recent developments in the biology of bone metastasis as they relate to breast cancer. New areas of study have suggested pathways that may be important in bone metastasis as well as in therapeutic targets. Level of evidence: V.

6. Ye X, Lee Y-C, Choueiri M, et al: Aberrant expression of katanin p60 in prostate cancer bone metastasis. *Prostate* 2012;72(3):291-300.

   This retrospective research study determined that katanin p60 is aberrantly expressed during prostate cancer progression and that this expression may aid prostate cancer metastasis by stimulating cell motility. Level of evidence: V.

7. Theriault RL, Theriault RL: Biology of bone metastases. *Cancer Control* 2012;19(2):92-101.

   This report described rapid growth in discoveries related to the pathophysiology of bone metastasis, specifically in breast and prostate cancers and multiple myeloma. Therapeutic targets were also described. Level of evidence: V.

8. Peng X, Guo W, Liu T, et al: Identification of miRs-143 and -145 that is associated with bone metastasis of prostate cancer and involved in the regulation of EMT. *PLoS One* 2011;6(5):e20341.

   This retrospective study identified microRNAs involved in prostate cancer. MicroRNAs 143 and 145 are associated with prostate cancer bone metastasis and may be involved in the epithelial mesenchymal transition. Level of evidence: V.

9. Casimiro S, Luis I, Fernandes A, et al: Analysis of a bone metastasis gene expression signature in patients with bone metastasis from solid tumors. *Clin Exp Metastasis* 2012;29(2):155-164.

   This retrospective study analyzed the expression of six metastasis-related genes in human bone metastasis. The genes' cooperative function in the bone microenvironment suggested an important role in vivo. Level of evidence: V.

10. Yin JJ, Selander K, Chirgwin JM, et al: TGF-beta signaling blockade inhibits PTHrP secretion by breast cancer cells and bone metastases development. *J Clin Invest* 1999;103(2):197-206.

11. Furugaki K, Moriya Y, Iwai T, et al: Erlotinib inhibits osteolytic bone invasion of human non-small-cell lung cancer cell line NCI-H292. *Clin Exp Metastasis* 2011; 28(7):649-659.

5: Metastatic Disease to Bone

This study found that erlotinib inhibits osteolytic tumor invasion in metastatic disease by supporting the activation of osteoclasts via inhibition of tumor growth in metastases. Osteolytic factors produced by tumor cells were described.

12. Coleman RE: Metastatic bone disease: Clinical features, pathophysiology and treatment strategies. *Cancer Treat Rev* 2001;27(3):165-176.

13. Fowler JA, Edwards CM, Croucher PI: Tumor-host cell interactions in the bone disease of myeloma. *Bone* 2011;48(1):121-128.

    Interactions of malignant plasma cells and cells within bone marrow, osteolytic bone disease, and cellular mechanisms and potential targets for therapy were discussed as they relate to multiple myeloma. Level of evidence: V.

14. Lentzsch S, Ehrlich LA, Roodman GD: Pathophysiology of multiple myeloma bone disease. *Hematol Oncol Clin North Am* 2007;21(6):1035-1049, viii.

    The potential mechanisms in the bone disease of multiple myeloma were discussed, with possible therapeutic targets. Level of evidence: V.

15. Abe M: Targeting the interplay between myeloma cells and the bone marrow microenvironment in myeloma. *Int J Hematol* 2011;94(4):334-343.

    Cellular interplay between multiple myeloma and the bone marrow mediates the progression of the disease. The authors of this review discussed the latest understanding of the mechanisms of interaction between the bone marrow and the plasma cells, which resulted in the vicious cycle. Level of evidence: V.

16. Wood SL, Brown JE: Skeletal metastasis in renal cell carcinoma: Current and future management options. *Cancer Treat Rev* 2012;38(4):284-291.

    Skeletal metastasis is relatively common in renal cell carcinoma and leads to complications. The authors of this review examined the pathways of metastasis and treatment of bone disease resulting from renal cancer metastasis. Level of evidence: V.

17. Woodward E, Jagdev S, McParland L, et al: Skeletal complications and survival in renal cancer patients with bone metastases. *Bone* 2011;48(1):160-166.

    Skeletal metastasis in renal cancer leads to skeletal complications. A large retrospective comparative study focused on the skeletal complications of renal cell carcinoma, with emphasis on spinal cord compression. Level of evidence: III.

18. Zhao FL, Guo W: Expression of stromal derived factor-1 (SDF-1) and chemokine receptor (CXCR4) in bone metastasis of renal carcinoma. *Mol Biol Rep* 2011;38(2):1039-1045.

    The authors of this retrospective study examined the roles of *SDF-1* and *CXCR4* in renal cell carcinoma metastasis. The data suggested that the expression of these genes is high in metastases and that their overexpression may play important roles in renal carcinoma bone metastasis. Level of evidence: II.

19. Weber KL, Doucet M, Price JE: Renal cell carcinoma bone metastasis: Epidermal growth factor receptor targeting. *Clin Orthop Relat Res* 2003;(415, Suppl) S86-S94.

20. Weber K, Doucet M, Kominsky S: Renal cell carcinoma bone metastasis—elucidating the molecular targets. *Cancer Metastasis Rev* 2007;26(3-4):691-704.

    Skeletal metastasis is a harbinger of a poor prognosis. The authors of this review discussed the roles of the EGFR and TGF-β pathways and the inhibition of these pathways, which leads to decreased bone destruction.

21. Mikami S, Katsube K, Oya M, et al: Increased RANKL expression is related to tumour migration and metastasis of renal cell carcinomas. *J Pathol* 2009;218(4):530-539.

    RANKL plays an important role in osteoclastogenesis. The authors of this study investigated the role of the RANK-OPG-RANKL system in renal carcinomas and suggested that this system is involved in bone metastases by stimulation of cancer cell migration.

22. Smit JW, van der Pluijm G, Vloedgraven HJ, Löwik CW, Goslings BM: Role of integrins in the attachment of metastatic follicular thyroid carcinoma cell lines to bone. *Thyroid* 1998;8(1):29-36.

23. Orita Y, Sugitani I, Toda K, Manabe J, Fujimoto Y: Zoledronic acid in the treatment of bone metastases from differentiated thyroid carcinoma. *Thyroid* 2011;21(1):31-35.

    Bisphosphonates often are administered to patients with osteolytic metastases. The authors of this retrospective study found that skeleton-related events were less common in patients with thyroid cancer who were treated with bisphosphonates. Level of evidence: III.

24. Heymann MF, Riet A, Le Goff B, Battaglia S, Paineau J, Heymann D: OPG, RANK and RANK ligand expression in thyroid lesions. *Regul Pept* 2008;148(1-3):46-53.

    The RANKL pathway is essential to bone metabolism. This retrospective study was the first to reveal RANKL expression in thyroid lesions, which may have a role in follicular and parafollicular malignancies. Level of evidence: V.

25. Sood SK, Balasubramanian S, Higham S, Fernando M, Harrison B: Osteoprotegerin (OPG) and related proteins (RANK, RANKL and TRAIL) in thyroid disease. *World J Surg* 2011;35(9):1984-1992.

    OPG, RANK, and RANKL are key to the development of bone metastasis. This retrospective study determined that nuclear expression of RANK in thyroid malignancy is a paradox that requires further investigation. Level of evidence: V.

26. Zhao XF, Young KH, Frank D, et al: Pediatric primary bone lymphoma-diffuse large B-cell lymphoma: Morphologic and immunohistochemical characteristics of 10 cases. *Am J Clin Pathol* 2007;127(1):47-54.

    Most primary bone lymphomas are of the diffuse large

B-cell type. Pediatric primary bone lymphomas are more variable. A retrospective study concluded that pediatric and adult diffuse large B-cell lymphomas are distinct entities. Level of evidence: V.

27. Shibata H, Abe M, Hiura K, et al: Malignant B-lymphoid cells with bone lesions express receptor activator of nuclear factor-kappa B ligand and vascular endothelial growth factor to enhance osteoclastogenesis. *Clin Cancer Res* 2005;11(17):6109-6115.

28. Horowitz MC, Fretz JA, Lorenzo JA: How B cells influence bone biology in health and disease. *Bone* 2010; 47(3):472-479.

The adaptive immune system, which responds to infection, is made up of B and T cells. The authors of this report discussed the relationship between the bone marrow microenvironment and B cells, with the effect of that relationship on the skeleton in health and disease. Level of evidence: V.

Chapter 32

Prediction of Impending Pathologic Fracture and Treatment Considerations in Patients With Metastatic Bone Disease

Kathleen S. Beebe, MD

Patient Survival

Metastatic bone lesions have serious effects on many patients' quality of life. Because of the severity of skeletal malignancies, it is important to properly assess which patients are suitable candidates for surgical intervention for impending pathologic fractures. The goals of treatment are to relieve pain, prevent fractures, preserve function, allow for early weight bearing, and provide an intervention that will last the patient's entire life span.[1]

Metastatic bone disease varies greatly among patients, and thus each patient's disease much be addressed individually. The prognoses of these lesions differ according to primary disease, location of metastasis, metabolic complications, and functional assessment. The ability to properly estimate the expected survival has great significance in the process of deciding the suitable method of fixation.

Primary Disease

Breast and prostate carcinomas are the most common causes of metastatic bone disease, followed by lung, kidney, and thyroid carcinomas.[2-4] The primary disease plays a vital role in assessing patients' length of survival. Patients who have longer survival times are better candidates for surgical interventions that may require longer postoperative healing times, whereas patients who are terminally ill may not benefit from surgery. Although survival rates may vary slightly depending on the location of osseous metastases, survival rates, in general, are longest for patients with primary carcinomas of the breast, prostate, and thyroid[5] (Table 1). With these patients, fixation methods that require bone healing or aggressive reconstruction can be an option in selected patients because these methods provide a more

stable and longer-lasting construct. The goal is to provide a construct that will survive the patient's life expectancy.

Metastatic Load

Although primary disease plays a vital role in life expectancy, factors such as metastatic load also affect the length of survival. Studies have shown that patients with bone metastases combined with visceral metastases have shorter mean lengths of survival than individuals with just osseous involvement. In 2005, researchers assessed 191 patients with metastatic skeletal involvement. They found that individuals who underwent surgery for metastatic bone disease without visceral metastases had longer median survival rates (25 months), whereas those with visceral involvement had shorter survival rates (6 months). In addition, the researchers found that the number of metastatic skeletal lesions also negatively affected survival rates.[6] These findings were similar to those found in previous studies.[1]

Table 1

Mean Survival by Tumor Histology in Patients Treated for Metastatic Spine Disease

Histology	Survival (months)
Thyroid	26
Breast	19
Prostate	18
Rectal	18
Renal	10
Lung	6
Unidentified carcinoma	5

Reproduced from Rose PS, Buchowski JM: Metastatic disease in the thoracic and lumbar spine: Evaluation and management. *J Am Acad Orthop Surg* 2011;19(1):37-48.

5: Metastatic Disease to Bone

Functional Assessment

Two functional assessment classification systems are the Eastern Cooperative Oncology Group scale and the Karnofsky performance scale. The Lansky score system has been adopted in addressing functional assessment in children. These systems can be used to quantify the functional status of patients with malignancies and assist in determining the eligibility for surgical intervention.

A 2005 study demonstrated significant improvement in Musculoskeletal Tumor Society functional scores for patients with nonspinal bony metastasis who received surgical intervention. Musculoskeletal Tumor Society scores rose from 7.9 preoperatively to 14.4 at 6 weeks and 17.5 at 3 months. The researchers demonstrated that improvement can be seen within 6 weeks postoperatively, and thus they recommended that patients who receive surgical intervention for bony metastases should have a life expectancy of at least 6 weeks for improvement in functional status to be visible.[7]

Metabolic Assessment

Patients with metastatic bone disease commonly have abnormal metabolic features. The most common complication in adults with osseous metastases is hypercalcemia of malignancy due to bone destruction from osteolytic metastases. In a study of 859 women with metastatic breast cancer of the bone, 19% were found to have hypercalcemia.[8] Although there are no clear criteria to determine which patients are suited for surgical treatment of an impending fracture with hypercalcemia, medical management and control of the hypercalcemia, in conjunction with treatments such as bisphosphonates, make the patient a more stable surgical candidate.

Recently, N-telopeptide of type I collagen (NTX) has been identified as a bone marker for skeletal metastases from the lung, breast, and prostate. Elevated urinary levels of NTX increased the risk of skeletal-related events (SREs), which included pathologic fractures, by two to three times. In addition, elevated NTX levels correlated with an overall decrease in rate of survival in individuals with bone metastasis from prostate or lung carcinomas.[9]

Roles of Pharmaceutical Therapies in the Prevention of Pathologic Fractures

Bisphosphonates

Bisphosphonates have been one of the key pharmaceutical treatments that assist in the prevention of pathologic fractures in patients with bone metastases. Within the class of bisphosphonates, zoledronic acid has been shown to effectively decrease the rate of SREs, including pathologic fractures. In a study of 773 patients, patients who were given a 4-mg infusion of zoledronic acid over 15 minutes every 3 weeks for 9 months had an overall pathologic fracture rate of 16%, compared with the placebo group, which had a pathologic fracture rate of 21%.[10]

Although the therapy dosage may vary slightly among practicing physicians, bisphosphonates have become a mainstay pharmaceutical agent in decreasing the risk of pathologic fracture, as well as for treatment of other SREs, including hypercalcemia of malignancy.[11] In addition, zoledronic acid has also demonstrated effectiveness in normalizing the levels of NTX. A large phase 3 study demonstrated normalization of NTX levels within 3 months of administration of zoledronic acid in 81% of breast cancer patients with bone metastases, 80% of non–small cell lung cancer patients with bone metastases, and 70% of hormone-refractory prostate cancer patients with bone metastases. In contrast, normalization of NTX levels in patients within the placebo group were between 8% and 17%.[12]

Recently, studies have examined atypical subtrochanteric fractures following long-term bisphosphonate use. Researchers stress the importance of close monitoring in patients with more than 5 years of bisphosphonate use. If these patients have thigh or groin pain, an immediate plain radiograph with AP and lateral views must be ordered to rule out possible fracture. When possible, it may also be advisable to allow these patients a drug holiday following 5 years of use.[13]

Denosumab

Denosumab is a human monoclonal antibody that binds to the receptor activator of nuclear factor-κ B ligand (RANKL). By binding to RANKL, denosumab inhibits the interaction between receptor activator of nuclear factor-κ B (RANK) and RANKL, which in turn decreases osteoclast activity, decreases bone resorption, and increases bone mass. In a phase 3, randomized, double-blind trial, denosumab was compared to zoledronic acid in the treatment of SREs in 1776 patients with bone metastases. Denosumab showed slightly superior effectiveness in decreasing the rate of SREs, including pathologic fractures.[14] With continued research, physicians may find more widespread use of denosumab, with or without bisphosphonates, in the prevention of pathologic fracture in patients with metastatic bone disease.

Other Alternatives to Open Surgery

Radiation Therapy

External beam irradiation is the most common treatment used for palliation of bone metastases. Studies have shown that external beam irradiation provides relief in patients with metastatic bone pain.[15]

Irradiation dosage varies among different metastatic diseases with target dosage limited by the bone and surrounding tissue. Pain relief can be delayed for up to 12 weeks, with some patients experiencing recurrence of pain within a few months.

Table 2				

Mirels Scoring System for Risk of Pathologic Fracture

Score (Points)	Site	Radiographic Appearance	Bone Width Involved	Pain
1	Upper extremity	Blastic	<1/3	Mild
2	Lower extremity non-peritrhchanteric)	Mixed (blastic-lytic)	1/3 - 2/3	Moderate
3	Peritrochanteric	(Lytic)	>2/3	Functional[a]

[a]Aggravated by function.
(Reproduced with permission from Bickels J, Dadia S, Lidar Z: Surgical management of metastic bone disease. *J Bone Joint Surg Am* 2009;91(6):1502-1516.)

Radiofrequency Ablation and Cryoablation

Another nonsurgical means of pain relief for patients with metastatic bone pain is focal ablative therapy, which includes radiofrequency ablation (RFA) and cryoablation. Focal ablative therapy for the purpose of pain improvement was used in patients who had moderate to severe pain, focal pain limited to one or two sites, and small lesions that were either osteolytic or mixed osteolytic/osteoblastic.[16]

RFA uses a radiofrequency probe placed directly at the lesion site, typically under CT guidance. The electrode provides 460-kHz frequency at a maximum power of 150 W. A study showed a clinically significant decrease in metastatic bone pain in patients for whom radiation therapy and chemotherapy were unsuccessful. These patients also experienced periods of relief.[16]

Cryoablation was initially limited to intraoperative use because of the large area necessary for the safe use of liquid nitrogen. With the development of cryoprobes and pressurized argon gas, cryoablation can be performed through a percutaneous technique. Unlike RFA, cryoablation allows for direct visualization of the zone of ablation using CT monitoring. Initial studies on cryoablation have shown metastatic bone pain relief results comparable to those found in multicenter RFA trials.[17]

Predicting Impending Pathologic Fractures

Classic Definition

Selected patients who are at high risk of subsequent pathologic fracture may be offered prophylactic fixation to preserve function and to have a more limited intervention than might be required after fracture. Successful execution, however, requires the ability to reliably predict fracture risk. Investigators have attempted to predict fracture risk in several ways; however, none has proved completely reliable.

The classic definition of an impending pathologic fracture consists of the following: lesions that measure at least 2.5 cm, lesions that occupy at least 50% of the bone diameter, and lesions accompanied by an adjacent fracture of the lesser trochanter or failure of radiation therapy. This system of classification has been shown to have low specificity in diagnosing impending pathologic fractures.[18]

Mirels Evaluation System

The Mirels scoring system was developed in 1989 as a screening tool for impending fractures in metastatic lesions of long bone and continues to be used. The system is based on a three-point scoring system in four criteria: site of lesion, nature of lesion, size of lesion, and pain (**Table 2**). Each category is equally weighed, and the overall score has a minimum of 3 and maximum of 12. An overall score of 7 or less is classified as low risk of fracture (5%) and would warrant medical management as the recommended treatment, whereas an overall score of 9 or greater poses a high risk of fracture (33%), and surgical intervention would be recommended. A score of 8 poses a 15% risk of fracture, with recommendation of surgery depending largely on the physician's clinical judgment.[19]

Although this system of evaluation is currently used, it has limitations. One limitation arises in the case of a patient who has a Mirels score of 8. If physicians were to prophylactically treat all patients with a score of 8, two thirds of patients would be inappropriately treated. An additional problem arises with interrater reliability. A study demonstrated significant variability in scoring among radiation and medical oncologists—specialists whom patients most often see before being seen by an orthopaedic surgeon.[20]

In addition, this system does not account for other factors that may contribute to impending pathologic fractures such as comorbidities, length of survival, functional assessment, and adjuvant therapy. In practice, the Mirels classification should be used with additional consideration of other factors to fully assess the need for surgical intervention. Examples of the clinical utility of the Mirels scoring system are shown in **Figure 1**.

Spine Fracture Risk Classification

The Tokuhashi classification system was developed in 1990 to determine the prognosis of metastatic spine tumors. Researchers examined six categories, with each category given a score of 0, 1, or 2. These categories

5: Metastatic Disease to Bone

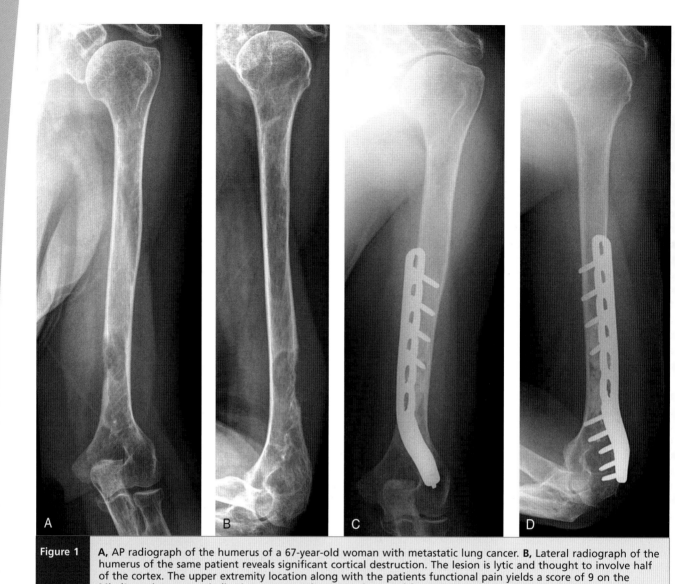

Figure 1   **A,** AP radiograph of the humerus of a 67-year-old woman with metastatic lung cancer. **B,** Lateral radiograph of the humerus of the same patient reveals significant cortical destruction. The lesion is lytic and thought to involve half of the cortex. The upper extremity location along with the patients functional pain yields a score of 9 on the Mirel's scoring system, indicating a graeter than 33% chance of fracture. **C** and **D,** Postoperative radiographs of the extremity after curetage, cementation, and plate fixation.

consisted of (1) general condition, (2) number of extraspinal bone metastases, (3) number of vertebral body metastases, (4) metastases to major internal organs, (5) primary site of malignancy, and (6) severity of spinal cord palsy.[21] In a retrospective study, researchers examined three criteria and created a scoring system similar to the Tokuhashi system. The Tokuhashi evaluation system was later revised to change the range of the category indicating the primary site of malignancy from 0–2 to 0–5.[22] Both systems have been used to identify survival rates and surgical suitability of individuals with spinal metastases.

Other Evaluation Systems
The authors of a 2004 study found that the Mirels scoring system overpredicted the risk of fractures. In a study of 110 patients with femoral metastases, the researchers examined the following risk factors: in-

creasing pain, size of lesion, radiographic appearance, localization, and transverse/axial/circumferential involvement. They found that axial cortical involvement of 30 mm or more on plain radiograph provided a simple and objective tool in identifying patients in need of prophylactic treatment[23] (**Figure 2**).

Imaging
The use of new imaging studies in assisting with identifying impending pathologic fractures has been limited. The authors of a 2011 study began to explore the use of new imaging techniques in identifying impending pathologic fractures. They examined the use of combined positron emission tomography (PET) and CT scanning (PET-CT) and MRI in multiple myeloma patients and found that PET-CT with a standardized uptake value (SUV) greater than 3.5 and MRI finding of diffuse or multifocal vertebral body involvement may

indicate impending pathologic fractures.[24] Although this study did not show statistically significant results because of the small sample size, it has provided the groundwork for future larger studies.

Principles of Treatment of Impending Pathologic Fractures

Perioperative Evaluation

A basic history and physical examination should be performed in all patients being evaluated preoperatively. Special emphases should be placed on the patient's previous and current treatments and medications, including chemotherapy and radiation therapy. A thorough social history should also be taken to evaluate the patient's and family's ability to care for the patient postoperatively. Counseling should be provided for the family and/or caretaker to equip them with realistic expectations regarding the postoperative needs of the patient. Additionally, all organ systems must be reviewed with foci on the cardiovascular and pulmonary systems.

Special attention must be given to educating the patient and family regarding the palliative nature of surgical intervention for impending fracture, and the acceptance of surgical risk in exchange for the possibility of preservation of function and pain relief. It is not intuitively obvious to the lay public that a patient with malignancy may undergo a surgical procedure that is not likely to affect the patient's longevity, and this point should be clarified as part of the informed consent process.

As for all patients with positive cardiac histories who undergo surgical procedures, a full cardiac workup should be completed for all patients with cardiac histories to appropriately stratify their risk class for perioperative cardiac mortality. Studies have shown that patients who undergo surgery within 3 months of their last myocardial infarction have reinfarction rates of 27% to 37%.[25] In 1990, a risk stratification aimed specifically for oncology patients was created.[26] Most patients with metastatic bone disease typically have electrolyte abnormalities. Hypercalcemia can be seen in up to 20% of patients with malignancy and can be fatal if left untreated. Serum calcium values greater than 14 mg/dL should be considered life threatening and should be treated immediately with rapid hydration and loop diuretics.[25]

Immediate Stability of Construct

A construct should provide immediate stability and allow full weight bearing. In most patients, physicians should avoid fixation methods that require bone healing, porous ingrowths, and bone grafting because of the limitations in activity that these constructs initially require for appropriate healing to occur. Whenever possible, priority should be given to providing immediate optimum functionality for patients with shortened life

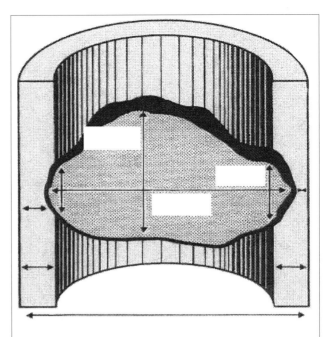

Figure 2 Measurements of metastatic lesions in the femur (mm): largest axial length of the entire lesion (L-lesion), largest transverse extension of the lesion (W-lesion), and largest axial cortical involvement (L-cort). Measurements of the femur (mm): largest transverse width of the bone (W-tot), maximal thickness of cortex without lesional involvement (C-tot), and minimal thickness of cortex with lesional involvement (C-lesion). (Reproduced with permission from Van der Linden YM, Dijkstra PD, Kroon HM, et al : Comparative analysis of risk factors for pathological fracture with femoral metastases. *J Bone Joint Surg Br* 2004;86[4]:568.)

expectancies. In addition, maximizing pain control should be the primary goal.

Polymethyl Methacrylate

Because of the importance of immediate stability following surgery, polymethyl methacrylate (PMMA) has become an important adjuvant in the treatment of impending fractures. PMMA has various properties that allow it to be used in conjunction with constructs, including its ability to conform to atypical cavities, immediate rigidity, and an exothermic reaction that has shown to cause local tumor necrosis.[27]

General Guidelines for Treatment

Before treatment of any lesion, an individualized treatment plan should be made considering diagnosis and surgical planning. Diagnoses of lesions are often made through biopsy and histologic confirmation. The surgical plan may vary according to primary disease, size of the metastatic lesion, and responsiveness to adjuvant therapy. For example, solitary metastatic lesions caused by renal cell carcinoma are typically resistant to irradiation and may require large resections and reconstructions to prevent local disease progression and complications, although some studies have shown that wide surgical excision does not improve survival.[28] Other tumors that are less responsive to adjuvant therapy may require debulking, PMMA, and plate fixation. Finally, when appropriate, surgeons should pursue more aggressive treatment options to avoid inadequate bone fixation and unwanted additional surgery. When in doubt, surgeons should maximize immediate mechanical stability and prevention of subsequent complications requiring revision surgery.

Postoperative Radiation Therapy Following Stabilization

Once an impending fracture has been stabilized, postoperative radiation therapy is usually used to improve function and decrease the failure rate. A study demonstrated that patients who underwent postoperative irradiation had higher rates of achieving normal function status with or without pain than those who did not receive irradiation following fixation of an impending fracture. The rates of achieving normal function status for patients who underwent postoperative irradiation and those who did not were 53% and 12%, respectively. The same study also showed an overall decrease in the failure rate in patients who underwent postoperative irradiation. In addition, postoperative irradiation helped slow the progression of the disease, as well as decrease remaining tumors that were unable to be removed intraoperatively.[29]

Location-Specific Treatment Method

Long Bone

Although different fixation methods exist for treating impending fractures in long bones, all methods should adhere to the following objectives: protect the long bone, provide immediate stabilization, and prevent future fractures. Fixation methods, either alone or in combination, can include PMMA, endoprostheses, various nailing systems, plates, and screws.

In the femur, treatment methods for impending fractures vary depending on the location of the lesion. Lesions in the femoral head or neck should be treated with replacement arthroplasty because of the high mechanical stress and limited healing found along the proximal femur. Reconstructive intramedullary nailing usually can be performed on impending subtrochanteric and diaphyseal fractures, stabilizing the lesion while guarding against fracture of potential subsequent, more proximal lesions. Larger lesions may require an open technique with debulking, PMMA, and fixation.[30]

Similar to methods used in the femur, fixation methods in the humerus differ according to the location of the lesion. In the proximal humerus, humeral endoprostheses are sometimes used because of the difficulties that result with the use of intramedullary nails or

plate fixation, although locking plate technology has extended the range of plating capability into the more proximal humerus. Impending fractures of the metadiaphysis or diaphysis can be treated with either intramedullary nailing or plate fixation. When plate fixation is used, at least three cortical screws are recommended in normal cortical bone.[31]

Spine

The spine is one of the most common sites of skeletal metastases, with approximately 70% of patients dying of malignancy having evidence of spinal metastases. However, prophylactic surgical treatment of spinal metastases is not done. Because of the risk involved in operating on spinal metastases, surgical intervention should be performed only when indicated.

Summary

The goal of surgical treatment is to provide palliative symptomatic relief and immediate function for patients with shortened life expectancies. When these goals cannot be met, the physician, patient, and family should discuss medical treatment, nonsurgical options, or best supportive care.

Acknowledgment

The author thanks John Hwang, MD, for his support and assistance.

Annotated References

1. Böhm P, Huber J: The surgical treatment of bony metastases of the spine and limbs. *J Bone Joint Surg Br* 2002;84(4):521-529.

2. Hage WD, Aboulafia AJ, Aboulafia DM: Incidence, location, and diagnostic evaluation of metastatic bone disease. *Orthop Clin North Am* 2000;31(4):515-528, vii.

3. Li S, Peng Y, Weinhandl ED, et al: Estimated number of prevalent cases of metastatic bone disease in the US adult population. *Clin Epidemiol* 2012;4:87-93.

   This study examines the prevalence of metastatic bone disease in the US population. Level of evidence: V.

4. Coleman RE: Clinical features of metastatic bone disease and risk of skeletal morbidity. *Clin Cancer Res* 2006;12(20 Pt 2):6243s-6249s.

5. Rose PS, Buchowski JM: Metastatic disease in the thoracic and lumbar spine: Evaluation and management. *J Am Acad Orthop Surg* 2011;19(1):37-48.

   This article provides a brief review of evaluation and management methods for metastatic disease in the thoracic and lumbar spine. Level of evidence: V.

6. Nathan SS, Healey JH, Mellano D, et al: Survival in patients operated on for pathologic fracture: Implications for end-of-life orthopedic care. *J Clin Oncol* 2005;23(25):6072-6082.

7. Talbot M, Turcotte RE, Isler M, Normandin D, Iannuzzi D, Downer P: Function and health status in surgically treated bone metastases. *Clin Orthop Relat Res* 2005;438:215-220.

8. Plunkett TA, Smith P, Rubens RD: Risk of complications from bone metastases in breast cancer: Implications for management. *Eur J Cancer* 2000;36(4):476-482.

9. Coleman R, Brown J, Terpos E, et al: Bone markers and their prognostic value in metastatic bone disease: Clinical evidence and future directions. *Cancer Treat Rev* 2008;34(7):629-639.

   This review article examines the correlation between biochemical bone markers and SREs in patients with metastatic bone disease. Bone markers may help identify patients who are at high risk for SREs or death. Level of evidence: V.

10. Rosen LS, Gordon D, Tchekmedyian S, et al: Zoledronic acid versus placebo in the treatment of skeletal metastases in patients with lung cancer and other solid tumors: A phase III, double-blind, randomized trial. The Zoledronic Acid Lung Cancer and Other Solid Tumors Study Group. *J Clin Oncol* 2003;21(16):3150-3157.

11. Major P, Lortholary A, Hon J, et al: Zoledronic acid is superior to pamidronate in the treatment of hypercalcemia of malignancy: A pooled analysis of two randomized, controlled clinical trials. *J Clin Oncol* 2001;19(2):558-567.

12. Lipton A, Cook R, Saad F, et al: Normalization of bone markers is associated with improved survival in patients with bone metastases from solid tumors and elevated bone resorption receiving zoledronic acid. *Cancer* 2008;113(1):193-201.

    This retrospective study showed that zoledronic acid normalized or maintained normal levels of NTX within 3 months of treatment in patients with bone metastases. Level of evidence: IV.

13. Yoon RS, Hwang JS, Beebe KS: Long-term bisphosphonate usage and subtrochanteric insufficiency fractures: A cause for concern? *J Bone Joint Surg Br* 2011; 93(10):1289-1295.

    The authors present a review of the most recent management and treatment methods for subtrochanteric insufficiency fractures following long-term bisphosphonate usage. Level of evidence: V.

14. Henry DH, Costa L, Goldwasser F, et al: Randomized, double-blind study of denosumab versus zoledronic acid in the treatment of bone metastases in patients with advanced cancer (excluding breast and prostate cancer) or multiple myeloma. *J Clin Oncol* 2011; 29(9):1125-1132.

    This randomized, double-blind study compared denosumab and zoledronic acid in patients with bone metastases. Denosumab was found to be as effective as zoledronic acid in preventing or delaying SREs in patients with metastases to the bone. Level of evidence: I.

15. Houston SJ, Rubens RD: The systemic treatment of bone metastases. *Clin Orthop Relat Res* 1995;312:95-104.

16. Callstrom MR, Charboneau JW, Goetz MP, et al: Painful metastases involving bone: Feasibility of percutaneous CT- and US-guided radio-frequency ablation. *Radiology* 2002;224(1):87-97.

17. Callstrom MR, Dupuy DE, Solomon SB, et al: Percutaneous image-guided cryoablation of painful metastases involving bone: Multicenter trial. *Cancer* 2013; 119(5):1033-1041.

    The authors present the results of the use of percutaneous cyroablation for painful metastatic bone tumors. Level of evidence: IV.

18. Keene JS, Sellinger DS, McBeath AA, Engber WD: Metastatic breast cancer in the femur: A search for the lesion at risk of fracture. *Clin Orthop Relat Res* 1986; 203:282-288.

19. Mirels H: Metastatic disease in long bones: A proposed scoring system for diagnosing impending pathologic fractures. *Clin Orthop Relat Res* 1989;249:256-264.

20. Damron TA, Morgan H, Prakash D, Grant W, Aronowitz J, Heiner J: Critical evaluation of Mirels' rating system for impending pathologic fractures. *Clin Orthop Relat Res* 2003;(Suppl 415):S201-S207.

21. Tokuhashi Y, Matsuzaki H, Toriyama S, Kawano H, Ohsaka S: Scoring system for the preoperative evaluation of metastatic spine tumor prognosis. *Spine (Phila Pa 1976)* 1990;15(11):1110-1113.

22. Tokuhashi Y, Matsuzaki H, Oda H, Oshima M, Ryu J: A revised scoring system for preoperative evaluation of metastatic spine tumor prognosis. *Spine (Phila Pa 1976)* 2005;30(19):2186-2191.

23. Van der Linden YM, Dijkstra PD, Kroon HM, et al: Comparative analysis of risk factors for pathological fracture with femoral metastases. *J Bone Joint Surg Br* 2004;86(4):566-573.

24. Mulligan M, Chirindel A, Karchevsky M: Characterizing and predicting pathologic spine fractures in myeloma patients with FDG PET/CT and MR imaging. *Cancer Invest* 2011;29(5):370-376.

    This retrospective study examined the use of PET-CT scans in discriminating between old and new pathologic spine fractures as well as the use of PET-CT and

MRI in combination to identify possible impending fractures. A PET-CT SUV greater than 3.5 as well as MRI findings of diffuse or multifocal vertebral body involvement may be indications for impending pathologic fractures in patients with multiple myeloma. Level of evidence: IV.

25. Bibbo C, Patel DV, Benevenia J: Perioperative considerations in patients with metastatic bone disease. *Orthop Clin North Am* 2000;31(4):577-595, viii.

26. Ewer MS, Ali MK: Surgical treatment of the cancer patient: Preoperative assessment and perioperative medical management. *J Surg Oncol* 1990;44(3):185-190.

27. Sim FH, Daugherty TW, Ivins JC: The adjunctive use of methylmethacrylate in fixation of pathological fractures. *J Bone Joint Surg Am* 1974;56(1):40-48.

28. Fuchs B, Trousdale RT, Rock MG: Solitary bony metastasis from renal cell carcinoma: Significance of surgical treatment. *Clin Orthop Relat Res* 2005;431:187-192.

29. Townsend PW, Rosenthal HG, Smalley SR, Cozad SC, Hassanein RE: Impact of postoperative radiation therapy and other perioperative factors on outcome after orthopedic stabilization of impending or pathologic fractures due to metastatic disease. *J Clin Oncol* 1994;12(11):2345-2350.

30. Swanson KC, Pritchard DJ, Sim FH: Surgical treatment of metastatic disease of the femur. *J Am Acad Orthop Surg* 2000;8(1):56-65.

31. Frassica FJ, Frassica DA: Metastatic bone disease of the humerus. *J Am Acad Orthop Surg* 2003;11(4):282-288.

Chapter 33

Surgical Management of Upper Extremity Bone Metastases: A Treatment Algorithm

Kevin A. Raskin, MD

Introduction

Metastatic disease to the upper extremity is a relatively common occurrence. Approximately 20% of patients with metastatic disease to bone will have an upper extremity metastasis. Within this group, the metastasis will be present in the humerus in more than 50% of cases. Although the upper extremity is non–weight bearing, its role in activities of daily living, including bathing, toileting, and eating, is critical to quality of life and patient integrity. Because metastatic disease in the skeleton commonly involves the lower extremities, competent and reliable upper extremities are needed for patients who rely on crutches or walkers for assistance with ambulation.

As with other skeletal sites, the common histologic subtypes present in the upper extremity are lung, breast, prostate, kidney, and thyroid carcinoma. Lung carcinoma has a predilection for metastasizing to the hand. A multidisciplinary team is imperative in managing this patient population. The surgical care for patients with bone metastases must be a collaborative effort, with medical and radiation oncologists sharing in the decision making. End-of-life discussions often are required to measure the extent of surgery to which a patient and the multidisciplinary team are willing to commit in an effort to treat a painful metastasis. The role of the orthopaedic surgeon caring for these patients should be carefully aligned with that of the other caregivers to provide thoughtful and appropriate care.

This chapter provides an algorithm (**Figure 1**) as a guide for decision making in the management of bone metastasis to the upper extremity. The algorithm is predicated on the presence of either metastatic cancer or a proximate history of cancer.[1] If, in the initial presentation, no documented history of cancer can be sub-

stantiated, the patient must undergo staging and biopsy to demonstrate the objective presence of metastasis.

Next, the presence or absence of a fracture is determined. If the patient has sustained a stable fracture with minimal bone loss or the patient has a short life span or poor performance status, the overall treatment recommendation would be immobilization and radiation as needed.[2] Conversely, in a patient who has sustained an unstable fracture, with significant structural bone loss and the patient's life span and performance status are amenable to surgery, surgery has been beneficial for improving function and relieving pain. The goal is to provide durable stability and ease symptoms with one procedure. Patients with impending fractures are approached similarly (**Figure 1**).

Humerus

The humerus is the site of most metastases to the upper extremity. A logical approach to surgical management is site-specific within the bone, with different considerations for the proximal humerus, humeral diaphysis, and distal humerus. **Figure 2** presents an algorithm for surgical management of metastatic disease in the humerus.

Proximal Humerus

Small proximal humeral lesions that occupy less than 50% of the bone stock and preserve the articular surface can be successfully treated with curettage and polymethyl methacrylate (PMMA) bone cement packing with or without application of a plate and screws (**Figure 2**). The addition of internal fixation in this location is based on the amount of bone loss and the bone's structural stability after curettage. These lesions often involve the proximal humeral metaphysis[3] (**Figure 3**).

When the lesion is large, more than 50% of the bone stock is lost, and/or the articular surface is lost, endoprosthetic replacement is recommended. If the greater and lesser tuberosities are intact, a standard cemented humeral hemiarthroplasty can be performed. If the tuberosities are effaced or deficient, a proximal humeral

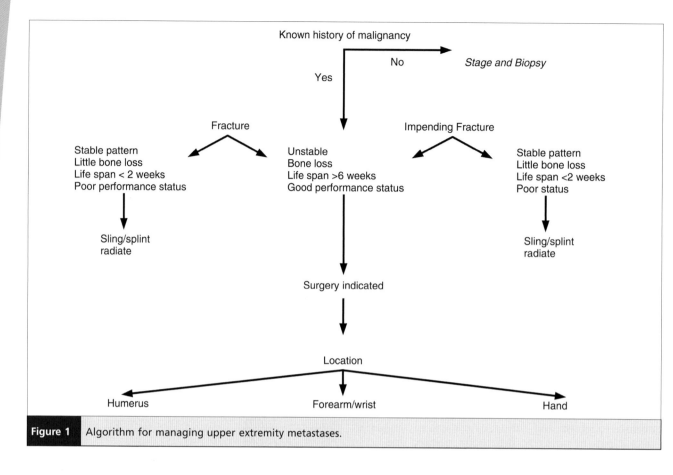

Figure 1 Algorithm for managing upper extremity metastases.

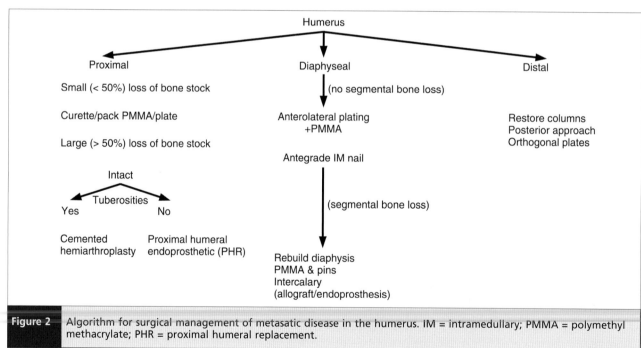

Figure 2 Algorithm for surgical management of metasatic disease in the humerus. IM = intramedullary; PMMA = polymethyl methacrylate; PHR = proximal humeral replacement.

segmental resection is recommended with a proximal humeral endoprosthetic hemiarthroplasty reconstruction (**Figure 4**). The standard endoprosthetic replacement provides a more favorable functional result where possible, because a proximal humeral replacement detaches soft tissues and can present problems of glenohumeral instability.[4,5]

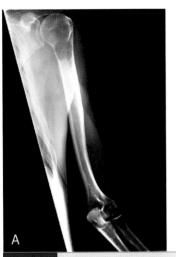
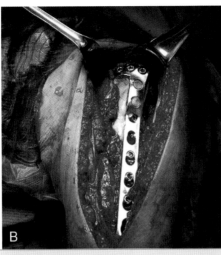
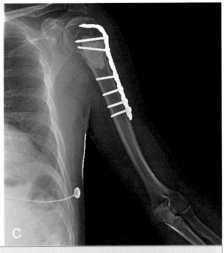

Figure 3   **A,** Radiograph of a metaphyseal lesion in the humerus involving approximately 50% of the bone stock. **B,** Intra-operative photograph showing the relationship of polymethyl methacrylate and internal fixation. **C,** Postoperative radiograph.

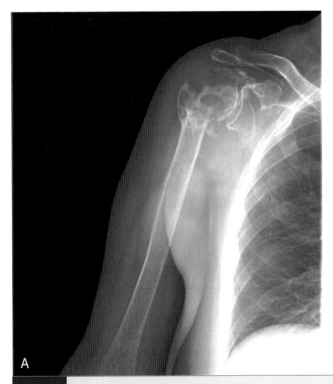
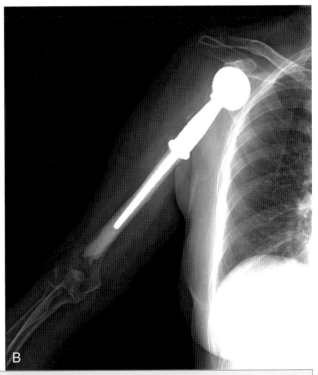

Figure 4   **A,** AP radiograph of a thyroid metastasis destroying both the proximal humerus and the greater and lesser tuberosities. **B,** Postoperative radiograph of a proximal humerus replacement.

Humeral Diaphysis

In the humeral diaphysis that has sustained no segmental bone loss, both anterolateral plating and antegrade intramedullary (IM) nailing (**Figure 5**) are well tolerated.[6] In radiosensitive lesions such as multiple myeloma and lung cancer, the IM nail is long enough to incorporate the entire bone length, and the addition of postoperative radiotherapy often enables long-lasting functional restoration and symptom relief. Conversely, tumors not generally considered responsive to radiation therapy, such as renal cell carcinoma or disease extending distally into the distal one sixth of the humerus (**Figure 6**), are often best treated with curettage, plate fixation, and PMMA packing to reduce the metastatic burden. In addition, large and destructive lesions of the humeral diaphysis in which segmental or large segment bone loss is present can be treated by modular intercalary devices or structural allografts. Structural allograft

5: Metastatic Disease to Bone

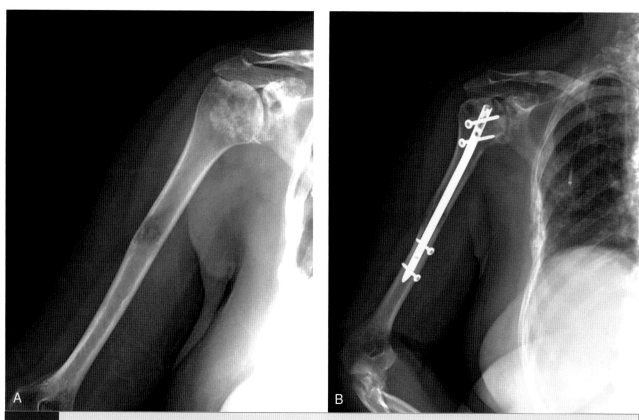

Figure 5   **A,** Preoperative radiograph of a diaphyseal metastases. **B,** Postoperative radiograph after antegrade intramedullary nailing.

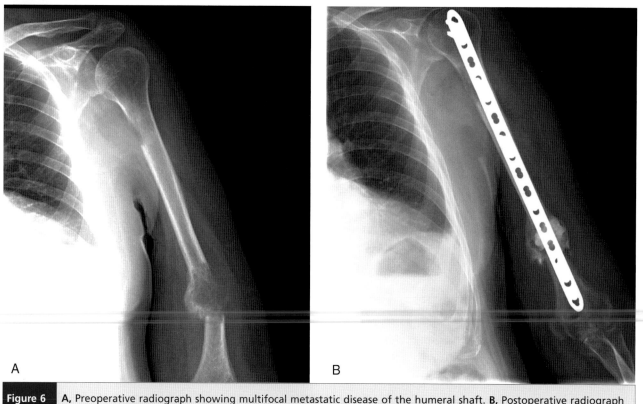

Figure 6   **A,** Preoperative radiograph showing multifocal metastatic disease of the humeral shaft. **B,** Postoperative radiograph showing use of a long plate with polymethyl methacrylate augmentation.

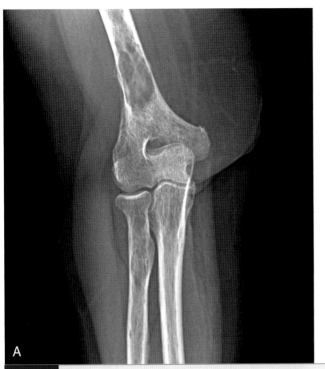
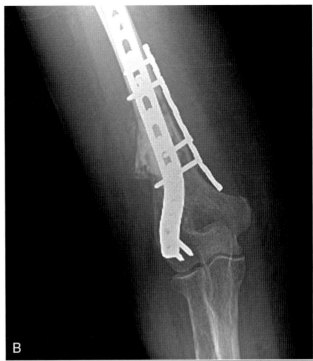

Figure 7 **A,** Preoperative AP radiograph of a distal humerus lesion. **B,** Postoperative image showing orthogonal plating with polymethyl methacrylate augmentation.

reconstruction can lead to additional complications, including infection, delayed union, or nonunion.[4]

Distal Humerus

The distal humerus does not tolerate a large metastatic burden. The supracondylar region of the humerus is a natural stress riser. A weakened cortex here secondary to metastatic carcinoma usually causes pain and presents a difficult surgical challenge. Fractures and impending fractures require a double plating technique and orthogonal plating through a posterior approach to restore the integrity of the medial and lateral columns of the distal humerus (**Figure 7**). PMMA augmentation with internal fixation is often a reliable and durable construct for pain relief and preservation of elbow function.[7] When significant bone loss precludes the use of internal fixation, modular endoprosthetic replacements can reconstruct the entire distal humeral segment. Additionally, a distal or proximal humeral endoprosthesis can be combined with an existing one to create a total humeral replacement if necessary.

Forearm, Wrist and Hand

An algorithm for decision making in the management of bone metastases to the forearm is presented in **Figure 8**. Overall metastases to the radius and ulna can be treated similarly. At their more substantial articular

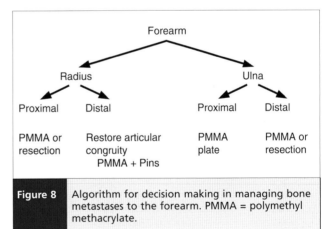

Figure 8 Algorithm for decision making in managing bone metastases to the forearm. PMMA = polymethyl methacrylate.

ends (proximal ulna and distal radius), an effort must be made to restore the articular congruity/stability with either PMMA packing alone or PMMA with internal fixation. In both the radius and ulna, plates and screws can be used as well as threaded and nonthreaded pins to bolster the articular surface. Conversely, at the radiocapitellar joint, proximal radius, and distal ulna, PMMA packing remains a mainstay of treatment, although resection in these areas is also a viable surgical tactic. Both the proximal radius and distal ulna can be resected with little postsurgical morbidity or dysfunction.

Metastatic disease to the bones of the hand is rare. Small, destructive lesions can be managed with curet-

5: Metastatic Disease to Bone

tage and PMMA packing alone. In the fingers where a large tumor is destructive not only of bone but also of soft tissues, ablative surgery such as ray amputation may be considered.

Summary

The approach to metastatic disease in the upper extremity can be simplified by adhering to basic principles; assessing patient performance status, appreciating the extent of bone loss, and planning for a durable postoperative construct. Surgery for these patients must be enduring.

Annotated References

1. Forsberg JA, Sjoberg D, Chen QR, Vickers A, Healey JH: Treating metastatic disease: Which survival model is best suited for the clinic? *Clin Orthop Relat Res* 2013;471(3):843-850.

   The authors compared three types of prognostic models to best determine 3- and 12-month survival after surgical intervention for skeletal metastases. The Artificial Neural Network model yielded the highest net benefit (highest discrimination), although all three models proved useful to varying degrees clinically. Level of evidence: II.

2. Evans AR, Bottros J, Grant W, Chen BY, Damron TA: Mirels' rating for humerus lesions is both reproducible and valid. *Clin Orthop Relat Res* 2008;466(6):1279-1284.

   The authors conducted an online survey of 39 physicians with 17 case histories and radiographs of 16 patients. Among this group, the Mirels criteria has a sensitivity 14.5% and a specificity of 82.9% at a rating of nine points or greater. In this study, the Mirels score was reproducible and deemed valid in the upper extremity. Level of evidence: III.

3. Spencer SJ, Holt G, Clarke JV, Mohammed A, Leach WJ, Roberts JL: Locked intramedullary nailing of symptomatic metastases in the humerus. *J Bone Joint Surg Br* 2010;92(1):142-145.

   The authors reviewed 35 patients (37 IM nails) with symptomatic metastases of the humeral shaft treated with locked antegrade nailing. Pain relief was excellent in 11.4% of patients, good in 82.9%, and fair in 5.7%. IM nailing effectively stabilizes and eases the pain associated with symptomatic pathologic humeral shaft fractures. Level of evidence: IV.

4. Siegel HJ, Lopez-Ben R, Mann JP, Ponce BA: Pathological fractures of the proximal humerus treated with a proximal humeral locking plate and bone cement. *J Bone Joint Surg Br* 2010;92(5):707-712.

   Use of locked plating combined with cement augmentation in 32 patients with pathologic humerus fractures resulted in a 94.6% Musculoskeletal Tumor Society functional score. Level of evidence: IV.

5. Wedin R, Hansen BH, Laitinen M, et al: Complications and survival after surgical treatment of 214 metastatic lesions of the humerus. *J Shoulder Elbow Surg* 2012;21(8, issue 8):1049-1055.

   Two hundred eight patients with 214 metastatic lesions of the humerus were treated surgically using IM nails (148), endoprostheses (35), plate fixation (21), or other means (10). Endoprostheses had the lowest failure rate (6%) compared to 10% seen with osteosynthesis devices. Among the osteosynthetic devices, plates failed more frequently than IM nails. Level of evidence: IV.

6. Piccioli A, Maccauro G, Rossi B, Scaramuzzo L, Frenos F, Capanna R: Surgical treatment of pathologic fractures of humerus. *Injury* 2010;41(11):1112-1116.

   The authors reviewed 87 pathologic fractures of the humerus. Proximal lesions involving the epiphysis were managed with resection and endoprostheses, and the remaining diaphyseal lesions all were treated with IM nails. The patients were scored postoperatively using the Musculoskeletal Tumor Society score: 73% for endoprostheses and 79.2% for locked IM nails. The authors concluded that the risk of endoprosthetic replacement for pathologic fractures of the proximal humerus is low with few complications, and IM nailing provided immediate pain relief and stability with little morbidity. Level of evidence: IV.

7. Weiss KR, Bhumbra R, Biau DJ, et al: Fixation of pathological humeral fractures by the cemented plate technique. *J Bone Joint Surg Br* 2011;93(8):1093-1097.

   A retrospective review of 63 patients who underwent intralesional curettage of a pathologic fracture of the humerus treated with intramedullary polymethyl methacrylate and plating is presented. Eighty-six percent had no or mild pain. The authors concluded that curettage with PMMA packing and plate fixation provides immediate rigidity and early return to function. Level of evidence: IV.

Chapter 34

Surgical Management of Lower Extremity Metastatic Disease

Howard J. Goodman, MD   Francis R. Patterson, MD

Introduction

The morbidity associated with osseous metastatic lesions of the pelvis and lower extremity can be devastating. Pain and decreased mobility can severely affect the quality of life of patients who are already undergoing other cancer treatments including radiation and chemotherapy. Because 40% of metastatic disease occurs in the pelvis and 25% in the femur, there is more opportunity for problems to occur that require surgical treatment. Many patients present with lower extremity pain and difficulty ambulating. Nonsurgical treatment can include bisphosphonates or denosumab, radiation, weight-bearing restrictions, and pain medications; however, surgery may be recommended in selected patients.

The goals of surgical treatment in lower extremity metastatic disease include stabilization of the bone, palliation of pain, and restoration of mobility. Without appropriate weight bearing, oncology patients can easily become even more deconditioned, leading to pulmonary complications, skin breakdown, and thromboembolic complications. It is important that impending fractures are evaluated for surgical stabilization.

Many different tools exist for determining whether particular lesions or selected patients will benefit from surgery.[1] Defects in the pelvis and periacetabular area can be classified by the size and location of the lesions. Long bone and periarticular lesions can be classified by the Mirels criteria, which estimate the risk of subsequent fracture, and recommendations for fixation. Fixation of pathologic fractures will help mobilize the patient. The patient's overall condition can be classified by the Eastern Cooperative Oncology Group performance status, which ranges from 0: fully active with no restrictions to 5: dead from disease. In general, patients who have a poor performance status because of ad-

vanced cancer will not benefit from surgical intervention. Regardless of the presurgical condition, patients with metastatic disease have higher complication rates, including increased intraoperative bleeding, failure of fixation, deep vein thrombosis, and other medical complications when compared with patients undergoing comparable procedures performed for nononcologic indications, and surgical decision making and informed consent should reflect these risks.

Global considerations in this population, such as the timing of surgery in patients receiving chemotherapy or radiation, often need to be addressed with a multidisciplinary team.[2,3] A discussion with the radiation oncologist will help identify relevant issues, including any previous treatment in the area that could impede osteosynthesis efforts, as well as the need for postoperative radiation. Postoperative radiation therapy generally commences after 2 to 3 weeks, when there has been appropriate soft-tissue healing, and is indicated in most patients who have not undergone preoperative radiation therapy. Close communication with the radiation oncologist will ensure that the entire surgical field is treated when necessary, including the whole bone if a long stem, long intramedullary rod, or reaming was used during surgery. Interventional radiologists may need to embolize lesions before surgery to prevent surgical bleeding in hypervascular tumors such as renal and thyroid metastases. Inferior vena cava filters can also be placed to prevent pulmonary embolism in selected high-risk patients, and in situations in which aggressive thromboembolic prophylaxis could cause significant wound morbidity, such as in the pelvis. Other medical specialists and an anesthesiologist need to be involved, because the patients are often malnourished and dehydrated in the perioperative period, or may have life-threatening conditions such as hypercalcemia that need to be treated before administration of anesthesia.

Finally, rehabilitation concerns need to be addressed. The patient should understand the postoperative weight-bearing status and the need for assistive devices or braces. Surgical interventions should be designed to allow full weight bearing in the early postoperative period. In patients with a decreased life span, surgery should not be performed if it will require them to reha-

Dr. Patterson or an immediate family member serves as an unpaid consultant to Merete and has received research or institutional support from Biomet and Synthes. Neither Dr. Goodman nor any immediate family member has received anything of value from or has stock or stock options held in a commercial company or institution related directly or indirectly to the subject of this chapter.

5: Metastatic Disease to Bone

bilitate longer than their anticipated survival. In addition, to the extent that other factors such as cancer fatigue and malnutrition diminish mobility, restoration of limb function might not return the patient to full function. By setting appropriate expectations in the patient with metastatic disease, appropriate stabilization and reconstruction can be achieved to restore a patient's mobility and function while affording appropriate pain relief.

Pelvis

The pelvis is second only to the spine in the occurrence of bony metastasis. These lesions can be divided into non–weight-bearing portions, such as the iliac wing and the pubis, from the weight-bearing columns and the periarticular area. Non–weight-bearing portions rarely require surgery, whereas selected patients may benefit from surgical intervention for lesions around the acetabulum.

Nonsurgical approaches in the pelvis including external beam radiotherapy, minimally invasive ablative therapies such as radiofrequency ablation, and cryotherapy may provide relief in selected patients, although they do not confer structural restoration.

After initial evaluation of location, the complex anatomy of the pelvis requires cross-sectional imaging. Judet views, often used in trauma evaluations around the acetabulum, generally underestimate the amount of bone loss around the hip joint. CT with three-dimensional reconstructions can help simplify the complexities of the lesion and the structural areas that might be affected. Recently developed three-dimensional modeling can also help plan for surgery and can be used to make physical models from which patient-matched custom implants can be manufactured. Typically, standard "off the shelf" implants and knowledge of various reconstructive options can minimize the need for more expensive custom implants, but in some patients with significant bone destruction and extended life expectancy, the expense can be justified.

Surgery in this area can be a difficult undertaking, requiring understanding of multiple approaches as well as implant possibilities. Preoperative planning is important to know locations of soft-tissue masses and their relationship to internal vital structures. Inferior vena cava filters should be considered if routine chemoprophylaxis for thrombosis is contraindicated. Epidural anesthesia can help with intraoperative and postoperative pain control, but can limit early mobilization. Appropriate fluid and blood management including other components (platelets and coagulation factors) should be available for surgery. Soft-tissue coverage can be tenuous, and plastic surgery consultation may be helpful. Placement in the intensive care unit should be considered for close postoperative management because of the massive fluid shifts that occur during this period. Physical therapists need to be carefully instructed on post-

operative care, because this may differ from that in conventional arthroplasty patients.

Nonacetabular Lesions

Fractures of the iliac wing or isolated ischial or pubic ramus fractures can often be treated nonsurgically. These lesions may not be structural, because they are not in the weight-bearing axis from the femur through the acetabulum to pelvic columns up to the sacrum. Because they are often nonstructural, the pain associated with them could be related to the tumor themselves, rather than weight-bearing, functional pain. For this reason, these lesions can also be treated with radiofrequency ablation,[4] embolization, and/or radiation. As the pain improves, treatment with chemotherapy and bisphosphonates can help reverse bone loss while allowing formation of new bone.

Refractory lesions can be treated with surgery with less morbidity than periacetabular lesions. Iliac wing lesions can be approached through the proximal portion of the iliofemoral or ilioinguinal approaches. Anterior ring surgery can be done via a Pfannenstiel incision. In general, no bony reconstruction is needed as long as the weight-bearing axis and columns are not affected. Soft-tissue reconstruction, by bringing muscular planes together and preventing abdominal or pelvic hernias, will minimize early wound healing problems as well as late morbidity from these hernias.

Periacetabular Lesions

Periacetabular lesions are perhaps the most troublesome lesions to treat in patients with multifactorial pain. After restricted weight bearing, modification of activity levels, administration of oral or transdermal medication, and radiation, selected patients with painful lesions, a good performance status, and a reasonable expected longevity can be offered more aggressive management. Recent advances have been made in less invasive percutaneous techniques, in conjunction with interventional radiologists, which may improve pain or function. Pathologic fractures remain a relative indication for surgical treatment in a patient whose performance status and prognosis do not contraindicate a large surgery. Osteosynthesis alone in patients with metastatic disease is often not sufficient, as lesions in metastatic bone are less likely to heal and are best treated in conjunction with arthroplasty and acetabular reconstruction. The goals of acetabular metastatic tumor treatment remain maintenance of ambulatory status and pain control. Nonnarcotic oral medications and community ambulation with or without an aide are reasonable goals, and the patient needs to be appropriately prepared. Furthermore, because of the extensive nature of these surgeries, surgeons generally confer with oncologists to ensure the patient will have sufficient life span to benefit from surgical intervention.

Once surgery is indicated, an anatomic approach to

characterizing the defects allows the surgeon to use a systematic way of choosing appropriate reconstruction. Assessing lesion location and size, and area of bone loss, will allow for a more appropriate restoration of mechanical stability. Reconstruction can be accomplished with standard arthroplasty components with cement augmentation, cement and Steinman pin fixation, antiprotrusio cages and triflanged reconstruction cages, or with a combination of techniques (**Figure 1**). Polymethyl methacrylate (PMMA) is most often used instead of bone graft because of its increased healing potential and immediate stability. Furthermore, recent advances have been made in less invasive techniques, in conjunction with interventional radiologists. The classification system used is the modified Harrington classification, based on the location of the lesion and the type of reconstruction needed. Type 0 nonarticular lesions are nonacetabular and do not penetrate the subchondral plate. They can be iliac, superior, ischial, or pubic, and are best treated by curettage, high-speed burr removal, and reconstruction with a combination of PMMA, Steinman pin, metallic mesh, and plates. Recent advances have also been made in percutaneous image-guided PMMA acetabuloplasty, with good pain relief and return to weight bearing.[5]

Type 1 lesions involve contained lesions about the acetabulum but retain an intact lateral cortex with superior and medial portions of the acetabulum untouched. Any standard approach that allows access to insert routine arthroplasty components can be used, with the caveat that complete exposure of the lesions should be possible. Cement augmentation in the lesions and rim-fitting acetabular cages are very useful and the most straightforward solution. Furthermore, trabecular metal can be used for a more immediate friction fit if all-cemented components are not used. Screws can also be used to help initial fixation. Cemented components are most often used due to decreased ingrowth potential after irradiation.

Type II lesions have a defect in the medial wall of the acetabulum. Routine acetabular components will not have enough support until the wall is reconstructed. After appropriate curettage and resection of tumor and nonviable bone, if the defect remains a type II and is not converted to a type III, reconstruction can be accomplished with mesh to support the medial wall and cementation. Steinman pins can be used in the pubis and ischium to further support an acetabular component. Antiprotrusio cups can also be used to distribute stresses away from the medial wall for a rim-loaded fit or screw fixation at the periphery, without the use of PMMA.

Type III lesions have loss of both the superior bone and the lateral cortex. These defects can be treated with the concept that the original acetabulum needs to be reconstructed, using cement to make up the area of the diseased bone. After resection, screws or Steinman pins can be placed through the defect into less involved areas of the pelvis to prepare for cementation, and an ac-

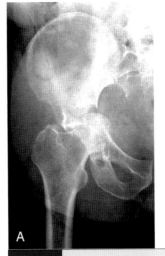 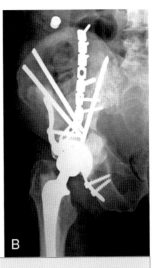

Figure 1 **A,** AP radiograph shows metastatic renal cell carcinoma lesion of the right acetabulum confirmed by percutaneous biopsy with pathologic fracture and protrusio deformity. **B,** Postoperative radiograph following complex reconstruction consisting of a total hip arthroplasty cemented into an antiprotrusio cage. Steinman pins and a reconstruction plate add support and disperse weight-bearing stresses to remaining pelvic bone.

etabular protrusio cup is then cemented over it. Cup-cage constructs can also be used with flanged cages supported by cement and an acetabular cup cemented into the cage. Screws can also be placed through the entire system for support. Depending on the amount of soft tissue released for exposure, a constrained liner can help reduce risk of dislocation.

Type IV lesions add inferior loss of bone, leading to pelvic discontinuity. Reconstruction of these defects are similar to that for type III; however, ischial fixation is needed. Some antiprotrusio cages have three flanges, with two flanges to the iliac wing and one to the ischium, fixed with either screws or slotted placement in a trough in the bone.

If enough nonviable bone has been resected, a type V defect is created, and several options are available. Resection arthroplasty without reconstruction remains an option, but involves the lowest ambulatory potential. Ischiofemoral fusion can be attempted to maintain stability and length, but this often devolves to a painful, unstable pseudarthrosis. An iliofemoral saddle prosthesis can be used for length-stable motion in the plane of the iliac wing, with long-term complications such as proximal migration and iliac wing fracture. If the patient has a longer life expectancy, acetabular allograft prosthetic composite can be considered.

By using the anatomic approach of classifying defects and reconstructing them according to recommendations by class, the most appropriate reinforced prosthetic construct can be accomplished.[6] In a recent review of outcomes after stabilization of metastatic disease, 63 acetabular reconstructions were performed in

5: Metastatic Disease to Bone

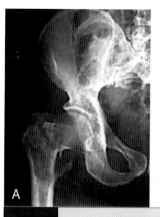
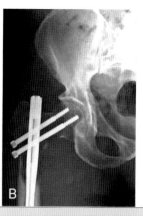
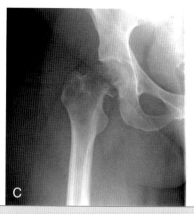
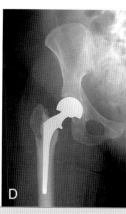

Figure 2 **A,** AP radiograph shows a metastatic lesion of the proximal femur with pathologic fracture and significant bone destruction. **B,** Postoperative AP radiograph following surgical management with reconstructive intramedullary femoral nail. This led to hardware failure and continued pain. **C,** AP radiograph of a different patient with proximal femoral head and neck lytic destruction with femoral neck fracture due to metastatic disease. **D,** Postoperative AP radiograph showing cemented hemiarthroplasty. The patient was able to bear weight immediately postoperatively. Treatment of pathologic fractures should allow for immediate weight bearing, and durability of the surgical fixation should be sufficient to minimize the need for future operations.

62 patients. One patient remained bed bound, and most of the other patients experienced improvement in functional scores. Four revisions were needed for dislocation, trochanteric fracture, and ischial fracture. The authors also noted that patients with metastases from breast cancer have the longest life expectancy, which should be considered before reconstruction is performed.

Femur

The femur is the long bone most commonly affected by metastatic disease. Because of the femur's importance in ambulation and mobility, any loss in its structural ability to bear weight will have a substantial effect on the patient's quality of life. The functional morbidity associated with a femur fracture is considerably higher than that in the upper extremity. Patients with a malignant diagnosis and unrelenting pain in the extremity or functional loss may benefit from stabilization of an impending or completed pathologic fracture in a manner that will allow for immediate weight bearing. Understanding the different life expectancies of patients with various diseases will help the orthopaedist choose the appropriate method of fixation. A surgery with the lowest chance of complication and the ability to bear weight immediately in the postoperative period is the best method of treating these patients. The greatest role for prophylactic fixation of metastatic disease is in the femur, where pain relief and function following prophylactic fixation are superior to results following fracture.

Femoral Head and Neck Lesions

Arthroplasty remains the mainstay of treatment of metastatic disease affecting the femoral neck and head.

Cemented hemiarthroplasty is an excellent method of resecting and replacing metastatic disease in this location. Fixation without resection will most likely lead to failure and need for revision to arthroplasty, so primarily replacing the bone is the most prudent course (**Figure 2**). Even with lesions in the femoral neck, a calcar-replacing femoral stem can lead to a lasting construct.

Controversies still exist regarding the use of hemiarthroplasty versus acetabular resurfacing. Hemiarthroplasty confers more inherent stability than total hips with fewer perioperative complications. In the absence of acetabular disease, resurfacing the socket is unlikely to add value in this patient population with limited longevity, and can lead to dislocation. The theoretical downside of developing arthritis over the subsequent 5 to 7 years is mitigated by decreased life expectancy.

Although a routine hemiarthroplasty has the tip of the stem in the proximal shaft, with metastatic disease it is imperative that femur radiographs or a whole bone MRI is obtained to determine the presence of more distal disease. Without knowing the extent of the metastatic lesions, a short implant might fail to protect other weakened areas of the bone. A stem that is the wrong length can also risk perforation of the anterior cortex. Knowing the locations of more distal lesions will also allow prophylaxis with the long stem or with a second, distally based device.

Cementation is necessary to treat the lesions and fill pathologic bone, while allowing immediate weight bearing. Complications of cemented long-stem hemiarthroplasties are rare,[7] but in a high-risk population can include cardiopulmonary issues, prolonged intubations, mental status compromises, and death. These complications are best minimized by appropriate medullary lavage, canal suctioning during cementation, use of low-viscosity PMMA, and slow, controlled insertion of the stem.[8,9]

Recent series of uncemented stems in the treatment of pathologic fractures or impending pathologic fractures have been reported with acceptable early outcomes.[10] Longer follow-up and analysis are necessary to determine if cementation should be performed routinely given the stability and pain relief historically associated with the use of PMMA in surgery for metastatic lesions. Adequate bone stock is necessary when considering this method of treatment.

Intertrochanteric/Subtrochanteric Lesions

Because the intertrochanteric portion of the proximal femur bears high stresses and is a common location for bony metastatic spread, surgery is often helpful and is dictated by the amount of bone loss. Segmental resection and replacement will allow for immediate weight bearing, although with the drawback of the need to reattach the abductors. If fracture with significant bone loss is present, or there is concomitant large disease load in the femoral neck and head, endoprosthesis is often indicated.[11] With metastatic disease, the soft-tissue envelope can often be spared and appropriate reconstruction can involve keeping most of the musculature surrounding the joint and proximal femur. Furthermore, if there is enough bone left from the greater trochanter, this (with the abductor mechanism and attached soft-tissue sleeve) can be attached to the prosthesis with cables, allowing for better mobility and decreased chance of a Trendelenberg gait.

In the absence of acetabular disease or previous hip arthritis, hemiarthroplasty is the best choice for the proximal femoral replacement. By avoiding placement of an acetabular cup, the prostheses will be less likely to dislocate, the procedure is easier to perform, and less surgical time is required. Special attention should also be given to keeping the joint capsule intact. When the abductor mechanism is compromised, even more stability can be applied by tying nonabsorbable suture in a purse-string through the capsule around the prosthetic femoral neck.

Cost analysis was recently conducted in a British tertiary musculoskeletal oncology unit for the expenditure for a proximal femoral replacement for metastatic disease.[12] They found that the average cost was £18,000 for the hospital stay, surgery, and implant. The conclusion was that although proximal femoral replacement is a clinically effective treatment of metastatic disease, current funding reimburses only approximately half of the associated costs.

If, however, sufficient bone stock remains, a piriformis entry or trochanteric entry femoral nail can stabilize the lesion, allowing for a shorter, more predictable surgery without the complications inherent in arthroplasty (**Figure 3**). The weight-bearing portion in the area of the calcar femorale should have adequate support to allow for ambulation. Life expectancy, which is often difficult to predict, needs to be considered when using proximal osteosynthesis instead of arthroplasty to avoid the potential complication of reoperation.

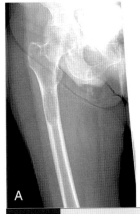
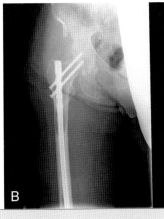

Figure 3 A 70-year-old woman presented with increasing pain with weight bearing. **A,** AP radiograph showing a lytic destructive lesion in the proximal femoral diaphysis. Biopsy confirmed metastatic lung cancer. **B,** AP radiograph following prophylactic stabilization of the lesion with an intramedullary nail. The patient underwent postoperative radiation therapy.

There is no role for sliding hip screw constructs in the management of proximal femur disease because they are associated with a high rate of failure and revision; healing lesions will continue to put more stress on the device, eventually leading to screw cutout and failure of fixation. The end of the plate can also create a stress riser in an area that potentially would be irradiated. These situations can lead to a revision surgery, often with endoprosthetic replacement, and the patient will be subject to additional morbidity from a potentially avoidable condition. In a purely subtrochanteric lesion without excessive bone loss, goals of early mobilization and immediate weight bearing remain paramount. Stabilizing the bone with locked intramedullary nailing has been shown to achieve these goals with a fairly uncomplicated surgery (**Figure 3**). Locking both proximally and distally allows for the greatest strength and longevity in a load-sharing device. Reconstruction nails or implants with fixation into the femoral neck and head allow for even more stability at both ends of the bone, as well as prophylaxis against the potential risk of fracture should subsequent femoral neck lesions develop with minimal extra morbidity. Augmentation can also be achieved with PMMA if appropriate, although with contemporary fixation devices the need for cement supplementation around intramedullary devices has decreased.

Femoral Shaft

The surgical management of large femoral shaft metastatic lesions can allow for continued weight bearing. Primarily cortically based lytic lesions are often seen in lung carcinoma, which is associated with a shorter life expectancy than metastases from breast or prostate disease. More central lesions also will cause substantial loss in structural integrity and are best treated by a

5: Metastatic Disease to Bone

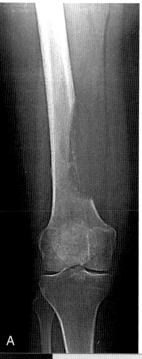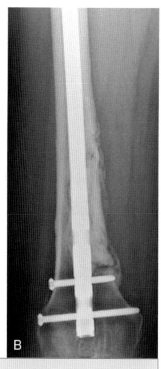

Figure 4 **A,** Radiograph of a distal femur metastatic lung lesion and impending pathologic fracture. **B,** Postoperative radiograph illustrating curettage followed by intramedullary prophylactic fixation and polymethyl methacrylate cement augmentation. This construct allowed immediate weight bearing with good pain relief. External beam radiation to the femur for the entire length of the femur was performed post-operatively to minimize risk of progression.

avoiding injury to the collateral ligaments and the quadriceps tendon that might prevent immediate mobilization.

Recent advances in osteosynthesis have allowed for the use of fixed-angle devices with locked screws.[14] These plates are primarily designed for use in osteoporotic fractures or with limited bone for fixation; however, they are highly applicable in metastatic bone, which presents similar fixation challenges. Recommendations for internal fixation include augmentation with PMMA and filling every hole in the plate to provide the stiffest construct and to retain fixation if disease progression occurs locally within the bone.

In patients whose metastatic disease has destroyed large portions of the distal femur, resection and endoprosthetic replacement offers a solution to allow for immediate weight bearing (**Figure 5**). Furthermore, because many patients are already at an advanced age, concomitant degenerative arthritic changes and metastatic deposits can be treated at the same time. If the cortical bone is preserved, primary components with metaphyseal sleeves, cement augmentation, and modular stems can keep the collateral ligaments intact. More aggressive lesions may require complete distal femoral replacement with a modular hinged system. Routine resurfacing of the patella is controversial.

Tibia

Metastatic disease of the tibia is encountered less frequently, but the goals of restoration of weight-bearing function and alleviation of pain are similar. As with the rest of the weight-bearing lower extremity, smaller lesions often become more symptomatic earlier and will need to be treated. Small, symptomatic lesions considered for surgery that do not affect the articular surface could be amenable to curettage and cement augmentation, most often with plate fixation for support (**Figure 6**). Arthroplasty is often preferred when the proximal tibial cartilage and subchondral plate are involved to provide immediate weight bearing and range of motion. Advances in arthroplasty, including metaphyseal cones and modular prostheses with long stems, add to the ability to augment fixation without resorting to proximal tibial replacement, with its inherent problems of reconstructing the extensor mechanism.

Tibial shaft metastatic lesions are treated with intramedullary nailing, with the largest-diameter nail available. Cement augmentation also can be used in larger defects. Large resections and intercalary prostheses are less often used, due to the increased soft-tissue loss and need for flap coverage. Palliation is best accomplished with immediate weight bearing with minimal surgical insult.

Fibular lesions are even more rare and usually best treated nonsurgically. When radiation is not appropriate or palliation fails, resection of the affected area can be indicated. Even the proximal tibia-fibular joint can be disrupted with minimal reconstruction of the lateral

large-diameter intramedullary nail, with or without tumor removal and cement augmentation. Because most nails currently can include large screws or blades into the femoral neck and head, adequate protection of the proximal femur is allowed without substantial addition of morbidity.

Recently, interest has turned toward the use of reaming and possible vascular dissemination of tumor cells during intramedullary nail placement. A concurrent reaming/aspiration device has been found to retrieve a significant amount of tumor volume during the reaming process.[13] Furthermore, because of the single reaming process, there is less manipulation of the canal and less possibility for extravasation of the tumor.

Distal Femur

In the distal portion of the femur, consideration is once again given to fixation versus arthroplasty. Defects in the metaphyseal supracondylar area may be best treated with curettage, cementation, and plate fixation while maintaining structural stability and allowing weight bearing. Distal femoral nails are less often used (**Figure 4**), with cement augmentation as necessary to enhance fixation. Special attention should be given to

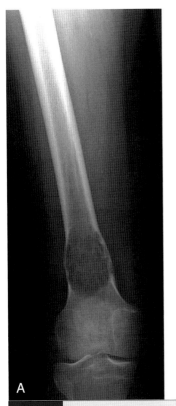
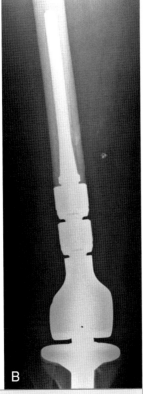
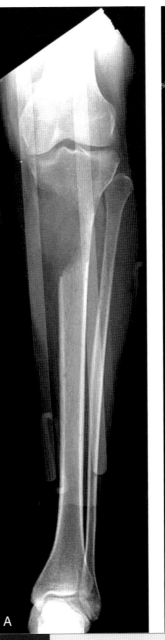
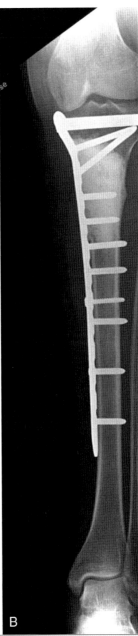

Figure 5 | **A,** AP radiograph of the distal femur shows an extensive lytic defect in the distal femoral metaphysis due to metastatic renal carcinoma. The patient experienced pain and was unable to bear weight. **B,** Postoperative radiograph following segmental distal femur replacement and endoprosthetic knee reconstruction with a rotating hinge knee. Note the intravascular coil used for preoperative embolization to minimize blood loss in this metastatic renal carcinoma lesion. If significant bone destruction is present and the metastatic lesion does not typically respond well to adjuvant treatments, as is this case with metastatic renal carcinoma, treatment should tend toward more durable reconstructions, and segmental resection with arthroplasty affords a more reliable pain control and return to function while minimizing the risk of reconstructive failure.

Figure 6 | **A,** Impending pathologic fracture through a metastatic breast carcinoma deposit in the proximal tibia. **B,** Curettage of the lesion followed by internal fixation of this impending pathologic fracture, with polymethyl methacrylate cement augmentation, allowed for immediate return to function and ambulation. Postoperative radiation was also used to minimize risk of progression.

ligaments. Shaft lesions can be resected with minimal morbidity, when necessary.

Ankle and Foot

In the setting of metastatic disease, lesions at the end of the tibia or fibula or in the bones of the foot are rare; when present they are most commonly seen in lung carcinoma, followed by genitourinary cancers. These lesions can be painful, and if the bone defect is small enough so as not to affect the structure of the bone, palliative radiation is usually effective. With hypervascular tumors, such as renal cell metastases, embolization can be used to treat painful lesions.

If a metastatic deposit is large enough to cause structural problems in this location, curettage with cementation will help control the lesions. Internal fixation will further strengthen the construct, especially if the cortex is sufficiently weakened. Periarticular lesions in the distal tibia and fibula are best treated this way, whereas bones such as the calcaneus (the most commonly af-

5: Metastatic Disease to Bone

fected bone in the foot, followed by the other tarsal bones) may require less invasive treatment. Refractory lesions of the metatarsals and phalanges may best be treated by amputation.

Summary

Metastatic disease in the lower extremities poses a unique challenge for the treating orthopaedist, by causing debilitating pain and limiting ambulation. Surgeons treating these patients should understand the patterns of weight bearing, the risk of pathologic fracture, and appropriate reconstructive techniques available. The goals of treatment must be kept in mind to avoid overtreatment. The patient's overall performance status, disease burden, and goals are incorporated into treatment planning. Prophylactic fixation of impending fractures leads to substantial reduction in morbidity associated with pathologic fractures, whereas complex periarticular reconstructions should be reserved for cases with significant bone loss and extended life expectancy.

Close communication with the team of medical oncologist, radiation oncologist, and physical therapist facilitates care coordination to allow for minimal time lost between continuing treatments. Surgical management allowing for immediate weight bearing, with stable fixation and cement augmentation as needed, usually provides appropriate palliation. With controlled pain and ambulatory status restored, patients with lower extremity metastatic disease can once more resume their quality of life.

Annotated References

1. Mac Niocaill RF, Quinlan JF, Stapleton RD, Hurson B, Dudeney S, O'Toole GC: Inter- and intra-observer variability associated with the use of the Mirels' scoring system for metastatic bone lesions. *Int Orthop* 2011;35(1):83-86.

   This study shows reproducibility in the Mirels scoring system with the same observer and between observers, although it does not address its validity. Level of evidence: II.

2. Bickels J, Dadia S, Lidar Z: Surgical management of metastatic bone disease. *J Bone Joint Surg Am* 2009; 91(6):1503-1516.

   This is a review article involving many newer techniques in evaluation and treatment in osseous bone metastases. Level of evidence: V.

3. Biermann JS, Holt GE, Lewis VO, Schwartz HS, Yaszemski MJ: Metastatic bone disease: Diagnosis, evaluation, and treatment. *J Bone Joint Surg Am* 2009; 91(6):1518-1530.

   This overview of diagnostic and staging studies and surgical management of bony metastatic disease also includes a discussion of pitfalls, as well as adjuvant and minimally invasive treatments. Level of evidence: V.

4. Hoffmann RT, Jakobs TF, Trumm C, Weber C, Helmberger TK, Reiser MF: Radiofrequency ablation in combination with osteoplasty in the treatment of painful metastatic bone disease. *J Vasc Interv Radiol* 2008; 19(3):419-425.

   Twenty-eight metastatic lesions in 22 patients were treated with radiofrequency ablation followed by PMMA injection. Mean visual analog scale score decreased after 24 hours and even more after 3 months, with most patients reducing the strength of narcotics used. Level of evidence: IV.

5. Sapkota BH, Hirsch AE, Yoo AJ, et al: Treatment of metastatic carcinoma to the hip with CT-guided percutaneous acetabuloplasty: Report of four cases. *J Vasc Interv Radiol* 2009;20(4):548-552.

   A procedure was described in which patients with painful, nonstructural lesions of the acetabulum that did not break into the joint were treated with percutaneous injection of PMMA into the lesion. All four patients had relief of pain and were able to resume weight-bearing activity. Level of evidence: IV.

6. Ghert M, Alsaleh K, Farrokhyar F, Colterjohn N: Outcomes of an anatomically based approach to metastatic disease of the acetabulum. *Clin Orthop Relat Res* 2007;459(459):122-127.

   A prospective analysis of 62 patients undergoing acetabular surgery for metastatic disease with approach and reconstruction dictated by lesion type is presented. Findings showed that this approach can improve function. Patients with breast cancer and no history of visceral metastasis had the longest survival. Level of evidence: II.

7. Randall RL, Aoki SK, Olson PR, Bott SI: Complications of cemented long-stem hip arthroplasties in metastatic bone disease. *Clin Orthop Relat Res* 2006; 443(443):287-295.

   The authors discussed the efficacy and safety of cemented long stem hemiarthroplasties, as well as the importance of modifying surgical and cementing techniques to avoid complications. Level of evidence: IV.

8. Camnasio F, Scotti C, Peretti GM, Fontana F, Fraschini G: Prosthetic joint replacement for long bone metastases: Analysis of 154 cases. *Arch Orthop Trauma Surg* 2008;128(8):787-793.

   The authors reported on 154 patients with 117 lower extremity prosthetic reconstructions for metastatic disease, showing better quality of life with few complications in selected populations. Level of evidence: III.

9. Alvi HM, Damron TA: Prophylactic stabilization for bone metastases, myeloma, or lymphoma: Do we need to protect the entire bone? *Clin Orthop Relat Res* 2013;471(3):706-714.

   This was a retrospective review of 96 patients treated with devices that covered the entire bone, regardless of disease in multiple areas. Findings showed only one patient with disease progression to a distant site in the same bone, with 12 patients having complications potentially related to the longer implants. Level of evidence: IV.

10. Thein R, Herman A, Chechik A, Liberman B: Uncemented arthroplasty for metastatic disease of the hip: Preliminary clinical experience. *J Arthroplasty* 2012; 27(9):1658-1662.

    Fifty-seven patients with extensive proximal femur metastases complicated by two early deep vein thromboses, two late deep vein thromboses, one pulmonary embolism, and four infections highlighted the increased surgical risks in this patient population compared to other surgical cohorts. Level of evidence: III.

11. Cannon CP, Mirza AN, Lin PP, Lewis VO, Yasko AW: Proximal femoral endoprosthesis for the treatment of metastatic. *Orthopedics* 2008;31(4):361.

    Fifty-seven patients with extensive proximal femur metastases complicated by two early deep vein thromboses, two late deep vein thromboses, one pulmonary embolism, and four infections highlighted the increased surgical risks in this patient population compared to other surgical cohorts. Level of evidence: III.

12. Ashford RU, Hanna SA, Park DH, et al: Proximal femoral replacements for metastatic bone disease: Financial implications for sarcoma units. *Int Orthop* 2010; 34(5):709-713.

    A cost analysis was performed for the implant, surgical, and early rehabilitative costs of inserting a proximal femoral replacement (mostly used for metastatic disease), and the reimbursement rates. Level of evidence: III.

13. Cipriano CA, Arvanitis LD, Virkus WW: Use of the reamer-irrigator-aspirator may reduce tumor dissemination during intramedullary fixation of malignancies. *Orthopedics* 2012;35(1):e48-e52.

    A novel study investigated how use of the reamer-irrigator-aspirator system can remove an average of 75 mL of tumorous marrow cells during intramedullary reaming. Level of evidence: IV.

14. Gregory JJ, Ockendon M, Cribb GL, Cool PW, Williams DH: The outcome of locking plate fixation for the treatment of periarticular metastases. *Acta Orthop Belg* 2011;77(3):362-370.

    The authors discussed the use of locked plating in pathologic bone with no implant failures or need for revisions. They supported the use of these implants with filling every hole and adding PMMA support. Level of evidence: III.

5: Metastatic Disease to Bone

Chapter 35

Evaluation and Treatment of Spinal Metastases

Michael J. Vives, MD   Saad B. Chaudhary, MD, MBA

Introduction

In 2008, approximately 12 million people in the United States had cancer. A diagnosis of cancer is made in more than 1.2 million people each year, according to American Cancer Society statistics. Approximately 40% of all patients with cancer eventually have spinal metastasis and related symptoms.[1] After the liver and the lung, the skeletal system is the most common site of metastases, and the spine is the most common site of bony metastases.[2] The primary cancer type and site dictate the incidence of spinal metastasis. Prostate, breast, and lung cancers account for most cancer diagnoses, and along with hematopoietic tumors, renal cancer, thyroid carcinoma, and melanoma account for almost all metastases to the spine.

At the time of death, as many as 80% of patients with cancer have evidence of spinal metastases as verified by postmortem examination.[3] However, only about one half of these patients had symptoms related to the spinal spread of their cancer. Symptoms can result from skeletal infiltration and destruction or neurologic compression. Clinically significant epidural compression requiring treatment develops only in approximately 20% of patients with metastatic disease to the spine and approximately 10% of all patients with cancer. Approximately 20,000 patients have metastatic epidural compression each year, and a larger number of patients require treatment of pain, fracture, or instability caused by spinal metastases.[4,5]

Spinal metastases can occur in a patient with an established diagnosis of cancer or as a newly diagnosed

malignancy. Disseminated spinal disease can result in morbidity and deterioration of functional status, thereby compromising quality of life and survivorship. It is critical to make an early diagnosis and institute a multidisciplinary care approach to maintain or restore the patient's neurologic function and quality of life.[6] As cancer care improves, the number of patients with spinal metastases will continue to increase. Enhanced diagnostic ability and superior systemic and surgical treatments have enabled spine surgeons to aggressively manage tumors and improve the short-term and long-term outcomes of many patients with spinal tumors.

Pathogenesis

Tumor cells are believed to spread to the spine hematogenously. Unlike the appendicular skeleton, the vertebral bodies contain active red bone marrow throughout life. This highly vascular sinusoidal system makes the spine vulnerable to cancer cells.[2] Several anatomic models exist for the metastatic spread of tumor cells. A valveless extradural venous plexus could account for the high rate of lumbar metastases in prostate cancer and the prevalence of thoracic metastases in breast cancer.[7] Another model of arterial spread of spinal metastases exists for lung cancer, in which the cancer cells are passed from the pulmonary vein to the left side of the heart and transmitted through the segmental arteries into the spine.[8] Many researchers believe that the tumor cells invade the vertebrae at the end plate junction, based on the location of the end arterioles, or from a posterocentral approach, often close to the base of a pedicle adjacent to the basivertebral veins. Although this theory supports the typical radiographic pattern of posterior vertebral body replacement or early destruction of the pedicle, it was refuted by an MRI-based retrospective review that evaluated the distribution of metastases as related to the proposed arteriovenous route of the spread.[9]

Improved molecular understanding has made it clear that factors other than vascular channels determine the location and predilection for tumor metastases. Tumor cells must dissociate from the primary lesion, penetrate through the extracellular matrix, and migrate through the hematogenous or lymphatic system before docking at the site of a distant metastasis. Here, the cells must rely on expression of surface proteins and adhesion molecules for selection of the new host site before the extracellular matrix is invaded and angiogenesis is initiated for successful metastasis.[10,11]

Despite this laborious process, spinal metastases are common and can result in significant morbidity. The clinical course depends on tumor histology and the location of spinal disease. The spinal region most commonly burdened with metastatic disease is the thoracic (70%), followed by the lumbar (20%) and cervical (10%) regions.[12] Given the small cross-sectional area of the spinal canal and the tenuous blood supply of the thoracic spine, it is fortunate that only a small group of patients with spinal metastases have significant progressive neurologic deterioration.

Clinical Evaluation

The clinical manifestations of spinal metastases range from an incidental asymptomatic finding to progressive neurologic deficit and paralysis. By far, the most common initial symptom is axial pain, which develops in 90% of patients with spinal metastases.[13] The hallmark of metastatic spinal pain is progressive, nonmechanical, and unrelenting pain. The pain usually is worse at night and generally has no associated antecedent trauma. However, the presence of mechanical pain or trauma does not preclude the presence of spinal malignancy.

Patients with metastatic spinal disease frequently have subtle signs of neurologic impairment, but these signs almost never precede axial pain. Neurologic signs and symptoms vary based on tumor location and characteristic. Eccentrically located tumors can often result in radiculopathy, and centrally positioned tumors with epidural compression can produce myelopathy or cauda equina symptoms. The presence of radiculopathy can assist the clinician in determining the vertebral levels involved. Usually the radiculopathy is present for weeks or longer before the development of long-tract signs that suggest spinal cord compression. Bowel and bladder involvement is a rare and late phenomenon that usually appears in patients with profound neurologic dysfunction.[2,14] Early neurologic signs often are overlooked or misdiagnosed, with resultant patient morbidity. The duration and rate of neurologic impairment has a significant effect on prognosis. Patients with a rapid onset of progressive neurologic deterioration (1 to 7 days) have a much worse prognosis than those with a slow course of neurologic impairment (7 to 14 days).[2,15,16]

A high index of suspicion and a thorough history and evaluation are imperative when the clinician evaluates a patient with risk factors for metastatic spinal disease. Neurologic status can be objectively characterized and followed using the American Spinal Injury Association scale, which has largely replaced the Frankel scale.

Diagnostic Strategy

One or more spinal lesions can appear in a patient with known metastatic disease, a history of nonmetastatic malignancy, or no known cancer diagnosis. Although metastatic tumors account for approximately 95% of all spinal lesions, it is imperative to differentiate them from the rare primary spinal lesion.[17] A thorough patient evaluation including history, physical examination, and imaging studies often must be supplemented with a biopsy to confirm the diagnosis of primary or metastatic disease and to delineate the specific tumor type.

A patient with established metastatic disease and spinal lesions typical for the disease process usually can be treated without first undergoing a biopsy. Staging is required before treating a patient with a history of localized nonmetastatic cancer who has single or multiple spinal lesions. Clinical and laboratory evaluation must be completed, with oncologic staging studies including CT of the chest, abdomen, and pelvis and a whole-body technetium Tc-99m bone scan; alternatively positron emission tomography can be performed. A biopsy is performed to obtain a histologic diagnosis. Staging studies can guide the site of the biopsy; the spinal lesion(s) or other appendicular lesion(s), including long bone lesions, may be technically easier and safer to obtain the biopsy specimen from than some spinal lesions. Treatment should not be initiated before confirmation of the source of the lesion.

A patient without an earlier diagnosis of malignancy may have spinal lesions. Spinal metastases must be strongly considered in such a patient because vertebral disease is the initial manifestation of malignancy in 20% of patients with spinal lesions.[18] Lung, prostate, breast, urologic, and gastrointestinal tract cancers are the most common pathologies that appear in such a manner.[19] An oncologic evaluation entailing a comprehensive clinical examination, laboratory tests, and staging imaging studies must be completed and followed by a histologic diagnosis after biopsy.

Image-guided biopsy has become the first-line approach for obtaining tissue from a lesion in the spine. Biopsy success has been correlated with a relatively large needle bore size and the type of skeletal response (lytic or blastic). The diagnostic accuracy of CT-guided spinal biopsy is approximately 93% for lytic lesions and 76% for blastic lesions, with a low complication rate.[20,21] The tissue should be sent for analysis of typical and atypical microorganisms. When necessary, open biopsy should be performed by the surgeon providing the definitive treatment to minimize tissue plane contamination and optimize the oncologic resection.

Patient Assessment and Imaging

A detailed history with a complete review of systems and family history of cancer should be the starting point of the evaluation. Inquiry should be made about routine age-appropriate screening studies for cancer, such as colonoscopy and mammography. The patient's history of tobacco use or occupational exposure to carcinogens should be assessed. A thorough examination of the spine should be performed, with an examination of potential primary tumor sites such as the thyroid gland, breast, prostate gland, and abdomen, if metastatic disease is suspected.

Upright biplanar plain radiographs are initially obtained. Radiographs can help delineate spinal alignment, stability, pathologic fractures, and possibly the presence of pathologic lesions. However, radiographs are not sufficiently sensitive for the reliable detection of early or small lesions. Lesions typically become visible on plain radiographs when 30% to 50% of the trabecular bone has been destroyed. Pedicle lysis, commonly known as the winking owl sign, is highly indicative of a tumor, but most radiographic findings are nonspecific for diagnosing tumor type.

CT often is obtained to define the bony anatomy and extent of destruction. Axial imaging combined with sagittal and coronal reconstruction can assist in defining any potential instability. CT lacks the sensitivity to be used as the primary imaging modality for the detection of metastatic spinal disease. CT was found to have sensitivity of 66% and diagnostic accuracy of 89% in detecting osseous spinal metastases.[22] Nonetheless, CT is invaluable in revealing skeletal detail, assessing stability, and planning surgery, and it is essential if the patient is unable to undergo MRI.

MRI provides the greatest soft-tissue detail, including epidural extension of disease. MRI is the most sensitive (98.5%) and specific (98.9%) imaging study for detecting spinal metastases.[22] MRI of the entire spine should be strongly considered because almost 15% of patients have clinically significant lesions at noncontiguous sites.[23] Tumors usually show a hypointense signal intensity on T1-weighted images and a hyperintense signal on T2-weighted sequences. Contrast enhancement with gadolinium does not help define intraosseous tumors but can be useful in evaluating epidural disease and the soft tissue surrounding the tumor. A combination of radiographs, MRI, and CT, including CT of the chest, abdomen, and pelvis, as well as a whole-body bone scan, must be obtained to assess for systemic disease burden.

Treatment Decision Making

The management of metastatic disease of the spine continues to evolve. During the past few decades of the 20th century, radiation therapy was considered to be the mainstay of treatment for patients with metastatic spinal lesions, including those with spinal cord compression. Comparative studies of surgical treatment and radiation found no advantage of surgical intervention. The standard surgical strategy involved posterior de-

compression of the neurologic elements by laminectomy, and stabilization with rigid instrumented constructs was infrequently used. These procedures provided poor decompression because most patients had significant vertebral body involvement and associated ventral compression of the neurologic elements. In the kyphotic thoracic spine, these factors limited the amount of indirect decompression achieved by a laminectomy, and the destabilizing nature of this method led to progressive postoperative deformity.

A focus on the need to treat the anterior pathology directly through an anterior or posterolateral approach, combined with the use of rigid instrumentation, has resulted in improved benefit after surgical management of spinal cord compression from metastatic disease. The field of radiation oncology also has advanced during the past two decades. High-precision targeting has led to improved treatment efficacy for lesions deemed radioresistant by conventional methods. As a result of these advances, several factors must be considered to determine the individualized treatment plan for a patient with metastatic spinal lesions. Although life expectancy plays a major role in the selection of a treatment strategy, the prediction of longevity for an individual patient remains imprecise and subject to error.[24] The indications for surgical intervention in metastatic disease of the spine include mechanical instability, significant deformity, symptomatic neurologic compression from retropulsed bony fragments, radiated lesions that continue to produce symptoms, and radioresistant tumors. A subset of patients with tumors of unknown origin require a surgical procedure to obtain tissue for diagnosis.

Scoring systems have been developed for use in estimating prognosis and making treatment decisions. One of the first to gain interest, the Tomita scoring system, uses three components: grade of malignancy, visceral metastasis, and bone metastasis.[25] More recently, the revised Tokuhashi scoring system was found to offer reasonable ability to predict survival. In addition to the domains considered by the Tomita system, the revised Tokuhashi system includes performance status, type and location of metastases, and Frankel-classified neurologic deficits.[26] As a general rule, a patient whose life expectancy exceeds 3 to 4 months may be a candidate for aggressive surgical intervention.

Radiotherapy

Conventional Radiotherapy

In the past, conventional external beam radiation was widely considered to be the mainstay treatment for metastatic disease of the spine. The current application of this modality is best assessed separately for two distinct groups of patients: those with spinal pain caused by metastatic disease in the absence of compression of the neurologic elements and those with neurologic deficit caused by compression of the spinal cord or nerve roots. Most patients with symptomatic spinal metastases without neurologic involvement are treated palliatively with conventional radiation. It is unclear whether any specific total dosage and fractionation schedule provides superior pain relief. The most common dosage is 30 to 35 Gy delivered in 5- to 10-Gy fractions. Patients with mechanical instability from a pathologic fracture are not well served by this approach.

For patients with spinal cord compression from epidural extension of tumor, the efficacy of conventional radiotherapy depends on several factors. Pretreatment neurologic status and favorable tumor histology (radiosensitivity) are the most important predictors of success. Patients with spinal cord compression but no neurologic deficit have an excellent chance of maintaining ambulatory ability. A meta-analysis of several studies found that fewer than 50% of patients with neurologic deficits will recover significant function.[27] The most important investigation on this subject was a multicenter level I study published in 2005, in which patients with metastatic spinal cord compression were treated with surgery followed by radiotherapy or with radiotherapy alone.[28] With the ability to walk as the primary end point, 84% of the surgically treated patients and 57% of those treated with radiation alone had favorable outcomes. In addition to radiosensitivity of the tumor, it is also important to determine whether neurologic compression is the result of retropulsed bone from pathologic fracture and instability. In such patients, surgery as the initial intervention, followed by postoperative radiation, has a significantly better outcome than the same treatment in reversed sequence.

Stereotactic Radiosurgery

Radioresistant tumors do not reliably respond to conventional radiotherapy. Conventional external beam radiation includes the tumor within a large field of normal tissue; in contrast, stereotactic delivery techniques allow high-precision targeting of tumors. In stereotactic radiosurgery, high-dosage radiation is delivered to a small target area with greater than 1-mm accuracy. This precision is accomplished using multiple beam positions (50 to 200) delivered in hypofractionated (1 to 3 sessions) doses. Pretreatment planning involves landmark or fiducial-based tracking obtained from CT fused with positron emission tomography or MRI. Real-time biplanar radiography is then used to confirm the calculated position during delivery.

Because of its precise, high-dosage delivery, stereotactic radiosurgery has better effectiveness against radioresistant tumors than conventional radiotherapy. Studies of this technique applied to spinal metastases from renal cell carcinoma, which are notably resistant to conventional radiotherapy, have found significant improvement in pain relief and local tumor control.[29] Further research is necessary to define the exact role of stereotactic radiosurgery in the treatment of such patients. A systematic review compared the available data on the treatment of solitary vertebral renal metastases by en bloc resection or stereotactic radiosurgery.[30]

Given that the ability of either local treatment to effect a cure in such patients is unpredictable, the review conclusion was based on local tumor control. The authors gave a weak recommendation based on the limited available evidence for considering stereotactic radiosurgery as a first-line treatment because it is less invasive than conventional radiotherapy and offers similar local control rates. Stereotactic radiosurgery also has been effective in treating patients with recurrent lesions after earlier spinal irradiation or surgery.[31] Because revision surgery in such patients is fraught with complexities and potential complications, the rationale for stereotactic radiosurgery is quite strong. The use of this technique as the primary intervention for patients with new-onset or progressive neurologic deficit has been limited, however. As a result of the time constraints created by the somewhat limited availability of the technology as well as the requirement for specialized pretreatment imaging and planning, surgical intervention may be the first-line treatment choice for some patients.

Surgical Treatment

The objectives of surgical treatment of spinal metastases include decompressing the neurologic elements, restoring mechanical stability, and decreasing pain. In general, anterior decompression and stabilization should be the surgical goal in the presence of anterior spinal cord compression or mechanical disruption of the anterior column. This goal can be accomplished using a variety of techniques; the choice depends on the location of the metastases and the surgeon's preference.

Cervical Spine

The occipitocervical junction, the subaxial cervical spine, and the cervicothoracic junction have distinct anatomic and biomechanical characteristics. Because the spinal canal in the upper cervical region is large, neurologic deficits are relatively uncommon. Pain and instability are more common indications for surgical management of metastatic disease in this region. For radiosensitive tumors, pain in the absence of instability can be treated with radiotherapy. Unstable, destructive lesions of the C2 body or the C1 lateral mass typically are managed with a posterior stabilization technique[32] (**Figure 1**).

The subaxial cervical spine is the cervical region predominantly affected by metastatic disease. The most common strategy for managing these lesions involves anterior corpectomy using a standard or modified Smith-Robinson approach. The reconstructive techniques range from the use of Kirschner wire–polymethyl methacrylate constructs to structural allografts and cage designs. An anterior cervical plate usually is used to increase stability if a strut graft or cage is used (**Figure 2**). Combined anterior-posterior surgical approaches should be considered if multilevel involvement or circumferential disease is present.

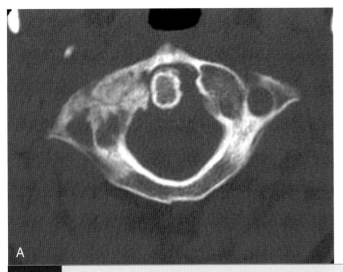

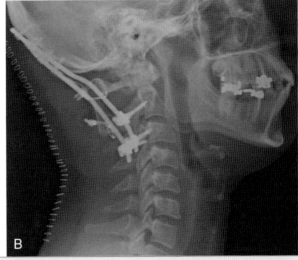

Figure 1   **A,** CT showing a lesion and fracture of the C1 lateral mass in a patient with metastatic breast cancer. **B,** Postoperative lateral radiograph showing posterior occipitocervical stabilization.

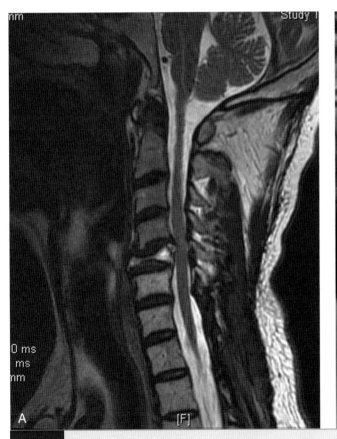

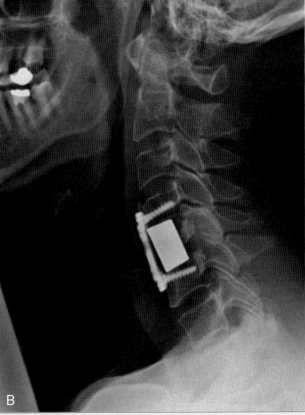

Figure 2   **A,** Sagittal MRI showing a pathologic fracture of C5 in a patient with metastatic breast cancer. **B,** Lateral radiograph after corpectomy and reconstruction using a porous tantalum spacer and an anterior cervical plate.

Neurologic involvement appears to be more common than pain as an indication for surgical intervention in studies on metastatic disease of the cervicothoracic junction.[33] Anterior approaches are viable for lesions involving the vertebral bodies of C7 or T1 because often they can be reached through a low cervical approach without the morbidity of splitting the manubrium. Given the biomechanical stresses in this transitional region, supplemental posterior stabilization should be considered.

5: Metastatic Disease to Bone

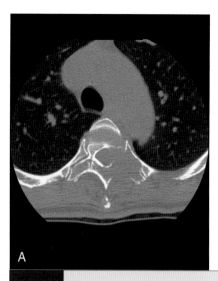
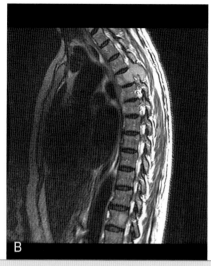
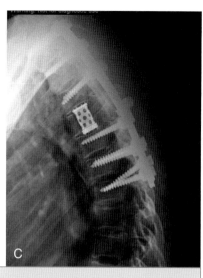

Figure 3 **A,** Axial CT showing an upper thoracic lesion in a patient with metastatic adenocarcinoma of the colon. **B,** Sagittal MRI showing the expansile nature of the lesion. **C,** Lateral radiograph after decompression through costotransversectomy with reconstruction using a cage and pedicle screw construct.

Thoracolumbar Spine

The thoracic and lumbar regions are the most common sites of symptomatic spinal metastasis, with axial pain being the predominant symptom.[34,35] A patient with a pathologic compression fracture may be a candidate for a minimally invasive cement augmentation procedure, such as vertebroplasty or kyphoplasty. The posterior wall of the vertebral body should be intact to minimize the risk of cement extrusion into the spinal canal. When vertebroplasty was introduced during the 1980s in France, it was commonly used to treat patients with myeloma and painful hemangioma. In North America, vertebroplasty has mostly been used to manage painful osteoporotic compression fractures. Two randomized placebo-controlled studies challenged the widespread belief that cement augmentation is effective for the treatment of painful osteoporotic compression fractures.[36,37] Uncontrolled studies of cement augmentation in spinal metastatic disease found that significant pain reduction was sustained for more than 1 year.[38] A multicenter prospective randomized study compared kyphoplasty and nonsurgical management in 134 patients with neoplastic disease.[39] The patients who were surgically treated had significant improvement in all Medical Outcomes Study 36-Item Short Form subscales at 1-month follow-up. Almost 60% of patients in the nonsurgical group were moved to the surgical treatment group because of ongoing symptoms, and the remaining patients had no improvement. The patients who underwent surgical treatment had outcomes similar to those of patients in the original kyphoplasty group.

A patient with a pathologic burst fracture involving retropulsed bone or tumor extension into the canal is best suited for open surgical treatment. Metastatic involvement of the vertebral body frequently results in ventral compression of the dura, and an anterior de-

compression and stabilization procedure is the most effective method of treating the pathology. In the upper thoracic spine (T2 through T5), an anterior approach is problematic. High thoracotomy is associated with morbidity from detachment of the periscapular musculature. Although a direct anterior approach can be achieved through sternotomy or manubriectomy, the presence of the heart and great vessels limits access to the spine in this region. The use of posterolateral approaches (transpedicular, costotransversectomy, and lateral extracavitary approaches) to the anterior column has become more widespread and increasingly is favored for treating pathology in this region of the thoracic spine. The sacrifice of one or more ipsilateral thoracic nerve roots facilitates ventral access with minimal functional consequence. The spinal cord can readily be seen for circumferential decompression. Reconstruction of the anterior column with a Kirschner wire–polymethyl methacrylate construct may suffice if the patient has a limited life expectancy. A patient with a more favorable prognosis can be considered for an anterior fusion construct involving a strut graft or cage (**Figure 3**). An expandable cage can be inserted using a posterolateral approach and dialed up to engage the corresponding end plates for stable seating. As surgeons have gained experience with the use of pedicle screws in the upper thoracic region, the addition of transpedicular fixation to the anterior construct increasingly is used to allow early mobilization with a decreased need for bracing.[40,41]

For thoracolumbar lesions below T6, anterior, posterior, and circumferential surgery may be viable options for selected patients. Clinical presentation, surgeon experience, and patient preference all should be considered. Lesions from the midthoracic level to the lumbosacral junction can be approached relatively easily through thoracotomy, thoracoabdominal, and retro-

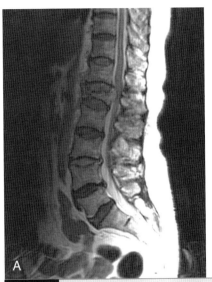
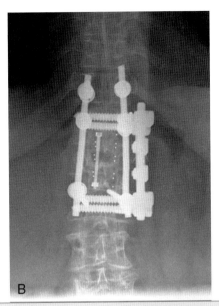
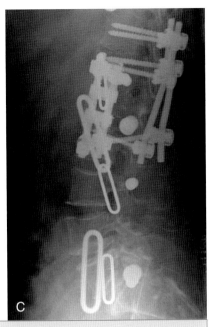

Figure 4   **A,** Sagittal MRI showing a pathologic fracture of L1 with neurologic involvement in a patient with metastatic breast cancer. AP **(B)** and lateral **(C)** radiographs after anterior-posterior decompression and fusion. The procedure was chosen because the patient had osteoporosis and a history of smoking.

peritoneal approaches. If a one-level lesion is treated with a load-sharing interbody device and anterior fixation, supplemental posterior stabilization may not be necessary. A patient with compromised cardiopulmonary physiology may not be able to tolerate an anterior approach, however, and a posterolateral approach to an anterior lesion may be preferable. In this region, unlike the upper thoracic spine, sacrifice of lumbar nerve roots carries substantial functional morbidity. As a result, a thorough decompression and reconstruction is more technically demanding. In vascular tumors, such as thyroid and renal cell carcinoma, preoperative embolization can significantly reduce surgical blood loss and therefore reduce associated morbidity.

A combined anterior-posterior approach occasionally may be necessary. A corpectomy and anterior reconstruction involving more than two levels in a patient with severe osteoporosis may benefit from the additional mechanical stability afforded by posterior fixation (**Figure 4**). Augmentation of screw purchase with polymethyl methacrylate also may need to be considered. The paucity of evidence to support the superiority of any of these strategies was highlighted in an extensive systematic review by the Spine Oncology Study Group.[42] No level I studies, only one level II study, and five level III studies were identified. The remaining 26 eligible studies were level IV. The authors concluded that very low quality evidence existed to support the superiority of one approach over another; the exception was the rationale for posterolateral management of upper thoracic lesions.

En bloc spondylectomy is commonly used for primary malignant tumors of the spine but occasionally is used to treat spinal metastatic disease. This strategy may offer a decreased likelihood of local recurrence compared with piecemeal corpectomy procedures, particularly in radioresistant/oligometastatic tumors such as renal cell carcinoma and sarcomas. Data do not clearly show improved survival compared with marginal resection, however. A systematic review found only six primary publications on the outcomes of en bloc resection of solitary renal cell metastases, with a total of only 15 patients.[30] In addition to weak supporting evidence, the drawbacks of these procedures include their technical demands and high rate of morbidity. Such an aggressive procedure is best considered for a patient with a solitary metastasis and a very favorable prognosis. As data are amassed on the performance of stereotactic radiosurgery, the role of en bloc treatment of spinal metastases may be further refined.

Outcome Measures

The literature on clinical outcomes for tumors of the spine is limited. In most studies, outcomes were reported as process variables such as survival, local recurrence, complications, and gross measures of function, such as ambulatory status. In a recent systematic review of clinical outcomes comparing surgery (with or without radiation) to radiation alone, the overall risk of complications was found to be 29% and was thought to be influenced by the systemic disease burden.[43] The common surgical complications included wound infection or dehiscence (8%); pneumonia, pleural effusion, or respiratory failure (4%); instrumentation failure (4%); thromboembolic disease (2%); and leakage of cerebrospinal fluid (2%).

During the past 20 years, a focus on health-related quality of life has led to the widespread use of patient self-assessment instruments that directly measure the value of care as perceived by the recipient. No disease-specific tool for metastatic spinal disease exists, but a recent analysis suggests that other patient self-assessment instruments should be used to foster a uniform and in-depth study of the treatment options.[44] As a generic tool, the Medical Outcomes Study 36-Item Short Form has been validated and is frequently used in research on metastatic disease of the spine. The Eastern Cooperative Oncology Group Performance Status instrument is well correlated with the universal framework of the International Classification of Functioning, Disability, and Health and therefore is a useful cancer-specific tool.

Summary

Cancer is diagnosed in more than 1 million people annually. Approximately 40% of all patients with cancer eventually have spinal metastases and related symptoms. After the liver and lung, the skeletal system is the most common site of metastases, and the spine is the most common site of bony metastases. Clinically significant epidural compression develops in approximately 20% of patients with metastatic disease of the spine and approximately 10% of all patients with cancer. The most common clinical manifestation of spinal metastasis is axial pain. The hallmark of metastatic spinal pain is progressive, nonmechanical, and unrelenting pain. Although metastatic tumors account for approximately 95% of all spinal lesions, it is imperative to differentiate them from the rare primary spinal lesion. This differentiation is accomplished by performing a thorough patient evaluation including history, physical examination, and imaging studies. Often, a biopsy must be performed to confirm the diagnosis of primary or metastatic disease and to delineate the specific tumor type.

Annotated References

1. Wong DA, Fornasier VL, MacNab I: Spinal metastases: The obvious, the occult, and the impostors. *Spine (Phila Pa 1976)* 1990;15(1):1-4.

2. Harrington KD: Metastatic disease of the spine. *J Bone Joint Surg Am* 1986;68(7):1110-1115.

3. Jaffe WL: *Tumors and Tumorous Conditions of the Bones and Joints.* Philadelphia, PA, Lea and Febiger, 1958.

4. Byrne T, Benzel E, Waxman S (eds): *Diseases of the Spine and Spinal Cord.* New York, NY, Oxford University Press, 2000.

5. Posner JB: Spinal metastases, in *Neurologic Complications of Cancer.* Philadelphia, PA: Davis Company, 1995.

6. Riley LH III, Frassica DA, Kostuik JP, Frassica FJ: Metastatic disease to the spine: Diagnosis and treatment. *Instr Course Lect* 2000;49:471-477.

7. Batson OV: The function of the vertebral veins and their role in the spread of metastases. *Ann Surg* 1940; 112(1):138-149.

8. Harada M, Shimizu A, Nakamura Y, Nemoto R: Role of the vertebral venous system in metastatic spread of cancer cells to the bone. *Adv Exp Med Biol* 1992;324: 83-92.

9. Yuh WT, Quets JP, Lee HJ, et al: Anatomic distribution of metastases in the vertebral body and modes of hematogenous spread. *Spine (Phila Pa 1976)* 1996; 21(19):2243-2250.

10. Choong PF: The molecular basis of skeletal metastases. *Clin Orthop Relat Res* 2003;(415, Suppl):S19-S31.

11. White AP, Kwon BK, Lindskog DM, Friedlaender GE, Grauer JN: Metastatic disease of the spine. *J Am Acad Orthop Surg* 2006;14(11):587-598.

12. Brihaye J, Ectors P, Lemort M, Van Houtte P: The management of spinal epidural metastases. *Adv Tech Stand Neurosurg* 1988;16:121-176.

13. Gilbert RW, Kim JH, Posner JB: Epidural spinal cord compression from metastatic tumor: Diagnosis and treatment. *Ann Neurol* 1978;3(1):40-51.

14. Constans JP, de Divitiis E, Donzelli R, Spaziante R, Meder JF, Haye C: Spinal metastases with neurological manifestations: Review of 600 cases. *J Neurosurg* 1983;59(1):111-118.

15. Jacobs WB, Perrin RG: Evaluation and treatment of spinal metastases: An overview. *Neurosurg Focus* 2001;11(6):e10.

16. Perrin RG, Laxton AW: Metastatic spine disease: Epidemiology, pathophysiology, and evaluation of patients. *Neurosurg Clin N Am* 2004;15(4):365-373.

17. Kelley SP, Ashford RU, Rao AS, Dickson RA: Primary bone tumours of the spine: A 42-year survey from the Leeds Regional Bone Tumour Registry. *Eur Spine J* 2007;16(3):405-409.

    The authors conducted a retrospective review of a tumor registry that revealed 2,750 incidences of bone or bonelike tumors, of which primary bone tumors of the spine constituted 4.6%. Multiple myeloma and plasmacytoma were the most common pathologies, followed by osteosarcoma.

18. Schiff D, O'Neill BP, Suman VJ: Spinal epidural metastasis as the initial manifestation of malignancy: Clinical features and diagnostic approach. *Neurology* 1997;49(2):452-456.

19. Destombe C, Botton E, Le Gal G, et al: Investigations for bone metastasis from an unknown primary. *Joint Bone Spine* 2007;74(1):85-89.

    In a retrospective review of 152 patients with metastatic spinal lesions from an unknown primary site, the authors found that the most common primary tumor site was the lung, followed by the prostate gland, the breast, the urologic system, and the gastrointestinal tract.

20. Lis E, Bilsky MH, Pisinski L, et al: Percutaneous CT-guided biopsy of osseous lesion of the spine in patients with known or suspected malignancy. *AJNR Am J Neuroradiol* 2004;25(9):1583-1588.

21. Nourbakhsh A, Grady JJ, Garges KJ: Percutaneous spine biopsy: A meta-analysis. *J Bone Joint Surg Am* 2008;90(8):1722-1725.

    The authors conducted a meta-analysis of the adequacy and complications associated with percutaneous spinal biopsies and found that needles with a larger diameter were correlated with improved adequacy and accuracy, but with an increased complication rate. The complication rate was 3.3% when using CT and 5.3% when using fluoroscopy.

22. Buhmann Kirchhoff S, Becker C, Duerr HR, Reiser M, Baur-Melnyk A: Detection of osseous metastases of the spine: Comparison of high resolution multi-detector-CT with MRI. *Eur J Radiol* 2009;69(3):567-573.

    The authors of this retrospective analysis of the detection of 639 vertebral bodies in 41 patients with a confirmed malignancy found that the sensitivity of MRI in detecting metastatic disease was 98.5%, compared with 66.2% for multidetector CT. The specificity was similar. CT provided excellent assessment of bony architecture.

23. Maranzano E, Trippa F, Chirico L, Basagni ML, Rossi R: Management of metastatic spinal cord compression. *Tumori* 2003;89(5):469-475.

24. Nathan SS, Healey JH, Mellano D, et al: Survival in patients operated on for pathologic fracture: Implications for end-of-life orthopedic care. *J Clin Oncol* 2005;23(25):6072-6082.

25. Tomita K, Kawahara N, Kobayashi T, Yoshida A, Murakami H, Akamaru T: Surgical strategy for spinal metastases. *Spine (Phila Pa 1976)* 2001;26(3):298-306.

26. Tokuhashi Y, Matsuzaki H, Oda H, Oshima M, Ryu J: A revised scoring system for preoperative evaluation of metastatic spine tumor prognosis. *Spine (Phila Pa 1976)* 2005;30(19):2186-2191.

27. Klimo P Jr, Thompson CJ, Kestle JR, Schmidt MH: A meta-analysis of surgery versus conventional radiotherapy for the treatment of metastatic spinal epidural disease. *Neuro Oncol* 2005;7(1):64-76.

28. Patchell RA, Tibbs PA, Regine WF, et al: Direct decompressive surgical resection in the treatment of spinal cord compression caused by metastatic cancer: A randomised trial. *Lancet* 2005;366(9486):643-648.

29. Gerszten PC, Burton SA, Ozhasoglu C, et al: Stereotactic radiosurgery for spinal metastases from renal cell carcinoma. *J Neurosurg Spine* 2005;3(4):288-295.

30. Bilsky MH, Laufer I, Burch S: Shifting paradigms in the treatment of metastatic spine disease. *Spine (Phila Pa 1976)* 2009;(34)Suppl:22:S101-S107.

    Based on a systematic review of the literature, the authors found that surgery followed by radiotherapy was strongly recommended for patients with high-grade spinal cord compression caused by metastatic disease. A weak recommendation was made that patients with solitary renal cell metastases undergo stereotactic radiosurgery.

31. Gerszten PC, Burton SA, Ozhasoglu C, Welch WC: Radiosurgery for spinal metastases: Clinical experience in 500 cases from a single institution. *Spine (Phila Pa 1976)* 2007;32(2):193-199.

    In a longitudinal cohort study, the authors reviewed 500 patients with spinal metastases who underwent radiosurgery. Long-term tumor control was achieved in 90% of patients in whom the radiosurgery was the primary treatment modality.

32. Fourney DR, York JE, Cohen ZR, Suki D, Rhines LD, Gokaslan ZL: Management of atlantoaxial metastases with posterior occipitocervical stabilization. *J Neurosurg* 2003;98(2)Suppl:165-170.

33. Placantonakis DG, Laufer I, Wang JC, Beria JS, Boland P, Bilsky M: Posterior stabilization strategies following resection of cervicothoracic junction tumors: Review of 90 consecutive cases. *J Neurosurg Spine* 2008;9(2):111-119.

    The authors retrospectively analyzed outcomes for 90 patients who were treated with a posterior approach for metastatic disease at the cervicothoracic junction. The rate of fixation failure was 12%.

34. Gokaslan ZL, York JE, Walsh GL, et al: Transthoracic vertebrectomy for metastatic spinal tumors. *J Neurosurg* 1998;89(4):599-609.

35. Holman PJ, Suki D, McCutcheon I, Wolinsky JP, Rhines LD, Gokaslan ZL: Surgical management of metastatic disease of the lumbar spine: Experience with 139 patients. *J Neurosurg Spine* 2005;2(5): 550-563.

36. Buchbinder R, Osborne RH, Ebeling PR, et al: A randomized trial of vertebroplasty for painful osteoporotic vertebral fractures. *N Engl J Med* 2009;361(6):557-568.

5: Metastatic Disease to Bone

The authors conducted a randomized double-blind study in which patients undergoing vertebroplasty for the treatment of osteoporotic compression fracture had outcomes similar to those of patients who underwent a sham procedure.

37. Kallmes DF, Comstock BA, Heagerty PJ, et al: A randomized trial of vertebroplasty for osteoporotic spinal fractures. *N Engl J Med* 2009;361(6):569-579.

The authors conducred a multicenter randomized double-blind study in which patients treated with vertebroplasty had similar improvement in pain and disability associated with osteoporotic compression fracture as patients who underwent a simulated procedure.

38. Fourney DR, Schomer DF, Nader R, et al: Percutaneous vertebroplasty and kyphoplasty for painful vertebral body fractures in cancer patients. *J Neurosurg* 2003;98(1)Suppl:21-30.

39. Berenson J, Pflugmacher R, Jarzem P, et al; Cancer Patient Fracture Evaluation (CAFE) Investigators: Balloon kyphoplasty versus non-surgical fracture management for treatment of painful vertebral body compression fractures in patients with cancer: A multicentre, randomised controlled trial. *Lancet Oncol* 2011;12(3):225-235.

The authors of this multicenter international study found that cancer patients with painful compression fracture who were randomly assigned to kyphoplasty showed more improvement at 1-month follow-up than those treated nonsurgically.

40. Fisher C, Singh S, Boyd M, et al: Clinical and radiographic outcomes of pedicle screw fixation for upper thoracic spine (T1-5) fractures: A retrospective cohort study of 27 cases. *J Neurosurg Spine* 2009;10(3):207-213.

The authors of this retrospective study of patients with upper thoracic fracture found that pedicle screw fixation was safe and effective.

41. Guzey FK, Emel E, Hakan Seyithanoglu M, et al: Accuracy of pedicle screw placement for upper and middle thoracic pathologies without coronal plane spinal deformity using conventional methods. *J Spinal Disord Tech* 2006;19(6):436-441.

42. Polly DW Jr, Chou D, Sembrano JN, Ledonio CG, Tomita K: An analysis of decision making and treatment in thoracolumbar metastases. *Spine (Phila Pa 1976)* 2009;34(22)Suppl:S118-S127.

A systematic review found very low quality evidence to support the superiority of one approach over another for surgical management of thoracolumbar metastases.

43. Kim JM, Losina E, Bono CM, et al: Clinical outcome of metastatic spinal cord compression treated with surgical excision ± radiation versus radiation therapy alone: A systematic review of literature. *Spine (Phila Pa 1976)* 2012;37(1):78-84.

The authors of this systematic review of English-language literature from 1970 to 2007 suggested that surgical tumor excision and instrumented stabilization improves clinical outcome more than radiation alone.

44. Street J, Berven S, Fisher C, Ryken T: Health related quality of life assessment in metastatic disease of the spine: A systematic review. *Spine (Phila Pa 1976)* 2009;34(22)Suppl:S128-S134.

The authors of this systematic review of the literature found that valid, reliable health-related quality-of-life measures exist for the assessment of oncology patients. A disease-specific tool for metastatic spinal disease awaits development.

Chapter 36

Disease-Specific Considerations in Metastatic Bone Disease

Robert H. Quinn, MD   Rajiv Rajani, MD

Introduction

Metastatic bony lesions have more similarities than differences. For the most part, surgical intervention is similar across the spectrum. However, several of the more common bony metastatic tumors exhibit differences in their clinical behavior and treatment susceptibility that warrant specific considerations.

Metastatic tumors differ by class in the areas of life expectancy, likelihood that a pathologic fracture will heal, and sensitivity to adjuvant treatment. Table 1 illustrates the differences in these parameters.[1] It is important to recognize that wide variations exist in individual patients, regardless of their primary tumor morphology.

Breast Cancer

According to recent data, an estimated 232,340 new cases of invasive breast cancer are expected to occur among women in the United States during 2013.[2] Breast cancer is the second most common malignancy in women, after skin cancer. An estimated 40,030 breast cancer deaths are expected in 2013. Breast cancer is the second leading cause of death from malignancy in women, after lung cancer. Death rates for breast cancer have steadily decreased in women since 1990, with larger decreases in younger women.

Bone metastases occur in 70% of patients with breast cancer and represent the most common cause of pathologic fractures.[3,4] Approximately one half of patients with metastatic bone disease are women with breast cancer. More than 50% of pathologic fractures are secondary to metastatic breast cancer.

Endocrine therapy is the initial treatment of choice for hormone receptor-positive breast cancer in patients

with metastatic bone disease. Premenopausal patients are usually treated with pharmacologic ovarian ablation achieved through the use of luteinizing hormone-releasing hormone agonists. Postmenopausal patients are generally treated initially with a selective estrogen receptor downregulator, or antiestrogen. Although the median duration of response to endocrine therapy is 15 months, many patients exhibit prolonged responses lasting several years.

For patients who demonstrate progressive disease on initial endocrine therapy, second-line and third-line agents are available and include progestins and aromatase inhibitors.

Human epidermal growth factor receptor 2 (HER2) targeting has shown promising results in selected patients.

Bisphosphonates are used in the treatment of metastatic bone disease to delay the time to the first skeletal-related event (SRE), reduce frequency of SREs, reduce bone pain, and improve quality of life. Denosumab is a fully human monoclonal antibody against the receptor activator of nuclear factor-κ B ligand (RANKL), which suppresses bone resorption. Denosumab has proven superior to zoledronic acid in delaying the first SRE with lower toxicity.

Patients with progressive disease after endocrine therapy, rapidly progressive and life-threatening disease, and estrogen-negative and progesterone-negative tumors are considered for cytotoxic chemotherapy.

In general, bony metastatic breast cancer tends to be relatively radiosensitive. Therefore, patients with bony lesions in the absence of either real or impending pathologic fracture are more likely to respond favorably to nonsurgical treatment than patients with tumors that are more resistant to radiation therapy. For patients with pathologic fractures or impending fractures, treatment with combined surgery and radiation is more likely to lead to fracture healing and less likely to demonstrate significant local disease progression. Surgical intervention (including the extent of tumor resection and defect reconstruction) therefore can often be less extensive than with more aggressive tumors. Figure 1 shows a pathologic fracture of the humerus secondary to metastatic breast carcinoma with demonstrable healing of the fracture 4 months after internal fixation

Table 1

Tumor Characteristics

Primary Tumor	Common Type of Bone Destruction	Fracture Healing (%)[a]	5-Year Relative Survival (%)[b]	Radiosensitivity [c]
Breast	Mixed	37	23.8	+++
Lung	Lytic	0	3.7	+
Thyroid	Lytic	?	53.9	+
Kidney	Lytic	44	11.6	-
Prostate	Blastic	42	27.8	+++
Melanoma	Lytic	?	15.1	+

[a]Data from Gainor and Buchert.[1] Question marks indicate tumors that were not included/analyzed.
[b]2002–2008 SEER (Surveillance, Epidemiology, and End Results) data.[2]
[c] +++, [very sensitive]; +, [marginally sensitive]; -, [minimally sensitive].

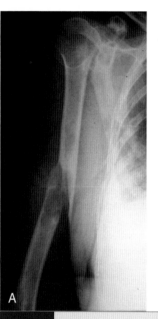
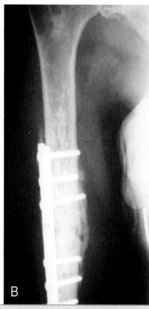

Figure 1 **A,** A preoperative radiograph shows a pathologic fracture of the humerus secondary to metastatic breast carcinoma. **B,** The fracture had demonstrable healing 4 months postoperatively.

with polymethyl methacrylate. In most series of patients with real or impending fractures in metastatic bone disease, those with metastatic breast cancer generally achieve the best results.

Prostate Cancer

An estimated 238,590 new cases of prostate carcinoma are expected to occur among men in the United States during 2013.[2] An estimated 29,720 prostate cancer deaths are expected to occur in 2013. Incidence rates are significantly higher in blacks than in whites. Since 2004, incidence rates have decreased by 2.7% per year

among men 65 years of age and older and have remained stable among men younger than 65 years. Prostate cancer death rates have been decreasing since the early 1990s in both blacks and whites. Although death rates have decreased more rapidly among black men than among white men, rates for blacks remain more than twice as high as those for whites. Prostate cancer death rates decreased 3.0% per year for white men and 3.5% per year for black men from 2004 to 2008. Prostate cancer rarely affects individuals younger than 45 years but increases almost exponentially between the ages of 50 and 80 years.

Patients with prostate cancer are treated with hormone manipulation as the first line of systemic therapy. Androgen deprivation therapy (ADT) includes surgical orchiectomy, administration of gonadotropin-releasing hormone agonists, and the use of antiandrogens. Concurrent use of bisphosphonate therapy has proven successful in managing the osteopenia associated with ADT and in delaying onset of the first SRE. Cytotoxic drugs and prednisone are used in patients with disease refractory to ADT.

Although as many as 85% of patients with advanced prostate cancer demonstrate bone metastasis, the incidence of pathologic fracture is far lower than with other forms of metastatic bone disease. This finding is likely secondary to the predominantly blastic nature of the disease. Nevertheless, bone pain is a significant problem in these patients. Metastases are seen most frequently in the spine and pelvis, likely secondary to dissemination of tumor cells through the Batson plexus of vertebral veins. Despite the frequency of spinal involvement, neurologic compromise as a result of pathologic fracture is rare.

Like metastatic breast carcinoma, metastatic prostate cancer tends to be very responsive to radiation therapy. Because of their blastic nature, with a concomitant lower risk of pathologic fracture and general responsiveness to hormonal manipulation and radiation therapy, metastatic skeletal lesions are usually treated nonsurgically, with good long-term results and a high rate of lesion and/or fracture healing. In some series, the longest survival rate after pathologic fracture occurs in patients with metastatic prostate cancer.

Lung Cancer

Approximately 228,190 new cases of lung cancer are expected to occur in the United States in 2013, accounting for about 14% of malignancy diagnoses.[2] The incidence rate has been declining in men over the past 20 years. In women, the rate has just begun to decrease after a long period of increase. Lung cancer accounts for the highest malignancy death rate. An estimated 159,480 lung cancer deaths, accounting for about 27% of all malignancy deaths, are expected to occur in 2013. Death rates began declining in men in 1991 and in women in 2003. The demographics of lung cancer and associated deaths are strongly correlated to cigarette smoking patterns in men and women.

Lung cancer is classified as small cell (15%) or non–small cell (85%). For localized non–small cell cancers, surgery and chemotherapy result in a 5-year survival rate of 52%. Unfortunately, only 15% of these patients have localized disease. Other patients are treated with a combination of chemotherapy, targeted therapy, and radiation therapy. The 5-year survival rate for all stages combined is 16%. In general, small cell cancers are more responsive to chemotherapy and radiation therapy.

Approximately 30% of lung cancer patients demonstrate bony metastatic disease. A small percentage of patients have bone lesions secondary to paraneoplastic syndromes (including oncogenic osteomalacia, which may be associated with pseudofractures), and these should not be confused with metastatic lesions.

Lung cancer patients overall have a shorter life span than patients with breast or prostate cancer, and therefore the necessity and magnitude of surgical intervention must be weighed accordingly. Bone lesions and pathologic fractures are less likely to heal with a combination of systemic chemotherapy and localized radiation therapy, when compared to lesions and fractures secondary to breast, prostate, or renal cancers. The method of surgical stabilization and treatment should not rely primarily on the patient's bone healing. The aim of surgery should be to create a durable construct that will have a high likelihood of lasting beyond the patient's predicted survival in the absence of any bony healing.

Renal Cell Cancer

An estimated 65,150 new cases of renal cell cancer are expected to be diagnosed in the United States in 2013.[2] An estimated 13,680 deaths from kidney cancer are expected to occur in 2013.

Surgery is the primary treatment of localized renal cell cancer. Kidney cancer tends to be resistant to both traditional chemotherapy and radiation therapy. Interleukin-2 and interferon-α have been used with limited success. Thalidomide has also shown effectiveness in some patients. Targeted therapies, including those aimed at the tumor's blood supply such as bevacizumab, have led to prolonged survival times in patients with metastatic disease.

Approximately 25% to 30% of patients with renal cell carcinoma develop bony metastases. Bone metastases from renal cell carcinoma are more likely to cause intractable pain and pathologic fracture than most other tumors. The hypervascularity associated with these tumors causes them to enlarge quickly, stretching the periosteum and destroying bone. The increased blood flow of the tumor also creates regional osteopenia, which further increases the weakness of the bone.

Surgical treatment of bony lesions from renal cell carcinoma is perhaps the most challenging aspect of metastatic bone disease management. Because these tumors are poorly responsive to systemic therapy and radiation therapy, surgical intervention is required more often than with other malignancies. Massive hemorrhage may occur. When surgery is indicated, extensive reconstruction is often required to create a construct durable enough to withstand potential tumor recurrence and last throughout the patient's remaining lifetime. In a 2007 study, the authors reported superior survival rates with clear-cell histologic subtype, bone-only metastases, and a solitary metastasis.[5]

Wide tumor resection is often advocated in renal cell carcinoma. This surgery allows for lower risk of local recurrence, more extensive reconstruction, and less blood loss. Reasonable evidence suggests that aggressive management of isolated metastasis can prolong patient survival and improve palliation.[6,7] These benefits are most likely to become manifest in patients who have a solitary metastasis occurring after a prolonged disease-free interval following treatment of a localized primary tumor. Figure 2 shows an isolated metastatic renal cell carcinoma treated with wide resection and reconstruction; 4 years postoperatively, the patient has no evidence of disease.

Hemorrhage remains a challenging problem in the treatment of these tumors. Tourniquets should be used in the rare instances in which the lesion is distal enough to allow successful application. Preoperative embolization has proven successful in decreasing intraoperative blood loss. Embolization is most effective when performed within 24 to 48 hours of surgery because these tumors quickly revascularize. Adequate replacement blood should be available during surgery regardless of whether embolization is performed.

Thyroid Cancer

An estimated 60,220 new cases of thyroid cancer are expected to be diagnosed in 2013 in the United States.[2] The male to female ratio is 1:4. Thyroid cancer is the

5: Metastatic Disease to Bone

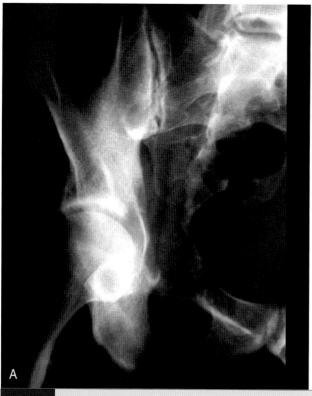
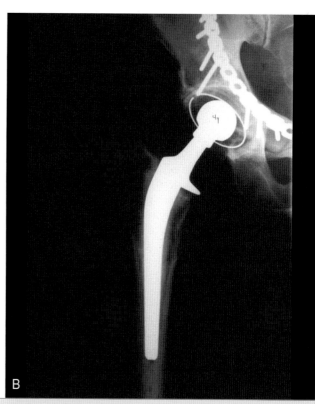

Figure 2 **A,** A solitary renal cell carcinoma metastasis in the right superior pubic ramus and the anterior column of the acetabulum is shown. **B,** A radiograph 4 years postoperatively shows no evidence of local recurrence.

fastest-increasing malignancy in both men and women. An estimated 1,850 deaths from thyroid cancer are expected in 2013 in the United States.

Most thyroid cancers are highly curable; however, approximately 5% represent more aggressive subtypes with metastatic potential. For most patients, surgery is the treatment of choice. Treatment with radioactive iodine (^{131}I) postoperatively may be recommended for more advanced disease. Hormone therapy is used to replace hormones normally produced by the thyroid gland after thyroidectomy and to prevent production of thyroid-stimulating hormone, decreasing the likelihood of recurrence.

The 5-year survival rate approaches 100% for localized disease, 97% for regional-stage disease, and 56% for distant-stage disease.[2] For all stages combined, survival is highest (almost 100%) for patients younger than 45 years.

Although thyroid cancer is the most common endocrine malignancy and one of the five most common malignancies metastasizing to bone, the actual number of patients with bone metastases is quite low in comparison to the other malignancies discussed previously. The incidence of bone metastasis has been reported at 5% to 10% for follicular thyroid cancer and less than 1% for papillary carcinoma. Metastases most often involve the axial skeleton. However, although the incidence of metastatic bone disease is relatively low, 78% of patients with bony metastasis will develop an SRE, and 65% of these will develop at least a second SRE.[8]

Radiation therapy alone is often successful in eradicating skeletal metastases, particularly well-differentiated tumors. In patients with multifocal metastatic disease from a primary tumor that exhibits iodine uptake, long-term palliation often results from systemic treatment with ^{131}I. However, prognosis is far worse with metastatic tumors that do not demonstrate uptake of iodine.

Of the five most common types of metastatic bone tumors, a solitary metastatic bone lesion is most common with thyroid cancer. Complete or definitive surgical management of these solitary lesions often results in cure, or at least substantial prolongation of survival, when compared to solitary lesions from breast, prostate, lung, or renal cancers.

Melanoma

Melanoma is expected to be diagnosed in about 76,690 persons in the United States in 2013, accounting for less than 5% of all skin cancer patients but the vast majority of skin cancer deaths.[2] An estimated 9,480 deaths are expected to occur in 2013.

Metastatic tumors are treated with combination chemotherapy, immunotherapy, and targeted therapy.

Metastatic bone lesions from melanoma are unusual but not rare. Because they are relatively resistant to radiation therapy, more aggressive definitive surgery or complete removal is generally warranted. Some evidence supports wide resection of isolated skeletal or soft-tissue metastases in an effort to prolong survival. A 2012 study showed a favorable prognostic effect with the following: a prolonged delay between diagnosis and surgery, radical excision, a solitary skeletal metastasis, radiation therapy, perioperative lactate dehydrogenase level ≤ 8 microkat/L, and preoperative hemoglobin level > 11.5 mg/dL.[9]

Summary

Metastatic bony lesions share many similarities, and surgical treatment of these lesions tends to be more similar than different. However, cancers commonly metastatic to bone do demonstrate important differences in their responses to adjuvant treatment, the propensity to demonstrate fracture healing, and prognosis.

Annotated References

1. Gainor BJ, Buchert P: Fracture healing in metastatic bone disease. *Clin Orthop Relat Res* 1983;178:297-302.

2. American Cancer Society: *Cancer Facts & Figures 2013*. Atlanta, GA, American Cancer Society, 2013.

   This source provides annual updates on malignancy statistics. Level of evidence: I.

3. Walkington L, Coleman RE: Advances in management of bone disease in breast cancer. *Bone* 2011;48(1):80-87.

   A comprehensive review of current strategies in the management of bone disease in breast cancer, including evidence-based recommendations for clinical practice, is presented. Level of evidence: I.

4. Coleman RE, Rubens RD: The clinical course of bone metastases from breast cancer. *Br J Cancer* 1987;55(1):61-66.

5. Lin PP, Mirza AN, Lewis VO, et al: Patient survival after surgery for osseous metastases from renal cell carcinoma. *J Bone Joint Surg Am* 2007;89(8):1794-1801.

   A retrospective review of 295 consecutive patients treated for metastatic renal cell carcinoma is presented. Patients demonstrated superior survival rates with clear-cell histologic subtype, bone-only metastases, and a solitary metastasis. Level of evidence: III.

6. Alt AL, Boorjian SA, Lohse CM, Costello BA, Leibovich BC, Blute ML: Survival after complete surgical resection of multiple metastases from renal cell carcinoma. *Cancer* 2011;117(13):2873-2882.

   A retrospective review of 887 patients who underwent nephrectomy for renal call carcinoma who developed multiple metastatic lesions is presented. The effect of complete metastatectomy on survival was evaluated. Complete resection of multiple renal cell carcinoma metastases was associated with a significant increase in long-term survival and should be considered when technically feasible in appropriate surgical candidates. Level of evidence: III.

7. Jung ST, Ghert MA, Harrelson JM, Scully SP: Treatment of osseous metastases in patients with renal cell carcinoma. *Clin Orthop Relat Res* 2003;409:223-231.

8. Farooki A, Leung V, Tala H, Tuttle RM: Skeletal-related events due to bone metastases from differentiated thyroid cancer. *J Clin Endocrinol Metab* 2012;97(7):2433-2439.

   The authors present a retrospective review of 245 differentiated thyroid cancer patients with bone metastasis. Occurences of SRE from initial diagnosis to final follow-up or death are reported. Level of evidence: III.

9. Wedin R, Falkenius J, Weiss RJ, Hansson J: Surgical treatment of skeletal metastases in 31 melanoma patients. *Acta Orthop Belg* 2012;78(2):246-253.

   The authors present a retrospective review of 31 patients with malignant melanoma surgically treated for 34 skeletal metastases. A prolonged delay between diagnosis and surgery, radical excision, a solitary skeletal metastasis, radiotherapy, a perioperative lactate dehydrogenase level ≤ 8 microkat/L ($p = 0.04$), and a preoperative hemoglobin level > 11.5 mg/dL ($p = 0.003$) had a favorable prognostic effect. A vertebral localization was unfavorable. Level of evidence: III.

Special Considerations in Tumor Management

SECTION EDITOR:

Ginger E. Holt, MD

Chapter 37

Pelvic Sarcoma Resection and Reconstruction

Peter C. Ferguson, MD, FRCSC

Introduction

Pelvic sarcomas pose significant challenges for the orthopaedic oncologist. The incidence of pelvic sarcomas has been gradually increasing since the early 1970s.[1] Chondrosarcoma and Ewing sarcoma in particular have a predilection to occur in this region, making the pelvis one of the more common locations for bone sarcomas. Pelvic and axial locations of some sarcomas portend a poorer prognosis than other sites. In Ewing sarcoma, for example, axial location is associated with a lower overall survival than appendicular location, along with large size, metastases at presentation, lack of definitive treatment, and positive surgical margins at surgical resection.[2] On multivariate analysis, axial location is still predictive of poorer outcome after adjustment for pretreatment variables. Although comparatively rare, osteosarcoma of the pelvis has a similar poor prognosis, with a 5-year event-free survival of 22% and 5-year overall survival of 47%, compared to 57% and 69%, respectively, for nonpelvic sites in a study in children.[3] In adults, the results are also poor, with a high rate of local recurrence and 5-year survival of less than 50%.[4,5] The pelvis is the second most common site of chondrosarcoma, after the femur. Although low-grade and intermediate-grade chondrosarcomas have a reasonably good prognosis in the pelvis, high-grade chondrosarcomas in this location have a poorer prognosis than those that arise in appendicular locations.[6]

There are many potential reasons for the pelvis to be associated with poorer oncologic outcomes. Because of local anatomy, these tumors are often in very close proximity to critical neurovascular, gastrointestinal, and genitourinary structures, and preservation of these structures may be associated with compromised margins, which can lead to local progression of disease and subsequently to metastasis development. Pelvic tumors also often attain a significant size before being detected,

which itself is predictive of poor outcome in most sarcomas. Complications of surgery are much higher in pelvic locations than in other sites, which may impair the patient's capacity to receive adjuvant treatments.

The concerning oncologic outcomes for pelvic sarcomas are rivaled by the significant reconstructive challenges in these patients. The role of the pelvis in transferring forces from the extremity to the spine on weight bearing necessitates a reliable and durable reconstruction that will last many years in the frequently young sarcoma patient. The complex and variable pelvic bony anatomy makes it difficult to use modular prostheses, which have proven so effective and have revolutionized limb salvage surgery in the appendicular skeleton. The proximity to gastrointestinal and genitourinary organs and mucosal surfaces as well as the prolonged surgical times involved in the extensive resections increases the incidence of surgical infections, which can be disastrous for massive pelvic reconstructions.

Anatomic Considerations in Pelvic Reconstruction

Reconstructive issues vary depending on the anatomic location of the sarcoma within the pelvis, according to the Enneking classification system (**Figure 1**).[7] Tumors arising superior to the acetabulum (type I) may be resected without compromising the hip joint, although they sometimes involve the sacroiliac joint and sacrum (type IV) and the combined type I-IV resection can compromise the stability of the pelvic ring. Tumors arising in the acetabulum (type II) necessitate consideration of reconstruction of the hip joint, which may be possible if the ilium is intact, but for tumors that extend above the acetabulum as well (type I-II), the reconstruction options become more limited. Tumors arising inferior to the acetabulum (type III) may not require any reconstruction at all, unless the tumor again extends into the acetabulum (type II-III) and above (type I-II-III).

Recent studies on pelvic sarcomas have focused on two major areas: first, the utility of image guidance to improve the resectability of these challenging tumors, and, second, the ongoing discussion regarding the optimal reconstructive techniques in the various anatomic

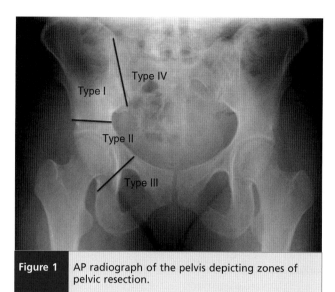

Figure 1 AP radiograph of the pelvis depicting zones of pelvic resection.

areas. There is currently no universal agreement on the latter issue, leaving individual surgeons to base their decisions on personal comfort and experience with the technique, availability of a multidisciplinary surgical team, and patient preference.

Computer-Assisted Navigation for Pelvic Sarcoma Resection

For all sarcomas, it is ideal to obtain negative surgical margins at the time of tumor resection to prevent local disease recurrence. Because of complex pelvic anatomy, attainment of adequate negative margins can prove difficult. The incidence of positive margins for resections of pelvic sarcomas in general has been reported to be between 30% and 35%.[8]

Using surgical navigation, some groups have been able to obtain adequate negative margins for all anatomic sites, with a corresponding decrease in local recurrence.[9-11] Furthermore, the ability to undertake an accurate reconstruction can be improved. When using allograft for reconstruction, the donor bone can be cut to resemble exactly the anatomy of the specimen that was resected.[12] Similarly, custom prostheses can be fabricated to exactly replicate the resected bone.[13]

One of the main disadvantages of the use of computer-assisted navigation is the prolongation of surgical time, which can increase the risk of surgical infections. One study showed that after six resections, including four pelvic tumors, one tumor in the proximal tibia, and one tumor in the proximal femur, the surgical time was lengthened by as little as 13 minutes, with a mean navigation time of 28 minutes.[10]

The application of computer-assisted navigation in pelvic sarcoma resection is in its infancy, with most publications consisting of isolated case reports or small case series.[11,12,14,15] It is readily apparent, however, that the ability to resect pelvic sarcomas using this tech-

nique has significantly improved, with an appreciable decrease in the incidence of positive margins. Further long-term follow-up in large patient series is needed to ensure that this improvement translates into an improvement in local recurrence for pelvic sarcomas, and to determine whether the ability to preserve more normal anatomy is associated with improved functional outcome.

Reconstruction After Resection of Pelvic Sarcomas

The Enneking classification of pelvic resections[7] has enabled musculoskeletal oncology surgeons to discuss the options for resection and reconstruction of the different anatomic regions in a common language. Although in some areas there is general consensus about the preferred management, significant controversy exists in others. Tumors arising in the iliac wing (type I), where the posterior column is unaffected by disease and where the sacrum is uninvolved, can be resected, and because the pelvic ring and acetabulum are maintained, no reconstruction need be undertaken.[16] Similarly, tumors in the ischiopubic region (type III) also do not involve the acetabulum, and despite the fact that the pelvic ring is disrupted, good function is usually obtained without any reconstruction.[16] In contrast, there continues to be significant discussion about the preferred reconstruction technique for two anatomic regions of the pelvis: the sacroiliac region and the acetabulum.

Iliosacral Reconstruction (Type I-IV)

Iliosacral reconstruction can also include tumors that are isolated to the iliac wing but require disruption of the pelvic ring. The proximal osteotomy can be done through the sacroiliac joint. The result of this resection is that the remaining pelvis on the ipsilateral side, including the acetabulum, can rotate proximally through the pubic symphysis, leading to significant limb-length discrepancy and marked alteration in gait. There are two general approaches to this situation. In the first, the defect is not reconstructed, and any functional deficit and limb-length discrepancy is managed by the patient nonsurgically (shoe lifts, gait accommodations). In the second, reconstruction of the defect is undertaken, generally using biologic reconstruction, to maintain leg length and function.

The option for resection without reconstruction was raised as a result of a direct comparison of two groups of patients in a case-control study.[17] Twelve patients without iliosacral reconstruction were compared with four patients who underwent reconstruction—one with contralateral iliac crest bone graft and three with irradiated allografts. Internal fixation was used in all four patients. Patients without reconstruction had shorter surgical time, less blood loss, fewer complications requiring secondary surgery, and were more likely to walk without assistive devices. They had similar func-

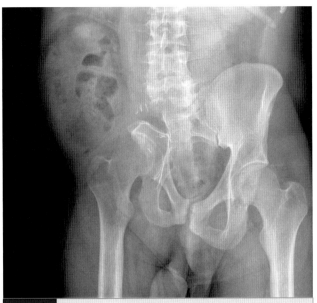

Figure 2 AP radiograph of the pelvis after type I-IV resection without reconstruction. The right hemipelvis has rotated through the symphysis, and the transected ilium has impacted on the sacrum.

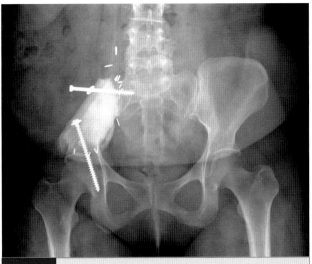

Figure 3 AP radiograph of the pelvis after type I resection reconstructed with allograft tibia filled with cement.

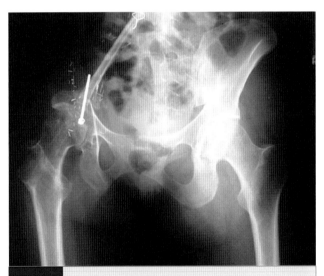

Figure 4 AP radiograph of pelvis after type I resection and reconstruction with vascularized fibular grafting.

tional outcome scores using the Toronto Extremity Salvage Score (TESS) as the group with reconstruction. Patients develop limb-length discrepancy, which often requires shoewear modifications, but the edge of the ilium often impacts on or fuses to the edge of the sacrum, resulting in long-term stability without risk of subsequent failure (**Figure 2**).

Other studies have suggested that the rates of surgical complications in patients without reconstruction are no lower than in patients with reconstruction, and that reconstruction has a clear benefit in terms of functional outcome. Patients in whom pelvic ring stability is restored have higher scores on all aspects of the Musculoskeletal Tumor Society (MSTS) functional score.[18] Reconstruction of the sacroiliac defect is usually undertaken using autograft or allograft. Structural allografts using tibia, femur, or humerus, sterilized with deep freezing or irradiation, can be affixed to the residual ilium and sacrum using lag screw or plate fixation (**Figure 3**).[19] These structural grafts act as struts to maintain the acetabulum at the proper level. Provided that union is obtained, a good functional outcome can be obtained, with an average MSTS score of 87% in one small series.[8] The nonunion rate has been reported to be 12%, which can lead to the necessity for further surgical intervention. To improve the potential for union, vascularized fibular grafting has been advocated by some authors (**Figure 4**). A "double-barreled" free fibular autograft using the ipsilateral fibula can be anastomosed to the superior gluteal, inferior gluteal, inferior epigastric, or external iliac vessels and fixed to the sacrum and residual acetabulum using internal fixation. Union is very reliable, with most studies reporting a 100% union rate.[20,21] In other studies, nonunion is predictive of poorer functional outcome.[22] Vascularized grafts can also be used in rare situations of ablative surgery, where a pedicled autogenous femoral graft has been used at the time of hindquarter amputation to provide spinopelvic stability.[23] To minimize the risk of nonunion and fatigue failure of the implanted allograft or autograft, one study assessed different instrumentation techniques using a finite element analysis model.[24] The stress transferred to the residual pelvis is substantially decreased using internal fixation, and the most stable fixation was found to be a double rod system, with bilateral L5-S1 pedicle screws and two iliac screws inserted into the residual ipsilateral ilium.

Several factors may play a role in the surgeon's decision whether to reconstruct the pelvic defect from a

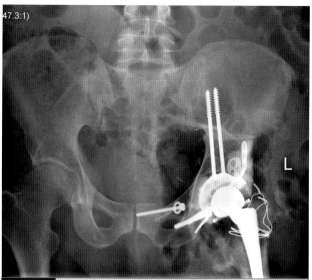

Figure 5 AP radiograph of the pelvis after type II resection and reconstruction with acetabular allograft and total hip replacement with reconstruction ring and constrained acetabular liner.

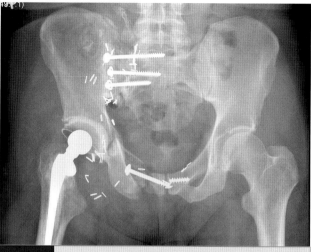

Figure 6 AP radiograph of the pelvis after type I-II-III resection and reconstruction with hemipelvic allograft and total hip replacement with cemented polyethylene acetabular implant.

type I-IV resection. Whether the apparent improved functional outcome justifies the extra surgical time and surgical risk is debatable. A well-executed reconstruction with stable internal fixation that achieves union appears to be associated with the best long-term result in this group of patients, and can be associated with high functional outcome scores and an activity level that is near normal.

Periacetabular Reconstruction

Reconstruction after resection of periacetabular sarcomas remains a significant challenge. Because of the necessity of restoring force transmission between the lower extremity and the axial skeleton, any reconstruction has to endure a significant amount of stress over the lifetime of the patient's weight bearing. The risk of complication remains significant, with studies reporting up to one major complication per patient, and functional outcome that is lower than in patients with type I-IV resections.[8] Infection, instability, neurovascular injury, nonunion, and prosthetic loosening are all prevalent complications in patients undergoing reconstruction for periacetabular sarcomas, and all detrimentally affect patient function. These results are reasonably consistent among all reported series of reconstruction techniques. As a result, no method of reconstruction is universally accepted as superior. These techniques can be grouped into biologic methods of reconstruction, using either allograft or pasteurized autograft with associated hip replacement, and endoprosthetic reconstruction using various devices that are currently available.

Reconstruction with hemipelvic allograft is advantageous in that if union is achieved, bone stock is restored for possible future reconstructions. The limitations of this technique include the poor availability of donor

bone in some regions and the potential for host-donor anatomic mismatch. After tumor resection, allograft pasteurized with either freezing or irradiation is cut to resemble the exact segment of bone that was resected, the allograft is inserted into the patient, and internal fixation is used to obtain rigid fixation. A solid compressive surface, as can be obtained with type II or type II-III resections, is ideal. A total hip replacement is usually then performed, although osteoarticular allograft of the acetabulum can be used.[8] In a comparison of patients with type II resections (**Figure 5**) versus type I-II and type I-II-III (**Figure 6**) resections reconstructed with allograft-prosthetic composites, patients with type II resections appear to have a lower rate of complications and better functional outcomes.[25] One possible reason for this finding is that in type II resections, a compressive force is applied to the allograft-host bone interface, whereas in the type I-II and type I-II-III resections, a shearing force is applied on weight bearing to the junction at the sacroiliac joint. This force could lead to a higher risk of nonunion. The incidence of nonunion, which can be subsequently managed by autologous morcellized bone grafting, can be as high as 10% to 15%.[8] The risk of infection is high, with 10 of 24 patients in one series developing deep infections of the allograft.[25] Prosthetic dislocation is similarly a significant problem, occurring in almost one fourth of patients.[8] Dislocation may be due to loss of proprioception as a result of the allograft reconstruction, or to subtle differences in anatomy of the allograft compared to the patient's native pelvis. Overall, the MSTS functional outcome scores for this technique are moderate, approximately 60% to 75% of normal. Despite a high risk of complications, patients with intact reconstructions that survive the complication function reasonably well.[8,25]

An alternative method of biologic reconstruction is the use of pasteurized autograft. In this technique, the

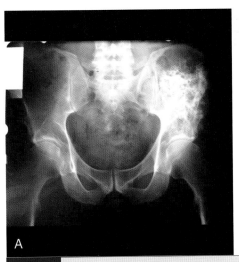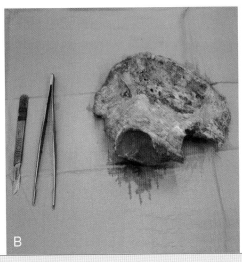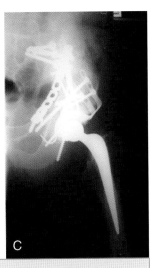

Figure 7   **A,** AP radiograph of the pelvis showing chondrosarcoma involving zones I and II. **B,** Gross specimen after tumor removal showing residual bone. The bone is then pasteurized. **C,** AP radiograph of left hip showing reimplanted pasteurized autograft and total hip replacement with reconstruction ring.

specimen is removed from the patient, and on a separate table, the tumor is then removed from the specimen grossly. For significant areas of bone destruction, cement can be inserted. The specimen is then pasteurized using irradiation, heat therapy, or cryotherapy to eliminate all remaining viable tumor cells. The specimen is then implanted back into the patient, with internal fixation and prosthetic reconstruction performed as noted for the allografts (**Figure 7**). The advantages of this technique are that it ensures a precise anatomic match of the autograft and the defect and that it does not rely on organ or tissue donation. Disadvantages include the potential for tumor reimplantation (although with the pasteurization techniques used, this concern is mainly theoretical) and the inability for the pathologist to assess tumor margins and chemotherapy response. The results of this technique are similar to that of allograft reconstruction, with one study reporting only 4 of 14 implanted autografts still intact.[26] Common causes for failure include infection, graft fracture, and prosthetic loosening, with rates of major complication anywhere from 30% to 60%.[27] The functional outcomes are also modest, with one study reporting seven patients ambulating without assistive devices or with one cane, and four patients ambulating with two crutches or using a wheelchair.[27]

Various forms of prostheses are available for reconstruction of periacetabular defects. These prostheses share the common challenge of biologic reconstructions with respect to force transmission during ambulation. The incidence of complications remains high,[28] and the cost of these prostheses can be significant, which may limit their application in some centers. Available implants include the saddle prosthesis, periacetabular replacement (PAR) endoprosthesis, the ice-cream cone endoprostheses, various other modular endoprostheses, and custom-designed implants.

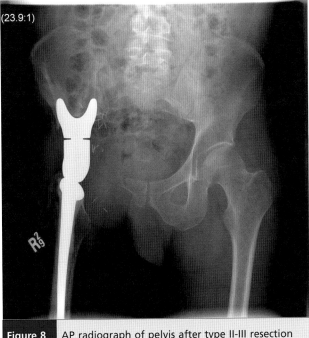

Figure 8   AP radiograph of pelvis after type II-III resection and reconstruction with saddle prosthesis.

The saddle prosthesis (**Figure 8**) relies on an intact ilium for fixation and is therefore applicable only for type II and type II-III resections. A notch is created in the iliac wing, and the saddle is seated in the notch, often fixed into place with soft-tissue repair using local tissues or synthetic materials such as aortic graft. Movement of the saddle on the iliac wing can allow flexion/extension, abduction/adduction, and rotation of the extremity. The modularity of this system is attractive because it can be used to replace various lengths of resected pelvis. In the early stages, infection remains a

6: Special Considerations in Tumor Management

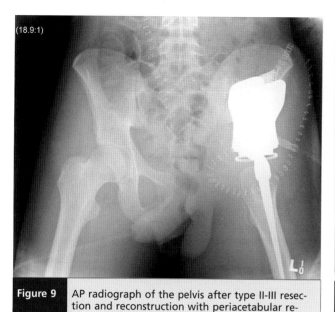

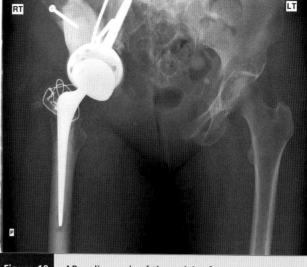

Figure 9 AP radiograph of the pelvis after type II-III resection and reconstruction with periacetabular replacement prosthesis.

Figure 10 AP radiograph of the pelvis after type II-III resection and reconstruction with an ice-cream cone endoprosthesis, supplemented with cement and screws.

significant risk, with rates between 30% and 40%.[29] Heterotopic ossification is also prevalent in up to 40% of patients. In the long term, the saddle prosthesis can wear away the iliac wing, resulting in proximal migration, progressive limb-length discrepancy, and potential fracture of the iliac wing. This problem can be overcome by applying a reconstruction plate to the iliac crest.[30] Final limb-length discrepancy up to 6 cm has been observed. Ambulatory status can be quite limited, with one study reporting that only 36% of patients ambulated without walking aids or with a single cane. Functional outcome scores are modest, ranging from 53% for the MSTS score and 65% for the TESS.[30] One small study has shown the complication rate to be highest for the saddle prosthesis compared to modular hemipelvic prostheses or pasteurized bone reconstruction.[31]

The PAR endoprosthesis can also be used for type II and type II-III resections (**Figure 9**). A component with flanges that sit on either side of the resected iliac wing is used, but it is bolted into place and supplemented with cement. In this prosthesis, the mobile interface is between a constrained liner attached to the iliac component and the femoral component, rather than between the prosthesis and the bone as in the saddle prosthesis. For this reason, iliac wear does not appear to be a problem. However, other complications are prominent, including infection in one third of patients and prosthetic instability in 15% of patients. The overall rate of major complication is greater than 50%, with an average MSTS functional score of 67% of normal.[32]

Another prosthetic option for reconstruction of type II and type II-III defects is the ice-cream cone endoprosthesis (**Figure 10**). The acetabular component of this system resembles an inverted ice-cream cone, with the long stem cemented into the intact supra-acetabular ilium, being careful not to traverse the sacroiliac joint,

which can be a source of postoperative pain. Threaded pins and cement can be used to supplement the fixation into the ilium. Various head and liner options, including resurfacing implants, constrained acetabular implants, and large femoral heads, have been used to attempt to obtain stability. The current follow-up for these prostheses is reasonably short. Complications include infection (11%) and instability (15%), with an overall complication rate of 37%. Functional outcome is reasonable, with a mean TESS score of 69%.[33] An acetabular implant with similar appearance, the pedestal cup, has shown similar promise in early studies and has the advantage of being modular with conventional hip replacement systems.[16] Modular systems are also available for reconstruction of larger defects, including those of the supra-acetabular ilium. Reconstruction of type I-II and type I-II-III defects can be performed using systems that rely on variable-length plate and screw attachments that are affixed to a more conventional acetabular implant. These systems allow for fixation to the contralateral superior pubic ramus and the residual iliac wing or sacral ala. Although series are small with short follow-up, complication rates (40%), gait status (75% using walking aids), and functional outcome scores (MSTS 62%) are comparable to reconstruction of smaller type II and type II-III defects.[34,35]

Custom pelvic endoprostheses can be designed and manufactured on the basis of imaging templates, where the surgeon indicates the expected level of resections, taking into account surgical margins. A disadvantage of this approach is that it does not account for any change in tumor dimensions in the interim period between imaging and surgical resection. Growth of some tumors can lead to resections that are larger than originally planned and subsequent mismatch of prosthesis and defect. These implants can be attached to the native pelvis

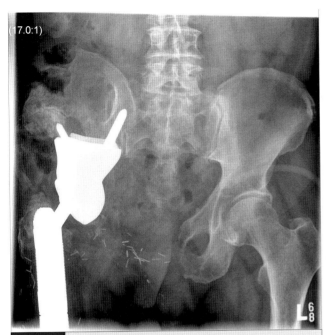

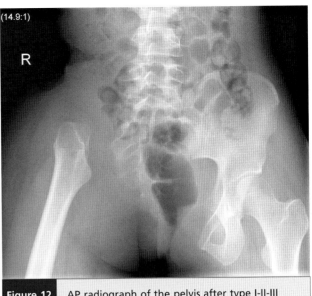

Figure 12   AP radiograph of the pelvis after type I-II-III resection without reconstruction. The flail hip has migrated proximally but is stable in soft tissues.

Figure 11   AP radiograph of the pelvis after type II-III resection and reconstruction with a custom prosthesis. The patient had a prior proximal femoral endoprosthesis.

using custom-designed intraosseous pins, screws, and cement (**Figure 11**). For defects that are impossible to reconstruct with the previously mentioned systems (type I-II and I-II-III), custom implants may be the only reconstruction option. The complication rates are similar to those of modular systems, with a 25% infection rate in one series, the highest of any anatomic area in the body.[36] The Modular Universal Tumour and Revision System (MUTARS) hemipelvic prosthesis uses stem fixation into any remaining ilium or sacrum with a wide collar at the interface, supplemented by screws. Mesh is used to secure fixation to the surrounding soft tissues and achieve stability of the prosthesis. Complications are frequent, with 75% of patients developing at least one complication, wound complications occurring in almost 50% of patients, and instability or prosthetic mechanical complications occurring in 25% of patients. The mean reported MSTS score is 50% of normal.[37]

The high complication and revision surgery rate, along with the generally poor or modest functional outcome scores in all methods noted previously, have led some physicians to advocate less extensive and nonanatomic reconstruction for large pelvic defects after sarcoma resection. Hip transposition involves attaching the femoral head to the residual sacral ala in the case of type I-II or type I-II-III resection. If intact bone remains inferiorly after type I-II resection, it is used to create a shelf of bone under which the femoral head can rest. In either situation, synthetic mesh is used to create pseudocapsule for the femoral head. The mesh is attached with suture anchors or transosseous sutures to the residual sacrum. The patient is kept on bed rest for a prolonged period to achieve fibrosis before mobilization with the new high hip center. By performing a hemiarthroplasty and affixing the prosthetic femoral head to the sacrum, the surgeon can even extend this technique to situations in which there is intra-articular extension of the tumor. The advantage of this technique is that the relative lack of large inanimate material leads to a smaller incidence of infection and other complications, although patients have to adjust to a significant limb-length discrepancy.[38]

The Friedman-Eilber resection arthroplasty, or flail-hip procedure, is undertaken by using multiple layers of soft-tissue closure over the residual proximal femur. The hip abductors and abdominal wall are sutured together, and mesh can be used to repair the adductors to the femur to prevent herniation of pelvic contents. The incidence of complications with this procedure is low, and functional outcome is quite reasonable, with one study reporting a mean MSTS score of 73% and seven of eight patients achieving independent ambulation status without pain or any assistive devices. Once again, the main drawback is a resultant significant limb-length discrepancy[39] (**Figure 12**).

Summary

The ideal solution for reconstruction after pelvic sarcoma resection has yet to be found. The simple fact that so many different techniques of reconstruction have been reported indicates that no single method has gained universal acceptance. There is general consensus that patients with type I, type I-IV, and type III resections do well, having good functional outcomes and little decline in function over time. In contrast, all series of patients with periacetabular sarcomas demonstrate high complication rates and comparatively poor functional outcomes, which continue to deteriorate over time. A recent trend toward less extensive bony reconstruction could improve some of these outcomes, with the expense of limb-length discrepancy and some gait disturbance. The use of image guidance in pelvic sarcoma surgery may allow for preservation of more intact bone and design of more anatomic prostheses, both of which could lead to improved patient function.

Annotated References

1. Jawad MU, Haleem AA, Scully SP: Malignant sarcoma of the pelvic bones: Treatment outcomes and prognostic factors vary by histopathology. *Cancer* 2011; 117(7):1529-1541.

    This Surveillance, Epidemiology, and End Results (SEER) database review of prognostic factors for 1185 patients with pelvic sarcoma reported osteosarcoma to have the worst 5-year survival at 19%. Level of evidence: II.

2. Weiss KR, Biau DJ, Bhumbra R, et al: Axial skeletal location predicts poor outcome in Ewing's sarcoma: A single institution experience. *Sarcoma* 2011;2011: 395180.

    This single-center study of prognostic factors for patients with Ewing sarcoma reported that axial location is an independent predictor of poor outcome on multivariate analysis with adjustment for pretreatment variables. Level of evidence: II.

3. Isakoff MS, Barkauskas DA, Ebb D, Morris C, Letson GD: Poor survival for osteosarcoma of the pelvis: A report from the Children's Oncology Group. *Clin Orthop Relat Res* 2012;470(7):2007-2013.

    This retrospective review of 1054 pediatric patients with osteosarcoma reported pelvic site to be associated with poorer 5-year overall survival than nonpelvic sites. Level of evidence: IV.

4. Guo W, Sun X, Ji T, Tang X: Outcome of surgical treatment of pelvic osteosarcoma. *J Surg Oncol* 2012; 106(4):406-410.

    This retrospective review of 19 patients with pelvic osteosarcoma reported a local recurrence rate of 26% and 5-year overall survival of 45%. Level of evidence: IV.

5. Fuchs B, Hoekzema N, Larson DR, Inwards CY, Sim FH: Osteosarcoma of the pelvis: Outcome analysis of surgical treatment. *Clin Orthop Relat Res* 2009; 467(2):510-518.

    This retrospective review of 43 patients with high-grade pelvic osteosarcoma to assess risk factors for recurrence showed local recurrence of 35% and a 5-year overall survival rate of 38%. Level of evidence: II.

6. Angelini A, Guerra G, Mavrogenis AF, Pala E, Picci P, Ruggieri P: Clinical outcome of central conventional chondrosarcoma. *J Surg Oncol* 2012;106(8):929-937.

    This review of 296 patients with chondrosarcoma showed that patients with high-grade tumors had significantly worse survival if the tumor was in the axial skeleton, including the pelvis. Level of evidence: II.

7. Enneking WF, Dunham WK: Resection and reconstruction for primary neoplasms involving the innominate bone. *J Bone Joint Surg Am* 1978;60(6):731-746.

8. Delloye C, Banse X, Brichard B, Docquier PL, Cornu O: Pelvic reconstruction with a structural pelvic allograft after resection of a malignant bone tumor. *J Bone Joint Surg Am* 2007;89(3):579-587.

    This retrospective review of patients with pelvic resections reconstructed with pasteurized allografts reported a high rate of complications, predominantly infection and nonunion. Outcomes are better in primary bone tumors. Level of evidence: IV.

9. Cheong D, Letson GD: Computer-assisted navigation and musculoskeletal sarcoma surgery. *Cancer Control* 2011;18(3):171-176.

    This retrospective review reported on a single center's experience with navigated musculoskeletal tumor resection and reconstruction. Accurate resection can be undertaken with a low rate of complications. Level of evidence: IV.

10. Wong KC, Kumta SM, Chiu KH, Antonio GE, Unwin P, Leung KS: Precision tumour resection and reconstruction using image-guided computer navigation. *J Bone Joint Surg Br* 2007;89(7):943-947.

    A series of six consecutive musculoskeletal tumor resections using navigation software showed minimal additional surgical time and all patients with negative margins. Level of evidence: IV.

11. Fehlberg S, Eulenstein S, Lange T, Andreou D, Tunn PU: Computer-assisted pelvic tumor resection: Fields of application, limits, and perspectives. *Recent Results Cancer Res* 2009;179:169-182.

    This article reviews the current status and applications of computer-assisted navigation in pelvic tumor resection. Level of evidence: V.

12. Docquier PL, Paul L, Cartiaux O, Delloye C, Banse X: Computer-assisted resection and reconstruction of pelvic tumor sarcoma. *Sarcoma* 2010;2010:125162.

    This article is a case report of resection of pelvic sarcoma and allograft modeling based on computer-assisted navigation to create an anatomic reconstruction. Level of evidence: V.

13. Wong KC, Kumta SM, Chiu KH, et al: Computer assisted pelvic tumor resection and reconstruction with a custom-made prosthesis using an innovative adaptation and its validation. *Comput Aided Surg* 2007; 12(4):225-232.

    This article is a case report of the manufacture of a

custom prosthesis using computer-assisted navigation software to virtually plan resection. Level of evidence: V.

14. Reijnders K, Coppes MH, van Hulzen AL, Gravendeel JP, van Ginkel RJ, Hoekstra HJ: Image guided surgery: New technology for surgery of soft tissue and bone sarcomas. *Eur J Surg Oncol* 2007;33(3):390-398.

    Two cases of pelvic sarcoma resected using navigation software demonstrate the feasibility of the procedure and the ability to obtain negative margins. Level of evidence: V.

15. Wu K, Webber NP, Ward RA, Jones KB, Randall RL: Intraoperative navigation for minimally invasive resection of periarticular and pelvic tumors. *Orthopedics* 2011;34(5):372.

    This case series describes technical aspects of computer-assisted navigation for minimally invasive pelvic tumor resection. Level of evidence: IV.

16. Dominkus M, Darwish E, Funovics P: Reconstruction of the pelvis after resection of malignant bone tumours in children and adolescents. *Recent Results Cancer Res* 2009;179:85-111.

    This review article discusses techniques of reconstruction in children and adolescents after pelvic sarcoma resection. Level of evidence: V.

17. Beadel GP, McLaughlin CE, Aljassir F, et al: Iliosacral resection for primary bone tumors: Is pelvic reconstruction necessary? *Clin Orthop Relat Res* 2005;438: 22-29.

18. Han I, Lee YM, Cho HS, Oh JH, Lee SH, Kim HS: Outcome after surgical treatment of pelvic sarcomas. *Clin Orthop Surg* 2010;2(3):160-166.

    This retrospective review of 44 patients with pelvic sarcomas reported a high complication rate of 50% and a higher functional outcome score if pelvis ring continuity and hip joint anatomy are restored. Level of evidence: IV.

19. Court C, Bosca L, Le Cesne A, Nordin JY, Missenard G: Surgical excision of bone sarcomas involving the sacroiliac joint. *Clin Orthop Relat Res* 2006;451:189-194.

20. Chang DW, Fortin AJ, Oates SD, Lewis VO: Reconstruction of the pelvic ring with vascularized double-strut fibular flap following internal hemipelvectomy. *Plast Reconstr Surg* 2008;121(6):1993-2000.

    This series of six patients with iliosacral resections reconstructed with vascularized double-strut fibular flaps showed 100% union at a mean of 2.5 months, and all patients were ambulatory. Level of evidence: IV.

21. Hubert DM, Low DW, Serletti JM, Chang B, Dormans JP: Fibula free flap reconstruction of the pelvis in children after limb-sparing internal hemipelvectomy for bone sarcoma. *Plast Reconstr Surg* 2010;125(1):195-200.

    This series of four pediatric patients with iliosacral resections reconstructed with vascularized fibular grafts showed 100% union and return to normal walking with long-term follow-up. Level of evidence: IV.

22. Sabourin M, Biau D, Babinet A, Dumaine V, Tomeno B, Anract P: Surgical management of pelvic primary bone tumors involving the sacroiliac joint. *Orthop Traumatol Surg Res* 2009;95(4):284-292.

    This retrospective review of 24 patients with iliosacral sarcoma resection and reconstruction reported that patients with union to have a significantly higher functional outcome than those with nonunion. Level of evidence: IV.

23. Mendel E, Mayerson JL, Nathoo N, Edgar RL, Schmidt C, Miller MJ: Reconstruction of the pelvis and lumbar-pelvic junction using 2 vascularized autologous bone grafts after en bloc resection for an iliosacral chondrosarcoma. *J Neurosurg Spine* 2011; 15(2):168-173.

    This article is a case report of hindquarter amputation with hemisacrectomy that was reconstructed with pedicled femoral and fibular autografts to provide pelvic stability. Level of evidence: V.

24. Jia YW, Cheng LM, Yu GR, et al: A finite element analysis of the pelvic reconstruction using fibular transplantation fixed with four different rod-screw systems after type I resection. *Chin Med J (Engl)* 2008; 121(4):321-326.

    This biomechanical study, which used finite element analysis of iliosacral resection, demonstrated the most stable construct to be bilateral lumbar pedicle screw fixation with dual rods and fibular graft. Level of evidence: N/A.

25. Beadel GP, McLaughlin CE, Wunder JS, Griffin AM, Ferguson PC, Bell RS: Outcome in two groups of patients with allograft-prosthetic reconstruction of pelvic tumor defects. *Clin Orthop Relat Res* 2005;438:30-35.

26. Jeon DG, Kim MS, Cho WH, Song WS, Lee SY: Reconstruction with pasteurized autograft-total hip prosthesis composite for periacetabular tumors. *J Surg Oncol* 2007;96(6):493-502.

    This review of 14 patients with periacetabular tumors reconstructed with autograft pasteurized by low-heat treatment and reimplanted reported that 5-year graft survival of 64.3%. Infection, fracture, and loosening were major complications. Level of evidence: IV.

27. Kim HS, Kim KJ, Han I, Oh JH, Lee SH: The use of pasteurized autologous grafts for periacetabular reconstruction. *Clin Orthop Relat Res* 2007;464:217-223.

    This retrospective series of 11 patients with periacetabular resections reconstructed with autograft pasteurized by low-heat treatment and reimplanted back into patients reported a 73% union rate and reasonable function. Level of evidence: IV.

28. Sherman CE, O'Connor MI, Sim FH: Survival, local recurrence, and function after pelvic limb salvage at 23

to 38 years of followup. *Clin Orthop Relat Res* 2012; 470(3):712-727.

Long-term assessment of patients with pelvic sarcoma shows a progressive decrease in functional outcome scores between 23 and 38 years after surgery. Level of evidence: IV.

29. Aljassir F, Beadel GP, Turcotte RE, et al: Outcome after pelvic sarcoma resection reconstructed with saddle prosthesis. *Clin Orthop Relat Res* 2005;438:36-41.

30. Kitagawa Y, Ek ET, Choong PF: Pelvic reconstruction using saddle prosthesis following limb salvage operation for periacetabular tumour. *J Orthop Surg (Hong Kong)* 2006;14(2):155-162.

31. Guo W, Li D, Tang X, Ji T: Surgical treatment of pelvic chondrosarcoma involving periacetabulum. *J Surg Oncol* 2010;101(2):160-165.

    This review of 45 patients with periacetabular chondrosarcoma showed that the complication rate is highest for saddle prosthesis. Level of evidence: IV.

32. Menendez LR, Ahlmann ER, Falkinstein Y, Allison DC: Periacetabular reconstruction with a new endoprosthesis. *Clin Orthop Relat Res* 2009;467(11):2831-2837.

    This retrospective review of 25 patients who underwent type II pelvic resection and reconstruction with PAR pelvic prostheses found the PAR prosthesis to be associated with a major complication rate of 56%. Level of evidence: IV.

33. Fisher NE, Patton JT, Grimer RJ, et al: Ice-cream cone reconstruction of the pelvis: A new type of pelvic replacement. Early results. *J Bone Joint Surg Br* 2011; 93(5):684-688.

    This retrospective review of 27 patients who underwent pelvic reconstruction with the ice-cream cone prosthesis reported a 37% complication rate, with instability being the most frequent complication. Level of evidence: IV.

34. Zhou Y, Duan H, Liu Y, Min L, Kong Q, Tu C: Outcome after pelvic sarcoma resection and reconstruction with a modular hemipelvic prostheses. *Int Orthop* 2011;35(12):1839-1846.

    This small series of eight patients with periacetabular sarcomas resected and reconstructed with modular hemipelvic prostheses demonstrated a low complication rate and no infection in the five surviving patients. Level of evidence: IV.

35. Guo W, Li D, Tang X, Yang Y, Ji T: Reconstruction with modular hemipelvic prostheses for periacetabular tumor. *Clin Orthop Relat Res* 2007;461:180-188.

    This retrospective review of 28 patients with periacetabular resections reconstructed with modular prostheses reported that a high number of patients died of disease, but the remaining patients had reasonable function. Level of evidence: IV.

36. Jeys LM, Kulkarni A, Grimer RJ, Carter SR, Tillman RM, Abudu A: Endoprosthetic reconstruction for the treatment of musculoskeletal tumors of the appendicular skeleton and pelvis. *J Bone Joint Surg Am* 2008; 90(6):1265-1271.

    This retrospective review of a single center's experience of 776 custom endoprostheses reported that the 28 pelvic prostheses had the highest infection rate at 25%. Level of evidence: IV.

37. Witte D, Bernd L, Bruns J, et al: Limb-salvage reconstruction with MUTARS hemipelvic endoprosthesis: A prospective multicenter study. *Eur J Surg Oncol* 2009; 35(12):1318-1325.

    This review of 40 patients with MUTARS custom pelvic endoprostheses showed a complication rate of 75%, with infection the most common complication. Level of evidence: IV.

38. Gebert C, Gosheger G, Winkelmann W: Hip transposition as a universal surgical procedure for periacetabular tumors of the pelvis. *J Surg Oncol* 2009;99(3): 169-172.

    This technical article explains the technique of hip transposition for periacetabular tumors. Level of evidence: V.

39. Schwartz AJ, Kiatisevi P, Eilber FC, Eilber FR, Eckardt JJ: The Friedman-Eilber resection arthroplasty of the pelvis. *Clin Orthop Relat Res* 2009;467(11):2825-2830.

    This retrospective review of eight consecutive patients who underwent resection of pelvic sarcomas without bony reconstruction demonstrated that seven of eight patients could walk without assistive devices. Level of evidence: IV.

Chapter 38

Proximal Femur Resection and Reconstruction

Christian M. Ogilvie, MD

Introduction

The proximal femur and femoral diaphysis are common sites for primary bone tumors including Ewing sarcoma, osteosarcoma, and chondrosarcoma. Additionally, metastatic bone disease will often affect the proximal femur. Carcinomas are the most common metastatic tumor in these patients and are generally treated with irradiation either instead of or after surgical management. In some patients with metastatic tumors who have massive bone loss and failed healing of pathologic fractures, replacement of bone may be the best option to relieve pain and improve function. Surgical treatment of these diseases as well as bone destruction due to neoplasia at the proximal femur can result in loss of metaphyseal bone and tendon attachments. Reconstruction at this site should address these soft-tissue deficits as well as provide skeletal stability.

Modular implants have become the standard endoprosthetic approach to reconstruct large bone defects. Allograft-prosthetic composite (APC) reconstructions are used in selected patients. Less common choices include resection only, arthrodesis, and, in the skeletally immature, rotationplasty.

Proximal femur replacement has enjoyed relatively good implant success. Loosening is less frequent than with cemented distal femur endoprostheses, and the failure rate from other causes has been relatively low compared to other megaprosthetic replacements. Dislocation has historically been a problem for these procedures, especially with loss of muscle about the hip, but has been 6% or lower with the use of meticulous soft-tissue reconstruction and a preference for hemiarthroplasty when possible.[1,2] One recent series of segmental proximal femur endoprostheses had a conversion rate from hemiarthroplasty to acetabular resurfacing of 5.8%, and 60% of the revisions were in teenagers.[1] High rates of revision for hemiarthroplasty have been noted in patients younger than 21 years.[3] Limp is common if not universal after these procedures.

Resection

When the proximal femur is resected, a posterolateral approach is used with the patient in the lateral position.[4] The extent of bone involvement must be determined with MRI and plain radiography to plan the distal resection level and assess whether any part of the greater trochanter can be left attached to the abductor tendons. This piece of greater trochanter provides length for the abductor mechanism and solid tissue to help anchor the abductors to the endoprosthesis. Hip joint involvement must be evaluated to determine if capsule can be spared and to plan the best hip reconstruction. Preserving the hip capsule to help secure a hemiarthroplasty is highly favored because the muscles that stabilize the hip are compromised. The extent of soft-tissue resection is determined by the extent of soft-tissue involvement as seen on MRI and by the need for negative or wide soft-tissue margins. In the setting of metastatic disease, negative soft-tissue margins may not be clinically relevant, and thus muscle and capsule should be spared as much as possible.

During the resection, several structures deserve particular attention once bone and soft-tissue resection decisions have been made. The sciatic nerve should be noted and protected. Branches of the lateral circumflex artery that supply the quadriceps muscle can be large and are more likely to be encountered if any part of the medial quadriceps needs to be resected. If the gluteus medius is compromised, the tensor fascia and the gluteus maximus are the remaining soft-tissue structures that cross the joint in this area and become important hip stabilizers. Reconstruction may involve suturing these muscles together and/or to the prosthesis.

Reconstruction Options

Proximal femur reconstruction may be done with an endoprosthesis or allograft, or both. Allograft use and success have been limited by availability, infection, and

Dr. Ogilvie or an immediate family member serves as a paid consultant to or is an employee of NuVasive, and serves as an unpaid consultant to Axial Biotec.

6: Special Considerations in Tumor Management

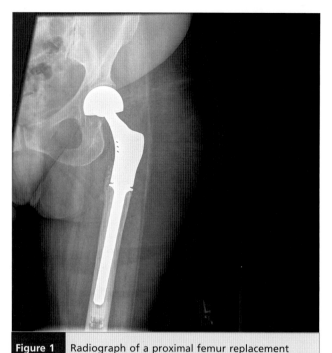

Figure 1   Radiograph of a proximal femur replacement shows a cemented stem and bipolar hemiarthroplasty.

Hip Choices

Hip dislocation after proximal femur replacement has been a problem in part because of the amount of soft-tissue release and resection. Hemiarthroplasty is commonly used in proximal femur replacement primarily to prevent dislocation. The low rate of conversion of hemiarthroplasty to total hip replacement may be related in part to compromised patient survival from the underlying conditions, patient populations with little baseline arthritis, and/or use in patients who have undergone larger surgeries with muscle loss who self-limit their activity.[8] However, use of a unipolar replacement, which has a low dislocation rate, has been associated with a high risk of acetabular revision in patients younger than 21 years, with no hip implant in that age group lasting longer than 11 years in one study.[3] Bipolar hip replacements or the more recently available large-head total hip replacements may provide more durability with acceptable stability in patients with longer life expectancy. Preservation of the acetabulum in growing children is still advocated because it allows for acetabular growth with the acknowledgment that these children will likely need revision surgery at some point.[9]

Stem Implantation

Once the method of hip reconstruction has been chosen and the size of the prosthesis has been determined, the prosthesis must be secured to the bone. Cemented stems have long been preferred. A recent series had a revision rate of only 4.7% for loosening or osteolysis.[1] Loosening of cemented stems has been more of a problem with the distal femur than with the proximal femur. Uncemented stems have been widely available and are often used when good bone stock permits use of a press-fit stem, in patients with relatively longer anticipated longevity, and in patients in whom postoperative radiation therapy is not anticipated. One recent series of 25 patients using conical fluted stems, including three proximal femur replacements, showed no loosening or subsidence at a mean of 2.5 years; however, marked stress shielding was observed in 20% of stems.[10] Although not specific to the proximal femur, a novel uncemented bone interface for these prostheses has been developed that statically loads the cut end of the bone, leading to hypertrophy instead of bone loss from stress shielding. This interface also encourages bone growth onto the implant interface, sealing it from wear debris, but the biggest advantage may be the long-term stability of a biologic attachment of bone to implant. These implants require good bone stock but need less length for attachment than a typical uncemented stem. Good early results in the distal femur have been reported,[11] but a proximal femur series has yet to be published. Although some innovations are becoming widespread, not all options for bone ingrowth, bone

delayed diaphyseal healing but have the advantage of providing soft-tissue attachments and the ability to size the allograft intraoperatively. Allografts are often used as part of an APC and can be used to salvage failed hip replacements and failed tumor megaprostheses. A recent study of APC use for total hip revision showed a rate of complications requiring revision of 26.5%, including 6.9% with deep infections. The 10-year survival of the APCs was 69%.[5] Another study of APCs for revision total hip replacement in patients with developmental dysplasia found 93% implant survival at 10 years.[6]

For patients with tumors who are undergoing segmental resection, another alternative is use of the patient's own bone (autoclaved or irradiated autograft) in the APC after the bone has been cleaned and irradiated during surgery. At one center where this technique was used to reconstruct the proximal femur, nonunion occurred in only 1 of 13 patients. The average time to heal was 20 weeks, and the mean Enneking score was 72.1%.[7]

Modular prostheses can require a minimum of 70 mm of resection from the proximal femur for implantation of the smallest construct (**Figure 1**). Smaller amounts of bone loss may be managed with the use of revision hip stems. It is helpful to keep the specimen on the back table when putting together trial prostheses to most accurately restore the correct length. With loss of muscle, soft-tissue tension becomes a less reliable determinant of limb length. Various commercial guides use markers in the pelvis and femur to help assess correct length. Modular prostheses allow for almost any length up to and including a total femur replacement. Some systems require a special linkage piece for the total femur that joins hip and knee joint attachments.

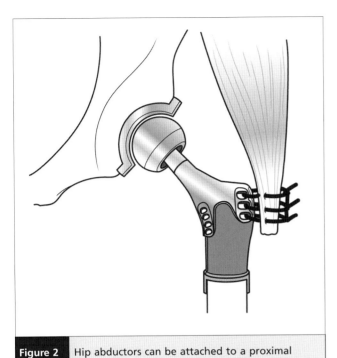

Figure 2 Hip abductors can be attached to a proximal femur replacement with 5-mm polyester sutures by passing them through the prosthesis and tying them through holes in the tendon or, if available, a shell of the greater trochanter with tendons attached.

implant interfaces, and prosthetic expansion are available in any one implant format.

Positioning of the stem of an implant should be given special consideration. After resection, the usual anatomic landmarks for rotation of a femoral implant are gone. The linea aspera is roughly posterior, but its relationship to true posterior varies throughout its course. Determining the best femoral anteversion by trial can be difficult because trials for cemented prostheses lack rotational stability, and implantation of an uncemented femoral stem first may limit the options for rotation, depending on the implant system. Rotation can be judged against the plane of knee flexion, and a jig has even been devised for this procedure to improve accuracy.[12]

Soft-Tissue Reconstruction

The abductor insertion is the most critical soft-tissue reconstruction for function and stability. If a shell of the greater trochanter can be spared and left on the abductor tendons, this method is preferred because it offers solid tissue to attach to the prosthesis. Various bone attachment methods, including wires, hooks, screws, and washers, are available, but three 5-mm polyester sutures also work well and can be applied with almost any system (**Figure 2**). Wrapping a prosthesis with mesh or a tube to assist soft-tissue reattachment has also been described. Recently, a small series

using an aortograft sleeve sutured around a proximal femur replacement showed encouraging functional results with no Trendelenburg gait or use of a cane.[13] This sleeve allows for attachment of abductors and other soft tissues such as the quadriceps. It is not clear, however, if this technique offers a consistent functional advantage over simple soft-tissue repair.[14]

Another helpful element of soft-tissue repair is capsular closure to prevent dislocation. Hip stability is a concern despite use of bipolar femoral heads because of the extensive soft-tissue release and the resection that is sometimes required. Use of 3-mm Dacron in a purse-string capsule repair was associated with only one dislocation in a series of 36 patients.[15]

Implant Surface Treatments

Many implant surface treatments that address common causes of failure in proximal femur replacements, including aseptic loosening and infection, are being used or studied. Hydroxyapatite coatings have been used in uncemented prostheses to encourage bone ingrowth and are available in some megaprosthetic stems.[16] Another material in common use for prostheses to promote tissue ingrowth is tantalum. One report describes its use in the proximal femur in a custom device with areas of tantalum on the surface of the body of the implant.[17] This encouraging report showed excellent function, but larger studies are needed to evaluate the true clinical potential. Tendon ingrowth into porous titanium has been promising in animal models and would seem to have a valuable application in the proximal femur.[18] To help combat infection, a surface treatment of silver ions on a titanium implant is currently available on one prosthesis. Silver has bactericidal properties and completely dissipates from the prosthesis over several months. These prostheses may have application particularly for primary procedures in patients at highest risk for infection and for revision implants, especially those done because of infection. The clinical outcomes of the use of silver on tumor prostheses have yet to be published.

Outcomes

Recent large series of proximal femur replacements demonstrated good implant survival and generally good function as well. Five-year implant survival in one group was 90% with mean Toronto Extremity Salvage Scores of 61%.[2] Implant survival in another current series was 93% at 5 years, 84% at 10 years, and 56% at 20 years, and the average Musculoskeletal Tumor Society (MSTS) score for all patients was 87% (range, 7 to 288 months).[1] In studies of patients with metastatic disease treated with proximal femur replacement, the function was good but inferior to that achieved in patients with primary tumors. This discrepancy between the two groups seems to be a reflection of differences in age and comorbidities.[19] Patients with metastatic disease may not regain ambulation because of other factors, and in fact, the rate of ambulation in this group decreases over time.[20]

Complications

Infection is considered the most devastating complication for a megaprosthesis, and most current series report rates of 6% to 7%. Revisions of a proximal femoral prosthesis can be managed as a two-stage exchange, but a spacer of that size is difficult to construct and may dislocate from the acetabulum. Use of a spacer can be attempted by coating a prosthesis or femoral nail with antibiotic-impregnated cement.[21] One-stage exchanges have been attempted with some success.[22]

Summary

Proximal femur replacement is a well-established treatment of tumors that provides excellent pain relief and good function in most patients. Current advances that may further improve implant longevity and patient function include surface treatments that promote muscle and tendon attachment as well as reduce the risk of infection. Innovation in bone implant interfaces may also reduce the aseptic loosening rate. Although some companies have worked together to combine technologies,[23] it may take time to combine all available advances into one implant. Remaining challenges include an optimal implant for growing children and the ideal hip bearing surface, especially in younger patients.

Annotated References

1. Bernthal NM, Schwartz AJ, Oakes DA, Kabo JM, Eckardt JJ: How long do endoprosthetic reconstructions for proximal femoral tumors last? *Clin Orthop Relat Res* 2010;468(11):2867-2874.

   One institution's experience with cemented bipolar proximal femur replacements is reviewed and includes primary tumors and metastatic disease. Level of evidence: IV.

2. Chandrasekar CR, Grimer RJ, Carter SR, Tillman RM, Abudu A, Buckley L: Modular endoprosthetic replacement for tumours of the proximal femur. *J Bone Joint Surg Br* 2009;91(1):108-112.

   This review of 100 consecutive patients with tumors of the proximal femur showed good function and a low complication rate. Level of evidence: IV.

3. Chandrasekar CR, Grimer RJ, Carter SR, Tillman RM, Abudu A, Jeys LM: Unipolar proximal femoral endoprosthetic replacement for tumour: The risk of revision in young patients. *J Bone Joint Surg Br* 2009; 91(3):401-404.

   Cemented unipolar proximal femur replacements were reviewed and demonstrated a markedly higher revision rate of the acetabulum in patients younger than 21 years. Level of evidence: IV.

4. Malawer MM, Sugarbaker PH: *Musculoskeletal Cancer Surgery: Treatment of Sarcomas and Allied Diseases*. Dordrecht, Netherlands, Kluwer, 2001, pp 626.

5. Babis GC, Sakellariou VI, O'Connor MI, Hanssen AD, Sim FH: Proximal femoral allograft-prosthesis composites in revision hip replacement: A 12-year follow-up study. *J Bone Joint Surg Br* 2010;92(3):349-355.

   The implant survival rate at 10 years of APC done for revision hips was 69%. Of 72 hips, 4 failed by loosening, 4 by allograft fracture, and 5 by infection. Severe bone loss was associated with worse outcome. Level of evidence: IV.

6. Sternheim A, Rogers BA, Kuzyk PR, Safir OA, Backstein D, Gross AE: Segmental proximal femoral bone loss and revision total hip replacement in patients with developmental dysplasia of the hip: The role of allograft prosthesis composite. *J Bone Joint Surg Br* 2012;94(6):762-767.

   APCs demonstrated good long-term outcomes in patients requiring revision total hip arthroplasty in patients who previously had developmental dysplasia of the hip. At 20 years implant, survivorship was 75.5%; 5 of 30 hips required implant removal for loosening and 1 for infection. Level of evidence: IV.

7. Chen CF, Chen WM, Cheng YC, Chiang CC, Huang CK, Chen TH: Extracorporeally irradiated autograft-prosthetic composite arthroplasty using AML extensively porous-coated stem for proximal femur reconstruction: A clinical analysis of 14 patients. *J Surg Oncol* 2009;100(5):418-422.

   APCs using extracorporally radiated autograft resulted in union in 12 of 14 cases. The average time to union was 20.3 weeks (range, 14 to 40). Level of evidence: IV.

8. Kabukcuoglu Y, Grimer RJ, Tillman RM, Carter SR: Endoprosthetic replacement for primary malignant tumors of the proximal femur. *Clin Orthop Relat Res* 1999;358:8-14.

9. van Kampen M, Grimer RJ, Carter SR, Tillman RM, Abudu A: Replacement of the hip in children with a tumor in the proximal part of the femur. *J Bone Joint Surg Am* 2008;90(4):785-795.

   Although unipolar hip replacements lasted at most only 10 years in children acetabular preservation to allow for growth was still thought to be important to facilitate likely future surgeries. Level of evidence: IV.

10. Bruns J, Delling G, Gruber H, Lohmann CH, Habermann CR: Cementless fixation of megaprostheses using a conical fluted stem in the treatment of bone tumours. *J Bone Joint Surg Br* 2007;89(8):1084-1087.

Short-term results (2.5 years) demonstrated no loosening in megaprostheses using a fluted conical stem. Level of evidence: IV.

11. Farfalli GL, Boland PJ, Morris CD, Athanasian EA, Healey JH: Early equivalence of uncemented press-fit and Compress femoral fixation. *Clin Orthop Relat Res* 2009;467(11):2792-2799.

    Femoral fixation was equivalent in uncemented stems and the Compress stem at 5 years. Most failures were because of aseptic loosening. Level of evidence: III.

12. Lackman RD, Torbert JT, Finstein JL, Ogilvie CM, Fox EJ: Inaccuracies in the assessment of femoral anteversion in proximal femoral replacement prostheses. *J Arthroplasty* 2008;23(1):97-101.

    A novel jig was described to measure anteversion for a proximal femur implant. The accuracy of attending surgeons and trainees was compared and found to be improved when using the jig. Level of evidence: II.

13. Henderson ER, Jennings JM, Marulanda GA, Groundland JS, Cheong D, Letson GD: Enhancing soft tissue ingrowth in proximal femoral arthroplasty with aortograft sleeve: A novel technique and early results. *J Arthroplasty* 2011;26(1):161-163.

    Proximal femurs were wrapped with an aortograft that provided extensive surface area for soft-tissue attachment. A larger study is needed to confirm any significant advantage over conventional techniques. Level of evidence: IV.

14. Ogilvie CM, Wunder JS, Ferguson PC, Griffin AM, Bell RS: Functional outcome of endoprosthetic proximal femoral replacement. *Clin Orthop Relat Res* 2004;426:44-48.

15. Henderson ER, Jennings JM, Marulanda GA, Palumbo BT, Cheong D, Letson GD: Purse-string capsule repair to reduce proximal femoral arthroplasty dislocation for tumor: A novel technique with results. *J Arthroplasty* 2010;25(4):654-657.

    A purse-string hip capsule repair around the head of a proximal femur replacement was described with a dislocation rate below historic controls. This may be especially useful in patients who lack a gluteus medius and a greater trochanter. Level of evidence: IV.

16. Blunn GW, Briggs TW, Cannon SR, et al: Cementless fixation for primary segmental bone tumor endoprostheses. *Clin Orthop Relat Res* 2000;372:223-230.

17. Holt GE, Christie MJ, Schwartz HS: Trabecular metal endoprosthetic limb salvage reconstruction of the lower limb. *J Arthroplasty* 2009;24(7):1079-1085.

    Early follow-up on several custom large implants with porous surfaces for bone and soft-tissue ingrowth showed good function. Although feasible to use these implants, any functional advantages to such an approach are not clear. Level of evidence: IV.

18. Reach JS Jr, Dickey ID, Zobitz ME, Adams JE, Scully SP, Lewallen DG: Direct tendon attachment and healing to porous tantalum: An experimental animal study. *J Bone Joint Surg Am* 2007;89(5):1000-1009.

    Ingrowth of tendon into titanium implants can be reproduced in a robust way in an animal model. It is not clear if a configuration of sufficient strength will be attainable in a human lower-extremity model.

19. Potter BK, Chow VE, Adams SC, Letson GD, Temple HT: Endoprosthetic proximal femur replacement: Metastatic versus primary tumors. *Surg Oncol* 2009; 18(4):343-349.

    Although both metastatic and primary tumor groups did well, patients with primary tumors had significantly better MSTS scores. This finding was attributed mostly to age. Resection length did not have a noted effect on function. Level of evidence: III.

20. Nakashima H, Katagiri H, Takahashi M, Sugiura H: Survival and ambulatory function after endoprosthetic replacement for metastatic bone tumor of the proximal femur. *Nagoya J Med Sci* 2010;72(1-2):13-21.

    In 40 patients treated with proximal femur replacement for metastatic disease, the survival rate at 6 months was 60%, and the rate of ambulation was 48%. Both rates decreased at 12 months. Ambulation time averaged 75.9% of survival time. Level of evidence: IV.

21. Rodriguez H, Ziran BH: Temporary antibiotic cement-covered gamma nail spacer for an infected nonunion of the proximal femur. *Clin Orthop Relat Res* 2007; 454:270-274.

    The authors used a cement-covered femoral nail followed by a proximal femoral replacement to treat an infected proximal femur. Level of evidence: V.

22. Funovics PT, Hipfl C, Hofstaetter JG, Puchner S, Kotz RI, Dominkus M: Management of septic complications following modular endoprosthetic reconstruction of the proximal femur. *Int Orthop* 2011;35(10):1437-1444.

    In a study of 170 consecutive patients with proximal femur replacements, 12 patients of 166 (7.2%) had infections. One-stage revision was successful in five of eight patients treated, whereas the remaining three patients required a second surgery to eradicate the infection. Level of evidence: IV.

23. Webber NP, Seidel M: Combining advanced technologies: The Compress-Repiphysis prosthesis for pediatric limb salvage. *Orthopedics* 2010;33(11):823.

    A successful case was described using one implant that combines a novel bone interface and novel expandable technologies from two companies using a custom connector. Level of evidence: V.

6: Special Considerations in Tumor Management

Chapter 39

Distal Femoral Resection and Reconstruction

Theresa Pazionis, MD, MA   Michelle Ghert, MD, FRCSC

Introduction

Primary bone malignancies such as osteosarcoma and Ewing sarcoma commonly occur in the distal femur (**Figures 1** and **2**). Prior to the advent of modern chemotherapy protocols and reconstruction options, the mainstay of surgical treatment of these malignancies was above-knee amputation. Currently, with advances in multimodal treatment, limb-sparing surgery and reconstruction with curative intent has become the standard of practice. Local recurrence rates after neoadjuvant chemotherapy and oncologic resection of distal femoral osteosarcoma with endoprosthetic reconstruction have been reported to be 5% to 10%.[1,2] Adequate surgical margins and good response to chemotherapy are essential in minimizing local recurrence.[3] Reconstruction is commonly achieved with the use of a modular replacement system, or, in very select populations, an allograft-prosthetic composite.

Although the primary indication for distal femoral resection and reconstruction is primary bone sarcoma, other indications include metastatic disease, trauma, and revision total knee arthroplasty in the setting of massive bone loss. Distal femoral resection and endoprosthetic or allograft reconstruction should be considered in all cases where the oncologic and functional outcomes are preferable to an above-knee amputation or rotationplasty. Although it is a viable option to restore function after an oncologic resection of the distal femur, rotationplasty is not discussed in this chapter. The reader should, however, be aware of rotationplasty as a surgical option when conventional limb salvage is not feasible. This chapter describes the perioperative considerations, reconstructive options, and observed outcomes of distal femoral resection and reconstruction with a focus on the population with primary bone sarcoma.

Dr. Ghert or an immediate family member serves as a board member, owner, officer, or committee member of the Musculoskeletal Tumor Society. Neither Dr. Pazionis nor any immediate family member has received anything of value from or has stock or stock options held in a commercial company or institution related directly or indirectly to the subject of this chapter.

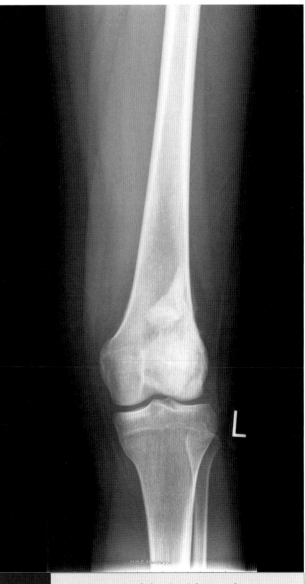

| **Figure 1** | AP radiograph of the distal femur of a 15-year-old girl shows osteosarcoma. Note the ectopic production of osteoid and lateral Codman triangle. |

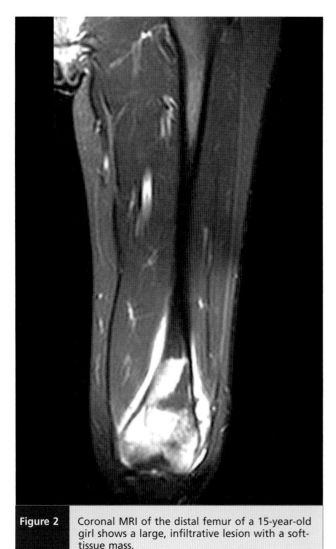

Figure 2 Coronal MRI of the distal femur of a 15-year-old girl shows a large, infiltrative lesion with a soft-tissue mass.

Indications for Distal Femoral Resection and Reconstruction

Indications for distal femoral resection and reconstruction are (1) primary bone sarcoma, (2) benign aggressive bone tumors or disease associated with distal femoral compromise where other treatment options are not feasible or would yield inferior oncologic and functional results (ie, circumferential bone loss), (3) metastatic disease limited to the distal femur where overall patient survival and function may be improved with an oncologic resection (ie, solitary bone metastasis from renal cell carcinoma),[4] (4) revision total knee arthroplasty in the setting of massive bone loss without infection, and (5) trauma in the setting of massive bone loss. Immediate reconstruction with an endoprosthetic device should not be attempted in a contaminated field; however, delayed reconstruction remains a useful salvage option if the distal femoral fragments are not amenable to repair.

Perioperative Considerations

Once sarcoma is suspected on the basis of radiographs, local cross-section imaging as well as systemic staging should be completed per existing guidelines, and a biopsy should be performed in accordance with the oncologic principles of biopsy, preferably by an orthopaedic oncologist. The tumor volume and extent of systemic disease should be evaluated both before and after neoadjuvant chemotherapy. With limb salvage as the current standard of care, patients who undergo above-knee amputation generally are those who have more extensive tumors such that the reconstructed limb would have inferior function to a prosthesis, or, rarely, have a preference for amputation.

Whether a pathologic fracture necessitated immediate amputation in the setting of a primary bone sarcoma was previously controversial. Primary bone tumors with pathologic femur fracture were found to have a poor prognosis with a 38% local recurrence rate in a population-based study.[5] In this study, the patients who underwent resection and reconstruction had a similar overall prognosis as those who underwent limb salvage. In a 2002 study, researchers reported a 5-year survival rate of 55% for osteosarcoma patients with a pathologic fracture compared to 77% for matched patients without a fracture.[6] However, the final surgical decision should be made after induction chemotherapy, and in the interim, fracture stability can be achieved with external immobilization. If radiographs show ossification of the fracture site after induction chemotherapy, it is reasonable to consider limb salvage. In the setting of benign aggressive tumors, a pathologic fracture does not necessitate wide resection and endoprosthetic reconstruction. A 2007 study reported similar functional and recurrence outcomes for patients with intra-articular pathologic fractures from giant cell tumor of bone treated with intralesional curettage versus wide resection and reconstruction.[7]

Surgical Technique: Distal Femoral Resection

The femur may be resected from a lateral, anterior, or medial approach. A medial approach is most commonly used and is described here. The patient should be positioned supine with a sandbag positioning device under the ipsilateral hip and the entire leg including the hip prepped and draped in a sterile manner. The planned excision should be considered on a patient-by-patient basis but classically begins at the medial thigh and extends past the knee using a medial parapatellar approach to below the pes anserinus. The approach begins with exploration of the popliteal fossa and demarcation of the tumor mass from the popliteal neurovascular structures. Distal femoral sarcoma resection should be performed in accordance with strict oncologic principles. The tumor should be removed en bloc with adequate soft-tissue and bony margins on the ba-

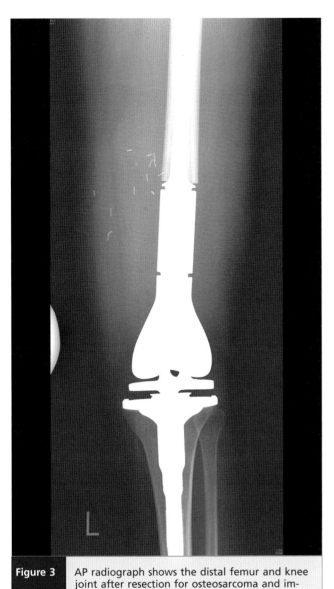

Figure 3 AP radiograph shows the distal femur and knee joint after resection for osteosarcoma and implantation of an uncemented modular prosthesis with a rotating-hinge knee.

sis of postchemotherapy imaging, with care taken to include the biopsy tract and other potentially contaminated tissues in the resection specimen. Intraoperative frozen sections of the proximal femoral margin should be sent for pathologic analysis to ensure a negative proximal margin before proceeding with skeletal reconstruction. Distal femoral reconstruction is then performed. Adequate soft-tissue coverage is ensured by medial gastrocnemius flap and/or sartorius flap reconstruction in selected patients if primary closure is not feasible. Rarely, free-tissue transfers may be considered to ensure coverage. The optimal duration of postoperative antibiotic therapy is controversial, and a multicenter randomized controlled trial currently in progress is aimed at determining the optimal duration. As background work for the trial, a survey of musculoskeletal oncologists was completed to determine practice patterns in postoperative antibiotic prophylaxis and identified widely disparate treatment patterns.[8]

Reconstruction Options

Available reconstructive options vary by extent of resection, soft-tissue loss, and skeletal maturity. Appropriate reconstructions should be considered on a patient-by-patient basis.

Endoprosthesis

When considering endoprosthetic reconstruction, the most commonly used endoprostheses are of a modular construction with a rotating-hinge knee prosthesis (**Figure 3**). These endoprostheses generally are used when the tumor morphology is such that preservation of the joint is not possible given the proximity of the tumor. One must also ensure that soft-tissue coverage of the prosthesis is adequate to prevent flap necrosis and exposure of the underlying hardware. Soft-tissue coverage of the distal femoral endoprosthesis is rarely insufficient, and can be augmented by local rotational flaps if required. The tibial component of a distal femoral endoprosthetic reconstruction for a joint-sacrificing resection, however, is more prone to wound complications due to its superficial location.[9] Several authors[9-12] have described the use of the medial gastrocnemius flap to augment coverage of the distal aspect of the prosthesis. For example, the authors of a 1999 study[9] reported that flap augmentation of the proximal tibial component of the endoprosthesis decreases approximate infection rates from 36% to 12%. The authors of a 2003 study[12] reported similar findings with a reduction of infection rates from 20% to 5% with the use of a medial gastrocnemius flap.

In a recently published 30-year observational study,[13] the overall survival rates of cemented modular rotating-hinge distal femoral endoprostheses at 10, 20, and 25 years were 77%, 58%, and 50%, respectively. Furthermore, these implants were shown to be superior to the custom-casted implants of earlier generations, with 15-year implant survival of 87% versus 51%. Early complications were observed in 88 of 186 patients and included mechanical failure, superficial infection or flap necrosis, local recurrence, transient peroneal nerve palsy, deep infection, cement extrusion into a vascular channel, patellofemoral subluxation, positive oncologic margins, and stress fracture. Observed reasons for late failure and revision include aseptic loosening and implant fatigue, and less commonly infection and local recurrence. Approximately 9% of the initial 186 patients required eventual amputation.

In the 30-year study,[13] the mean Musculoskeletal Tumor Society (MSTS) functional score for modular component implants was 86.7% with mean flexion to 110°, mean passive extension of 1.3°, and a mean extension lag of 6.9°. Flexion contracture was observed in 7 of 160 patients with an observed mean of 10°. Patients

6: Special Considerations in Tumor Management

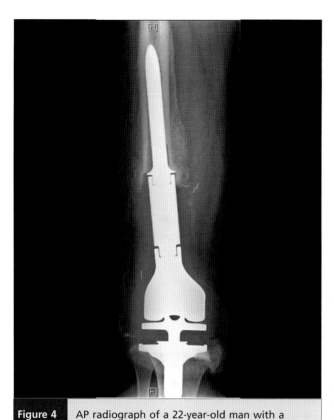

Figure 4 AP radiograph of a 22-year-old man with a history of limb-sparing surgery for osteosarcoma shows a deep prosthetic infection. Note the loosening of the femoral stem with surrounding reactive bone matrix.

generally lead unrestricted lives with only some limitations of kneeling, running, and contact sports. Furthermore, the authors of a 2011 study[14] compared the functional outcomes of total femur, proximal femur, and distal femur replacements. In their analysis, no significant differences in Toronto Extremity Salvage Score were observed between rotating-hinge and fixed-hinge distal femoral reconstructions.

Advances in implant biomechanics continue to reduce revision rates for mechanical failure, but deep endoprosthetic infection continues to be a leading cause of revision (**Figure 4**). Common causative organisms include coagulase-negative staphylococcus, *Staphylococcus aureus*, and *Staphylococcus epidermidis*.[15] The prevention of surgical site infection remains a major challenge in tumor surgery. It is widely accepted that oncology patients are at an increased risk relative to conventional arthroplasty patients of developing postoperative infections, given their immunocompromised status following chemotherapy and radiation treatment, and the magnitude of the bone and soft-tissue removal. A systematic review of studies reporting infection rates for endoprosthetic reconstruction after resection of lower extremity primary bony tumors reported a 9% weighted mean for deep infection.[16] This infection rate is significantly higher than the 1% infection rate commonly reported for conventional knee and hip arthroplasties.[17,18] Prophylactic perioperative antibiotic regimens vary tremendously, as reported in a survey of members of the MSTS and the Canadian Orthopaedic Oncology Society.[8]

In a series of 428 patients with distal femoral resection and endoprosthetic reconstruction, the authors reported a 9.6% deep infection rate at 13 months.[19] Aseptic loosening and infection were the predominant modes of failure and cause for revision. Interestingly, the fixed-hinge prosthesis has been largely replaced by the rotating-hinge prosthesis with a hydroxyapatite collar in the study population, reducing risk of revision by 52%.

Surgical methodology and extent of resection have also been shown to be important predictors of implant longevity. The authors of a 2012 study comment that the bone to stem ratio is a significant predictor of aseptic failure.[20] Intuitively, implants that more completely fill the canal (resulting in a higher bone to stem ratio) are inherently more stable than those with a lower bone to stem ratio. Remaining femoral bone stock has also proven to be a predictor of implant longevity; the authors of a 2011 study found that resection of more than 40% of the femur is correlated with accelerated mechanical implant failure.[21] The authors of a biomechanical study found that newer uncemented stems exhibit acceptable initial stability with respect to axial compression, lateral bending, torsional stiffness, and torque to failure compared to an older cemented prosthesis.[22] Interestingly, the authors of this study also reported that cylindrical reaming in the femoral diaphysis is associated with a significantly higher torque to failure compared to flexible reaming.

Stem fixation techniques vary and include cemented stems, uncemented press-fit stems, and compression-based press-fit stems (Biomet; **Figures 5** and **6**). The advantage of cemented femoral stems is that they allow immediate weight bearing and strength; however, bony ingrowth does not occur through the cement, and loosening becomes a significant mode of failure. For nonpalliative reconstructions, press-fit stems have also become common for treatment, although the fixation type is considered on a patient-by-patient basis. Uncemented press-fit stems do allow for bony ingrowth; however, they require an initial caution period of 6 to 12 weeks to optimize bony ingrowth. Compression-based press-fit stems exhibit higher failure rates within the first year after implantation; however, if they succeed, they tend to have a longer expected life span than the press-fit stem. In a 2009 study comparing press-fit stems with compression-based press-fit stems, survival rates in the press-fit group were 85% at 5 years and 71% at 10 years, with the predominant mode of failure being aseptic loosening mostly occurring in the long term.[23] Interestingly, stems with diameter less than 13.5 mm and those with a diaphyseal/stem coefficient greater than 2.5 mm showed shorter survival than larger stems. The compression-based press-fit stem exhibited slightly higher survival at 5 years (88%), and most failures occurred within 1 year by either failure of

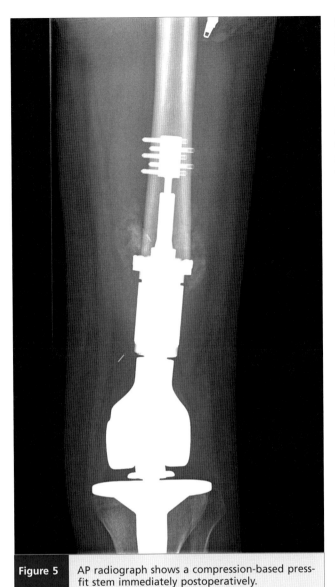

Figure 5 AP radiograph shows a compression-based press-fit stem immediately postoperatively.

femoral fixation or fracture. No failures of compression-based press-fit stems were observed in this study after the first year, and if the implants survived, no differences in prosthetic function were observed. Pros and cons of each implant type should be considered given the preference, activity level, and compliance of a patient receiving the implant to optimize function over the expected life span.

Implant Coatings

There has been ongoing investigation into the effect of prosthetic coatings on decreasing infection rates without compromising implant longevity. Silver-coated endoprosthetics are commercially available, and retrospective cohort studies suggest a correlation between surgical site silver ion concentration and infection rates.[24] More recently, iodine-coated endoprosthetics have become a topic of interest. Although FDA approval is currently pending, cohort studies from Kanazawa, Japan[25] suggest promising results for the use of these implants in preventing and treating endoprosthetic infection in immunocompromised hosts. Currently there is no level I evidence to support the exclusive use of either of these implant types, and further research must be conducted.

Reconstructions

Allograft-prosthetic composite is a less common reconstructive option in the distal femur. It is very rarely used for primary reconstruction after distal femoral resection in the adult population; however, it can be useful as a revision option for a failed endoprosthesis when the remaining host bone is insufficient because of osteolysis or aseptic loosening. Another reconstructive alternative is total femoral endoprosthetic reconstruction. However, if the hip joint and abductors are fully functional, preservation of these structures is optimal.

Allograft

The authors of a study examining a series of 96 patients with osteoarticular allograft reconstruction following resection of a tumor in the distal femur concluded that allograft reconstruction may be considered in selected patients where the articular cartilage can be safely preserved and the healing time required for the allograft would not compete with the timing of any required chemotherapy.[26] These reconstructions are not without complications, with 14% of patients experiencing nonunions, 12% experiencing postoperative arthritis, 7% experiencing instability, 6% experiencing infection, and 6% experiencing bone resorption. Significant differences were observed in both infection rates (13% versus 2%) and nonunion rates (23% versus 6%) between patients receiving chemotherapy compared to those not receiving chemotherapy. Overall final results were slightly better in the nonchemotherapy group, with 70% reporting good or excellent results and 4% reporting poor results, whereas in the chemotherapy group 53% reported good or excellent results and 10% reported poor results.

Fibular Grafting

Vascularized fibular grafting, either series-connected double-strut or allograft composite, are options for reconstructing massive juxta-articular defects. Series-connected double-strut vascularized fibular grafting has been shown to yield good results, with 93% of patients achieving union.[27] However, an external fixator was used for stabilization for 1 year in this series, which may be undesirable to patients when immediate unimpeded weight bearing is feasible with endoprosthetic reconstruction. The authors of a 2010 study described vascularized fibular grafts for reconstruction of distal femoral defects.[28] On a patient-by-patient basis, external fixation, plating, or intramedullary nailing was used as adjunct stabilization. Although all patients in the study achieved union, protective braces were used for more than 1 year, and subjective knee stiffness was a concern. Final mean ranges of motion were 96.9° ±

6: Special Considerations in Tumor Management

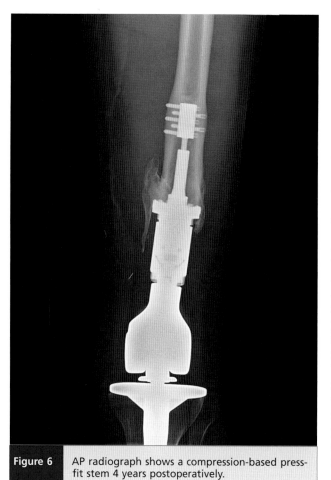

Figure 6 | AP radiograph shows a compression-based press-fit stem 4 years postoperatively.

come a trend toward improved outcomes for robot-assisted resections and allograft-prosthetic reconstructions, but further research needs to be conducted before conclusions can be drawn.

Summary

Distal femoral resection and reconstruction is most commonly performed for primary bone sarcoma; however, other indications include benign aggressive tumors, metastatic bone disease in selected patients, and bone loss due to failed arthroplasty or trauma. Local recurrence rates are low with wide resection and reconstruction of primary bone sarcomas of the distal femur following neoadjuvant chemotherapy. In skeletally mature patients, endoprosthetic reconstruction provides an immediately stable reconstruction, but infection rates are high, and mechanical failures result in the need for revision in many patients. More recent endoprosthetic designs could result in longer-term implant survival. The options of allograft-prosthetic composite reconstruction or allograft alone are losing popularity because of the high risks of nonunion, fracture, and infection. Computer-assisted navigation could improve union rates in these patients. In skeletally immature patients, rotationplasty, amputation, and expandable prostheses remain viable reconstruction options; however, high mechanical failure rates have been reported for expandable prostheses.

36.0° for knee flexion and −5.0° ± 10.0° for extension. Internal fixation was suggested as preferable to external fixation where feasible.

Computer-Assisted Navigation

Computer-assisted resection of primary bone tumors has attracted significant recent interest. In two separate studies, researchers simulated manual and computer jig-assisted tumor resections in a cadaveric model, as well as manual and haptic robot-assisted resections.[29,30] They found that both computer-assisted custom resection jigs and haptic robot-assisted resections increase accuracy of tumor resection compared to traditional manual methods. These results are the first of their kind and have the potential to reduce bone loss without compromising oncologic outcomes. The researchers postulated that nonunion rates with traditional allograft reconstruction are approximately 20% and that increasing the contact area between host bone and allograft is paramount in minimizing nonunion rates. They used a cadaver model in which haptic robot technology and the traditional manual method of cutting allograft to fill a resection defect were compared. They found 24% contact between host bone and allograft in the manual method and 76% contact in the haptic model. With increasing use of robotic technology may

Annotated References

1. Bickels J, Wittig JC, Kollender Y, et al: Distal femur resection with endoprosthetic reconstruction: A long-term followup study. *Clin Orthop Relat Res* 2002;400: 225-235.

2. Katagiri H, Cannon SR, Briggs TW, Cobb J, Witt J, Pringle J: Local recurrence of osteosarcoma: Survival rate and management. *J Bone Joint Surg Br* 2003;85-B(suppl 1):50.

3. Bacci G, Longhi A, Fagioli F, Briccoli A, Versari M, Picci P: Adjuvant and neoadjuvant chemotherapy for osteosarcoma of the extremities: 27 year experience at Rizzoli Institute, Italy. *Eur J Cancer* 2005;41(18): 2836-2845.

4. Fottner A, Szalantzy M, Wirthmann L, et al: Bone metastases from renal cell carcinoma: Patient survival after surgical treatment. *BMC Musculoskelet Disord* 2010;11:145.

   A retrospective review of 101 patients surgically treated for skeletal metastases of renal cell carcinoma between 1980 and 2005 showed that patients with a solitary metastasis or a limited number of resectable metastases are candidates for wide resections to achieve local control and improve survival.

5. Godley K, Watts AC, Robb JE: Pathological femoral fracture caused by primary bone tumour: A population-based study. *Scott Med J* 2011;56(1):5-9.

   This population-based study identified 84 patients with malignant primary bone tumor of the femur and pathologic fracture between 1960 and 2004. Despite improvements in chemotherapy and surgical technique over the study period, these patients have a poor prognosis, and attempts at limb salvage did not alter prognosis.

6. Scully SP, Ghert MA, Zurakowski D, Thompson RC, Gebhardt MC: Pathologic fracture in osteosarcoma: Prognostic importance and treatment implications. *J Bone Joint Surg Am* 2002;84-A(1):49-57.

7. Deheshi BM, Jaffer SN, Griffin AM, Ferguson PC, Bell RS, Wunder JS: Joint salvage for pathologic fracture of giant cell tumor of the lower extremity. *Clin Orthop Relat Res* 2007;459(459):96-104.

   This retrospective review compared outcomes of 139 patients with giant cell tumor of weight-bearing bones with or without pathologic fracture. Although trends toward lower rates of 5-year metastatic-free survival and higher rates of arthrofibrosis were identified in the pathologic fracture group, it is reasonable to attempt joint salvage in these patients.

8. Hasan K, Racano A, Deheshi B, et al: Prophylactic antibiotic regimens in tumor surgery (PARITY) survey. *BMC Musculoskelet Disord* 2012;13(1):91.

   A cross-sectional survey of MSTS members showed variable practices in prophylactic antibiotic prescription, with most surgeons employing a first-generation cephalosporin for at least 24 hours postoperatively. The inconsistency in prescribing practices as well as overwhelming surgeon interest supported the rationale for a randomized multicenter clinical trial.

9. Grimer RJ, Carter SR, Tillman RM, et al: Endoprosthetic replacement of the proximal tibia. *J Bone Joint Surg Br* 1999;81(3):488-494.

10. Malawer MM, Price WM: Gastrocnemius transposition flap in conjunction with limb-sparing surgery for primary bone sarcomas around the knee. *Plast Reconstr Surg* 1984;73(5):741-750.

11. Anract P, Missenard G, Jeanrot C, Dubois V, Tomeno B: Knee reconstruction with prosthesis and muscle flap after total arthrectomy. *Clin Orthop Relat Res* 2001; 384:208-216.

12. Buchner M, Zeifang F, Bernd L: Medial gastrocnemius muscle flap in limb-sparing surgery of malignant bone tumors of the proximal tibia: Mid-term results in 25 patients. *Ann Plast Surg* 2003;51(3):266-272.

13. Schwartz AJ, Kabo JM, Eilber FC, Eilber FR, Eckardt JJ: Cemented distal femoral endoprostheses for musculoskeletal tumor: Improved survival of modular versus custom implants. *Clin Orthop Relat Res* 2010;468(8): 2198-2210.

   This three-decade retrospective review of 254 patients with distal femoral endoprosthetic reconstruction suggests that cemented modular rotating-hinge distal femoral endoprostheses demonstrated improved survivorship compared with older custom-casted implant designs.

14. Jones KB, Griffin AM, Chandrasekar CR, et al: Patient-oriented functional results of total femoral endoprosthetic reconstruction following oncologic resection. *J Surg Oncol* 2011;104(6):561-565.

   Outcomes of total femoral replacement, proximal femoral replacement, and distal femoral replacement were compared. No significant difference was found between fixed-hinge and rotating-hinge prostheses, or between hemiarthroplasty and total hip arthroplasty. Total femoral replacement carried a poor functional prognosis overall, with additive functional impairments conferred from both proximal and distal femoral replacement.

15. Jeys L, Grimer R: The long-term risks of infection and amputation with limb salvage surgery using endoprostheses. *Recent Results Cancer Res* 2009;179(II):75-84.

   Limb salvage surgery with endoprosthetic reconstruction when possible is the current standard of treatment in tumor surgery, with local recurrence and deep prosthetic infection being the leading causes of secondary amputation. A periprosthetic infection rate of 10% is quoted, with most infections occurring postoperatively within 12 months and coagulase-negative staphylococcus being the most common causative organism.

16. Racano A, Pazionis T, Farrokhyar F, Deheshi B, Ghert M: High infection rate outcomes in long-bone tumor surgery with endoprosthetic reconstruction in adults: A systematic review. *Clin Orthop Relat Res* 2013; 471(6):2017-2027.

   In this systematic review of infection rates and antibiotic regimens in tumor surgery with endoprosthetic reconstruction, average infection rates are shown to be 10% compared to 1%, as cited for conventional arthroplasty. Long-term antibiotic prophylaxis may decrease the rate of infection; however, larger-scale trials are needed to draw definitive conclusions. Level of evidence: IV.

17. Blom AW, Taylor AH, Pattison G, Whitehouse S, Bannister GC: Infection after total hip arthroplasty: The Avon experience. *J Bone Joint Surg Br* 2003; 85(7):956-959.

18. Jämsen E, Huhtala H, Puolakka T, Moilanen T: Risk factors for infection after knee arthroplasty: A register-based analysis of 43,149 cases. *J Bone Joint Surg Am* 2009;91(1):38-47.

   An analysis of results from the Finnish arthroplasty registry quoted infection rates from conventional total knee arthroplasty at approximately 1%. Male patients, those with rheumatoid arthritis, and those with a previous fracture at the joint in question have an increased risk of postoperative infection. The authors recommended combining intravenous antibiotic prophylaxis with antibiotic-impregnated cement in revision arthroplasty.

6: Special Considerations in Tumor Management

19. Myers GJ, Abudu AT, Carter SR, Tillman RM, Grimer RJ: Endoprosthetic replacement of the distal femur for bone tumours: Long-term results. *J Bone Joint Surg Br* 2007;89(4):521-526.

    Function and implant longevity were compared between patients with either a fixed-hinge or rotating-hinge distal femoral replacement in a 335-patient series. The study suggested that a cemented, rotating-hinge prosthesis with a hydroxyapatite collar offers the best chance of long-term prosthetic survival. Infections remain a serious problem irrespective of implant design.

20. Song WS, Kong CB, Jeon DG, et al: The impact of amount of bone resection on uncemented prosthesis failure in patients with a distal femoral tumor. *J Surg Oncol* 2011;104(2):192-197.

    The outcomes of 117 patients who underwent intra-articular resection and cementless modular prosthetic reconstruction from a distal femoral tumor were examined. Infection was found to be the predominant cause of implant failure, with femoral resection of more than 40% also significantly correlated with implant failure.

21. Bergin PF, Noveau JB, Jelinek JS, Henshaw RM: Aseptic loosening rates in distal femoral endoprostheses: Does stem size matter? *Clin Orthop Relat Res* 2012; 470(3):743-750.

    Analysis of the characteristics and longevity of 104 distal femoral replacements implanted between 1985 and 2008 showed that of stem size, bone diaphyseal width, and resection percentage of the femur, only the bone-to-stem ratio independently predicted aseptic failure. The authors suggested that selecting a stem that fills the femoral canal may increase implant longevity.

22. Ferguson PC, Zdero R, Schemitsch EH, Deheshi BM, Bell RS, Wunder JS: A biomechanical evaluation of press-fit stem constructs for tumor endoprosthetic reconstruction of the distal femur. *J Arthroplasty* 2011; 26(8):1373-1379.

    This biomechanical study showed that newer uncemented stems exhibit acceptable initial results with respect to axial compression, lateral bending, torsional stiffness, and torque to failure compared to the older cemented prosthesis. This study also reported that cylindrical reaming in the femoral diaphysis is associated with a significantly higher torque to failure compared to flexible reaming.

23. Farfalli GL, Boland PJ, Morris CD, Athanasian EA, Healey JH: Early equivalence of uncemented press-fit and Compress femoral fixation. *Clin Orthop Relat Res* 2009;467(11):2792-2799.

    The fixation of intramedullary uncemented press-fit stems was compared with that of the compression-based press-fit uncemented press-fit stem. In the press-fit group, the predominant mode of failure was aseptic loosening, mostly in the long term, whereas the compression-based press-fit stem exhibited slightly higher survival at 5 years with most failures occurring within 1 year by either failure of femoral fixation or fracture. No compression-based press-fit stem failures were observed after the first year. Among surviving implants, no differences in prosthetic function were observed.

24. Hussmann B, Johann I, Kauther MD, Landgraeber S, Jäger M, Lendemans S: Measurement of the silver ion concentration in wound fluids after implantation of silver-coated megaprostheses: Correlation with the clinical outcome. *Biomed Res Int* 2013;2013:763096.

    In patients who underwent reconstruction with a silver-coated megaprosthesis, the concentration of silver ions was measured both in the surgical site as well as in patient blood samples. Patients who showed an increased silver concentration in the blood postoperatively presented a lower silver concentration in the wound fluids and a delayed decrease in C-reactive protein levels. There were significantly fewer reinfections and shorter hospitalization in comparison with a group that did not receive a silver-coated megaprosthesis.

25. Tsuchiya H, Shirai T, Nishida H, et al: Innovative antimicrobial coating of titanium implants with iodine. *J Orthop Sci* 2012;17(5):595-604.

    Patients with postoperative infection or compromised status were treated using iodine-supported titanium implants. These implants were shown to be associated with effective infection prevention and treatment with no evidence of cytotoxicity or mechanical implant failure.

26. Mnaymneh W, Malinin TI, Lackman RD, Hornicek FJ, Ghandur-Mnaymneh L: Massive distal femoral osteoarticular allografts after resection of bone tumors. *Clin Orthop Relat Res* 1994;303:103-115.

27. Liang K, Cen S, Xiang Z, Zhong G, Yi M, Huang F: Massive juxta-articular defects of the distal femur reconstructed by series connected double-strut free-vascularized fibular grafts. *J Trauma Acute Care Surg* 2012;72(2):E71-E76.

    This study is a retrospective review of 19 patients who underwent free-vascularized fibular grafting to treat massive juxta-articular defects of the distal femur. Results suggested that reconstruction of huge femoral defects by series-connected, double-strut, free-vascularized fibular grafting provides good results in achieving bone union, reducing the stress fracture rate, and achieving leg length equality.

28. Coulet B, Pflieger JF, Arnaud S, Lazerges C, Chammas M: Double-barrel fibular graft for metaphyseal areas of reconstruction around the knee. *Orthop Traumatol Surg Res* 2010;96(8):868-875.

    This study described free-vascularized fibular grafting for reconstruction of distal femoral defects. External fixation, plating, or intramedullary nailing was used as adjunct stabilization. Although all treatments achieved union, protective braces were used for more than 1 year, and concerns surrounding subjective knee stiffness remained. Internal fixation was suggested to be preferable to external fixation where feasible.

29. Khan F, Lipman JD, Healey JH, Pearle AD: Abstract:

Haptic robot-assisted surgery substantially improves contact area for structural bone allograft reconstructions. *Annual Meeting Proceedings*. Rosemont, IL, American Academy of Orthopaedic Surgeons, 2012, p 1181.

This abstract reported a novel technique of haptic robot-assisted surgery to reconstruct defects after primary bone sarcoma resection with structural allograft. The study showed significantly increased contact between host bone and allograft in the robot-assisted group compared to the manual group, suggesting that further development of this technology may yield substantial clinical utility.

30. Khan F, Pearle AD, Lipman JD, Healey JH: Haptic robot-assisted surgery substantially improves accuracy of wide resection of bone tumors. *Annual Meeting Proceedings*. Rosemont, IL, American Academy of Orthopaedic Surgeons, 2012, p 1184.

This abstract reported use of haptic robot-assisted technology as a method of improving accuracy of resections of primary bone tumors compared to the traditional manual method. The haptic robot-assisted technique was found to be significantly more accurate in terms of maximum deviation from the preoperative plan than the manual technique, suggesting substantial possible clinical utility in achieving oncologic margins while maximizing residual available bone stock.

Chapter 40

Proximal Tibial Resection and Reconstruction

Robert K. Heck Jr, MD   Patrick C. Toy, MD

Resection

The proximal tibia is second to the distal femur as the most common site of primary bone sarcomas. As for any patient with a neoplastic process, oncologic cure is the priority, with preservation of function being of secondary importance. However, the proximal tibia presents challenges unique to this particular anatomic location when an adequate resection, subsequent limb salvage, and function are considered. Although amputation is a simple and effective way to obtain negative oncologic margins, the advent of adjuvant chemotherapy has provided an opportunity to consider limb salvage as a viable option. Successful limb salvage is difficult because of factors in this anatomic location that are independent of the tumor characteristics, including the superficial location of the bone, the difficulty of achieving adequate soft-tissue coverage after resection, preservation of neurovascular structures, and reconstruction of the extensor mechanism of the knee.

Limb Salvage Versus Amputation

Limb salvage of the proximal tibia is considered a reasonable option when the tumor can be resected with negative margins and when the appropriate neurovascular structures, adequate distal tibial bone, and soft-tissue coverage remain. Limb-salvage techniques with wide resection should be considered for benign aggressive tumors (giant cell tumors), some low-grade bone sarcomas (low-grade osteosarcoma), and most high-grade bone sarcomas. With high-grade bone sarcomas, the timing of resection depends on the treatment protocol involving neoadjuvant chemotherapy. Factors that determine limb salvage feasibility include the patient's ability to tolerate and recover from a surgical procedure, the location of the biopsy site, the extraosseous

extension and potential involvement of neurovascular structures, the ability to reconstruct the extensor mechanism, soft-tissue coverage, and the patient's functional demands.

Negative margins are technically easier to achieve with amputation. Although indications are gradually changing, traditionally amputation has been considered a better option than limb salvage in patients with pathologic fracture, a poorly placed biopsy site, soft-tissue compromise, or infection. Newer techniques of bone fixation and soft-tissue management have made these relative indications for amputation, and limb-salvage procedures may be more appropriate.

Skeletally immature patients present a challenge because the proximal tibial physis usually is sacrificed during the resection. Expandable prostheses have been introduced as a potential solution to minimize problems related to limb-length discrepancy. If oncologically possible, an amputation in a skeletally immature patient should be completed at the level of the knee joint to preserve the distal femoral physis.

Potential Complications

The surgeon performing the biopsy should follow proper techniques to avoid oncologic compromise, and usually should be the same individual who will be involved in the definitive resection. An errantly placed biopsy incision could result in the inability to perform a successful resection if vital structures (patellar tendon, joint, neurovascular structures) are contaminated. Because the anteromedial aspect of the tibia is subcutaneous, the biopsy should be in this location whenever possible. The biopsy track and a cuff of normal tissue must be resected with the tumor specimen to achieve adequate margins.

Compared with other anatomic sites where sarcomas occur relatively frequently, the proximal tibia is in a superficial location, a difference thought to be a significant factor in the higher rate of infection following reconstruction and the potential compromise of limb retention. The risk of infection is further increased when adjuvant chemotherapy is part of the treatment protocol. Rotation of the medial gastrocnemius flap anteriorly has become a routine part of reconstruction to

Dr. Heck or an immediate family member has received royalties from DePuy and Wright Medical Technology, and serves as a paid consultant to or is an employee of DePuy and Wright Medical Technology. Neither Dr. Toy nor any immediate family member has received anything of value from or has stock or stock options held in a commercial company or institution related directly or indirectly to the subject of this chapter.

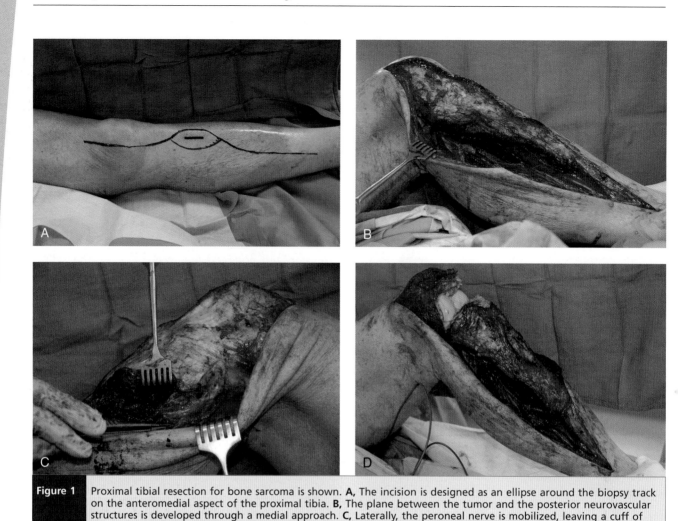

Figure 1 Proximal tibial resection for bone sarcoma is shown. **A,** The incision is designed as an ellipse around the biopsy track on the anteromedial aspect of the proximal tibia. **B,** The plane between the tumor and the posterior neurovascular structures is developed through a medial approach. **C,** Laterally, the peroneal nerve is mobilized, leaving a cuff of muscle to serve as a margin around the proximal tibia. **D,** The patellar tendon is released from its insertion, and a circumferential capsulotomy is made. The final step of the resection is osteotomy of the tibia distal to the tumor.

minimize this problem. This flap also serves to help anchor the patellar tendon to allow restoration of the extensor mechanism. The union achieved between the patellar tendon and rotational flap will eventually allow some active extension at the knee, but extensor lag is common after this method of reconstruction.

Technique

The resection technique is illustrated in **Figure 1**. A longitudinal incision that forms an ellipse around the biopsy scar is made, usually in the anteromedial tibia. Large fasciocutaneous flaps are raised both medially and laterally, and the posterior neurovascular structures are evaluated. The trifurcation of the popliteal artery into the anterior tibial artery, the posterior tibial artery, and the peroneal artery begins at the inferior border of the popliteus muscle. The popliteus muscle covers the posterior surface of the tibia and often acts as an effective barrier to tumor extension posteriorly. As a result, the neurovascular structures often are preserved. The anterior tibial artery and vein pass anteriorly through the interosseous membrane and may be sacrificed in the resection, if necessary, without vascular

compromise to the limb distally. The posterior tibial vessels must be preserved for limb viability.

For intra-articular resections, the ligaments of the knee are divided and the patellar tendon is released from the tibial tubercle without contamination. The level of the tibial diaphyseal osteotomy is determined on the basis of preoperative MRI. The proximal tibiofibular joint is resected as part of the specimen, along with a short segment of the proximal fibula. The common peroneal nerve rarely is involved with the tumor and must be identified and protected. The specimen is delivered en bloc and is evaluated by a pathologist to determine margin status.

If preoperative MRI studies indicate that adequate margins can be obtained, an attempt may be made to preserve the knee joint. An intercalary resection, rather than resection through the joint, can be done by making an osteotomy just distal to the proximal tibial articular surface. Intercalary reconstruction usually is done with a size-matched proximal tibial allograft with its associated patellar tendon. When technically possible and safe from an oncologic standpoint, this technique can be used to achieve a more durable and better-functioning reconstruction compared to techniques necessitated by joint sacrifice.

Reconstruction

Reconstruction after wide resection of proximal tibial sarcomas can be extremely challenging. Historically, complication rates in this location have been relatively high compared to oncologic reconstructions in other locations because of two major factors: wound complications and extensor reconstruction challenges. The proximal tibia can be replaced with an allograft, a tumor prosthesis, or an allograft-prosthetic composite (APC). Each of these options is associated with advantages as well as complications specific to each type of reconstruction. Fortunately, with modern surgical techniques, most patients are able to retain a functional limb.

Soft-Tissue Reconstruction

Soft-tissue coverage in this area usually is tenuous after wide resection of the proximal tibia. Because most proximal tibial sarcomas have extension into the soft tissues, and because there is naturally little soft tissue anteriorly, limited tissue is available for coverage of the skeletal reconstruction after wide resection. Most patients also are undergoing chemotherapy, making wound complications frequent and the risk of infection high. A deep infection can be devastating, often leading to amputation of the limb. Reconstruction of the knee extensor mechanism also poses unique challenges. Resection of sarcomas of the proximal tibia usually requires resection of the tibial tubercle and a portion of the patellar tendon as well. Secure reattachment of the extensor mechanism can be difficult and frequently results in quadriceps weakness and an extensor lag, although modern surgical techniques, such as the routine use of a gastrocnemius flap, have helped to partially overcome some of these problems.[1,2] The gastrocnemius flap improves soft-tissue coverage and facilitates wound healing, thus decreasing the infection rate; it also provides a biologic attachment for the patellar tendon.

Osteoarticular Allograft

An osteoarticular allograft provides restoration of the tibial joint surface as well as attachments for the ligaments and joint capsule. Major advantages of an osteoarticular allograft are the ability to provide a secure attachment of the extensor mechanism to the allograft patellar tendon and complete preservation of the distal femur, which can be extremely important for pediatric patients in whom preservation of the distal femoral physis will minimize future limb-length discrepancy.

The first step in osteoarticular allograft reconstruction is locating an allograft that matches the size of the tibia that will be resected. Ideally, the joint surfaces should match as closely as possible. It is acceptable for the allograft joint surface to be slightly larger than that of the resected bone, but it should not be smaller. After resection of the proximal tibia, the allograft is opened onto the field. It should be cut to match the length of the resected specimen. In pediatric patients, the allograft can be cut slightly longer (1 cm) to provide some additional length to compensate for the lost physis. An attempt to gain too much length can cause injury to neurovascular structures and increase the risk of wound healing complications. Host knee ligaments are repaired to the allograft ligaments using nonabsorbable sutures. The diaphyseal graft-host junction is then fixed with compression plating along the lateral surface. The patellar tendon is repaired with the knee in full extension. Care should be taken to close the wound without tension. Use of a medial gastrocnemius flap can help with soft-tissue coverage as well as with healing of the extensor mechanism. Postoperatively, the knee usually is braced in full extension for 6 weeks to protect the extensor repair. The brace is then adjusted gradually over the next 6 weeks to slowly allow progressive flexion. Touch-down weight bearing is recommended until union is evident at the graft-host junction.

Although this technique has the potential to restore adequate knee function, complications are frequent and may be prohibitive. Infection rates have been reported to range from 12% to 25%.[3-8] The risk of infection can be minimized by attention to tension-free soft-tissue closure, use of a gastrocnemius flap to improve coverage, perioperative antibiotic prophylaxis, and postoperative wound care. Fracture of bulk allografts has been reported in 13% to 80% of patients depending on the technique.[3,4,6-10] The risk of fracture can be minimized by protecting as much of the allograft as possible with metal implants. Even with prophylactic fixation, however, subchondral fractures still are common, usually requiring treatment by placement of arthroplasty implants. Finally, delayed union or nonunion of the graft-host junction is common, occurring in 11% to 50% of patients.[4,6,9-11] This risk can be minimized by maximizing graft-host contact and using rigid internal fixation. Some authors have recommended primary autogenous bone grafting of the graft-host junction at the index procedure. Unfortunately, however, because most patients undergoing this procedure are also undergoing intense chemotherapy regimens, complication rates remain high.

Tumor Prosthesis

To overcome some of the shortfalls of osteoarticular allografts, some surgeons prefer using a tumor prosthesis to reconstruct the proximal tibia (**Figure 2**). These prostheses are produced by multiple orthopaedic manufacturers and are readily available. The implants are modular, and are assembled in the operating room to the desired specifications after resection of the proximal tibia. Most tumor prostheses use a rotating hinge to replace the knee joint. Compared to a fixed hinge, a

6: Special Considerations in Tumor Management

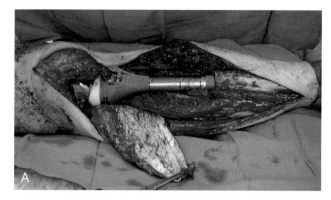

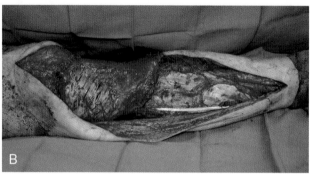

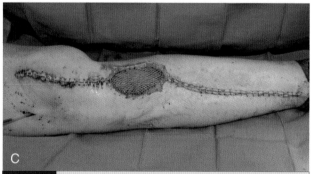

Figure 2 Skeletal and soft-tissue reconstruction following proximal tibial resection is shown. **A,** A proximal tibial tumor prosthesis has been implanted. The patellar tendon is attached to the prosthesis with heavy nonabsorbable sutures. A medial gastrocnemius flap has been prepared. **B,** The gastrocnemius flap is repaired to the patellar tendon and to the remaining anterior and lateral compartment musculature. The flap will augment the extensor mechanism and provide soft-tissue coverage for the prosthesis. **C,** The wound is closed, and the residual defect is treated with a split-thickness skin graft.

rotating hinge decreases the torsional stresses at the bone-implant interface and lessens the risk of aseptic loosening.[2,12] In general, tumor prostheses are less bulky than allografts, allowing wound closure with less tension, which, theoretically, could lessen the risk of infection. Despite smaller dimensions, prostheses are mechanically superior to allograft bone. Although allograft fractures are common, mechanical failure of modern prostheses is relatively rare, although stem fractures and mechanical failure of the rotating-hinge

mechanism occasionally occur. The prosthesis can be fixed to bone with a cemented stem or through a porous ingrowth surface. Recently, in hopes of decreasing the risk of aseptic loosening, a new method of fixation that uses a compression device to promote osseointegration was developed.[13] This device also has the advantage of requiring less residual host bone to achieve secure fixation. Finally, compared with allograft reconstruction, tumor prostheses have the advantage of allowing the patient earlier full weight bearing and quicker rehabilitation because there is no need to wait for union of a graft-host junction. Patients with cemented prostheses can bear weight as tolerated right away. Some surgeons opt for protected weight bearing for 6 weeks after use of press-fit stems.

The largest disadvantage of a tumor prosthesis is difficulty with reconstruction of the extensor mechanism.[1,2,14] Most prostheses have holes or a metal bar for reattachment of the patellar tendon. Some prostheses have a porous coating in this area. The patellar tendon can be secured to the porous coating in hopes of achieving stable soft-tissue ingrowth. Regardless of the method of fixation of the patellar tendon to the prosthesis, failure of the extensor mechanism is likely unless biologic healing is achieved. To achieve biologic healing, use of a gastrocnemius flap is considered mandatory by most surgeons who use tumor prostheses to reconstruct the proximal tibia. After the patellar tendon has been secured to the prosthesis with heavy nonabsorbable sutures, the gastrocnemius flap is laid across the repair and secured to the tendon and to the remaining anterior compartment musculature and fascia to provide a continuous biologic extensor mechanism. The wound is closed over the muscle repair without tension. Split-thickness skin grafting usually is required to avoid tension on the closure. The knee is held in full extension for 6 weeks postoperatively. Protected gradual flexion is then progressed for the next 6 weeks. Using this method, extensor function usually is satisfactory with minimal lag (**Figure 3**).

Infection is a potentially devastating complication. Older series reported infection rates as high as 40%.[12,15-18] The risk of infection can be minimized with use of a gastrocnemius flap to improve soft-tissue coverage, a tension-free closure, perioperative antibiotics, and postoperative wound care. Using current techniques, reported infection rates range from 12% to 18%.[12,16,19-21] Infections can be treated with staged revision, but recurrent infection is common and amputation sometimes is necessary.

Polyethylene wear is an issue for patients with prosthetic reconstructions. Historically, polyethylene particles could travel the entire length of the prosthesis to the prosthesis-bone interface, where they could cause massive osteolysis, with subsequent bone loss and aseptic loosening. Most modern tumor prostheses, however, are constructed with a porous collar around the base of the stem. This porous collar allows extracortical bone bridging, which could theoretically enhance the stabil-

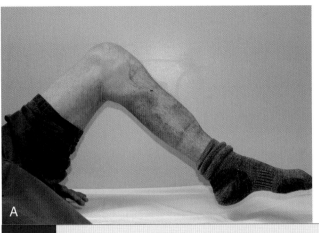
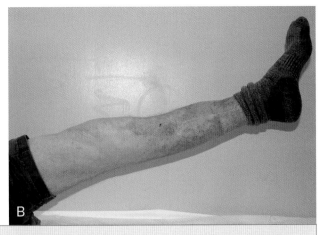

Figure 3 **A** and **B,** At 1 year following proximal tibial resection and endoprosthetic reconstruction, active knee range of motion is from 90° of flexion to full extension. The patient is pain free and ambulates without an assistive device.

ity of the stem.[2,12,18] Whether mechanical stability is enhanced by the porous collar is debatable. What has become apparent, though, is that ingrowth into the porous collar (either bone or fibrous tissue ingrowth) acts as a biologic purse string that protects the prosthesis-bone interface from potentially damaging polyethylene particles. Although particulate wear debris appears to be a waning problem, mechanical failure of polyethylene bushings in the hinge continues to be relatively common,[20,21] but these bushings are relatively easy to replace.

Compared with historical controls, rates of aseptic loosening have dramatically decreased, probably because of multiple factors. Controlling polyethylene-induced osteolysis likely plays a significant role. Stem fixation into the bone also has improved. Modern cementing techniques (vacuum mixing, canal preparation, and cement pressurization) have led to good results in studies with medium-term and long-term follow-up.[12,18,20] Likewise, aseptic loosening is relatively uncommon with modern porous-coated stems, as well as with compressive osseointegration fixation.[13] Finally, use of a rotating hinge (as opposed to a fixed hinge) decreases the mechanical stresses at the bone-implant interface and likely has contributed to decreased rates of aseptic loosening.[12] Currently, 10-year survival rates of 75% to 86% are being reported for proximal tibial prosthetic reconstruction using modern designs and surgical techniques.[12,15,20]

A disadvantage of using a proximal tibial tumor prosthesis rather than an osteoarticular allograft involves violation of the distal femoral physis. Proximal tibial tumor prostheses use a rotating-hinge mechanism to replace the knee joint, and for most currently used prostheses, fixation requires placement of a stem through the distal femoral physis. In skeletally immature patients, this placement can further contribute to a progressive limb-length discrepancy. Specially designed expandable prostheses are currently available and are discussed in chapter 43.

Allograft-Prosthetic Composite

An APC reconstruction combines the main advantages of an allograft (secure patellar tendon fixation) with the biggest advantage of a prosthesis (reliable reconstruction of a stable joint with no risk of subchondral fracture).

The APC reconstruction technique has many variations. A standard total knee prosthesis can be used if the allograft ligaments can provide stability. More often, however, a rotating-hinge prosthesis is used to provide more reliable stability. The allograft can be secured to the host bone by compression plating, or a long-stem prosthesis can be used to span the entire length of the allograft and secure the APC into the host bone (**Figure 4**). The stem must be cemented into the allograft, but can be fixed into the host bone with cemented or press-fit techniques. If the stem is cemented into the host bone, care should be taken to make sure that there is no cement in the graft-host junction, which could lead to nonunion. When the APC has been secured to the host bone and the femoral implant has been placed, the prosthetic knee joint is reduced, and the extensor mechanism is repaired with the knee in full extension. A gastrocnemius flap can then be used to augment the extensor repair, soft-tissue coverage, and closure.

Postoperatively, the knee is maintained in full extension for 6 weeks to protect the extensor mechanism repair. The period of full extension is followed by progressive protected flexion. Depending on the method of fixation at the graft-host junction, weight bearing usually is protected until some evidence of bone healing is observed. The most common complications are nonunion (20% to 27%) and infection (8% to 24%).[14,22-26]

Other Options

When the proximal tibial joint surface can be preserved while still obtaining an adequate surgical resection margin, the defect usually is reconstructed with an intercalary allograft. The reconstruction technique is similar to that of an osteoarticular allograft with the exception

6: Special Considerations in Tumor Management

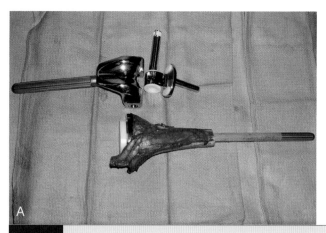
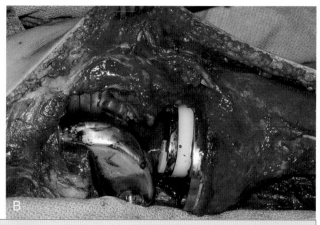

Figure 4 APC reconstruction following proximal tibial resection is shown. **A,** An APC was constructed by cementing a long-stem constrained prosthesis into a proximal tibial allograft that was cut to match the resulting defect after tumor resection. The APC tibial stem will be fixed with a press-fit technique into the host tibia. **B,** The APC has been implanted, and the allograft tendon has been repaired to the host tendon. A gastrocnemius flap can be used to augment the repair and improve soft-tissue coverage.

that the patient's own joint surface is preserved and is repaired to the proximal portion of the allograft with multiple screws. This technique has the potential to preserve a more natural and durable joint with less risk of developing secondary degenerative changes; however, complications, including nonunion and infection, are frequent.[27]

Other reconstruction options have been reported but are used less frequently. Intercalary reconstructions using vascularized fibular grafts or extracorporeally irradiated autografts have been described. Extracorporeally irradiated autografts also have been used as osteoarticular grafts or as part of allograft-prosthetic-composite reconstructions.[28] Vascularized fibular grafts have been used in conjunction with allograft "shells" to reconstruct the proximal tibia.[29] Each of these options, although less well studied, has potential merit depending on the resources available at each institution and the clinical scenario.

Summary

The proximal tibia is a relatively common location for primary bone sarcomas. The anatomy of this area makes wide resection and reconstruction of proximal tibial tumors very challenging. Historically, most patients with proximal tibial sarcomas were treated with amputation. Currently, multiple options for reconstruction are available, including allografts, tumor prostheses, and allograft-prosthetic-composite reconstructions. Fortunately, with modern surgical techniques, most patients with proximal tibial sarcomas are candidates for limb salvage and are able to retain a functional limb.

Annotated References

1. Malawer MM, McHale KA: Limb-sparing surgery for high-grade malignant tumors of the proximal tibia: Surgical technique and a method of extensor mechanism reconstruction. *Clin Orthop Relat Res* 1989;239: 231-248.

2. Eckardt JJ, Matthews JG II, Eilber FR: Endoprosthetic reconstruction after bone tumor resections of the proximal tibia. *Orthop Clin North Am* 1991;22(1):149-160.

3. Brien EW, Terek RM, Healey JH, Lane JM: Allograft reconstruction after proximal tibial resection for bone tumors: An analysis of function and outcome comparing allograft and prosthetic reconstructions. *Clin Orthop Relat Res* 1994;303:116-127.

4. Clohisy DR, Mankin HJ: Osteoarticular allografts for reconstruction after resection of a musculoskeletal tumor in the proximal end of the tibia. *J Bone Joint Surg Am* 1994;76(4):549-554.

5. Lord CF, Gebhardt MC, Tomford WW, Mankin HJ: Infection in bone allografts: Incidence, nature, and treatment. *J Bone Joint Surg Am* 1988;70(3):369-376.

6. Mankin HJ, Doppelt SH, Sullivan TR, Tomford WW: Osteoarticular and intercalary allograft transplantation in the management of malignant tumors of bone. *Cancer* 1982;50(4):613-630.

7. Mankin HJ, Gebhardt MC, Jennings LC, Springfield DS, Tomford WW: Long-term results of allograft replacement in the management of bone tumors. *Clin Orthop Relat Res* 1996;324:86-97.

8. Muscolo DL, Ayerza MA, Farfalli G, Aponte-Tinao LA: Proximal tibia osteoarticular allografts in tumor

limb salvage surgery. *Clin Orthop Relat Res* 2010; 468(5):1396-1404.

Complications of 52 reconstructions included infection (13), fracture (3), and articular collapse (4). The overall rate of graft survival without removal or conversion to APC was 57% at 5 and 10 years, with excellent functional results and minimal extensor lag. Level of evidence: IV.

9. Campanacci L, Manfrini M, Colangeli M, Alí N, Mercuri M: Long-term results in children with massive bone osteoarticular allografts of the knee for high-grade osteosarcoma. *J Pediatr Orthop* 2010;30(8): 919-927.

    Nine of 10 graft-host junctions healed primarily in an average of 13 months (9 to 19 months). There were no deep infections; 8 of 10 allografts fractured. Overall rates of graft survival were 45% at 5 years and 20% at 10 years. Level of evidence: IV.

10. Donati D, Di Liddo M, Zavatta M, et al: Massive bone allograft reconstruction in high-grade osteosarcoma. *Clin Orthop Relat Res* 2000;377:186-194.

11. Hornicek FJ, Gebhardt MC, Tomford WW, et al: Factors affecting nonunion of the allograft-host junction. *Clin Orthop Relat Res* 2001;382:87-98.

12. Myers GJ, Abudu AT, Carter SR, Tillman RM, Grimer RJ: The long-term results of endoprosthetic replacement of the proximal tibia for bone tumours. *J Bone Joint Surg Br* 2007;89(12):1632-1637.

    The rate of revision at 15 years was 75% with fixed-hinge design and 30% with rotating-hinge design. Aseptic loosening at 10 years occurred in 46% with fixed-hinge design and 3% with rotating-hinge design; the infection rate decreased from 40% to 18% with a gastrocnemius flap. Level of evidence: IV.

13. O'Donnell RJ: Compressive osseointegration of tibial implants in primary cancer reconstruction. *Clin Orthop Relat Res* 2009;467(11):2807-2812.

    Early and midterm data were presented for 16 patients with proximal tibial reconstruction with tumor prostheses using compressive osseointegration technology. Complications included three deep infections, one of which necessitated amputation, but only one case of aseptic loosening. Level of evidence: IV.

14. Biau D, Faure F, Katsahian S, Jeanrot C, Tomeno B, Anract P: Survival of total knee replacement with a megaprosthesis after bone tumor resection. *J Bone Joint Surg Am* 2006;88(6):1285-1293.

15. Cho WH, Song WS, Jeon DG, Kong CB, Kim JI, Lee SY: Cause of infection in proximal tibial endoprosthetic reconstructions. *Arch Orthop Trauma Surg* 2012;132(2):163-169.

    Sixteen patients of 62 (26%) who had reconstruction of the proximal tibia with a tumor prosthesis had deep infections. Resection of more than 37% of the tibia was found to be the only statistically significant risk factor. Level of evidence: IV.

16. Grimer RJ, Carter SR, Tillman RM, et al: Endoprosthetic replacement of the proximal tibia. *J Bone Joint Surg Br* 1999;81(3):488-494.

17. Jeon DG, Kawai A, Boland P, Healey JH: Algorithm for the surgical treatment of malignant lesions of the proximal tibia. *Clin Orthop Relat Res* 1999;358:15-26.

18. Malawer MM, Chou LB: Prosthetic survival and clinical results with use of large-segment replacements in the treatment of high-grade bone sarcomas. *J Bone Joint Surg Am* 1995;77(8):1154-1165.

19. Flint MN, Griffin AM, Bell RS, Ferguson PC, Wunder JS: Aseptic loosening is uncommon with uncemented proximal tibia tumor prostheses. *Clin Orthop Relat Res* 2006;450:52-59.

20. Schwartz AJ, Kabo JM, Eilber FC, Eilber FR, Eckardt JJ: Cemented endoprosthetic reconstruction of the proximal tibia: How long do they last? *Clin Orthop Relat Res* 2010;468(11):2875-2884.

    Overall prosthetic survival in 52 patients at 5, 10, 15, and 20 years was 94%, 86%, 66%, and 37%, respectively. The mean Musculoskeletal Tumor Society (MSTS) functional score was 24.6 (82%) at the most recent follow-up. Level of evidence: IV.

21. Wu CC, Henshaw RM, Pritsch T, Squires MH, Malawer MM: Implant design and resection length affect cemented endoprosthesis survival in proximal tibial reconstruction. *J Arthroplasty* 2008;23(6):886-893.

    In 44 consecutive patients, complications occurred in 26 patients (61%) and included 13 mechanical failures, seven deep infections, and six wound complications. Overall prosthetic survival was 72% at 5 years and 53% at 10 years. Level of evidence: IV.

22. Biau DJ, Dumaine V, Babinet A, Tomeno B, Anract P: Allograft-prosthesis composites after bone tumor resection at the proximal tibia. *Clin Orthop Relat Res* 2007;456:211-217.

    Complications were frequent in 26 patients with irradiated APCs for reconstruction of the proximal tibia: seven fractures, seven occurrences of aseptic loosening, six occurrences of partial resorption, six infections, and six extensor mechanism disruptions. Mean survival of the reconstructions was 102 months. Level of evidence: IV.

23. Donati D, Colangeli M, Colangeli S, Di Bella C, Mercuri M: Allograft-prosthetic composite in the proximal tibia after bone tumor resection. *Clin Orthop Relat Res* 2008;466(2):459-465.

    In 62 patients, the 5-year survival rate of the reconstruction was 73% with an average MSTS functional score of 90%. A high infection rate (24%) led the authors to caution against use of APCs in patients who are receiving chemotherapy. Level of evidence: IV.

24. Gilbert NF, Yasko AW, Oates SD, Lewis VO, Cannon CP, Lin PP: Allograft-prosthetic composite reconstruc-

6: Special Considerations in Tumor Management

tion of the proximal part of the tibia: An analysis of the early results. *J Bone Joint Surg Am* 2009;91(7): 1646-1656.

In this study of 12 patients, the mean MSTS score was 24.3 (81%), and extensor function was excellent with minimal lag. There were no nonunions at graft-host junctions, and there was only one infection, which was treated successfully with retention of the APC. Level of evidence: IV

25. Gitelis S, Piasecki P: Allograft prosthetic composite arthroplasty for osteosarcoma and other aggressive bone tumors. *Clin Orthop Relat Res* 1991;270:197-201.

26. Harris AI, Poddar S, Gitelis S, Sheinkop MB, Rosenberg AG: Arthroplasty with a composite of an allograft and a prosthesis for knees with severe deficiency of bone. *J Bone Joint Surg Am* 1995;77(3):373-386.

27. Muscolo DL, Ayerza MA, Aponte-Tinao LA, Ranalletta M: Partial epiphyseal preservation and intercalary allograft reconstruction in high-grade metaphyseal osteosarcoma of the knee. *J Bone Joint Surg Am* 2004;86-A(12):2686-2693.

28. Kim J-D, Lee GW, Chung SH: A reconstruction with extracorporeal irradiated autograft in osteosarcoma around the knee. *J Surg Oncol* 2011;104(2):187-191.

Of 23 reconstructions, consisting of 14 distal femur and 9 proximal tibia reconstructions, 18 used osteoarticular grafts and 5 used autograft-prosthetic composites. The complication rate was high (87%) and included six nonunions, five deep infections, four joint instabilities, and two fractures. Level of evidence: IV.

29. Innocenti M, Abed YY, Beltrami G, Delcroix L, Manfrini M, Capanna R: Biological reconstruction after resection of bone tumors of the proximal tibia using allograft shell and intramedullary free vascularized fibular graft: Long-term results. *Microsurgery* 2009; 29(5):361-372.

In this study, primary union was achieved in 91% of patients, full weight bearing was achieved at an average of 21.6 months, and the average MSTS score was 27.3. Ten patients (47.6%) had 14 local complications: six fractures, one infection, four occurrences of wound dehiscence, two local recurrences, and one occurrence of peroneal nerve palsy. Level of evidence: IV.

Chapter 41

Upper Extremity Resection and Reconstruction

Kelly C. Homlar, MD   Jennifer L. Halpern, MD

Introduction

Skeletal sarcomas are commonly seen in the proximal upper extremity and much less commonly in the distal upper extremity. All suspected skeletal sarcomas should be appropriately staged and biopsied (preferably by or after discussion with the treating orthopaedic oncologist), and then the patient should be referred for appropriate chemotherapy on the basis of discussion and recommendations from a multidisciplinary tumor board. At the time of surgery, an oncologically sound resection is the first and foremost concern; only after resection has been successfully accomplished can reconstruction begin.

With advances in chemotherapy and imaging, limb salvage surgery is now possible in 90% to 95% of patients with primary bone sarcomas, with limb salvage being comparable to amputation in terms of disease-free interval and long-term survival with only a slight increase in local recurrence rates.[1-3] With patients experiencing longer survival times, it is important that a durable reconstruction be attained.

Reconstruction can generally be thought of in the broad categories of arthrodesis, allograft, autograft, or arthroplasty. Historically, as alternatives to amputation or arthrodesis, three primary means of reconstruction have been used after periarticular tumor resection: osteoarticular allograft, allograft-prosthetic composite (APC), and endoprosthesis. Table 1 shows the advantages and disadvantages of each method of reconstruction. Diaphyseal sarcomas of both the humerus and the forearm are often amenable to intercalary resection. Options for reconstruction following intercalary resection include intercalary allograft, vascularized fibular graft, extracorporally irradiated autograft, segmental prosthesis, and bone transport. Options for reconstruction following scapulectomy, resection of the proximal humerus, diaphyseal humerus, distal humerus/elbow, and forearm are discussed in this chapter.

Scapulectomy

The scapula is a less common location for skeletal sarcoma; however, Ewing sarcoma, osteosarcoma, and chondrosarcoma, among others, are all found in this location. The first total scapulectomy for neoplastic disease was by performed in 1856 and has since become an accepted technique for the treatment of primary malignant bone tumors.[4-6] The Malawer classification of shoulder girdle resections was proposed in 1991 (Figure 1).[7] Scapulectomies can be partial (type II), complete intra-articular (type III), complete extra-articular (type IV), or complete extra-articular in a more traditional Tikhoff-Linberg-type procedure (type VI). This classification scheme was modified by the Musculoskeletal Tumor Society (MSTS)[8] (Figure 2).

Challenges following scapulectomy include attempts to maintain the mobility and stability of the shoulder joint as well as an acceptable cosmetic result because scapulectomy leads to loss of the normal shoulder contour. The functional goal following reconstruction after scapulectomy is to provide a stable base against which the patient can position the arm in space as elbow, wrist, and hand function is typically preserved.

The patient is typically positioned in the lateral decubitus position with the entire forequarter draped free. The incision can vary, but commonly begins at the inferior angle of the scapula, continues obliquely along the scapular spine toward the acromion process where it then crosses in strap fashion to the anterior shoulder and then can be continued distally along the deltopectoral interval if needed.[4,5] The biopsy site is excised en bloc with the tumor specimen. All muscular attachments are divided approximately 1 cm away from bone through normal tissue, beginning from the inferior angle and elevating the scapula away from the chest wall. Only after an oncologically sound resection is confirmed can reconstruction begin.

Options after total scapulectomy include humeral suspension to the remaining clavicle or reconstruction with allograft or endoprosthesis. Humeral suspension involves suspending the native humerus or proximal humerus endoprosthesis to the remaining clavicle. Following this method of reconstruction, shoulder abduction ranges from 30° to 45°. Complications include

6: Special Considerations in Tumor Management

Table 1

Pros and Cons of Reconstructive Methods Following Periarticular Tumor Resection

Method	Pros	Cons
Osteoarticular allograft	Preservation of bone stock Soft-tissue attachments (theoretically improving joint stability, muscle function, range of motion)	Transmission of infectious diseases (such as HIV, hepatitis C, cytomegalovirus) Allograft fracture Allograft-host nonunion Subchondral collapse or degeneration of the allograft, causing osteoarthritis Technically challenging procedure Availability of appropriately sized allografts Delayed weight bearing
Endoprosthesis	Immediate weight bearing Modularity Shortened surgical time	Concerns related to durability/longevity Aseptic loosening No anatomic soft-tissue attachments
Allograft-prosthetic composite	Preservation of bone stock Soft-tissue attachments Prevention of late subchondral collapse/arthritis seen in allografts	Allograft fracture Allograft-host nonunion Transmission of infectious disease Aseptic loosening, wear Technically challenging procedure

---

deep infection (5.0% to 12.5%), periprosthetic fracture (10.5%), subluxation of endoprosthesis, and traction neuralgia or paresthesias if the humerus is not adequately suspended.[9-12] Reconstruction with scapular endoprosthesis involves laying the prosthesis in place, careful tenodesis of the latissimus dorsi, rhomboids, trapezius, and deltoid over the prosthesis, and articulation with a proximal humerus prosthesis (most recently in a constrained implant design).[13,14] Complications include dislocation, infection, aseptic loosening, and periprosthetic fracture. Reconstruction with scapular allograft involves using an osteoarticular allograft with soft-tissue reattachments preserved and careful repair of remaining host muscle back to donor tissue. Complications include infection, dislocation, and allograft fracture/resorption.[15]

Based on current literature, reconstruction with allograft or endoprosthesis could provide an additional 20° to 40° of abduction/forward flexion (40° to 60° versus 20° to 45°), and improved cosmesis, however, is associated with additional complications such as aseptic loosening, dislocation, periprosthetic fracture, and allograft fracture/resorption, etc.[4,5,9-15] The treating surgeon must carefully consider the risks and benefits when deciding whether to proceed with reconstruction.

Proximal Humerus

The proximal humerus is a common location for skeletal sarcoma, representing the third most common location for osteosarcoma and a common location for chondrosarcoma. The challenge following resection of proximal humeral lesions is replication of normal shoulder anatomy. The glenohumeral joint is a ball-

and-socket joint that allows numerous degrees of freedom, lending itself to tremendous mobility and thus requiring significant stability. Commonly, the rotator cuff is resected with the tumor, and occasionally the deltoid or axillary nerve must be sacrificed, having a significant effect on shoulder function.

At the time of biopsy of a proximal humerus sarcoma, the extended deltopectoral incision should be marked out, with the actual biopsy taking place slightly lateral to the interval to position the biopsy tract through the anterior portion of the deltoid muscle and not through the true deltopectoral interval. This technique helps contain any postbiopsy hematoma to the deltoid and avoid contamination of the cephalic vein or pectoralis major, or spread onto the chest wall.

In the preoperative workup, it is important to determine whether the tumor extends into the glenohumeral joint and thus whether intra-articular or extra-articular resection is required. Routes of intra-articular tumor spread include direct extension through articular cartilage or capsule, extension of tumor along the long head of the biceps tendon, and hematoma from pathologic fracture. Contraindications to limb salvage are tumor invasion of the brachial plexus/axillary artery and extensive invasion of the chest wall.

With the Malawer classification of shoulder girdle resections (**Figure 1**), resections of the proximal humerus are typically classified as type I (intra-articular proximal humeral resection) or type V (extra-articular humeral and glenoid resection). This classification scheme was modified by the MSTS[8] (**Figure 2**). In both classifications, *A* denotes that the abductor mechanism is intact, and *B*, that the abductor mechanism is disrupted. The status of the abductor mechanism is key in decision making because allograft or endoprosthesis

---

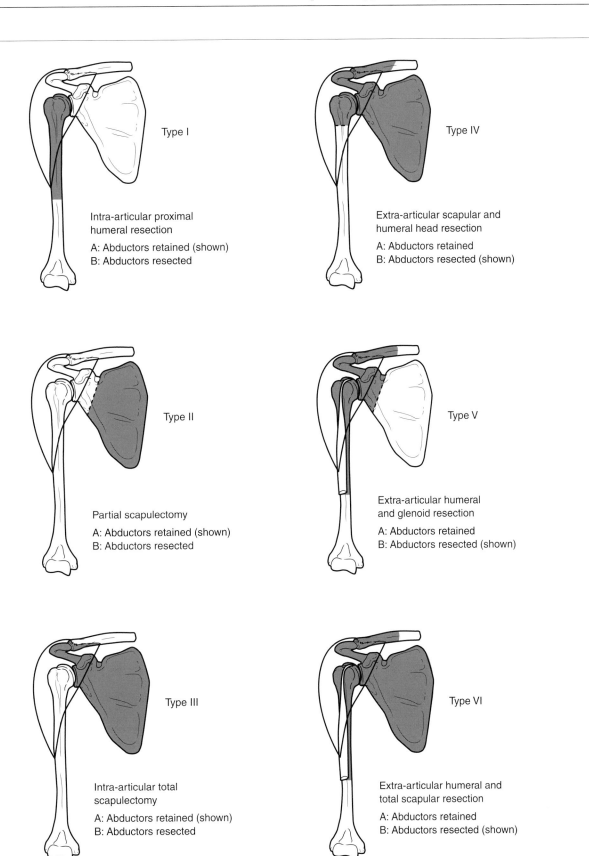

Type I

Intra-articular proximal
humeral resection

A: Abductors retained (shown)
B: Abductors resected

Type IV

Extra-articular scapular and
humeral head resection

A: Abductors retained
B: Abductors resected (shown)

Type II

Partial scapulectomy

A: Abductors retained (shown)
B: Abductors resected

Type V

Extra-articular humeral
and glenoid resection

A: Abductors retained
B: Abductors resected (shown)

Type III

Intra-articular total
scapulectomy

A: Abductors retained (shown)
B: Abductors resected

Type VI

Extra-articular humeral and
total scapular resection

A: Abductors retained
B: Abductors resected (shown)

Figure 1   Shoulder girdle resections according to Malawer.

6: Special Considerations in Tumor Management

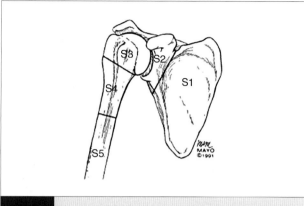

| Figure 2 | Illustration of the Musculoskeletal Tumor Society classification of skeletal resections about the shoulder girdle. S1 = blade or spine of the scapula, S2 = acromion-glenoid cavity complex, S3 = proximal epiphysis of the humerus, S4 = proximal metaphysis of the humerus, S5 = proximal diaphysis of the humerus. (Reproduced with permission from the Mayo Foundation for Medical Education and Research, Rochester, MN.) |

Table 2

Reconstruction Algorithm Following Shoulder Girdle Resections

Type of Resection	Method of Osseous Reconstruction
S1	None
S2	Primary arthrodesis
S12	None
S1234	Spacer cemented into humeral canal distally and sutured to chest wall proximally
S234 or S2345	
Older, inactive patients	Spacer cemented into humeral canal distally and anchored to remaining scapula proximally
Younger, active patients	Arthrodesis with intercalary allograft and vascularized fibular graft
S34A or S345A	Osteoarticular allograft or allograft-prosthetic composite
S34B or S345B	
Older, inactive patients	Proximal humeral replacement prosthesis
Younger, active patients	Arthrodesis with intercalary allograft and vascularized fibular graft

(Reproduced with permission from O'Connor MI, Sim FH, Chao EY: Limb Salvage for neoplasms of the shoulder girdle: Intermediate reconstructive and functional results. J Bone Joint Surg 1999;134(3):252-257.)

may be chosen if it is intact or arthrodesis if it is disrupted. A suggested reconstructive algorithm based on the type of resection was proposed in 1996[9] (**Table 2**).

Extra-articular Resection (Malawer Type V)

Limb salvage surgery of the shoulder girdle began with the description of the interscapulothoracic resection, known as the Tikhoff-Linberg procedure, in 1922 and 1928.[16] The Tikhoff-Linberg procedure is an en bloc extra-articular resection including the proximal humerus, entire scapula, lateral two thirds of the clavicle, rotator cuff, deltoid, coracobrachialis, and proximal biceps. This procedure resulted in a fully functional hand and forearm, but a flail shoulder. Modifications include removal of only the glenoid portion of the scapula when possible; use of alternative incisions; and addition of a spacer or prosthetic reconstruction of the humerus, which is then suspended from the remaining scapula and clavicle.[10,17-19] Following this method of reconstruction, shoulder abduction ranges from 30° to 45°. The overall complication rate is high (up to 47%). Complications include deep infection (5.0% to 12.5%), periprosthetic fracture (10.5%), subluxation of endoprosthesis, and traction neuralgia or paresthesias if the humerus is not adequately suspended.[9-12] Because of the extensive soft-tissue resection required for extra-articular resections, it is sometimes necessary to add a rotational latissimus dorsi or pectoralis major flap for coverage of the spacer or endoprosthesis.

Arthrodesis can also be performed following extra-articular proximal humerus resection.[9,20] This procedure may be favorable in a young patient who wants to return to strenuous activity. The goal is to provide a stable, painless base against which the hand can be po-

sitioned in space. Techniques include allograft arthrodesis, vascularized fibular grafting, and a combination of the two. The arm is positioned where the hand can easily reach the mouth without excessive scapular winging with the arm at the side, approximately 15° to 30° abduction, 15° to 30° forward flexion, and 20° to 50° internal rotation (the exact position is much debated). Several methods of fixation are described, but the most common probably is the use of a long plate contoured along the scapular spine, over the acromion, and extending down the humerus in addition to screws placed through the humeral head into the glenoid. Patients are immobilized in either a sling or shoulder spica cast for several weeks. Some motion of the arm is maintained through the thoracoscapular articulation, approximately 45° to 60° of forward flexion and abduction, although internal and external rotation is severely limited. The overall complication rate is high, with reports of up to 43% of patients requiring a second major surgical procedure. Complications include nonunion (0% to 40%), fracture (4% to 40%), and infection (0% to 37.5%).[9,20]

Another option is the clavicula pro humero procedure. This procedure was originally described for the treatment of phocomelia in 1963 but was reported after shoulder girdle resections of malignant tumors in 1992.[21] The clavicle is cut at the sternoclavicular joint, the sternocleidomastoid and trapezius muscles are released, and the entire clavicle is rotated down to meet the residual humerus, pivoting on the acromioclavicular joint. The mean length of clavicle available is 13.5 cm, and thus the planned resection length must be considered. The arm is immobilized in a sling for 3 weeks, after which passive and active motion are initiated. Using the clavicle as a vascularized autograft improves union rates and avoids the risk of disease transmission with allograft. Stability is provided by the intact acromioclavicular joint. The overall complication rate is high, with a revision rate as high as 67%. Complications include hardware failure, nonunion (14% to 27%), fracture (0% to 27%), and deep infection (0% to 27%).[11,21,22]

Intra-articular Resection (Malawer Type I)

In the case of intra-articular resection, reconstruction options include osteoarticular allograft, APC, and endoprosthesis. In type Ib resections in which the deltoid is removed, arthrodesis can be considered.

Osteoarticular allografts are requested so that donor tendon and ligaments remain attached (**Figure 3**). Proponents of osteoarticular allografts suggest that the ability to repair the remainder of the rotator cuff musculature and deltoid back to corresponding tissue on the allograft provides superior stability and muscle force for abduction and forward flexion of the shoulder. Although some patients obtain greater than 90° of abduction, pooled data from the available literature show a mean abduction and forward flexion of approximately 45°, similar to results obtained with endoprosthesis and APC. Rates of dislocation were not improved and were actually higher in pooled data when compared with endoprosthesis and APC (21% versus 6% and 14%, respectively). Additional risks with the use of allografts include transmission of infectious diseases (HIV, hepatitis C, cytomegalovirus), allograft fracture (35% in pooled data), allograft-host nonunion (11% in pooled data), deep infection (8% in pooled data), and subchondral collapse or degeneration of the allograft articular surface causing pain (19% to 50%).[11,23-27] Postoperatively, prolonged immobilization and weight-bearing restrictions are required to allow for allograft-host junction healing. Although restrictions are not typically maintained this long, the process of allograft healing can last longer than 1 year.[28] Despite these concerns, osteoarticular allograft remains a popular choice in reconstruction, especially in the pediatric population, in which concern regarding the long-term durability of endoprostheses and the desire to preserve bone stock exist.

APC reconstruction uses an osteoarticular allograft; however, the articular surface is removed and replaced with a standard joint-replacing prosthesis. APCs are thought to maintain the advantages of allografts in preserving bone stock and providing donor soft-tissue attachments for repair, while preventing the complica-

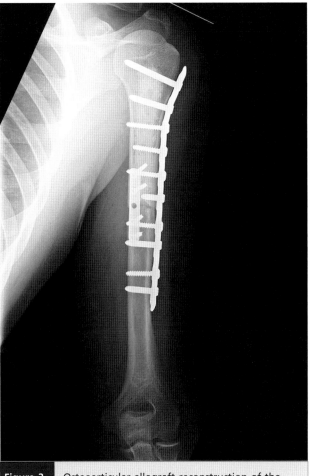

Figure 3 Osteoarticular allograft reconstruction of the proximal humerus. Note the cement filling of the graft to reduce fracture risk.

tions of subchondral collapse and articular surface degeneration. APCs still have the risk of allograft fracture (2% in pooled data), nonunion (11% in pooled data), and deep infection (5% in pooled data). Additionally, like endoprostheses, APCs carry the risk of aseptic loosening (5% in pooled data).[25,26,29]

Endoprosthetic reconstruction replaces the entire resected bone with a segmental implant, with soft tissues reattached through suture holes in the implant designed for this purpose (**Figure 4**). Some implants now offer porous tantalum metal at sites of tissue reattachment in the hope of improving tissue incorporation. Whereas these prostheses were previously custom ordered, they are now modular, allowing for intraoperative adjustments to accommodate tumor progression or to maximize joint stability. Endoprostheses have the advantage of immediate weight bearing; however, concerns exist as to their durability and longevity. Endoprostheses have a risk of aseptic loosening (4% in pooled data) and deep infection (1.4% in pooled data). The overall revision rate was found to be 11%, compared with 22% for osteoarticular allografts.[11,25,26,30,31]

6: Special Considerations in Tumor Management

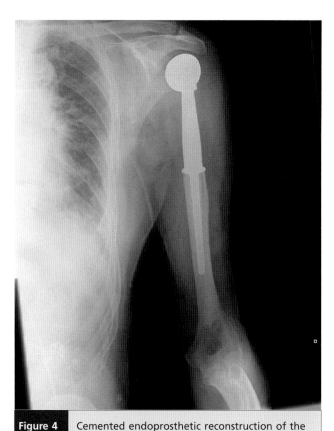

Figure 4 Cemented endoprosthetic reconstruction of the proximal humerus.

Humeral Diaphysis

Diaphyseal sarcomas are commonly amenable to intercalary resection. Options for reconstruction following intercalary resection include intercalary allograft, vascularized fibular autograft, extracorporally irradiated autograft, segmental prosthesis, and bone transport. Because intercalary resection does not involve the adjacent joint, the patient's function is typically better than that following periarticular resection.

Intercalary allografts have the advantage of being generally readily available (except for extremes of sizes such as in very young children) and technically straightforward without donor site morbidity. A disadvantage is that long periods of protected weight bearing may be required, with allograft-host junctions requiring 9 to 12 months to heal.[28] Additional risks include transmission of infectious diseases, allograft fracture (7% to 19%), allograft-host junction nonunion (15% to 50%), and deep infection (12% to 14%).[32-36] Data evaluating intercalary allografts in all long bone locations show overall 5-year survivorship between 79% and 84%.[19,32-35] Most failures occur in the first 3 to 4 years, after which the allograft appears to become a durable construct. Several studies have investigated ways to decrease allograft fracture, including limiting the number of screw holes within the allograft, filling the allograft with cement, and using one long plate (as opposed to a

plate at each junction) or intramedullary nail (although a nail exhibits less compression at junction and is less stable rotationally).[22,33,37,38] Adjuvant chemotherapy has been shown to increase the risk of allograft nonunion.[39] Overall revision rates for intercalary allografts in all locations were 37% to 47%, with most revision procedures performed to bone graft the allograft-host junctions.[32,33,37]

Vascularized fibular autografts avoid the risk of transmission of infectious diseases and theoretically have higher rates of graft incorporation (though still having a nonunion rate of 33% at initial attempt). Union occurs at an average of 6 months, requiring prolonged periods of no weight bearing and protected activity. Other disadvantages include a fracture rate even in the non–weight-bearing upper extremity of 14% to 57%, donor site morbidity in 12% to 30% of patients, prolonged surgical times and hospital length of stay, and rarely compartment syndrome following ischemia from thrombosis at the site of end-to-end arteriorrhaphy. The vascularized fibular autograft can be used alone or in conjunction with an allograft via an intramedullary or onlay technique.[40-48]

Intercalary diaphyseal endoprostheses have the advantages of immediate stability and early weight bearing, with fixation (when cemented) not being affected by chemotherapy or irradiation. The reconstruction tends to be less technically demanding, requiring less surgical time. Most implants require approximately 5 cm of intramedullary canal remaining at each end to accept standard stems. Ten-year implant survival rates of intercalary endoprostheses at all long bone locations range from 63% to 68%. Risks include aseptic loosening (4% to 33%), periprosthetic fracture (3% to 11%), and deep infection (3% to 5%).[49-53]

In areas where allograft is not readily available or is culturally unacceptable, extracorporeally irradiated or pasteurized autograft has been used. The bone invaded by sarcoma is immediately irradiated or pasteurized and then placed back into the patient as autograft. Advantages include ensurance of size match and avoidance of immunologic response or transmission of infectious disease. Local recurrence rates of 0% to 12% are similar to those reported with other methods of reconstruction. The risks are similar to those of allograft and include nonunion (4% to 32%), fracture (10% to 20%), and deep infection (0% to 29%).[33,54-56]

Bone transport also has been described as a reconstruction option for intercalary defects. Advantages include the fact that it is a biologic option avoiding autograft donor site morbidity and allograft infectious or immunologic risks, and that it offers the potential for early weight bearing. It is, however, a slow and tedious process, requiring approximately 30 days per centimeter of transported bone. Several techniques can be used, including shortening-distraction or docking. Risks include fracture through regenerated bone or around fixator hardware (13%), skin complications (20%), and infection (6%).[57-60]

Distal Upper Extremity (Distal Humerus and Forearm)

Primary sarcomas of bone in the distal upper extremity are rare, and therefore the outcomes following tumor resection and reconstruction are anecdotal, with limited retrospective reviews of small numbers of appropriate patients. For example, over a 23-year period, one institution reported only 101 primary sarcomas of the hand and forearm. Of these, 85 were soft-tissue sarcomas, with a predominance of fibrosarcoma, rhabdomyosarcoma, epithelioid sarcoma, synovial cell sarcoma, and liposarcoma. In the 15 primary bone tumors, chondrosarcoma, Ewing sarcoma, and osteosarcoma were most common. Of interest, 5-year survival rates for patients with distal upper extremity osteosarcoma and Ewing sarcoma are 86.2% and 84.1%, respectively.[61] Limb salvage in the distal upper extremity to treat these tumors is challenging because of the limited local soft tissues. Large resections and reconstructions often require tissue transport for coverage. Tumors can cross compartments more readily. Critical nerves are often involved.

Similar to the proximal upper extremity, reconstruction options in the elbow and forearm include arthroplasty, intercalary/osteoarticular allograft, intercalary/osteoarticular autograft (often free fibular transfer with or without fasciocutaneous flap), or resection and conversion to a one-bone forearm, among others. Although amputation outcomes are not discussed here, ablative surgery is also a viable option.

Distal Humerus

The prevalence of distal humeral primary bone tumors is approximately 1%.[62] Reconstructive options include modular elbow arthroplasty and osteochondral allograft.

Modular elbow arthroplasty is an effective means of reconstruction associated with acceptable functional and oncologic outcomes.[63] In a series of 38 patients treated with modular elbow arthroplasty, local control was achieved in all patients. Functional outcomes were also good with mean MSTS scores of 78% and mean Inglis-Pellicci scores of 84. The primary complication encountered was postoperative infection. Sixteen percent of patients developed a deep infection at a mean of 11 months, and therefore required a one-stage or two-stage revision. However, infection rates involving endoprostheses about the elbow vary, and rates as low as 0% have even been reported. Aseptic loosening can occur.[64]

Osteoarticular allograft reconstruction is considered a viable option in elbow reconstruction, especially in younger patients in whom the insertion of an endoprosthesis is trying to be avoided. As expected, hemiarticular allografts and total elbow osteoarticular allografts generate very different postoperative functional scores. In one study, "14 of 16 patients [treated with hemiarticular allografts] were able to return to their preoperative level of occupational function. . . . For the three

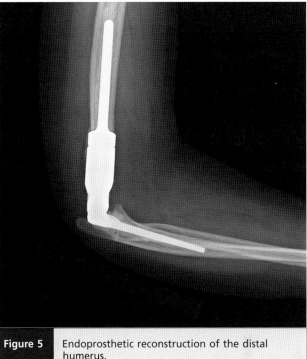

patients who had total elbow allograft reconstructions, all had degenerative changes develop after surgery"[65] (**Figure 5**). The perioperative and postoperative complications included infection, allograft-host junction nonunion, dislocation, instability, and nerve palsy.

APCs have also been used in tumors about the elbow.[62,63] The proposed benefits of APCs are that the allografts have intact soft-tissue attachments and preserve bone stock. Specific to the elbow, the triceps insertion and flexor-pronator and extensor origins are intact. In a small retrospective series, patients demonstrated an arc of motion between 95° and 130°, and good or excellent Mayo Elbow Performance Index scores.[62]

Forearm
Intercalary Allograft

Intercalary allograft reconstruction following large-segment radial or ulnar resections is an option. As described previously, allograft reconstruction complications primarily include allograft-host junction nonunions or allograft fracture.[32-36,66] Functional outcomes are improved in the case of intercalary as opposed to osteoarticular allografts.[66]

Free Fibular Transfer/Tissue Transfer

Typical vascularized flaps used in forearm reconstruction include gracilis flaps (as an example of functional muscle transfer), radial forearm flaps (ipsilateral or contralateral), latissimus flaps, groin flaps, and free vascularized fibular grafts.[67] Free flaps are beneficial in that they do not require tissue from a limb already compromised by tumor resection, and also in that a

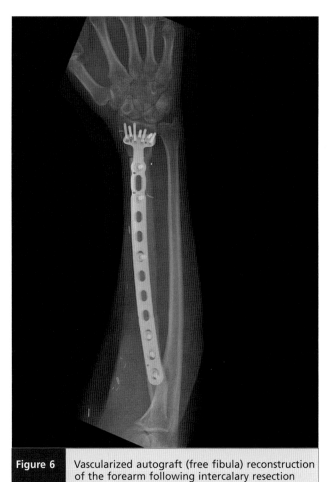

Figure 6 | Vascularized autograft (free fibula) reconstruction of the forearm following intercalary resection of the radius.

larger volume of tissue is available for use. Vascularized free fibular grafts can be used for reconstruction of diaphyseal defects (**Figure 6**) and even osteoarticular defects (distal radius).[40,41,68] The obvious problem with free tissue transfer is the risk of microvascular anastomotic failure, leading to flap death. Free flap survival in the setting of forearm and hand sarcoma in one study was reported as 100%, although some of those patients did require venous thrombectomy for flap rescue.[67] The same study demonstrated bony union in all four patients who required a free vascularized osteocutaneous fibula flap. Pedicled flaps, such as the radial forearm flap, are preferred if the appropriate arterial supply is intact.

A distinction between allograft and vascularized autograft healing has been studied in a canine model.[68] Conventional grafts were noted to heal by creeping substitution, whereas vascularized fibular grafts maintained their normal structure and were "hypertrophied by subperiosteal new bone formation."[68] The vascularized graft was stronger at earlier time points, although between 6 months and 1 year, both grafts resembled the bone they replaced.

One-Bone Forearm

The creation of a one-bone forearm sacrifices rotation of the forearm, but also may allow for primary closure. In addition, if both bones of the forearm are resected, allograft reconstruction could potentially require healing at four allograft-host junction sites. Therefore, creation of a one-bone forearm has been described as a reasonable option. In this procedure, a single bony bridge is created. For example, one technique involves preserving the ulna at the elbow and the distal radius at the wrist.[69] The forearm is typically placed in slight pronation.

Summary

Skeletal sarcomas are commonly seen in the proximal upper extremity and much less commonly in the distal upper extremity. Reconstruction following tumor resection can be achieved in a variety of ways, all with relative advantages and disadvantages. The treating surgeon must take into account the physiology and functional demands of the patient, the biology of the tumor, and the expected bone and soft-tissue loss with resection when deciding which method of reconstruction will best serve the patient.

Annotated References

1. Eilber FR, Mirra JJ, Grant TT, Weisenburger T, Morton DL: Is amputation necessary for sarcomas? A seven-year experience with limb salvage. *Ann Surg* 1980;192(4):431-438.

2. Rao BN, Champion JE, Pratt CB, et al: Limb salvage procedures for children with osteosarcoma: An alternative to amputation. *J Pediatr Surg* 1983;18(6):901-908.

3. Rougraff BT, Simon MA, Kneisl JS, Greenberg DB, Mankin HJ: Limb salvage compared with amputation for osteosarcoma of the distal end of the femur: A long-term oncological, functional, and quality-of-life study. *J Bone Joint Surg Am* 1994;76(5):649-656.

4. Papaioannou AN, Francis KC: Scapulectomy for the treatment of primary malignant tumors of the scapula. *Clin Orthop Relat Res* 1965;41(41):125-132.

5. Rodriguez JA, Craven JE, Heinrich S, Wilson S, Levine EA: Current role of scapulectomy. *Am Surg* 1999;65(12):1167-1170.

6. Volpe CM, Pell M, Doerr RJ, Karakousis CP: Radical scapulectomy with limb salvage for shoulder girdle soft tissue sarcoma. *Surg Oncol* 1996;5(1):43-48.

7. Malawer MM, Meller I, Dunham WK: A new surgical classification system for shoulder-girdle resections: Analysis of 38 patients. *Clin Orthop Relat Res* 1991;267:33-44.

8. Enneking W, Dunham W, Gebhardt M, Malawar M, Pritchard D: A system for the classification of skeletal resections. *Chir Organi Mov* 1990;75(Suppl 1): 217-240.

9. O'Connor MI, Sim FH, Chao EY: Limb salvage for neoplasms of the shoulder girdle: Intermediate reconstructive and functional results. *J Bone Joint Surg Am* 1996;78(12):1872-1888.

10. Voggenreiter G, Assenmacher S, Schmit-Neuerburg KP: Tikhoff-Linberg procedure for bone and soft tissue tumors of the shoulder girdle. *Arch Surg* 1999;134(3): 252-257.

11. Rödl RW, Gosheger G, Gebert C, Lindner N, Ozaki T, Winkelmann W: Reconstruction of the proximal humerus after wide resection of tumours. *J Bone Joint Surg Br* 2002;84(7):1004-1008.

12. Meller I, Bickels J, Kollender Y, Ovadia D, Oren R, Mozes M: Malignant bone and soft tissue tumors of the shoulder girdle: A retrospective analysis of 30 operated cases. *Acta Orthop Scand* 1997;68(4):374-380.

13. Pritsch T, Bickels J, Wu CC, Squires MH, Malawer MM: Is scapular endoprosthesis functionally superior to humeral suspension? *Clin Orthop Relat Res* 2007; 456(456):188-195.

14. Wittig JC, Bickels J, Wodajo F, Kellar-Graney KL, Malawer MM: Constrained total scapula reconstruction after resection of a high-grade sarcoma. *Clin Orthop Relat Res* 2002;397:143-155.

15. Mnaymneh WA, Temple HT, Malinin TI: Allograft reconstruction after resection of malignant tumors of the scapula. *Clin Orthop Relat Res* 2002;405:223-229.

16. Linberg BE: Interscapulo-thoracic resection for malignant tumors of the shoulder joint region. *J Bone Joint Surg Am* 1928;10:344-349.

17. Capanna R, van Horn JR, Biagini R, Ruggieri P, Ferruzzi A, Campanacci M: The Tikhoff-Linberg procedure for bone tumors of the proximal humerus: The classical "extensive" technique versus a modified "transglenoid" resection. *Arch Orthop Trauma Surg* 1990;109(2):63-67.

18. Ham SJ, Hoekstra HJ, Eisma WH, Schraffordt Koops H, Oldhoff J: The Tikhoff-Linberg procedure in the treatment of sarcomas of the shoulder girdle. *J Surg Oncol* 1993;53(2):71-77.

19. Marcove RC, Lewis MM, Huvos AG: En bloc upper humeral interscapulo-thoracic resection: The Tikhoff-Linberg procedure. *Clin Orthop Relat Res* 1977;124: 219-228.

20. Fuchs B, O'Connor MI, Padgett DJ, Kaufman KR, Sim FH: Arthrodesis of the shoulder after tumor resection. *Clin Orthop Relat Res* 2005;436:202-207.

21. Winkelmann WW: Clavicula pro humero—a new surgical method for malignant tumors of the proximal humerus. *Z Orthop Ihre Grenzgeb* 1992;130(3):197-201.

22. Tsukushi S, Nishida Y, Takahashi M, Ishiguro N: Clavicula pro humero reconstruction after wide resection of the proximal humerus. *Clin Orthop Relat Res* 2006;447(447):132-137.

23. DeGroot H, Donati D, Di Liddo M, Gozzi E, Mercuri M: The use of cement in osteoarticular allografts for proximal humeral bone tumors. *Clin Orthop Relat Res* 2004;427:190-197.

24. Gebhardt MC, Roth YF, Mankin HJ: Osteoarticular allografts for reconstruction in the proximal part of the humerus after excision of a musculoskeletal tumor. *J Bone Joint Surg Am* 1990;72(3):334-345.

25. Homlar KC, Halpern JL, Schwartz HS, Holt GE: Surgery in bone sarcoma—allograft versus megaprothesis, in Bhandari M, ed: *Evidence-Based Orthopedics*. Chichester, England, Wiley-Blackwell, 2012, pp 1097-1107.

This chapter reviews available literature comparing allograft, APC, and endoprosthesis in the proximal humerus and proximal tibia. Raw data were collected from all studies meeting search criteria, and analysis of pooled data was used to compare complications, oncologic outcomes, and functional outcomes.

26. Potter BK, Adams SC, Pitcher JD Jr , Malinin TI, Temple HT: Proximal humerus reconstructions for tumors. *Clin Orthop Relat Res* 2009;467(4):1035-1041.

Forty-nine patients underwent proximal humerus resection for primary malignancy, metastatic disease, and benign aggressive lesions. Revision surgery was most common for osteoarticular allograft, followed by APC, then endoprosthesis. At a median follow-up of 98 months, MSTS scores averaged 79% for APC, 71% for osteoarticular allograft, and 69% for endoprosthesis. Allograft fracture occurred in 53% of osteoarticular allografts. Level of evidence: IV.

27. Thompson RC Jr , Pickvance EA, Garry D: Fractures in large-segment allografts. *J Bone Joint Surg Am* 1993;75(11):1663-1673.

28. Enneking WF, Campanacci DA: Retrieved human allografts: A clinicopathological study. *J Bone Joint Surg Am* 2001;83-A(7):971-986.

29. Abdeen A, Hoang BH, Athanasian EA, Morris CD, Boland PJ, Healey JH: Allograft-prosthesis composite reconstruction of the proximal part of the humerus: Functional outcome and survivorship. *J Bone Joint Surg Am* 2009;91(10):2406-2415.

In this study, 36 patients underwent APC reconstruction of the proximal humerus. Findings included 10-year implant survival in 88%, revision in 8%, nonunion in 11%, aseptic loosening in 8%, dislocation in 3%, a mean abduction of 50°, a mean forward flexion

6: Special Considerations in Tumor Management

of 65°, and a mean MSTS score of 26. Level of evidence: IV.

30. Cannon CP, Paraliticci GU, Lin PP, Lewis VO, Yasko AW: Functional outcome following endoprosthetic reconstruction of the proximal humerus. *J Shoulder Elbow Surg* 2009;18(5):705-710.

    In this study, 83 patients had endoprosthetic reconstruction of the proximal humerus with a revision rate of 2%, deep infection in 2%, dislocation in 6%, a mean abduction of 41°, a mean forward flexion of 42, and a mean MSTS score of 18.9. Level of evidence: IV.

31. Jeys LM, Kulkarni A, Grimer RJ, Carter SR, Tillman RM, Abudu A: Endoprosthetic reconstruction for the treatment of musculoskeletal tumors of the appendicular skeleton and pelvis. *J Bone Joint Surg Am* 2008; 90(6):1265-1271.

    In this study, 103 patients had endoprosthetic reconstruction of the proximal humerus with a revision rate of 17%, local recurrence in 6%, aseptic loosening in 7%, implant fracture in 1.8%, and dislocation in 1%. Level of evidence: IV.

32. Ortiz-Cruz E, Gebhardt MC, Jennings LC, Springfield DS, Mankin HJ: The results of transplantation of intercalary allografts after resection of tumors: A long-term follow-up study. *J Bone Joint Surg Am* 1997; 79(1):97-106.

33. Chen TH, Chen WM, Huang CK: Reconstruction after intercalary resection of malignant bone tumours: comparison between segmental allograft and extracorporeally-irradiated autograft. *J Bone Joint Surg Br* 2005;87(5):704-709.

34. Donati D, Di Liddo M, Zavatta M, et al: Massive bone allograft reconstruction in high-grade osteosarcoma. *Clin Orthop Relat Res* 2000;377:186-194.

35. Mankin HJ, Gebhardt MC, Jennings LC, Springfield DS, Tomford WW: Long-term results of allograft replacement in the management of bone tumors. *Clin Orthop Relat Res* 1996;324:86-97.

36. Mankin HJ, Springfield DS, Gebhardt MC, Tomford WW: Current status of allografting for bone tumors. *Orthopedics* 1992;15(10):1147-1154.

37. Gerrand CH, Griffin AM, Davis AM, Gross AE, Bell RS, Wunder JS: Large segment allograft survival is improved with intramedullary cement. *J Surg Oncol* 2003;84(4):198-208.

38. Vander Griend RA: The effect of internal fixation on the healing of large allografts. *J Bone Joint Surg Am* 1994;76(5):657-663.

39. Hornicek FJ, Gebhardt MC, Tomford WW, et al: Factors affecting nonunion of the allograft-host junction. *Clin Orthop Relat Res* 2001;382:87-98.

40. Bernd L, Sabo D, Zahlten-Hinguranage A, Niemeyer P,

Daecke W, Simank HG: Experiences with vascular pedicled fibula in reconstruction of osseous defects in primary malignant bone tumors. *Orthopade* 2003; 32(11):983-993.

41. Pollock R, Stalley P, Lee K, Pennington D: Free vascularized fibula grafts in limb-salvage surgery. *J Reconstr Microsurg* 2005;21(2):79-84.

42. Aberg M, Rydholm A, Holmberg J, Wieslander JB: Reconstruction with a free vascularized fibular graft for malignant bone tumor. *Acta Orthop Scand* 1988; 59(4):430-437.

43. Ceruso M, Falcone C, Innocenti M, Delcroix L, Capanna R, Manfrini M: Skeletal reconstruction with a free vascularized fibula graft associated to bone allograft after resection of malignant bone tumor of limbs. *Handchir Mikrochir Plast Chir* 2001;33(4):277-282.

44. de Boer HH, Wood MB, Hermans J: Reconstruction of large skeletal defects by vascularized fibula transfer: Factors that influenced the outcome of union in 62 cases. *Int Orthop* 1990;14(2):121-128.

45. Gao YH, Ketch LL, Eladoumikdachi F, Netscher DT: Upper limb salvage with microvascular bone transfer for major long-bone segmental tumor resections. *Ann Plast Surg* 2001;47(3):240-246.

46. Hsu RW, Wood MB, Sim FH, Chao EY: Free vascularised fibular grafting for reconstruction after tumour resection. *J Bone Joint Surg Br* 1997;79(1):36-42.

47. Minami A, Kutsumi K, Takeda N, Kaneda K: Vascularized fibular graft for bone reconstruction of the extremities after tumor resection in limb-saving procedures. *Microsurgery* 1995;16(2):56-64.

48. Shea KG, Coleman DA, Scott SM, Coleman SS, Christianson M: Microvascularized free fibular grafts for reconstruction of skeletal defects after tumor resection. *J Pediatr Orthop* 1997;17(4):424-432.

49. Aldlyami E, Abudu A, Grimer RJ, Carter SR, Tillman RM: Endoprosthetic replacement of diaphyseal bone defects: Long-term results. *Int Orthop* 2005;29(1):25-29.

50. Abudu A, Carter SR, Grimer RJ: The outcome and functional results of diaphyseal endoprostheses after tumour excision. *J Bone Joint Surg Br* 1996;78(4):652-657.

51. Ahlmann ER, Menendez LR: Intercalary endoprosthetic reconstruction for diaphyseal bone tumours. *J Bone Joint Surg Br* 2006;88(11):1487-1491.

52. Hanna SA, Sewell MD, Aston WJ, et al: Femoral diaphyseal endoprosthetic reconstruction after segmental resection of primary bone tumours. *J Bone Joint Surg Br* 2010;92(6):867-874.

Twenty-three patients underwent endoprosthetic replacement of the femoral diaphysis after segmental resection for primary bone tumor. At a mean follow-up of 97 months, the overall revision rate was 22% and the reoperation rate was 26%. Complications included deep infection (4%), breakage of prosthesis (8%), periprosthetic fracture (4%), and aseptic loosening (4%). Sixteen of 23 patients retained their prostheses with a mean MSTS score of 87%. Level of evidence: IV.

53. Sewell MD, Hanna SA, McGrath A, et al: Intercalary diaphyseal endoprosthetic reconstruction for malignant tibial bone tumours. *J Bone Joint Surg Br* 2011; 93(8):1111-1117.

Eighteen patients underwent intercalary endoprosthetic replacement after excision of a malignant bone tumor. At mean follow-up of 58.5 months, 10-year implant survival was 63%. Complications included revision to proximal tibia replacement (22%), aseptic loosing (22%), periprosthetic fracture (11%), and infection (5%). Level of evidence: IV.

54. Manabe J, Ahmed AR, Kawaguchi N, Matsumoto S, Kuroda H: Pasteurized autologous bone graft in surgery for bone and soft tissue sarcoma. *Clin Orthop Relat Res* 2004;419:258-266.

55. Hong A, Stevens G, Stalley P, et al: Extracorporeal irradiation for malignant bone tumors. *Int J Radiat Oncol Biol Phys* 2001;50(2):441-447.

56. Uyttendaele D, De Schryver A, Claessens H, Roels H, Berkvens P, Mondelaers W: Limb conservation in primary bone tumours by resection, extracorporeal irradiation and re-implantation. *J Bone Joint Surg Br* 1988;70(3):348-353.

57. Tsuchiya H, Tomita K, Minematsu K, Mori Y, Asada N, Kitano S: Limb salvage using distraction osteogenesis: A classification of the technique. *J Bone Joint Surg Br* 1997;79(3):403-411.

58. Green SA, Jackson JM, Wall DM, Marinow H, Ishkanian J: Management of segmental defects by the Ilizarov intercalary bone transport method. *Clin Orthop Relat Res* 1992;280:136-142.

59. Jarka DE, Nicholas RW, Aronson J: Effect of methotrexate on distraction osteogenesis. *Clin Orthop Relat Res* 1998;354:209-215.

60. Subasi M, Kapukaya A, Kesemenli C, Balci TA, Buyukbayram H, Ozates M: Effect of chemotherapeutic agents on distraction osteogenesis: An experimental investigation in rabbits. *Arch Orthop Trauma Surg* 2001;121(7):417-421.

61. Bryan RS, Soule EH, Dobyns JH, Pritchard DJ, Linscheid RL: Primary epithelioid sarcoma of the hand and forearm: A review of thirteen cases. *J Bone Joint Surg Am* 1974;56(3):458-465.

62. Schwab JH, Healey JH, Athanasian EA: Wide en bloc extra-articular excision of the elbow for sarcoma with complex reconstruction. *J Bone Joint Surg Br* 2008; 90(1):78-83.

This study was a retrospective review of five patients treated with APC using a pedicled latissimus dorsi flap. No local wound complications or infections were seen. The functional results were excellent in four patients and good in one. Level of evidence: IV.

63. Weber KL, Lin PP, Yasko AW: Complex segmental elbow reconstruction after tumor resection. *Clin Orthop Relat Res* 2003;415:31-44.

64. Funovics PT, Schuh R, Adams SB Jr, Sabeti-Aschraf M, Dominkus M, Kotz RI: Modular prosthetic reconstruction of major bone defects of the distal end of the humerus. *J Bone Joint Surg Am* 2011;93(11):1064-1074.

Twenty-seven patients underwent distal humeral reconstruction with endoprosthesis following tumor resection. At an overall follow-up of 28 months, 11% had deep infection and 3% had aseptic loosening with a mean MSTS score of 81%. Average elbow range of motion for the tumor group (total humerus and distal humerus included) was 8° to 105°. Level of evidence: IV.

65. Kharrazi FD, Busfield BT, Khorshad DS, Hornicek FJ, Mankin HJ: Osteoarticular and total elbow allograft reconstruction with severe bone loss. *Clin Orthop Relat Res* 2008;466(1):205-209.

Nineteen patients underwent osteoarticular allograft reconstruction of the distal humerus after tumor resection (3 complete, 16 hemiarticular). At a mean follow-up of 9 years, 10.5% had deep infection, 5% had host-allograft nonunion, 5% had dislocation, and 10.5% had nerve palsy. Average active range of elbow motion was flexion from 27° to 115°, pronation of 76°, and supination of 57°. All three patients who underwent a complete elbow allograft reconstruction experienced development of a Charcot-like joint 5 to 8 years after surgery. Level of evidence: IV.

66. van Isacker T, Barbier O, Traore A, Cornu O, Mazzeo F, Delloye C: Forearm reconstruction with bone allograft following tumor excision: A series of 10 patients with a mean follow-up of 10 years. *Orthop Traumatol Surg Res* 2011;97(8):793-799.

This study is a retrospective review of 10 patients who had tumors requiring segmental resection of the ulna or radius, which were reconstructed with bone allograft or osteochondral allograft. Allograft fracture was the most common complication. Intercalary allograft had fewer complications and better functional MSTS scores compared to osteochondral allograft reconstruction. There were no infections. Level of evidence: IV.

67. Muramatsu K, Ihara K, Doi K, Hashimoto T, Taguchi T: Sarcoma in the forearm and hand: Clinical outcomes and microsurgical reconstruction for limb salvage. *Ann Plast Surg* 2009;62(1):28-33.

6: Special Considerations in Tumor Management

This study was a retrospective review of 19 patients with soft-tissue or osseous sarcoma, of whom 12 received microvascular reconstruction (free tissue transfer). All flaps survived, and no postoperative wound infections were reported. In four patients with osseous sarcoma, free vascularized osteocutaneous fibula flaps were used to reconstruct radial or ulnar defects. Bony union was achieved in all patients. Level of evidence: IV.

68. Brown KL: Limb reconstruction with vascularized fibular grafts after bone tumor resection. *Clin Orthop Relat Res* 1991;262:64-73.

69. Kesani AK, Tuy B, Beebe K, Patterson F, Benevenia J: Single-bone forearm reconstruction for malignant and aggressive tumors. *Clin Orthop Relat Res* 2007;464: 210-216.

Four patients underwent single-bone forearm reconstruction following resection of malignant forearm lesions requiring extensive bone resection. Two patients received a distal radius allograft, 1 received vascularized free fibula autograft, and 1 underwent centralization of the ulna. Radiocarpal arthrodesis was performed in 3 patients. At follow-up of 12-82 months, the average MSTS score was 26 out of 30. Complications included host allograft nonunion in 2, superficial infection, and acute carpal tunnel syndrome. Level of evidence: IV.

Chapter 42

Concepts in Bone Grafting, Allografts, and Tissue Processing

Herbert S. Schwartz, MD

Introduction

Successfully managing bone defects remains a considerable challenge in orthopaedic practice. Bone grafting to fill skeletal defects is a common option for skeletal reconstruction that offers good long-term biologic outcomes in selected skeletal defects. The goals of bone grafting are simple, and may include fusion, union, and segmental defect repair. Bone grafting is governed by the same biologic principles as grafting of other tissues. The positive outcome of bone incorporation depends on the vascular status of the recipient site and the type of bone graft materials used. The size, shape, and biomechanical properties of the graft must also be considered.

The goals of this chapter are to describe the biology of bone grafts, allografts, and bone graft substitutes and help the surgeon to better understand how they are processed. Several synonyms are used to describe bone grafting and the process of bone incorporation. For the purpose of this chapter, transplantation is defined as the transfer of bone tissue from one part of the body to another or from one individual to another. Transplantation and grafting can mean the same thing. Orthotopic transplantation is the transfer of tissue from a donor into its anatomically normal position in the body of the recipient. Bone autografting involves bone transplantation between skeletal sites in the same individual. Allograft transplantation is the placement of tissue from one individual into another individual of the same species and is also called an allogeneic graft or homograft.

Definitions

Bone formation follows similar biologic pathways in processes referred to as osteogenesis, osteoinduction,

and osteoconduction. Osteogenesis is the formation of new bone by cells derived from precursors such as mesenchymal stem cells or preosteoblasts after proliferation and differentiation. Osteogenesis occurs when cellular elements of the donor bone survive transplantation and then synthesize new bone at a recipient site. For example, harvested pelvic bone marrow can be inserted into a tibial nonunion. Osteoinduction is the process in which transplanted tissue induces mesenchymal stem cells from the recipient site microenvironment to differentiate into bone-forming osteoblasts. Osteoinduction occurs when stimulatory molecules such as inflammatory cytokines, growth factors, and bone morphogenetic proteins (BMPs) in the grafting material recruit bone-forming precursor cells. For practical purposes, a material is termed osteoinductive when ectopic bone formation occurs in an athymic nude mouse or other animal. Many manufacturers claim osteoinduction on the basis of ectopic bone formation in a preclinical animal model; however, translating this scenario to the human is imprecise. Osteoconduction occurs when the transplanted bone graft acts as a conduit to facilitate bone healing in a passive manner through its structure. The effectiveness of an osteoconductive material depends on factors such as porosity and surface roughness. The terms osteogenesis, osteoinduction, and osteoconduction often overlap because an ideal grafting material would provide signaling molecules, bone-forming cells, and a scaffold. For example, fresh autogenous bone graft has the capability of supporting new bone via osteogenesis, osteoinduction, and osteoconduction. Bone marrow aspirate alone, in contrast, lacks an osteoconductive scaffold. Osteoconductive materials are often used when filling a large skeletal defect beyond critical size (approximately 5 cm in long bones), which would not otherwise easily heal. Osteoinduction implies a mechanism by which mesenchymal tissue is induced to change its cellular structure to become osteogenic; that is, to form bone, and is used when the recipient site is well vascularized.[1] Osteogenic tissue has the intrinsic capacity to form bone via the presence of contained mesenchymal stem cells but has size and volume restrictions.

Dr. Schwartz or an immediate family member has received non-income support (such as equipment or services), commercially derived honoraria, or other non–research-related funding (such as paid travel) from the Musculoskeletal Transplant Foundation and serves as a board member, owner, officer, or committee member of the American Board of Orthopaedic Surgery.

6: Special Considerations in Tumor Management

Bone Graft Biology

Autograft bone that has been severed from its vascular supply becomes necrotic after transplantation.[2] Osteocytes are normally able to survive by diffusion over a distance of approximately 100 μm. The peripheral cells of the graft are more easily affected by diffusion and thus survive to proliferate, whereas the more centrally located cells die within 2 hours.[3-5] The necrotic portion of the transplant acts as a scaffold and facilitates new bone formation on it via osteoconduction. The transplanted osteocytes secrete proteins, creating osteoinduction that stimulates nearby mesenchymal cells to begin the process of osteogenesis. Osteogenesis is ultimately dependent on vascularity. Capillaries must grow into the transplant from the surrounding soft tissues, which typically occurs 2 or 3 days after transplantation. New blood vessels penetrate older haversian canals and marrow spaces of the necrotic bone. As revascularization takes place, the transplanted necrotic bone is gradually resorbed by recruited osteoclasts. The dynamic interplay between bone resorption and bone formation in which new bone is laid down upon old bone is termed creeping substitution.[6] As the graft becomes incorporated and new bone is annealed directly on the trabeculae of the necrotic bone histologically, the admixture of these two elements becomes visible. The new bone is subjected to stress and undergoes the process of active remodeling.

Autografts can be of cancellous bone or cortical bone. They are repaired in similar but not identical ways.[7] Both cancellous bone and cortical bone initially have bone marrow areas revascularized. Cancellous bone then has deposition of new bone onto the preexisting trabeculae. This new bone thickens the trabeculae and encroaches on the marrow, increasing the radiodensity of the transplanted graft and yielding greater strength. The third step, which begins only after deposition is well advanced, involves the gradual removal of the necrotic central bone during the process of remodeling. Ultimately the cancellous graft is replaced by new bone in approximately 6 to 12 months.[8]

Nonvascularized autogenous cortical bone grafts also have their marrow areas revascularized as the initial step. However, the second step in cortical autogenous graft incorporation is resorption of the necrotic matrix within the graft. This step actually enlarges the haversian canals, making the graft less radiodense and weakening it, in contrast to the annealing and strengthening of cancellous autografts. After resorption completely removes dead osteons, new living bone begins to internally grow, returning radiodensity and strength to the construct.[9] Repair of cortical grafts is therefore less complete than repair of cancellous grafts, because interstitial lamellae remain buried in the depths of the graft and can be histologically seen as isolated islands of necrotic matrix. Consequently, the repair of cortical grafts requires 1 to 2 years to reach a steady state in which there may only be a 1:1 ratio of new bone to host

bone.[8] Nonvascularized cortical grafts provide immediate structural support but become weaker over time because of resorption and revascularization.[10]

Fresh allograft bone transplants are infrequently performed because of timing, cost, and immunobiology. When they are performed, often osteochondral allografts are used. The biology of fresh allograft bone transplantation is complex, and the procedures are performed without immunosuppressive drugs. The cells that try to proliferate in the transplant, immediately following the transplantation, trigger an immunologic rejection response that often stops osteoblast proliferation. This interaction evokes a granulomatous inflammatory response that may destroy the host-to-transplant neovascularization, impeding bone formation. In a series of experiments to investigate the fate of large bone allografts, researchers found that allografts were often poorly incorporated into the host bone and were vulnerable to infection and fatigue fractures.[11]

The transplantation of fresh-frozen skeletal allografts typically avoids the immunologic rejection phenomenon and is far more commonly performed, such as during reconstruction of bone defects following tumor resection. The immunogenic antigens on cell surfaces within the bone marrow are often destroyed in processing.[12] The antigens on the collagen matrix of cortical bone are only weakly antigenic. Thus, the biology of repair is analogous to the incorporation of cortical autografts although it is significantly prolonged, and, in fact, full graft incorporation may never completely occur.[13,14] The histologic features of allograft incorporation vary as a function of genetic disparity. In allograft incorporation using a fibular allograft in dogs, the indolently accepted graft with moderate genetic disparity is repaired via routine union of the allograft to the host by callus formed periosteally and endosteally.[7] Incorporative creeping substitution of new bone on necrotic bone is limited.[15,16] Clinically, the repair course is characterized by nonunion or delayed union and an increase in fatigue fractures.[17,18] There is considerably less internal repair than is seen with autografts. Callus typically forms and bridges the transplanted segments; however, the allografts are structurally weak.

Bone Banking

Human allograft tissue used for bone banking is not a commodity. Bone transplants are gifts donated by families of the deceased to benefit others. Bone banking organizations face ethical and financial challenges because they must function as both charities and businesses.[19] Some bone banks are for profit, but most are not-for-profit organizations. Selected banks have their own organ procurement organization responsible for tissue recovery, and other banks work with associated organ procurement organizations. It is illegal in the United States and most countries to buy or sell human tissue; however, it is permissible to pay service fees to individuals who procure human tissue during recovery. Nonprofit tissue banks often convert revenue into research, development, education, or donor family support services. Tissue processing is regulated under strict guidelines established by the American Association of Tissue Banks (AATB)[20] and the FDA. Most tissue banks adhere to these standards or exceed them.

Several milestones in the history of tissue transplantation using skeletal allografts have led to current state-of-the-art bone recovery and processing methods. As a result of the increasing needs of wounded World War II veterans, the US Navy Tissue Bank in Bethesda, Maryland, was founded in 1949. A sterile system for recovering bone from cadavers in operating rooms was developed, and freeze-drying was used to improve storage and increase availability of allograft bones.[21] In 1955, the reduction of antigenicity of bone transplants by low-temperature preservation began. In 1984, the first standards for tissue banking were published by the AATB. In 1989, the AATB Training and Certification Program for tissue banks began.[20] In 1993, the FDA began inspections of tissue banks for accreditation. Approximately 100 accredited tissue banks now exist in the United States, with approximately 8 of them accounting for 90% of musculoskeletal allograft production.

The strict criteria used to accept a donor's tissue for processing and distribution are listed at the Centers for Disease Control and Prevention website, www.CDC.gov. Donors are excluded from having their tissue processed when they present a high lifestyle risk, test positive for HIV, are found on autopsy to have occult diseases such as malignancy, are determined by positive culture to harbor infection, or test positive for hepatitis or syphilis. The donor's medical history is obtained to screen for systemic disease, malignancy, and infection.[22] The donor is tested for syphilis, hepatitis B and C, and HIV using nucleic acid testing.

Infectious disease testing regulations have evolved as technology has improved and the FDA has established increasingly rigid standards. HIV-1 and HIV-2 testing now almost exclusively occurs by nucleic acid-amplification testing (NAT) with a window period of 7 days when seroconversion is possible. The window period is defined as the time between infection and the time the virus is detectable by the screening test. Hepatitis C NAT testing also has a window period of 7 days. NAT testing has dramatically improved the infection-free transplantation of bone grafts.

The American Academy of Orthopaedic Surgeons (AAOS) sponsored an allograft safety symposium in 2008.[23] Since 1980, more than 10 million musculoskeletal allografts were implanted in the United States following AATB guidelines. Historically, the following infections related to musculoskeletal allografts have been documented: 1 tuberculosis infection in 1953, 10 bacterial infections (plus another 14 in non-AATB tissue banks), 1 hepatitis B infection in 1954, 7 hepatitis C infections before NAT, and 4 HIV infections before NAT. There have been no reported cases of disease transmission from demineralized bone matrix (DBM) usage.[23] With modern techniques, the risk of HIV transmission is currently estimated to be 1 in 1.6 million. The risk of hepatitis C transmission in fresh-frozen allograft is estimated to be 1 in 100,000. The risk of hepatitis B transmission in musculoskeletal fresh-frozen allograft transplants is 1 in 63,000. Clinically, however, the largest US musculoskeletal bone banks have reported only three patient infections out of 5.2 million tissue grafts distributed, none of which required graft removal.[24-26] For comparison, the risks of an infectious agent being transmitted from donor to recipient per unit of blood transfusion are as follows: HIV (HIV-1 or HIV-2), 1 in 2 million; human T-lymphotropic virus (HTLV-1 or HTLV-2), 1 in 3 million; hepatitis B, 1 in 250,000; and hepatitis C, 1 in 1.5 million.[26]

Allograft Recovery and Processing

Successful skeletal allograft transplantation is optimized when the tissue form is ethically harvested and the infection risk is minimized, and retains its unprocessed biologic and mechanical characteristics. The structural and biologic properties of allografts are determined by the recovery, processing, and sterilization methods. Different techniques influence the biologic and mechanical properties of each graft. An understanding of these processes allows identification of a suitable bone graft for allogeneic transplantation.

Skeletal and soft-tissue allografts can be recovered from the donor by either of two mechanisms: aseptic or clean-room. Aseptic procurement occurs immediately upon donation from a patient declared brain dead. Allograft tissues are obtained under the strict aseptic conditions of a sterile operating-room environment and processed accordingly. Clean-room procurement refers to patients whose tissues are harvested in a delayed fashion but less than 24 hours after death (asystole) and have been refrigerated for less than 12 hours. Sterile techniques practiced in an operating room are not used during clean-room harvesting. The bacterial burden of the allograft is minimized when using aseptic harvesting techniques. The FDA requires that each lot of DBM be categorized by batch and processed on the basis of the identity of the donor. Pooled lots make it difficult or impossible to trace the location of an intended donor, thus increasing infection risk.

After procurement, bone graft tissue must be processed before distribution and surgical implantation. The graft is débrided of unnecessary or unneeded soft tissues. In some instances, tendon insertions are retained. Lavage washing and ultrasound are performed to remove fat, marrow elements, blood, and other cells. Ethanol is used to denature proteins and destroy bacteria. Topical antibiotics supplement this process. This mechanical cleansing process differs slightly from tissue bank to tissue bank. DBM is created from allograft cortical bone after acid extraction.[27]

6: Special Considerations in Tumor Management

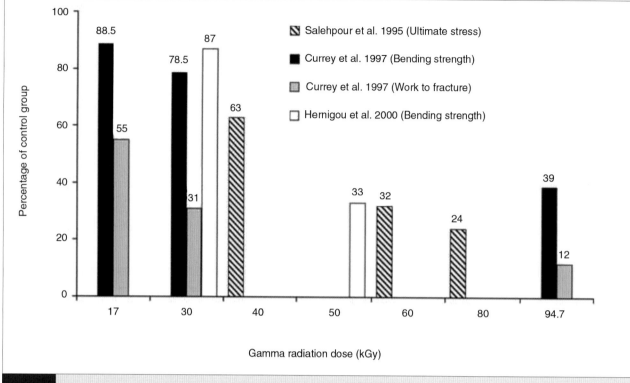

Figure 1 Dose-dependent loss of allograft biomechanical strength resulting from irradiation. Values from the literature show a general trend for dose-dependent degradation of mechanical properties of allograft bone after gamma irradiation. For comparison, degradation of mechanical properties is shown as percentage reduction compared to control specimens, and the mechanical variable measured is indicated in parentheses. (Reproduced with permission from Nguyen H, Morgan DA: Sterilization of allograft bone: Effects of gamma irradiation on allograft biology and biomechanics. *Cell Tissue Bank* 2007;8:93-105.)

Many tissue banks process human tissue using proprietary methods of sterilization to enhance risk-free transplantation. Irradiation is a common method used to lower the bacterial bioburden on tissues and in high doses can overcome contamination that occurs when the allograft is not harvested immediately in an aseptic environment. Often gamma irradiation is delivered in doses ranging from 10 to 25 kGy as a final step, called terminal sterilization. When higher doses of irradiation are administered, the mechanical properties and osteoinductive properties of the transplanted tissue diminish in a dose-dependent fashion[28-31] (**Figure 1**). This finding is especially true for soft-tissue allografts.[32] Other banks use low-dose irradiation on allograft tissue (less than approximately 17 kGy) in an effort to preserve mechanical strength and osteoinductivity, although a strict dose-dependent relationship for these lower irradiation levels has not been established.[30,33-35] Historically, the bacterial bioburden was determined by culturing preprocessing swabs in a qualitative fashion, resulting in bacterial detection in about 20% to 25% of infected donors. Newer techniques use quantitative tissue biopsy to calculate bacterial levels with approximately 70% detection accuracy. Bacterial levels above a threshold often result in donor rejection. Swabbing the allograft at the time of implantation has been proven to be unreliable in predicting clinical infection.[36]

Tissue banks must balance donor supply with market demand. Tissue banks may offer allograft products labeled as either aseptic or sterile. If the final product is labeled as aseptic, it is defined as the allograft tissue passing United States Pharmacopeia (USP) <71> sterility standards, implying minimal bacterial bioburden and little, if any, irradiation delivered during processing. USP <71> refers to sterility standards published in the 71st chapter of USP version 30.[37] It explains the methods and machine protocols required to ensure product asepsis, and outlines procedures and requirements for compounding sterile preparations. The sterility tests in USP <71> seek to deny the presence of viable forms of bacteria, fungi, and yeasts in or on an article. The USP rules were initially created for quality assurance in the pharmaceutical industry in 1980. Now, however, newer rules apply to ensure sterility of many tissue products. Sterile labeling, by contrast, implies contamination to less than 1 in 1 million parts, suggesting that terminal high-dose irradiation was used. Bone irradiation is not virucidal for HIV. In general, aseptic tissue receives less processing alteration compared to terminally sterilized tissue forms.

Grafts are prepared for distribution typically in one of three ways: either fresh, fresh-frozen, or freeze dried. Fresh allografts are rarely used in transplantation because of timing constraints, likelihood of rejection, and cost. When they are used, they are often used for osteoconductive reconstruction around the knee or ankle with the potential of filling defects with viable bone and cartilage cells. Fresh-frozen grafts are frozen at −80°C immediately after harvest. They have a shelf life of 3.5 years. Fresh-frozen allografts are used to reconstruct large skeletal defects. Specialized cryopreservatives may enhance articular cartilage survival in the allograft. Fresh-frozen allografts are the most common method of tissue preservation used for both bone and soft-tissue specimens. Freeze-drying removes more than 94% of the water content by lyophilization and significantly prolongs room temperature shelf life. Unfortunately, freeze-drying significantly weakens the bone and reduces mechanical strength and biologic activity.

Bone Graft Substitutes

Bone graft substitutes are a wide grouping of products that can be allograft tissue forms or synthetic.[38-41] DBM has both osteoinductive and osteoconductive potential. Osteoinduction occurs via endochondral ossification.[42] It is very difficult to prove clinical superiority of one product over another with objective scientific or clinical evidence. The many biologic variables, costs, and numbers are too great to establish a product's superiority. Often investigators use preclinical and small clinical in vitro series to document osteoinductive potential or fusion rates in an attempt to demonstrate the clinical value of a product. Lot variability, rodent type, outcome measures, and observer bias can affect results. Proprietary data provided by various vendors can be difficult to validate, thereby making choosing a superior product difficult.[43] Various reported studies suggest certain products have higher concentration of BMPs, but they change in amount from donor to donor and from lot to lot, and also have varying pH levels and sterility, storage, processing, carrier, and handling properties—all of which make it very difficult to characterize product efficacy.[33,44-47]

Synthetics such as calcium sulfate are considered to be biocompatible, and the product most readily dissolves in only 6 to 17 weeks.[48,49] Calcium phosphate ceramics are hard, porous, and brittle. They allow for attachment, proliferation, and migration of osteoblasts to make bone apposed to the ceramic. Resorption is product dependent. Ceramics have many pros: low infection rates, abundant supply with multiple shapes, and long shelf life. However, they often exhibit suboptimal handling and uniform osteoconductivity. A pore size of 300 to 500 μm is thought to be ideal for bone ingrowth.[50,51] Hydroxyapatite is a crystalline form of calcium phosphate bone with such a pore size. Calcium phosphate cements are useful because of the material's compressive biomechanical strength, and newer products are more resistant to sheer forces, which enables drilling of screws and filling of metaphyseal defects.[52] If osteoin-

Table 1

Examples of Bone Graft Substitutes

Bone Graft Substitute Type	Product	Manufacturer
Synthetic		
Ceramic (CaPO$_4$)	Vitoss	Stryker
	Norian SRS	Synthes
	ProOsteon	Biomet
	BoneSource	Stryker
	CopiOs	Zimmer
Plaster (CaSO$_4$)	Osteoset	Wright
Factor based (rhBMP-2)	Infuse	Medtronic
Polymer	Healos	DePuy
	OsteoScaf	Tissue Regeneration Therapeutics
Allograft based		
Demineralized bone matrix	AlloFuse	Allosource
	DBX	Musculoskeletal Transplant Foundation
	Opteform	Exactech
	Grafton	Medtronic
	Allomatrix	Wright
	BioSet	Regeneration Technologies Inc.
	InterGro	Biomet
	Accell TBM	Integra
	Optium	LifeNet Health
Cell containing	Trinity Evolution	Musculoskeletal Transplant Foundation
	NuVasive	AlloSource

duction occurs with calcium phosphate biomaterials, it is thought to occur by an intramembranous mechanism.[53,54]

BMP-2 and BMP-7 have been shown in randomized prospective controlled trials to be growth factors able to induce bone formation in tibial nonunions equal to autograft. They can also induce or accelerate bone healing in fresh tissue fractures, although at higher concentrations than physiologic doses.[55-58] BMP-2 is manu-

6: Special Considerations in Tumor Management

factured by recombinant technology, incurring high expense. Meta-analyses have identified at least 17 clinical trials demonstrating successful BMP usage, inducing significantly fewer nonunions in lumbar spine fusions than with the use of autografts.[59-61] However, recent studies raise serious concerns about the safety and efficacy of recombinant human BMP-2. The role of growth factor augmented bone healing, especially when used in supraphysiologic doses and/or in off-label situations, is evolving.[62,63]

Allograft tissue containing potential living cells and/or stem cells is a novel product that supposedly has DBM properties without carriers, available in a user-friendly tissue form. This product purportedly offers osteoinductive and osteogenic potential. Unpublished clinical trials are commencing based on early in vitro experimentation.[64,65] This product is currently classified as a human cell and tissue product (HCT/P) by the FDA. Market examples of bone graft substitutes are shown in **Table 1**.

Summary

Before selecting a particular bone graft for an individual patient and clinical situation, the surgeon must first determine the size, strength, and structure of graft that is required. Filling a void in the metaphysis of a long bone is different from a shaft defect larger than 5 cm using allograft whose strength may have been compromised during sterilization. Next, the amount of biologic activity remaining in the graftable tissue should be determined. Tissue processing affects active protein concentration in the allograft and must be balanced against infection risk. The age of the donor may also have profound effects on its biologic behavior once transplanted. In addition, the surgeon should assess the quality and character of the neovascularization potential in the recipient site, because mesenchymal stem cell recruitment and cell proliferation are dependent on this factor.

Annotated References

1. Blokhuis TJ, Arts JJ: Bioactive and osteoinductive bone graft substitutes: Definitions, facts and myths. *Injury* 2011;42(suppl 2):S26-S29.

   A review of bone graft substitutes and their bone biology is presented.

2. Chase SW, Herndon CH: The fate of autogenous and homogenous bone grafts. *J Bone Joint Surg Am* 1955; 37-A(4):809-841.

3. Laursen M, Christensen FB, Bünger C, Lind M: Optimal handling of fresh cancellous bone graft: Different preoperative storing techniques evaluated by in vitro osteoblastlike cell metabolism. *Acta Orthop Scand* 2003;74(4):490-496.

4. Marx RE: Bone and bone graft healing. *Oral Maxillofac Surg Clin North Am* 2007;19(4):455-466, v.

   Bone graft biology is reviewed and its regenerative properties are discussed.

5. Samartzis D, Shen FH, Goldberg EJ, An HS: Is autograft the gold standard in achieving radiographic fusion in one-level anterior cervical discectomy and fusion with rigid anterior plate fixation? *Spine (Phila Pa 1976)* 2005;30(15):1756-1761.

6. Phemister DB: The fate of transplanted bone and regenerative power of its various constituents. *Surg Gynecol Obstet* 1914;19:303-333.

7. Dell PC, Burchardt H, Glowczewskie FP Jr: A roentgenographic, biomechanical, and histological evaluation of vascularized and non-vascularized segmental fibular canine autografts. *J Bone Joint Surg Am* 1985; 67(1):105-112.

8. Enneking WF, Burchardt H, Puhl JJ, Piotrowski G: Physical and biological aspects of repair in dog cortical-bone transplants. *J Bone Joint Surg Am* 1975; 57(2):237-252.

9. Hammack BL, Enneking WF: Comparative vascularization of autogenous and homogenous-bone transplants. *J Bone Joint Surg Am* 1960;42-A:811-817.

10. Stevenson S: Biology of bone grafts. *Orthop Clin North Am* 1999;30(4):543-552.

11. Enneking WF: Histological investigation of bone transplants in immunologically prepared animals. *J Bone Joint Surg Am* 1957;39-A(3):597-615.

12. Beebe KS, Benevenia J, Tuy BE, DePaula CA, Harten RD, Enneking WF: Effects of a new allograft processing procedure on graft healing in a canine model: A preliminary study. *Clin Orthop Relat Res* 2009; 467(1):273-280.

   A new cleansing procedure, intended to reduce viral bioburden on transplanted bone allografts, was found not to affect graft healing.

13. Bonfiglio M, Jeter WS: Immunological responses to bone. *Clin Orthop Relat Res* 1972;87:19-27.

14. Burchardt H, Glowczewskie FP, Enneking WF: Allogeneic segmental fibular transplants in azathioprine-immunosuppressed dogs. *J Bone Joint Surg Am* 1977; 59(7):881-894.

15. Heyligers IC, Klein-Nulend J: Detection of living cells in non-processed but deep-frozen bone allografts. *Cell Tissue Bank* 2005;6(1):25-31.

16. Tsiridis E, Upadhyay N, Giannoudis P: Molecular aspects of fracture healing: Which are the important molecules? *Injury* 2007;38(suppl 1):S11-S25.

   Current knowledge on molecules involved in the chain

of events that contribute to promoting and inhibiting fracture healing and the signal pathways involved is summarized.

17. Enneking WF, Campanacci DA: Retrieved human allografts: A clinicopathological study. *J Bone Joint Surg Am* 2001;83-A(7):971-986.

18. Wheeler DL, Enneking WF: Allograft bone decreases in strength in vivo over time. *Clin Orthop Relat Res* 2005;435:36-42.

19. Wilson K, Lavrov V, Keller M, Maier T, Ryle G: Human corpses harvested in multimillion-dollar trade. *Sydney Morning Herald*, 17 July 2012. http://www.smh.com.au/opinion/political-news/human-corpses-harvested-in-multimilliondollar-trade-20120717-2278v.html. Accessed July 20, 2012.

The unethical, for-profit aspects of tissue harvesting are discussed.

20. http://www.aatb.org. Accessed August 12, 2012.

Public information detailing the accreditation requirements for approved tissue banks in the United States.

21. Tomford WW: Bone allografts: Past, present and future. *Cell Tissue Bank* 2000;1(2):105-109.

22. Tomford WW: Transmission of disease through transplantation of musculoskeletal allografts. *J Bone Joint Surg Am* 1995;77(11):1742-1754.

23. Joyce MJ, Greenwald AS, Boden S, Brubaker S, Heim CS: Musculoskeletal Allograft Tissue Safety. AAOS Annual Meeting, San Francisco, California, 2008.

This AAOS symposium presents a review of the history of allograft safety.

24. Lietman SA, Tomford WW, Gebhardt MC, Springfield DS, Mankin HJ: Complications of irradiated allografts in orthopaedic tumor surgery. *Clin Orthop Relat Res* 2000;375:214-217.

25. Mankin HJ, Gebhardt MC, Jennings LC, Springfield DS, Tomford WW: Long-term results of allograft replacement in the management of bone tumors. *Clin Orthop Relat Res* 1996;324:86-97.

26. Squires JE: Risks of transfusion. *South Med J* 2011;104(11):762-769.

This review article discusses disease transmission risks after blood transfusion.

27. Einhorn TA, Lane JM, Burstein AH, Kopman CR, Vigorita VJ: The healing of segmental bone defects induced by demineralized bone matrix: A radiographic and biomechanical study. *J Bone Joint Surg Am* 1984;66(2):274-279.

28. Currey JD, Foreman J, Laketić I, Mitchell J, Pegg DE, Reilly GC: Effects of ionizing radiation on the mechanical properties of human bone. *J Orthop Res* 1997;15(1):111-117.

29. Hernigou P, Gras G, Marinello G, Dormont D: Inactivation of HIV by application of heat and radiation: Implication in bone banking with irradiated allograft bone. *Acta Orthop Scand* 2000;71(5):508-512.

30. Nguyen H, Morgan DA, Forwood MR: Sterilization of allograft bone: Effects of gamma irradiation on allograft biology and biomechanics. *Cell Tissue Bank* 2007;8(2):93-105.

The dose-dependent effects of gamma radiation on bone mechanics are graphically displayed.

31. Salehpour A, Butler DL, Proch FS, et al: Dose-dependent response of gamma irradiation on mechanical properties and related biochemical composition of goat bone-patellar tendon-bone allografts. *J Orthop Res* 1995;13(6):898-906.

32. Rappé M, Horodyski M, Meister K, Indelicato PA: Nonirradiated versus irradiated Achilles allograft: In vivo failure comparison. *Am J Sports Med* 2007;35(10):1653-1658.

Ninety patients receiving Achilles tendon allografts for anterior cruciate ligament reconstruction were reviewed. Half of the allografts were radiated for terminal sterilization and the other half were not. Nonradiated grafts were superior, having only a 2.4% catastrophic failure rate vs. 33% in the radiated group *p* <0.01. Level of evidence: III.

33. Balsly CR, Cotter AT, Williams LA, Gaskins BD, Moore MA, Wolfinbarger L Jr: Effect of low dose and moderate dose gamma irradiation on the mechanical properties of bone and soft tissue allografts. *Cell Tissue Bank* 2008;9(4):289-298.

Low-dose radiation used for allograft sterilization may do so without compromising significant functional or mechanical properties.

34. Jinno T, Miric A, Feighan J, Kirk SK, Davy DT, Stevenson S: The effects of processing and low dose irradiation on cortical bone grafts. *Clin Orthop Relat Res* 2000;375:275-285.

35. Mitchell EJ, Stawarz AM, Kayacan R, Rimnac CM: The effect of gamma radiation sterilization on the fatigue crack propagation resistance of human cortical bone. *J Bone Joint Surg Am* 2004;86-A(12):2648-2657.

36. van de Pol GJ, Sturm PD, van Loon CJ, Verhagen C, Schreurs BW: Microbiological cultures of allografts of the femoral head just before transplantation. *J Bone Joint Surg Br* 2007;89(9):1225-1228.

Positive bone allograft cultures taken at implantation probably represent contamination as they do not result in higher postoperative infection rates. Level of evidence: III.

37. Kupiec TC: Quality-control analytical methods: A discussion of United States Pharmacopeia Chapter 71 Ste-

6: Special Considerations in Tumor Management

rility Tests. *Int J Pharm Compd* 2007;11(5):400-403.

The methodology used in a compounding pharmacy, which adheres to strict guidelines during processing, is reviewed.

38. Beaman FD, Bancroft LW, Peterson JJ, Kransdorf MJ: Bone graft materials and synthetic substitutes. *Radiol Clin North Am* 2006;44(3):451-461.

39. Calori GM, Mazza E, Colombo M, Ripamonti C: The use of bone-graft substitutes in large bone defects: Any specific needs? *Injury* 2011;42(suppl 2):S56-S63.

    Review of retrospective studies comparing the osteoconductive properties of various bone graft substitutes. Resorption times have the greatest variability. Level of evidence: III.

40. Gazdag AR, Lane JM, Glaser D, Forster RA: Alternatives to autogenous bone graft: Efficacy and indications. *J Am Acad Orthop Surg* 1995;3(1):1-8.

41. Giannoudis PV, Dinopoulos H, Tsiridis E: Bone substitutes: An update. *Injury* 2005;36(suppl 3):S20-S27.

42. Reddi AH: Cell biology and biochemistry of endochondral bone development. *Coll Relat Res* 1981;1(2):209-226.

43. Bhattacharyya T, Tornetta P III, Healy WL, Einhorn TA: The validity of claims made in orthopaedic print advertisements. *J Bone Joint Surg Am* 2003;85-A(7):1224-1228.

44. Bae HW, Zhao L, Kanim LE, Wong P, Delamarter RB, Dawson EG: Intervariability and intravariability of bone morphogenetic proteins in commercially available demineralized bone matrix products. *Spine (Phila Pa 1976)* 2006;31(12):1299-1306, discussion 1307-1308.

45. Peterson B, Whang PG, Iglesias R, Wang JC, Lieberman JR: Osteoinductivity of commercially available demineralized bone matrix: Preparations in a spine fusion model. *J Bone Joint Surg Am* 2004;86-A(10):2243-2250.

46. Wildemann B, Kadow-Romacker A, Haas NP, Schmidmaier G: Quantification of various growth factors in different demineralized bone matrix preparations. *J Biomed Mater Res A* 2007;81(2):437-442.

    Three different DBM commercially available products were quantified for eight growth factor concentrations. Ten lots of each product were analyzed. BMP-2 was high in all. TGF-β1 was selectively higher in one product, whereas the other growth factors were found in similar concentrations.

47. Wildemann B, Kadow-Romacker A, Pruss A, Haas NP, Schmidmaier G: Quantification of growth factors in allogenic bone grafts extracted with three different methods. *Cell Tissue Bank* 2007;8(2):107-114.

    The extraction method used to detect protein in sterilized bone allografts is technique dependent. Guanidine hydrochloride extraction results in the highest amount of protein in the supernatants.

48. LeGeros RZ: Properties of osteoconductive biomaterials: Calcium phosphates. *Clin Orthop Relat Res* 2002;395:81-98.

49. Peters CL, Hines JL, Bachus KN, Craig MA, Bloebaum RD: Biological effects of calcium sulfate as a bone graft substitute in ovine metaphyseal defects. *J Biomed Mater Res A* 2006;76(3):456-462.

50. Hannink G, Arts JJ: Bioresorbability, porosity and mechanical strength of bone substitutes: What is optimal for bone regeneration? *Injury* 2011;42(suppl 2):S22-S25.

    This review article discusses the role of physical properties of calcium phosphate preparations on bioavailability.

51. Kuboki Y, Jin Q, Kikuchi M, Mamood J, Takita H: Geometry of artificial ECM: Sizes of pores controlling phenotype expression in BMP-induced osteogenesis and chondrogenesis. *Connect Tissue Res* 2002;43(2-3):529-534.

52. Hak DJ: The use of osteoconductive bone graft substitutes in orthopaedic trauma. *J Am Acad Orthop Surg* 2007;15(9):525-536.

    This review article discusses the use of bone graft substitutes in skeletal defects caused by injury.

53. Kuboki Y, Saito T, Murata M, et al: Two distinctive BMP-carriers induce zonal chondrogenesis and membranous ossification, respectively; geometrical factors of matrices for cell-differentiation. *Connect Tissue Res* 1995;32(1-4):219-226.

54. Sasano Y, Ohtani E, Narita K, et al: BMPs induce direct bone formation in ectopic sites independent of the endochondral ossification in vivo. *Anat Rec* 1993;236(2):373-380.

55. Drosos GI, Kazakos KI, Kouzoumpasis P, Verettas DA: Safety and efficacy of commercially available demineralised bone matrix preparations: A critical review of clinical studies. *Injury* 2007;38(suppl 4):S13-S21.

    A summary of clinical applications of various DBM preparations is presented.

56. Friedlaender GE, Perry CR, Cole JD, et al: Osteogenic protein-1 (bone morphogenetic protein-7) in the treatment of tibial nonunions. *J Bone Joint Surg Am* 2001;83-A(Pt 2, suppl 1):S151-S158.

57. Govender S, Csimma C, Genant HK, et al; BMP-2 Evaluation in Surgery for Tibial Trauma (BESTT) Study Group: Recombinant human bone morphogenetic protein-2 for treatment of open tibial fractures: A prospective, controlled, randomized study of four hundred and fifty patients. *J Bone Joint Surg Am* 2002;84-A(12):2123-2134.

58. Kanakaris NK, Lasanianos N, Calori GM, et al: Application of bone morphogenetic proteins to femoral nonunions: A 4-year multicentre experience. *Injury* 2009; 40(suppl 3):S54-S61.

   In this case series, femoral nonunions were treated with BMP-7 without adverse effects. Level of evidence: IV.

59. Agarwal R, Williams K, Umscheid CA, Welch WC: Osteoinductive bone graft substitutes for lumbar fusion: A systematic review. *J Neurosurg Spine* 2009; 11(6):729-740.

   The authors conducted a systematic review to compare the efficacy and safety of osteoinductive bone graft substitutes using autografts and allografts in lumbar fusion in prospective clinical trials. BMP-2 may be an effective alternative to iliac crest bone graft. Level of evidence: III.

60. Berven S, Tay BK, Kleinstueck FS, Bradford DS: Clinical applications of bone graft substitutes in spine surgery: Consideration of mineralized and demineralized preparations and growth factor supplementation. *Eur Spine J* 2001;10(Suppl 2):S169-S177.

61. Hsu W, Fuchs D, Anderson P: A meta-analysis of fusion rates from bone graft substitutes in a rodent posterolateral spine arthrodesis model. *Spine J* 2011; 11(suppl 10):S59-S60.

   Significant variables are reviewed that help create posterolateral spinal fusion in rabbits. Proper thresholds for bone graft volume and animal weight are outlined.

62. Carragee EJ, Chu G, Rohatgi R, et al: Cancer risk after use of recombinant bone morphogenetic protein-2 for spinal arthrodesis. *J Bone Joint Surg Am* 2013;95(17): 1537-1545.

   The authors reviewed publically available data from several institutions and evaluated the risk of new cancers in patients receiving high dose rhBMP-2 for spinal fusion. The authors concluded there was an increased risk of cancer in the BMP-2 group compared to iliac crest bone graft supplemented spine fusions. It is puzzling that approximately half of the new cancers identified in the BMP-2 group had sun-exposure-related, nonmelanoma skin carcinomas. Although it is possible that the local administration of growth factor in the spine somehow stimulated accelerated skin growth, the possibility of selection bias must be considered. Level of evidence: II.

63. Mesfin A, Buchowski JM, Zebala LP, et al: High-dose rhBMP-2 for adults: Major and minor complications. A study of 502 spine cases. *J Bone Joint Surg Am* 2013;95(17):1546-1553.

   A level IV study examined the use of high dose BMP-2 in spinal surgery at one institution and any associated outcome complications. The authors identified an 11% to 12% medical and surgical complication rate at follow-up. No correlation between BMP-2 dosage and cancer was found.

64. Lohmann CH, Andreacchio D, Köster G, et al: Tissue response and osteoinduction of human bone grafts in vivo. *Arch Orthop Trauma Surg* 2001;121(10):583-590.

65. Seebach C, Schultheiss J, Wilhelm K, Frank J, Henrich D: Comparison of six bone-graft substitutes regarding to cell seeding efficiency, metabolism and growth behaviour of human mesenchymal stem cells (MSC) in vitro. *Injury* 2010;41(7):731-738.

   This in vitro study determined that processed human cancellous allograft is a suitable biocompatible scaffold for ingrowing mesenchymal stem cells.

6: Special Considerations in Tumor Management

Chapter 43

Surgical Management of Sarcomas in Skeletally Immature Patients

Antoinette W. Lindberg, MD   Stephanie E. W. Punt, BS   Janet F. Eary, MD   Ernest U. Conrad III, MD

Introduction

The immature skeleton adds a unique challenge to oncologic surgical interventions. The resection of bone sarcomas requires accommodating skeletal growth, planning for a life expectancy that exceeds average implant survival, and striving for levels of postoperative activity that are equivalent to that of the patient's peers. Surgeons should be completely aware of the issues regarding growth and the expectations that parents have for their children's treatment. Approximately two thirds of lower extremity growth occurs in the distal femur and proximal tibia, where most primary bone malignancies occur.[1] The onset of puberty (age 10 to 14 years) is a critical milepost signaling the beginning of the last skeletal growth phase. Ten-year-old children have 10% to 20% of their overall skeletal growth and 15% to 25% of their femoral growth remaining (Figure 1). Girls 8 to 10 years of age have 6 to 10 cm of remaining distal femoral and proximal tibial growth, and boys 10 to 12 years of age have 9 to 12 cm remaining. This remaining growth makes surgical decisions for younger patients with osteosarcoma or Ewing sarcoma more challenging than decisions for older patients.[2]

Patterns of Growth and Effects of Chemotherapy and Radiation Therapy

With the success of preoperative neoadjuvant chemotherapy and improvements in imaging, resection of an immature physis adjacent to the primary tumor is less common today than in the past. Systemic and local

treatments such as chemotherapy and radiation therapy can transiently or permanently disrupt chondrocyte proliferation at the physis. Tumor necrosis secondary to preoperative chemotherapy and radiation therapy allows a closer surgical margin and sparing of the adjacent physis, with what appears to be minimal increased risk. Precise guidelines for adequate margins in pediatric osteosarcoma and Ewing sarcoma remain controversial (Figure 2).

Weighing the indications and guidelines for the adequacy of osseous tumor resection margins and assessing these margins through preoperative imaging after neoadjuvant chemotherapy represent the most important and most challenging preoperative decisions that must be made for young patients who will undergo limb salvage—especially for those younger than 10 to 12 years, who are at risk for loss of their growth plates.

Physeal Biology: Growth Patterns

Pressure epiphyses, or normal growth plate physes, account for the majority of vertical height and are found near major joints. Traction epiphyses, such as the greater trochanter and the tibial apophysis, do not involve the joint and serve as major muscle insertion points. The growth plate is composed of chondrocytes in various stages of differentiation with the end result of skeletal growth by enchondral ossification.[3,4] This region is composed of three zones: the resting, proliferative, and hypertrophic zones. In the resting or reserve zone, chondrocytes rarely divide, and nutrients are stored. In the proliferative zone, chondrocytes rapidly divide and arrange themselves vertically in columns. In the hypertrophic zone, chondrocytes enlarge and proceed to proliferate. Because of its increased cellular division, the proliferative zone is at greater risk of being affected by adjuvant chemotherapy and radiation therapy. Regulation via feedback loops of parathyroid hormone-related protein (PTHrP), which in turn regulates Indian hedgehog (Ihh), is responsible for chondrocyte proliferation and maturation, and the rate at which this process occurs.[5] Vascular endothelial growth factor (VEGF) is found in hypertrophic chondrocytes and assists with chondrocyte apoptosis, angiogenesis, and subsequent ossification. Chondrocytes undergoing

Dr. Lindberg or an immediate family member is an employee of Oppo Medical. Dr. Conrad or an immediate family member serves as a paid consultant to Zimmer; serves as an unpaid consultant to Stryker; and has received nonincome support (such as equipment or services), commercially derived honoraria, or other non–research-related funding (such as paid travel) from LifeNet Health Northwest Tissue Division. Neither of the following authors nor any immediate family member has received anything of value from or has stock or stock options held in a commercial company or institution related directly or indirectly to the subject of this chapter: Ms. Punt and Dr. Eary.

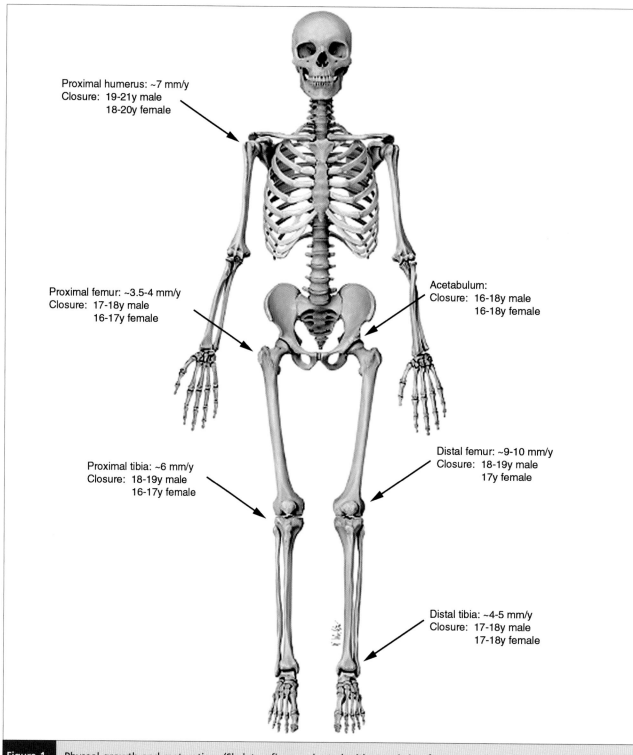

Proximal humerus: ~7 mm/y
Closure: 19-21y male
18-20y female

Proximal femur: ~3.5-4 mm/y
Closure: 17-18y male
16-17y female

Acetabulum:
Closure: 16-18y male
16-18y female

Distal femur: ~9-10 mm/y
Closure: 18-19y male
17y female

Proximal tibia: ~6 mm/y
Closure: 18-19y male
16-17y female

Distal tibia: ~4-5 mm/y
Closure: 17-18y male
17-18y female

Figure 1   Physeal growth and maturation. (Skeleton figure adapted with permission from Conrad EU: *Orthopaedic Oncology: Diagnosis and Treatment.* New York, NY, Thieme, 2008. Data from Rathjen KE, Birch JG: Physeal injuries and growth disturbances, in Beaty JH, Kasser JR, eds: *Rockwood and Wilkins' Fractures in Children*, ed 6. Philadelphia, PA, Lippincott Williams & Wilkins, 2006, pp 99-104; Anderson M, Messner MB, Green WT: Distribution of lengths of the normal femur and tibia in children from one to eighteen years. *J Bone Joint Surg Am* 1964;46:1197-1202.)

apoptosis express transforming growth factor-β (TGF-β), which regulates the hypertrophic zone and maintains physis height during growth.[6] Researchers have suggested that following a growth plate injury, an inflammatory phase is initiated and growth plate cells differentiate toward hypertrophy.[3] If disruption of the growth plate circulation or bone bridge formation occurs via trauma or surgical intervention, angular growth deformities or limb-length discrepancies can result.[7] Multiple methods of predicting limb-length discrepancy at skeletal maturity have been developed for use in pediatric orthopaedics and include the arithmetic method, the growth-remaining method, the Paley multiplier method, and the straight-line graph method.

Arithmetic Method
The arithmetic method is the simplest method for calculation of limb-length discrepancy because it does not require any special charts or graphs. It uses a child's chronologic age and assumes that boys reach skeletal maturity at age 16 years and girls reach skeletal maturity at age 14 years. The method also operates on the assumption that the distal femoral physis grows at a rate of 10 mm/y; the proximal tibia, at 6 mm/y; and the proximal femur and distal tibia, at 4 mm/y.[2] The arithmetic method is the preferred method of most oncologic surgeons because of its simplicity, but it is less accurate for children who are not in their last few years of growth.[8]

Growth-Remaining Method
The growth-remaining method relies on extensive longitudinal data collected in the earlier half of the 20th century. Benefits of this method include the use of skeletal (as opposed to chronologic) age and the ability to factor growth percentile into the prediction, but it does require the use of specific charts.[2,9]

Paley Multiplier Method
The Paley multiplier method was developed using the data from the charts used for the growth-remaining method, but rather than requiring the use of the actual charts, it is based on a table of "multipliers" and can use as few as one data point to predict discrepancy. For example, a 4-year-old boy has reached 50% of adult leg length; therefore, the multiplier would be 2.[10] The Paley multiplier method is recommended for limb salvage patients younger than 10 years because of the need for more accurate future growth predictions.

Straight-Line Graph Method
The straight-line graph method uses the data from the growth-remaining method in a complex system of graphs and charts. Benefits of the system include the use of skeletal age and growth percentiles, but the accuracy of the system is reliant on multiple data points.[11] Incorporation of this method into computer programs has greatly improved the method's ease of use.

Limitations of the Limb-Length Discrepancy Prediction Methods
Applying any of the four main limb-length discrepancy prediction methods is challenging for patients undergoing limb salvage surgery for sarcoma. None of the four methods takes into account any effects of chemother-

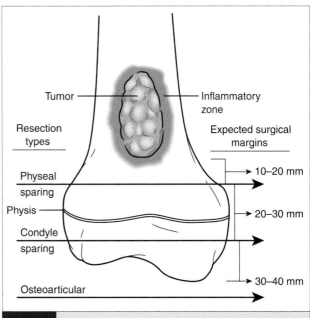

| **Figure 2** | Distal femoral resections are shown. Expected surgical margins are indicated for each resection type: physeal resection, condyle-sparing resection, and osteoarticular resection. |

apy, radiation therapy, or decreased nutrition, all of which can affect children undergoing sarcoma treatment. Each of these factors can affect not only the rate of growth in the physes, but also the age of skeletal maturity. Furthermore, three of the four methods are largely based on data collected from children in the Boston area in the 1940s, and may not accurately reflect current growth of children in various parts of the world (Tables 1 and 2).

Effects of Chemotherapy on the Pediatric Patient and the Physis
The effects of chemotherapy on the growing immature physis have been well documented in multiple studies demonstrating the negative transient effect of doxorubicin, methotrexate, and most of the other agents associated with current neoadjuvant protocols for sarcoma therapy in children. These agents typically affect chondrocytic proliferation in the proliferative zone. Although the effects may be transient, they are relatively immediate and are associated with decreased bone formation and an increased risk of fracture and other significant secondary bone effects.[6,12] Growth plate proliferation is affected by the direct effect of chemotherapy agents on the chondrocyte proliferation and by the depressive effects of chemotherapy and malnutrition on different regulatory pathways involving growth hormone-releasing hormone (GHRH), insulin-like growth factor 1 (IGF1), vitamin D, and alkaline phosphatase.[13] The authors of a 1993 study[14] examined distal femur growth plates of patients treated for osteosarcoma with neoadjuvant chemotherapy. They found

Table 1

Comparative Femoral Growth by Sex and Age

	Girls						Boys					
Age, y	6	8	10	12	14	16	6	8	10	12	14	16
Femoral length, cm	28.5	32.7	36.7	40.7	43.1	43.6	28.1	32.3	36.3	40.1	44.2	46.7
Growth, cm[a]	15.1	10.9	6.9	2.9	0.5	–	19.2	15.0	11.0	7.2	3.1	0.6
Growth, %[a]	34.6	25.0	15.8	6.7	1.2	–	40.6	38.7	23.3	15.2	6.6	1.3

[a]Compares difference with femoral length at 16 years of age for girls and 18 years for boys.[2]

Table 2

Predicted Leg-Length Discrepancy—Arithmetic Method[a]

	Girls							Boys						
Age, y	6	8	10	12	14	16	18	6	8	10	12	14	16	18
Distal femur growth remaining, cm	8.0	6.0	4.0	2.0	0.5	–	–	10.0	8.0	6.0	4.0	2.0	–	–
Proximal tibia growth remaining, cm	4.0	3.0	2.0	1.0	–	–	–	5.0	4.0	3.0	2.0	1.0	–	–
Total growth remaining, cm	12.0	9.0	6.0	3.0	0.5	–	–	15.0	12.0	9.0	6.0	3.0	–	–
Femur length, cm	28.5	32.7	36.7	40.7	43.1	43.6	43.6	28.1	32.3	36.3	40.1	44.2	46.7	47.3

[a]Assumes distal femur growth of 1.0 cm/y and proximal tibia growth of 0.5 cm/y; assumes growth ends at 14 years of age for girls and 16 years of age for boys.[7]

histologic evidence to support the presence of partial growth arrest, but confirmed that bone growth can resume after chemotherapy has ceased. Because current chemotherapy protocols for osteosarcoma and Ewing sarcoma involve chemotherapy agents that inhibit proliferating chondrocytes and reduce growth, better studies to assess the effects of chemotherapy and specific regimens are advised.[15,16]

Effects of Radiation Therapy on the Physis

The effects of radiation therapy at dosages given for osseous sarcoma may lead to a partial, if not complete, physeal compromise. These effects can occur even after moderate irradiation doses (20 Gy) in younger children and require longer follow-up and continuing assessments.[6] Radiation therapy is more commonly used for pediatric Ewing sarcoma and soft-tissue sarcomas than for osteosarcoma. The effects of radiation therapy on the growth plate have been well studied and include rapid and significant effects on the physis that are likely to be permanent, especially in younger children. Decreased skeletal growth is more evident when irradiation is used on patients younger than 10 years and is dose dependent.[17] Radiation therapy causes hypovascularity and cytotoxic effects in the chondrocyte population through downregulation. Cellular apoptosis increases, leading to decreased skeletal growth.[7,13] Radiation therapy to the axial skeleton appears to have an even greater effect on the spine and cranial axis

growth. Postoperative wound healing is affected by preoperative radiation therapy and has a well-established risk of complications involving at least 25% to 30% of adolescent and adult patients.[18]

Studies of radioprotectors involve mostly animal models, with only early preclinical work on patients. Amifostine and other radioprotectors (selenium, misoprostol) have shown protective effects on chondrocytic proliferation and subsequent longitudinal growth in animal models.[19] Radioprotectors are not currently in clinical use for pediatric sarcoma therapy.

Limb Salvage Surgery

Indication, Surgical Risk, Preoperative Assessment, and Obtaining Consent

The decision to perform limb salvage in a child younger than 10 years involves the need to accommodate skeletal growth or the appropriate selection and communication of alternative surgical solutions such as rotationplasty or amputation. Success with skeletal growth from an implant after a limb-sparing procedure is usually achieved with an expandable implant. These implants have historically had a relatively high failure rate in expansion that varies by the implant type, although greater success has been reported more recently.[20,21]

For children younger than 8 years, rotationplasty should be considered as an equal if not superior surgical option if the patient requires distal femoral physeal resection. Rotationplasty has been used for many years in Europe for most young patients with osseous sarcomas. In a rotationplasty procedure, tumor resection takes place in the distal femur or proximal tibia. The lower extremity, including the ankle, is rotated 180°, and the ankle serves as the new functioning knee; the gastrocnemius and soleus act as "knee" extensors, and the anterior leg muscles act as "knee" flexors. A prosthesis is fitted to the remaining foot and allows the extremity to function with remaining "knee" function[22-24] (**Figure 3**).

For patients 10 to 12 years of age, the decisions are more controversial, and surgical choices depend on patient age. Remaining growth in the lower extremity for this age group ranges from 2.9 to 6.9 cm for girls and from 7.2 to 11.0 cm for boys.[1,2] Patients older than 12 years have a lower extremity growth potential of approximately 3.0 cm (5.0%) for girls and approximately 6.0 cm (9.2%) for boys. These patients will have greater success with physeal arrest or expandable implants, and, as adolescents, are more likely to be resistant to the cosmetic issues of rotationplasty.[2]

Most important, pediatric limb salvage patients and their families should understand the surgical risks, required rehabilitation, and functional expectations (**Table 3**). The limitations involve restrictions during the postoperative period, the length of the postoperative rehabilitation time (allograft versus implant), and the permanent functional limitations associated with an implant or an allograft reconstruction. This understanding is critical in allowing for adequate bony healing and postoperative care that will assist with regaining function and avoiding joint stiffness.[25,26] In cases in which a limb salvage procedure is not possible, amputation should be considered as a treatment option if it can provide local control. Amputations avoid many of the leg-length issues of limb salvage and can allow for comparable or superior tumor control. Childhood amputations, however, also present challenges such as bony overgrowth and subsequent revision surgeries or difficult prosthetic fittings. Autogenous epiphyseal transplants harvested from the amputated limb, or osteochondral or synthetic caps placed over the residual limb's medullary canal, have reduced bone overgrowth complications.[27,28]

The preoperative consent process for limb salvage in children is demanding because parents have high expectations for their children. The consent process involves reviewing every detail of every complication, the length of recovery (allografts require 6 to 18 months to heal), and the expectations for growth and physical activity. Parents of limb salvage patients should be required to sign a surgical consent document that lists all complications item by item (**Table 3**). The majority of pediatric limb salvage patients in North America receive preoperative chemotherapy on a Children's Oncology Group protocol, and families receive abundant printed protocol information at the beginning of chemotherapy treatment.[15] They may expect similar preoperative in-

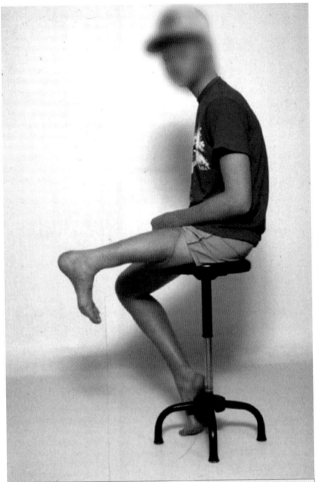

Figure 3 A patient who underwent rotationplasty demonstrates the matched height of the native knee and the ankle that serves as the new "knee" on the other side. Functionally, the gastrocnemius and soleus act as "knee" extensors, and the anterior leg muscles act as "knee" flexors. (Courtesy of Herbert S. Schwartz, MD, Nashville, TN.)

formation for the surgical treatment. Discussions about the procedure should be documented in the clinical notes over multiple visits, and a detailed copy of the reviewed information about the procedure and complications should be included in the medical record.

Postoperative complications include issues with (1) inadequate tumor control or margins, (2) possible neurovascular injury, (3) wound complications and revisions, (4) postoperative infections, (5) delayed healing, (6) loss of fixation (allograft) and implant failure, and (7) the need for additional procedures (**Table 3**). Amputation and death should also be documented as risks with all high-grade tumor patients. A fellow, resident, nurse, or social worker in the room can help facilitate and document the conversation. Older children should be present and engaged in discussions about the surgery and the postoperative plan and should be given the opportunity to have their questions answered. Also, parents who do not normally accompany the patient to

Table 3

Limb Salvage Complications

Possible Allograft Complications	Possible Oncologic Implant Complications
Wound complications (10%)—requires revision, incision and drainage, or washout and antibiotics	**Wound complications (10%)**—requires revision, incision and drainage, or washout and antibiotics
Deep infection (5% to 10%)—requires washout and/or possible graft removal or spacer and intravenous antibiotics	**Infection (5%)**—may develop deep infection and require washout or implant exchange and 6 to 12 weeks of intravenous antibiotics and revision
Fixation revision (10% to 20%)—required for graft fixation failure; usually associated with delayed union of graft	**Revision surgery (10%)**—for various implant failures
Possible nonunion or delayed union (10% to 20%)—at graft junction site	**Fixation problems (10% to 15%)**—aseptic loosening at stem requires revision
Tumor recurrence (5% to 10%)—usually requires amputation	**Tumor recurrence (5% to 10%)**—usually requires amputation
Joint stiffness (10% to 15%)—may require surgical manipulation or surgical release	**Joint stiffness (10% to 15%)**—may require surgical manipulation or surgical release
Neurovascular injury (10% to 15%)—usually peroneal nerve; usually recovers spontaneously	**Neurovascular injury (10% to 15%)**—usually peroneal nerve; usually recovers spontaneously
Contaminated surgical margins (5%)—documented in final pathology report and requires consideration of a second revision procedure	**Contaminated surgical margins (5%)**—documented in final pathology report and requires consideration of a second revision procedure
Chronic pain—variable and related to graft healing and patient	**Chronic pain**—variable and related to implant healing and patient
Limb-length discrepancy—dependent on age and growth plate status	**Limb-length discrepancy**—dependent on age and growth plate status
Second surgery (20% to 30%)—may be required for any of the preceding complications	**Second surgery (20% to 30%)**—may be required for any of the preceding complications

routine visits (such as those who are at work during doctor visits, or noncustodial parents) should be encouraged to participate in person for major discussions about surgery and its complications.

Managing Limb-Length Discrepancies

Many different methods are used to address limb-length discrepancy related to the treatment of pediatric sarcoma around the knee, including methods to address the problem more proactively as well as those that address the discrepancy later.[29]

Conservative Measures

The simplest method of addressing limb-length discrepancy is with a shoe lift. Shoe lifts are made in various sizes and are built into and onto a patient's shoes. Shoe lifts do not require surgical procedures but have limitations in how large a discrepancy they can correct; also, many patients may find them cosmetically unacceptable.

Intraoperative Lengthening

After tumor resection, the limb reconstruction can be done in a way that lengthens the limb a very limited amount through the placement of an implant or allograft that is longer than the resected bone. However, this method is limited to 5 to 15 mm of lengthening because of restrictions of the surrounding soft-tissue envelope and the neurovascular bundle.

Contralateral Epiphysiodesis

Arresting the physes of the contralateral leg is a good option for addressing ultimate limb-length discrepancy, regardless of the reconstructive procedures elected following the tumor resection. This method must be considered and performed before a child reaches skeletal maturity to allow continued growth of the remaining physes on the treated leg. Depending on the number of physes arrested and the timing of epiphysiodesis, a discrepancy of several centimeters can be addressed with this relatively small procedure, but at the expense of the child's overall height at skeletal maturity. Epiphyseodeses usually are performed 1 to 2 years after limb salvage in children 10 to 14 years of age.

Expandable Oncologic Endoprosthesis

Newer generations of expandable endoprostheses have been developed specifically to address the issue of limb-length discrepancy after limb salvage surgery. Earlier iterations of expandable implants required open surgical procedures to lengthen the implants, but newer versions can be lengthened using electromagnetic devices and noninvasive means. There are significant limits regarding how much these devices can lengthen (4 to 6 cm), and for some younger children, a revision to a second expandable implant may be necessary to fully address the ultimate limb-length discrepancy. Furthermore, many patients will also require revision to a

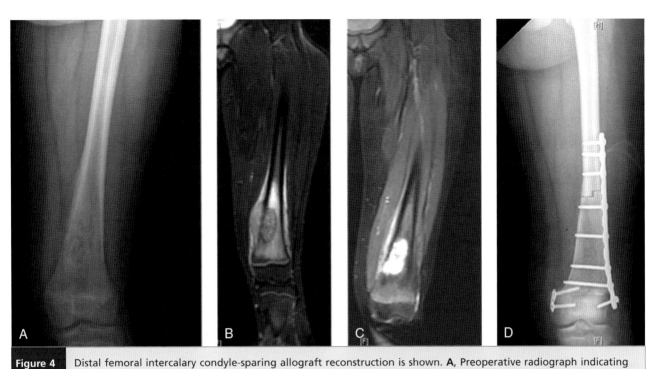

Figure 4 Distal femoral intercalary condyle-sparing allograft reconstruction is shown. **A,** Preoperative radiograph indicating osteosarcoma of the distal femur. **B,** Prechemotherapy staging MRI. **C,** Preoperative/postchemotherapy MRI showing focal response. **D,** Postoperative radiograph of intercalary condyle-sparing allograft.

standard adult-sized implant after reaching skeletal maturity or as a result of complications with the expandable implant.[20]

Distraction Osteogenesis

In patients for whom the discrepancy is projected to be greater than 2 cm and shortening of the contralateral limb is not desirable, distraction osteogenesis can be a consideration. Bone lengthening is accomplished with an osteotomy and gradual lengthening through the use of an Ilizarov-style external fixator. This procedure is largely limited by the amount of remaining viable bone that is suitable for distraction osteogenesis as well as the many potential complications. Distraction osteogenesis also requires a significant time commitment from both patient and provider because the procedure requires 6 to 12 months to complete. The entire course of lengthening requires multiple surgical procedures and a significant risk of pin sepsis and postoperative fractures. These risks are magnified in a patient undergoing chemotherapy, and the procedure has been infrequently used in pediatric sarcoma because of the complexity.[30]

Criteria for Adequate Bony Resection Margins

Adequate resection margins are the most important goal for a successful tumor resection procedure. Resections should be based on careful preoperative assessment of the response to preoperative chemotherapy. Careful review of MRI and positron emission tomography (PET) imaging should assess the extent of tumor

involvement, soft-tissue involvement, tumor inflammation, and proposed bony surgical margins. The assessment of the neoadjuvant chemotherapy response with a comparison of MRI and PET is an essential part of planning surgical margins in all patients, because a good response to chemotherapy can allow for closer surgical margins (**Figure 4**). In a tumor resection in the distal femur, the closest margin is typically at the distal femoral epiphysis or distal femoral condyles (**Figure 2**). Very close margins (<1.0 cm), however, are at higher risk for tumor contamination and subsequent tumor recurrence, whereas wide margins (≥ 1.0 cm) with a cuff of normal tissue are at less risk of tumor recurrence.[31] Evidence-based guidelines for determining the adequacy and quality of a tumor margin are limited, making the planning of margins a substantial challenge.

Evaluation of prechemotherapy and postchemotherapy imaging can make an important contribution to the assessment of tumor response and margin planning. On T2-weighted MRI, the increased signal surrounding the tumor indicates inflammation and edema at the tumor interface with surrounding tissues. With effective neoadjuvant therapy, this zone can disappear to form a thin tumor capsule that could allow for a closer margin of resection.[32] Increasing data on the assessment of treatment response to neoadjuvant chemotherapy and radiation therapy using fluorodeoxyglucose PET show that a significant decrease in tumor fluorodeoxyglucose uptake is predictive of survival.[33,]

Pediatric patients younger than 10 years are more likely to benefit from chemotherapy for osteosarcoma and Ewing sarcoma because they are more likely to have

6: Special Considerations in Tumor Management

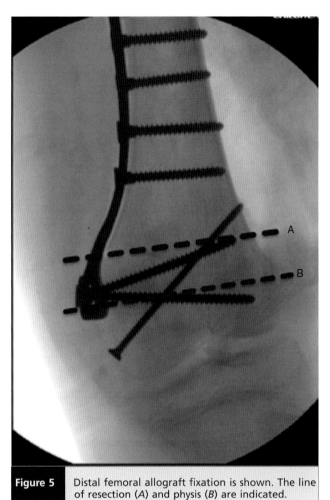

Figure 5 | Distal femoral allograft fixation is shown. The line of resection (*A*) and physis (*B*) are indicated.

a better treatment response than patients older than 14 years.[15] As a result, younger patients are more likely to be better candidates for narrower bony resection margins than patients who are in their mid-to-late teens.

Criteria for acceptable or successful bony margins are difficult to interpret from the literature.[34,35] The authors of a 2009 study[25] evaluated differences in margin width between condyle-sparing resections reconstructed with allografts and larger condylar resections reconstructed with endoprosthetic implants. In general, oncologic implant reconstructions had wider bony margins than the condyle-sparing and physeal-sparing procedures. Margins for intercalary allograft condyle-sparing resections ranged from 10 to 15 mm and were associated with a slightly higher incidence of local recurrence than margins for implants.

Allograft Versus Modular Oncologic Implants

Intercalary cadaveric allografts are used for physeal-sparing and condyle-sparing resections (**Figure 2**). Allografts are affixed to the remaining adjacent bone with a plate and screws or an intramedullary rod. If radiographic evidence of bony healing is not apparent at the osseous junction 8 to 10 months postoperatively, revi-

sion of fixation and autogenous bone grafting should be considered.[36] Plate fixation achieves better stability in the short term and more rapid allograft union but has a risk of late failure of the hardware. For physeal-sparing allografts that include distal fixation compressing or crossing the physis, this distal fixation should be removed 3 to 6 months postoperatively to allow for the potential resumption of physeal growth (**Figure 5**). Allograft incorporation usually requires anywhere from 6 to 18 months for evidence of radiographic healing, depending on the location (diaphyseal versus metaphyseal).

The incidence of revision for allograft complications ranges from 10% at 5 years to 30% at 10 years, with revision occurring most commonly for bony nonunions or fractures.[37-39] Painful allograft nonunions or fractures that have not yet healed at 12 to 18 months are unlikely to heal at the bony junction, and revision to an oncologic implant should be considered (**Figure 6**). Amputations are indicated for most tumor local recurrences and on rare occasions for allograft or neurovascular complications. Most limb salvage series demonstrate an overall risk of revision to amputation of approximately 5% to 10%.[40,41]

Modular oncologic implants are chosen for reconstruction of most osteoarticular or osteochondral resections involving the adjacent joint, because osteochondral allografts have a higher failure rate in the distal femur. Ligament instability (anterior cruciate ligament and medial collateral ligament) and poor cartilage viability are typical reasons for distal femoral osteochondral allograft failure and have led to a preference for implants. Oncologic implant reconstructions allow the patient to fully bear weight by 3 months postoperatively, whereas allograft reconstructions heal slowly and require weight-bearing restrictions for at least 6 to 12 months. Allografts also carry slightly higher infection and tumor recurrence risks[39-41]

Cemented or uncemented oncologic implant stems can be used to reconstruct osteoarticular or osteochondral resections; the use of uncemented stems has recently increased because of late failures with cemented implants. In North America, failure rates for oncologic implants are 10% to 15% at 5 years and 20% to 30% at 10 years. Most of these failures occur secondary to aseptic loosening at the stem. The risk of aseptic loosening is higher in children than in adults and appears in multiple series to be decreased with the use of uncemented stem techniques.[42]

Surgical Options—Age Versus Anatomic Location

Distal Femur Resections

Distal femur resections represent 50% to 60% of all osseous tumor procedures in most published series. These resections can be performed at one of three levels of the distal femur, and each requires varying methods of reconstruction (**Figure 2**). Physeal-sparing and condyle-sparing procedures involve reconstruction of the femur with a distal intercalary allograft (**Figure 7**). Osteoarticular reconstruction of the femur requires use of an oncologic total knee replacement. A physeal-sparing resection is of greatest significance to patients younger than 10 years, who may have a limb-length discrepancy of 6 to 8 cm, depending on the degree of skeletal immaturity. Intercalary allografts are the best reconstruction choice for physeal-sparing intercalary resections because the allograft can be tailored to fit the remaining bone and heals well to the adjacent distal femoral metaphysis and femoral condyles. Achieving fixation of the graft to the distal femoral condyles with minimal risk of arresting of the distal femoral physis is a challenge, requiring temporary crossing condylar screws or plate fixation with a temporary transverse epiphyseal screw (**Figure 5**).

Distal femur osteoarticular reconstruction is best achieved with a traditional oncologic distal femoral implant if the child is older than 12 years. If a patient is younger than 8 years, an expandable implant is a consideration, but carries a high risk for residual limb-length discrepancy and also the potential for chronic pain or stiffness. In patients 10 to 12 years of age, reconstruction with an expandable implant is easier than in their younger counterparts, depending on growth potential. Use of expandable implants requires that the patient and family understand that there may still be a need for contralateral epiphysiodesis to achieve more equal leg length and that expandable implants are at higher risk than traditional implants for failure or additional procedures.[43] The reliability and hardware durability of expandable implants has been suboptimal, with 50% to 75% of patients in many series left with more than 2 cm of length discrepancy and implant failures seen in more than 50% of patients.[20,44]

Rotationplasty Versus Expandable Implants

Rotationplasty is an excellent alternative to reconstructing a distal femur in patients younger than 8 to 10 years if the following criteria are met:

(1) The patient's distal femur tumor requires resection of the adjacent distal femoral physis.

(2) The patient and his or her parents are accepting of the cosmetic and psychologic issues of having a shortened limb with a reversed foot (watching videos of patients with rotationplasty, or, ideally, meeting a rotationplasty patient in person can greatly facilitate understanding of the procedure and its potential outcome) (**Figure 3**).

Rotationplasty is very durable and usually has postoperative function that approaches a below-knee amputation. Expandable oncology implants are an alternative to rotationplasty for patients younger than 10 years but need to be considered with an understanding that multiple surgical procedures will be required to achieve the expected lengthening goal.[23,24,45]

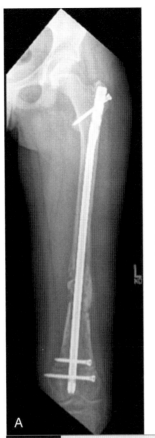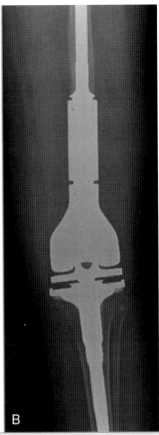

Figure 6 A failed distal femoral allograft (**A**) was revised to a distal femoral oncologic implant (**B**) secondary to allograft nonunion.

Proximal and Midshaft Femur Resections

Proximal femur Ewing sarcoma and osteosarcoma resections are reconstructed by using femoral implants or alloprosthetic composite implants with bipolar or total hip configurations. Postoperative hip dislocation risk can be minimized by the intimal use of a bipolar implant and careful gluteal reattachment to the greater trochanter with robust nonabsorbable surgical sutures or a cable grip system. Use of a synthetic sleeve wrapped around the implant (Dacron or GORE-TEX) is recommended to improve soft-tissue attachment to the implant. Suturing tendons directly onto the implant is often insufficient for long-term gluteal attachment. Loss of the gluteal attachment at the greater trochanter has been associated with greater risk of dislocation, abductor weakness, and a Trendelenburg gait.

Growth issues in the acetabulum are minimized by the fact that relatively early skeletal maturation occurs at the acetabular triradiate growth plate. The ischium, ilium, and pubis converge to create the triradiate growth plate, and they begin to fuse at 12 to 14 years of age. Interstitial growth of this cartilage accounts for the changes in acetabular height and width, whereas the femoral head influences the acetabular depth and cuplike shape.[1] Vertical growth and height achieved at

6: Special Considerations in Tumor Management

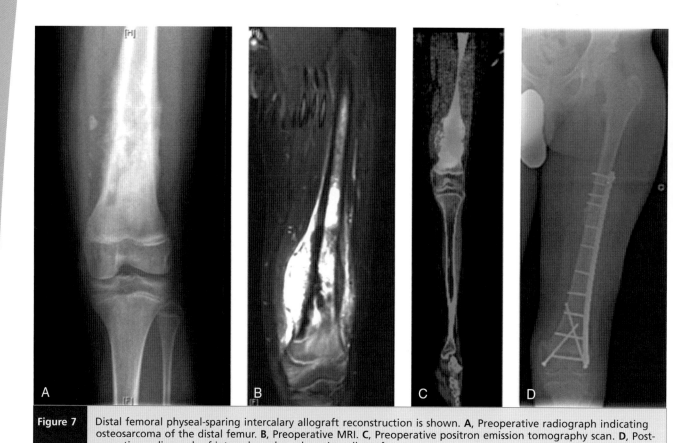

Figure 7 Distal femoral physeal-sparing intercalary allograft reconstruction is shown. **A,** Preoperative radiograph indicating osteosarcoma of the distal femur. **B,** Preoperative MRI. **C,** Preoperative positron emission tomography scan. **D,** Postoperative radiograph of intercalary physeal-sparing allograft.

the triradiate physis per year are not described in the literature. Surgical trauma can disrupt the triradiate growth plate, leading to disparate growth or deformity in the acetabulum and therefore increasing the risk for hip subluxation and the need for additional surgical interventions.[46]

Midshaft resections of the femur are the easiest to plan because they usually do not encroach upon an adjacent physis. These resections may be reconstructed with a locked intramedullary rod and intercalary femoral allograft. The ability to achieve interlocking fixation at the proximal and distal ends of the diaphyseal allograft with proximal and distal step cuts assists with rotational stability and bony healing. In patients younger than 10 years, diaphyseal resection of the femur or tibia can be reconstructed with an autogenous nonvascularized fibular graft with successful graft healing and remodeling to a relatively normal diaphyseal diameter and shape. Vascularized fibular grafts are an alternative reconstruction option for patients of any age but require 3 to 5 hours of additional surgical time to reconstruct a vascular blood supply for the bone graft. In older patients with longer (> 16 cm) resections, an intercalary allograft is a better choice for reconstruction because of the high incidence of vascularized autograft fracture, especially with grafts longer than 10 to 12 cm. Autogenous fibular grafts in younger patients should be harvested from the ipsilateral mid-

fibula, and the graft should not exceed 10 to 14 cm in length.

Proximal Tibial Resections

Proximal tibial resections for osteogenic sarcoma and Ewing sarcoma are best reconstructed with a proximal tibial allograft in patients younger than 12 years. A proximal tibial osteochondral allograft avoids disruption of the distal femoral physis and allows continued distal femoral growth. The patient's own menisci can be used to "resurface" the tibial allograft plateau, minimizing problems with graft chondrolysis. Ligament reconstructions should be carefully performed and protected by bracing for 6 months postoperatively to avoid joint laxity. Achieving bony healing with tibial allografts can occur more slowly than with femoral allografts because of a reduced blood supply in the tibial shaft, which should be protected with a patellar tendon-bearing knee brace for at least 6 to 12 months. Epiphyseal arrest of the contralateral leg should be done for all proximal tibial resections approximately 1 to 2 years after resection. Children with more than 2.0 cm of predicted shortening (boys younger than 10 years and girls younger than 8 years) even after contralateral epiphysiodesis should be considered for an expandable implant or rotationplasty. Proximal tibial resection and endoprosthetic reconstruction is the preferred reconstruction method in patients older than 12 years with a

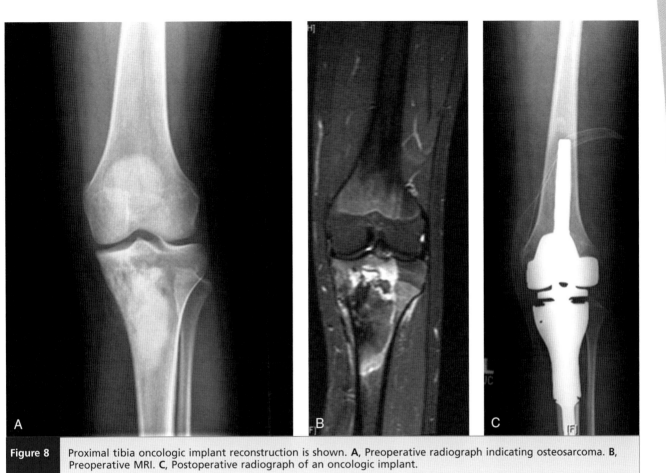

Figure 8 Proximal tibia oncologic implant reconstruction is shown. **A,** Preoperative radiograph indicating osteosarcoma. **B,** Preoperative MRI. **C,** Postoperative radiograph of an oncologic implant.

minimal predicted limb-length discrepancy (**Figure 8**). Those reconstructions carefully reattach the infrapatellar tendon to the oncologic implant with soft-tissue reinforcement with adjacent tibial fascia or a medial gastrocnemius rotational flap. Alloprosthetic implants represent a reasonable alternative for proximal tibial reconstruction but add allograft fractures as a risk.

Midshaft and Distal Tibial Resections

Midshaft and distal tibial resections are less common and are performed for both osteosarcoma and Ewing sarcoma. Plate fixation is preferred for most tibial allografts because of a need for superior graft fixation to achieve bony union in the tibia. A postoperative patellar tendon-bearing brace is strongly advised because of the need for prolonged protected weight bearing (6 to 12 months) in the tibia. Distal tibial allograft reconstruction can usually be achieved, but below-knee amputation often provides improved outcomes given the rate of allograft nonunion or postoperative infection in this location.

Humeral Resections

In patients younger than 10 years, humeral resections typically occur in the proximal humerus for either Ewing sarcoma or osteosarcoma, whereas distal humeral resections typically occur for Ewing sarcoma. Eighty percent of humeral growth occurs at the proximal

physis, and humeral length discrepancies after humeral resection are well tolerated without specific efforts to correct the subsequent discrepancy in length.[47]

Limb-length discrepancies of 4 cm or greater are better tolerated in the humerus than in the lower extremity and may not require attempts at lengthening. The reconstructive challenge with proximal humeral resections involves rotator cuff reattachment, which is often unsuccessful with tendon attachment directly onto the implant. Augmenting the reconstruction with a Dacron or GORE-TEX sleeve to the humeral head may lower the risk of shoulder instability and improve postoperative function. Muscle transfers (such as pectoralis or latissimus) have been described for rotator cuff deficiency, but have not gained popularity for oncologic reconstruction after proximal humeral resection.

Proximal humeral resection may also be performed with a resection that spares the articular surface and cuff attachments and employs an intercalary allograft (**Figure 9**). The humerus can be lengthened up to 1 cm at the time of reconstruction by using an allograft segment longer than the resected bone if the expected humeral length discrepancy is greater than 3 to 4 cm. Humeral discrepancies of 4 to 6 cm can occur in younger children (10 to 12 years of age) and, although not desirable, are tolerated well. As a general rule, contralateral humeral epiphysiodesis is not performed for upper

6: Special Considerations in Tumor Management

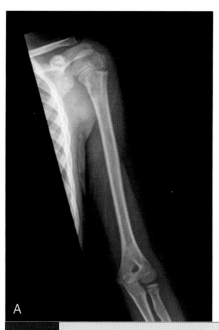
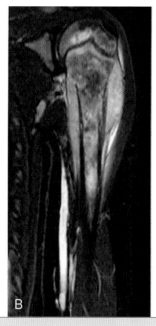
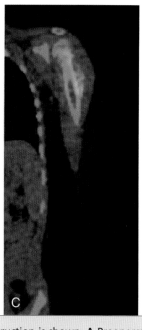
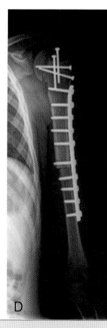

Figure 9   A proximal humerus articular-sparing intercalary allograft reconstruction is shown. **A** Preoperative radiograph indicating Ewing sarcoma. **B**, Preoperative MRI. **C**, Preoperative positron emission tomography (PET) scan. **D**, Postoperative radiograph of the intercalary articular-sparing allograft.

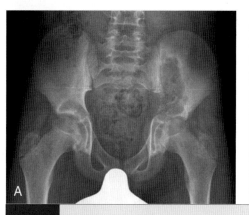
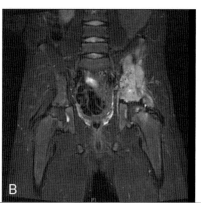
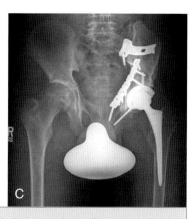

Figure 10   Allograft-prosthetic composite reconstruction of the left hemipelvis is shown. **A**, Preoperative radiograph indicating Ewing sarcoma of the left hemipelvis. **B**, Preoperative MRI. **C**, Postoperative radiograph of an allograft-prosthetic composite.

extremity length discrepancies. Distal humeral reconstruction in patients younger than 12 years is also well tolerated with minimal resultant limb-length discrepancy and can be accomplished with an osteochondral allograft or an oncologic total elbow implant. Total elbow oncology implants used for distal humeral resection require special implants, which have a high failure rate at the ulnar stem from aseptic loosening.

Pelvic Resections
Pelvic and sacral tumors represent the most challenging resections for osseous sarcomas. Pelvic involvement occurs in approximately 26% of patients with Ewing sarcoma and fewer than 10% of patients with osteosarcoma.[15,48] Local control with radiation therapy is an

option with Ewing sarcoma; however, surgical versus nonsurgical treatment of pelvic Ewing sarcoma remains an unresolved question without definitive scientific evidence to endorse either approach over the other.

Pelvic resections are well defined by the original Enneking classification (type I, posterior; type II, acetabulum; and type III, anterior obturator. Resections involving a crossover of these resection types are called combinations.)[49] The most significant factor predicting surgical challenges and higher complication rates is the inclusion of an acetabular resection (**Figure 10**). Complications vary by the type of resection, as do the length of surgery, the amount of surgical blood loss, and postoperative function. Choices of reconstruction range from no reconstruction (flail limb) to nonanatomic endoprosthetic implants (saddle prosthesis) or composite pelvic allograft/total hip combinations. The risks of postoperative infection (20% to 25%), local recurrence, neurovascular injury, and massive intraoperative blood loss are the most critical surgical risks.[50] The most crucial aspects of surgery are the control of the external iliac vessels during surgical exposure and perioperative blood loss. The lack of adequate large vessel control is associated with a higher risk of massive intraoperative hemorrhage and perioperative death.

Treatment of pelvic osteosarcoma has not routinely used adjuvant radiation therapy because it is relatively ineffective for this tumor subtype. However, Ewing sarcoma is a relatively radiosensitive tumor, and radiation therapy can be used preoperatively or postoperatively and even considered in lieu of surgery for local control. Growth issues do not preclude hemipelvic resections unless the patient is younger than 10 years. Patients younger than 10 years who require an acetabular resection for Ewing sarcoma should be considered for radiation therapy for local control, especially if they have demonstrated an excellent response to chemotherapy. Patients without a good response to neoadjuvant chemotherapy are poor candidates for nonsurgical local control and may require a hemipelvectomy to gain adequate tumor control. Nonsurgical therapy, however, carries a theoretically higher risk of local recurrence.

Future Directions/Summary

Future directions for the treatment of pediatric sarcoma patients include three promising areas for advancement: (1) improved assessment and confirmation of surgical margins, (2) development of more sophisticated oncologic implant and allograft reconstructions, and (3) improved methods to resume or reproduce skeletal growth. In the near future, improvements in the intraoperative assessment of surgical tumor margins could involve the ability to visualize more closely the adequacy of surgical margins. Immunofluorescence imaging techniques or other intraoperative real-time assessment tools of critical tumor margins will facilitate that process. Integration of quantitative MRI and PET may also allow for assessment of tumor cell viability at the margins of resection, and current studies are investigating the role of intraoperative navigation systems in the planning and attainment of adequate surgical margins.[51] New pediatric oncologic implants should allow for the successful reattachment of the rotator cuff, gluteal muscles, and patellar tendon to improve postoperative functional incomes and activity potential. As technology continues to advance, the options for robust expandable implants that allow for lengthening over time should improve. Ideally, these implants should allow for modularity, large growth capacity, noninvasive lengthening, and durability that meets or exceeds current adult oncologic implants. A biologic alternative for compensating for lost physeal growth could include the use of transplanted physeal cartilage if techniques to preserve and stimulate donor chondrocytes can be perfected. Biologic techniques could also become useful in augmenting diaphyseal allograft reconstructions. One example would be a collagen matrix incorporating osteoblastic stem cells to be used in conjunction with allografts to allow for bony union within 3 to 4 months rather than 6 to 12 months.

Limb salvage for sarcoma patients gained popularity in the 1970s and 1980s with the success of chemotherapy regimens. Although adult surgical resections have shown good success, the focus is now on developing better reconstruction options for children. The greatest challenges remaining in pediatric oncologic limb salvage currently involve improvements in perioperative imaging and developments in expandable implants and more durable reconstructions. With advances in technology and biologic research, these improvements will likely be accomplished in the near future.

Annotated References

1. Dimeglio A: Growth in pediatric orthopaedics. *J Pediatr Orthop* 2001;21(4):549-555.

2. Anderson M, Messner MB, Green WT: Distribution of lengths of the normal femur and tibia in children from one to eighteen years. *J Bone Joint Surg Am* 1964;46:1197-1202.

3. Pichler K, Schmidt B, Fischerauer EE, et al: Behaviour of human physeal chondro-progenitorcells in early growth plate injury response in vitro. *Int Orthop* 2012;36(9):1961-1966.

   This article provides an account of growth plate response to injury and proposed inflammation mechanisms of action after injury. Level of evidence: III.

4. Olsen BR, Reginato AM, Wang W: Bone development. *Annu Rev Cell Dev Biol* 2000;16:191-220.

5. Karp SJ, Schipani E, St-Jacques B, Hunzelman J, Kronenberg H, McMahon AP: Indian hedgehog coordinates endochondral bone growth and morphogenesis via parathyroid hormone related-protein-dependent and -independent pathways. *Development* 2000;127(3):543-548.

6. van Leeuwen BL, Kamps WA, Jansen HW, Hoekstra HJ: The effect of chemotherapy on the growing skeleton. *Cancer Treat Rev* 2000;26(5):363-376.

7. Wattenbarger JM, Gruber HE, Phieffer LS: Physeal fractures, part I: Histologic features of bone, cartilage, and bar formation in a small animal model. *J Pediatr Orthop* 2002;22(6):703-709.

8. Menelaus MB: Correction of leg length discrepancy by epiphysial arrest. *J Bone Joint Surg Br* 1966;48(2):336-339.

9. Green WT, Anderson M: Experiences with epiphyseal arrest in correcting discrepancies in length of the lower extremities in infantile paralysis; a method of predicting the effect. *J Bone Joint Surg Am* 1947;29(3):659-675.

10. Paley D, Bhave A, Herzenberg JE, Bowen JR: Multiplier method for predicting limb-length discrepancy. *J Bone Joint Surg Am* 2000;82-A(10):1432-1446.

11. Moseley CF: A straight-line graph for leg-length discrepancies. *J Bone Joint Surg Am* 1977;59(2):174-179.

12. Glasser DB, Duane K, Lane JM, Healey JH, Caparros-Sison B: The effect of chemotherapy on growth in the skeletally immature individual. *Clin Orthop Relat Res* 1991;262:93-100.

13. Krasin MJ, Constine LS, Friedman DL, Marks LB: Radiation-related treatment effects across the age spectrum: Differences and similarities or what the old and young can learn from each other. *Semin Radiat Oncol* 2010;20(1):21-29.

    The authors compared and contrasted radiation effects across different organ systems in both children and adults. Level of evidence: III.

14. Bar-On E, Beckwith JB, Odom LF, Eilert RE: Effect of chemotherapy on human growth plate. *J Pediatr Orthop* 1993;13(2):220-224.

15. Hawkins DS, Bölling T, Dubois S, et al: Ewing's sarcoma, in Poplack D, Pizzo PA (eds): *Principles and Practice of Pediatric Oncology*, ed 6. Philadelphia, PA, Lippincott Williams & Wilkins, 2010, pp 87-1014.

    The authors of this chapter outlined the current treatment approaches and reconstruction techniques used for pediatric patients with Ewing sarcoma.

16. Messerschmitt PJ, Garcia RM, Abdul-Karim FW, Greenfield EM, Getty PJ: Osteosarcoma. *J Am Acad Orthop Surg* 2009;17(8):515-527.

    The authors described treatment and surgical options for patients with osteosarcoma. Level of evidence: IV.

17. Margulies BS, Horton JA, Wang Y, Damron TA, Allen MJ: Effects of radiation therapy on chondrocytes in vitro. *Calcif Tissue Int* 2006;78(5):302-313.

18. O'Sullivan B, Davis AM, Turcotte R, et al: Preoperative versus postoperative radiotherapy in soft-tissue sarcoma of the limbs: A randomised trial. *Lancet* 2002;359(9325):2235-2241.

19. Damron TA, Spadaro JA, Horton JA, Margulies BS, Strauss JA, Farnum CE: Novel radioprotectant drugs for sparing radiation-induced damage to the physis. *Int J Radiat Biol* 2004;80(3):217-228.

20. Henderson ER, Pepper AM, Marulanda G, Binitie OT, Cheong D, Letson GD: Outcome of lower-limb preservation with an expandable endoprosthesis after bone tumor resection in children. *J Bone Joint Surg Am* 2012;94(6):537-547.

    The authors described good functional outcome rates with expandable endoprostheses; however, high revision rates remain a central issue for this reconstructive method. Level of evidence: IV.

21. Saghieh S, Abboud MR, Muwakkit SA, Saab R, Rao B, Haidar R: Seven-year experience of using Repiphysis expandable prosthesis in children with bone tumors. *Pediatr Blood Cancer* 2010;55(3):457-463.

    The authors analyzed their experience with the Repiphysis expandable prosthesis, describing outcomes and complications. High complication rates are experienced, but achieving comparable leg length in both extremities has been relatively successful. Level of evidence: IV.

22. Forni C, Gaudenzi N, Zoli M, et al: Living with rotationplasty—quality of life in rotationplasty patients from childhood to adulthood. *J Surg Oncol* 2012;105(4):331-336.

    The authors analyzed the Mental Component Summary scale and quality of life scores for adults who underwent rotationplasty for osteosarcoma as children compared to controls. Level of evidence: III.

23. Van Nes CP: Rotation-plasty for congenital defects of the femur: Making use of the ankle of the shortened limb to control the knee joint of a prosthesis. *J Bone Joint Surg Br* 1950;32-B(1):12-16.

24. Taminiau AH, Van der Eijken JW, Van Bockel JH, Sobotka MR, Obermann WR, Taconis WK: *New Developments for Limb Salvage in Musculoskeletal Tumors*. Tokyo, Japan, Springer-Verlag, 1989, pp 133-152.

25. Zimel MN, Cizik AM, Rapp TB, Weisstein JS, Conrad EU III: Megaprosthesis versus Condyle-sparing intercalary allograft: Distal femoral sarcoma. *Clin Orthop Relat Res* 2009;467(11):2813-2824.

    The authors compared the use of allografts to modular oncologic implants and found that at 2, 5, and 10 years, both groups experienced similar risk of local tumor recurrence. Level of evidence: IV.

26. Morgan HD, Cizik AM, Leopold SS, Hawkins DS, Conrad EU III: Survival of tumor megaprostheses replacements about the knee. *Clin Orthop Relat Res* 2006;450(450):39-45.

27. Tenholder M, Davids JR, Gruber HE, Blackhurst DW: Surgical management of juvenile amputation overgrowth with a synthetic cap. *J Pediatr Orthop* 2004;24(2):218-226.

28. Benevenia J, Makley JT, Leeson MC, Benevenia K: Primary epiphyseal transplants and bone overgrowth in childhood amputations. *J Pediatr Orthop* 1992;12(6):746-750.

29. Stanitski DF: Limb-length inequality: Assessment and

treatment options. *J Am Acad Orthop Surg* 1999;7(3): 143-153.

30. McCoy TH Jr, Kim HJ, Cross MB, et al: Bone tumor reconstruction with the Ilizarov method. *J Surg Oncol* 2013;107(4):343-352.

    The authors summarized their experience with the Ilizarov method of distraction osteogenesis for limb reconstruction after tumor resection. Level of evidence: IV.

31. Rougraff BT, Simon MA, Kneisl JS, Greenberg DB, Mankin HJ: Limb salvage compared with amputation for osteosarcoma of the distal end of the femur: A long-term oncological, functional, and quality-of-life study. *J Bone Joint Surg Am* 1994;76(5):649-656.

32. Fernebro J, Wiklund M, Jonsson K, et al: Focus on the tumour periphery in MRI evaluation of soft tissue sarcoma: Infiltrative growth signifies poor prognosis. *Sarcoma* 2006;2006:21251.

33. Eary JF, O'Sullivan F, Powitan Y, et al: Sarcoma tumor FDG uptake measured by PET and patient outcome: A retrospective analysis. *Eur J Nucl Med Mol Imaging* 2002;29(9):1149-1154.

34. Ozaki T, Hillmann A, Hoffmann C, et al: Significance of surgical margin on the prognosis of patients with Ewing's sarcoma: A report from the Cooperative Ewing's Sarcoma Study. *Cancer* 1996;78(4):892-900.

35. Gherlinzoni F, Picci P, Bacci G, Campanacci D: Limb sparing versus amputation in osteosarcoma: Correlation between local control, surgical margins and tumor necrosis. Istituto Rizzoli experience. *Ann Oncol* 1992; 3(suppl 2):S23-S27.

36. Dubousset J, Missenard G, Kalifa CH: Management of osteogenic sarcoma in children and adolescents. *Clin Orthop Relat Res* 1991;270:52-59.

37. Frisoni T, Cevolani L, Giorgini A, Dozza B, Donati DM: Factors affecting outcome of massive intercalary bone allografts in the treatment of tumours of the femur. *J Bone Joint Surg Br* 2012;94(6):836-841.

    The authors reviewed patients with femoral tumors reconstructed with allografts and reported outcomes and complications. Level of evidence: IV.

38. Ogilvie CM, Crawford EA, Hosalkar HS, King JJ, Lackman RD: Long-term results for limb salvage with osteoarticular allograft reconstruction. *Clin Orthop Relat Res* 2009;467(10):2685-2690.

    The authors reviewed extremity osteoarticular allograft reconstructions and evaluated function and complication rates. Level of evidence: IV.

39. Mankin HJ, Gebhardt MC, Jennings LC, Springfield DS, Tomford WW: Long-term results of allograft replacement in the management of bone tumors. *Clin Orthop Relat Res* 1996;324:86-97.

40. Campanacci L, Manfrini M, Colangeli M, Alí N, Mercuri M: Long-term results in children with massive bone osteoarticular allografts of the knee for high-grade osteosarcoma. *J Pediatr Orthop* 2010;30(8): 919-927.

    The authors reviewed pediatric high-grade osteosarcoma cases, which were treated with resection and reconstructed with an osteoarticular allograft. With good function outcomes and an acceptable graft survival at 5 years, the authors concluded that allografts may represent a viable reconstruction option. Level of evidence: IV.

41. Scharschmidt T, Cohen A, Thomas N, Ching R, Conrad E: Torsional stability of uncemented femoral stems in oncologic reconstructions. *Orthopedics* 2011; 34(2):96.

    The authors evaluated initial stability of stem design by torsional load to failure through the use of image analysis. Level of evidence: III.

42. Muscolo DL, Ayerza MA, Aponte-Tinao LA: Survivorship and radiographic analysis of knee osteoarticular allografts. *Clin Orthop Relat Res* 2000;373:73-79.

43. Futani H, Minamizaki T, Nishimoto Y, Abe S, Yabe H, Ueda T: Long-term follow-up after limb salvage in skeletally immature children with a primary malignant tumor of the distal end of the femur. *J Bone Joint Surg Am* 2006;88(3):595-603.

44. Schindler OS, Cannon SR, Briggs TW, Blunn GW: Stanmore custom-made extendible distal femoral replacements: Clinical experience in children with primary malignant bone tumours. *J Bone Joint Surg Br* 1997;79(6):927-937.

45. Veenstra KM, Sprangers MA, van der Eyken JW, Taminiau AH: Quality of life in survivors with a Van Ness-Borggreve rotationplasty after bone tumour resection. *J Surg Oncol* 2000;73(4):192-197.

46. Bucholz RW, Ezaki M, Ogden JA: Injury to the acetabular triradiate physeal cartilage. *J Bone Joint Surg Am* 1982;64(4):600-609.

47. Pritchett JW: Growth plate activity in the upper extremity. *Clin Orthop Relat Res* 1991;268:235-242.

48. Marina N, Gebhardt M, Teot L, Gorlick R: Biology and therapeutic advances for pediatric osteosarcoma. *Oncologist* 2004;9(4):422-441.

49. Enneking WF, Dunham W, Gebhardt MC, Malawar M, Pritchard DJ: A system for the functional evaluation of reconstructive procedures after surgical treatment of tumors of the musculoskeletal system. *Clin Orthop Relat Res* 1993;286:241-246.

50. Angelini A, Drago G, Trovarelli G, Calabrò T, Ruggieri P: Infection after surgical resection for pelvic bone tumors: An analysis of 270 patients from one institution. *Clin Orthop Relat Res* 2013 Aug 24 [Epub

ahead of print].

The authors evaluated the frequency of infection after the resection of pelvic bone tumors with and without reconstruction. They found that infection remains a common complication of pelvic resections and occurs more frequently in the reconstructed pelvis. Level of evidence: IV.

51. Ieguchi M, Hoshi M, Takada J, Hidaka N, Nakamura H: Navigation-assisted surgery for bone and soft tissue tumors with bony extension. *Clin Orthop Relat Res* 2012;470(1):275-283.

The authors evaluated the accuracy and the efficiency of surgical navigation for limb salvage surgery and concluded that when used in conjunction with skin fiducial markers, this computer system helped surgeons achieve reliable and accurate resections. Level of evidence: IV.

Chapter 44

Amputations

Kurt R. Weiss, MD   Richard L. McGough III, MD   Mark A. Goodman, MD

Introduction

Before the advent of modern medical and surgical oncologic treatments, amputation was the only surgical option thought to provide acceptable pathologic margins for bone and soft-tissue tumors. Advances in orthopaedic surgery, oncology, radiology, and pathology have produced better systemic oncologic treatments, modular reconstruction systems, and more precise measurements of disease burden. These factors have contributed to the dramatic increase in the prevalence of limb-sparing surgery.[1] However, in many instances, amputation of the affected limb is the safest and most reasonable surgical option. This chapter explores fundamental concepts of amputation in the setting of orthopaedic oncology. After a review of nomenclature and indications, upper extremity and lower extremity amputations are discussed. Finally, a practical discussion on postoperative management of patients who have undergone amputation will provide the reader with tools to encourage the patient's physical and psychological adaptation.

Nomenclature

Amputations should be described on the basis of the anatomic structure(s) transected during the procedure. For example, transtibial is preferable to below-the-knee, and transhumeral is preferable to above-the-elbow. Technically, a transmetatarsal amputation is below the knee and a forequarter amputation is above the elbow. Both of these examples illustrate that incomplete descriptions of the amputation level can be misleading. Second, the use of the word stump should be discouraged as a descriptor of the most distal portion of the remaining limb. Physical medicine and rehabilitation physicians, prosthetists, and physical therapists are all accustomed to using the term residual limb.[2] This far more accurate and sensitive term should be embraced by orthopaedic surgeons as well.

Dr. Weiss or an immediate family member serves as an unpaid consultant to Eleison Pharmaceuticals. Neither of the following authors nor any immediate family member has received anything of value from or has stock or stock options held in a commercial company or institution related directly or indirectly to the subject of this chapter: Dr. McGough and Dr. Goodman.

Indications

The author of a 1991 article[3] suggested four questions that guide the decision of whether limb-sparing surgery or amputation is the most appropriate for a particular patient: (1) Will survival be the same? (2) How do immediate and late complications compare? (3) How does function compare? (4) Does limb-sparing surgery impart improved psychosocial/quality-of-life outcomes? This last question is revisited at the end of the chapter, but the first three can be used to build a framework for decision making. Generally, indications for amputation surgery fall into three general categories: anatomic, reconstructive, or palliative.

Anatomic indications include instances when a malignant process involves major neurovascular structures that preclude reconstruction and/or the ability to achieve acceptable oncologic margins. Common areas where this occurs include the popliteal fossa, the antecubital fossa, the brachial plexus, and the sciatic notch. Reconstructive indications are encountered when postoperative function is expected to be superior with amputation compared with limb salvage. The most common examples of this indication are with tumors of the foot and ankle. Because of this area's comparatively small volume, malignant lesions tend to obliterate the typical anatomic barriers to tumor growth. The functional demands of the foot and ankle (stability, durability, functional weight bearing) are often better served with amputation than with limb salvage.[4,5] Finally, amputations may be performed for palliative reasons. The patient's disease may be voluminous or advanced to the point where a limb-sparing procedure is impractical. For example, a patient with widely metastatic carcinoma and debilitating pain may benefit more from an amputation than from an extensive limb-sparing procedure from which the patient will derive little functional gain (**Figure 1**).

General Surgical Considerations

Regardless of the site of the amputation, some general principles apply to all patients. Appropriate oncologic margins are the first priority in any musculoskeletal oncology procedure. Major vessels should be ligated twice to prevent catastrophic blood loss. Similarly, if a tourniquet is used, it should be deflated, and meticulous hemostasis should be obtained before closure. The liberal

6: Special Considerations in Tumor Management

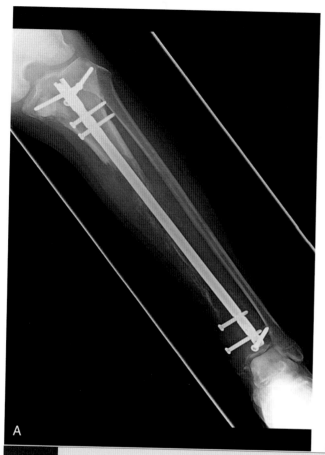
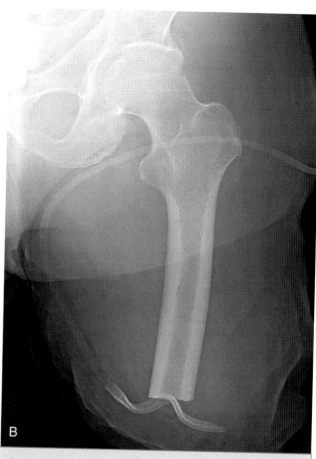

Figure 1 **A,** The tibia of a patient with metastatic renal cancer is shown. Despite initial rigid fixation with adequate bone stock, chemotherapy, and irradiation, the patient's disease and pain progressed dramatically. **B,** The patient underwent a palliative transfemoral amputation and experienced substantial pain relief.

use of drains should be encouraged.[5,6] These measures will help decrease the incidence of hematoma formation and wound complications. Large nerves should be ligated to avoid bleeding from the vasa nervorum, which can be quite large. Nerves should be gently retracted, cut with a fresh blade, and allowed to retract into the proximal soft tissues. Infiltration of large peripheral nerves with local anesthesia may help with postoperative pain control. Finally, and perhaps most important, meticulous soft-tissue handling is essential for a successful amputation outcome and a functional residual limb. Skin and soft-tissue flaps should be carefully planned and constructed. If necessary, a plastic and reconstructive surgery consultation should be obtained. Flaps should be kept as thick as possible without excessive dissection. It is essential that wounds be closed without undue tension on the soft tissues. This point is of heightened importance in patients with malignancy, many of whom require postoperative chemotherapy and/or radiation therapy treatments. A wound complication can delay essential adjuvants, and an improperly constructed amputation flap might not withstand the rigors of adjuvant therapy.

Upper Extremity Amputations

As with tumors in other anatomic locations, modern orthopaedic implants, microvascular techniques, and nerve grafting have encouraged limb-sparing surgery in the upper extremity. However, amputation as a primary oncologic procedure still plays a prominent role in the treatment of upper extremity tumors.

Hand

The hand is a common location for primary and secondary malignant tumors and benign-aggressive lesions. Metastatic disease, although more common in the lower extremity, can also occur in the hand. Examples of primary and secondary malignant tumors, benign-aggressive lesions, and metastatic disease include, respectively, epithelioid sarcoma, secondary chondrosarcoma, giant cell tumor, and metastatic lung cancer. Adequate ablation and disease-free margins are always the primary concern, whereas preservation of anatomy and restoration of function are secondary considerations. Metallic implants for the hand are limited, but microvascular transfers can sometimes obviate the need for amputation.

Phalangeal tumors, or tumors involving the soft tissue overlying the phalanges, are treated with disarticulation or amputation proximal to the tumor, allowing for adequate bone and/or soft-tissue margins. In most patients the healing potential of the hand is excellent. Fish-mouth incisions are useful distal to the metacarpophalangeal joints.[7] They are easy to design and tend to heal well while preserving some degree of palmar sensitivity. The metacarpophalangeal joints do not accommodate fish-mouth incisions, so palmar or dorsal "racquet" incisions are more useful. Soft-tissue flaps based on either the radial or ulnar neurovascular bundles are very serviceable, but only if the tumor resection will allow for clear margins. Tumors involving the index ray or phalanges are best treated by ray resection. The pinch function of the index finger is easily taken over by the long finger, so complex reconstruction of the index finger is misguided. Resections of the distal phalanx of the thumb leave a useful digit and do not require further reconstruction, although prostheses have been made for this resection level. Amputations of the proximal phalanx of the thumb have been treated with microvascular toe-to-hand transfer with good results.[8] Patients accommodate well to the absence of one thumb and do not always require this complex reconstruction.

More proximal tumors of the metacarpal rays and soft tissues are treated by ray amputation. This procedure removes the ray and soft tissues back to the carpal articulation. Multiple rays can be resected at one time to obtain good tumor margins. Preserving two rays may yield a good functional result. Keeping the fourth and fifth rays will allow for power grip with the involved hand, although pinch grip is sacrificed. Conversely, keeping the thumb and index rays will permit normal pinch grip but limited power grip. The authors of a 2010 study described their success with double ray amputations.[9] Although functionally inferior to single ray amputations, the authors reported that key, tip, and tripod pinch could be preserved, and the operated hand was able to assist in bimanual activities. A hand with a lobster claw composed of the first and fifth rays can be useful for moderate pinch and power grip and is clearly useful. Restoration of the thumb ray by vascular transplant can be helpful but should be avoided in cases in which the thenar musculature is resected with the tumor. Patients can accommodate thumb loss despite conventional teachings.

Wrist Disarticulation

For tumors involving the entire hand, tumors that have recurred despite adequate initial surgery, and proximal hand tumors, wrist disarticulation is the amputation of choice. Anterior and posterior flaps work very well. Amputation is performed through the radiocarpal articulation. No benefit is derived from leaving carpal bones, because these can contract into a disadvantageous position. Pronation and supination of the forearm is preserved through the distal radioulnar joint and

the forearm musculature. A standard transforearm prosthesis can be very functional. The ultimate length of the arm with the prosthesis is longer than the uninvolved side, but this result produces neither functional nor cosmetic problems (as it would in the lower extremity). Sophisticated myoelectric hands are in development and may hold promise of a more normal functional outcome at this level.

Forearm

The function regained when an amputation is done below the elbow but proximal to the wrist (transforearm) is dependent on residual limb length and remaining muscular attachments. Very long residual forearms have nearly full pronation and supination and a large contact area to support a prosthesis. At the midforearm, the pronator quadratus and a portion of the pronator teres are sacrificed, and some pronation strength is therefore lost. The amputation is usually done with dorsal and volar flaps and can usually accommodate the sleeve and harness of a transforearm prosthesis. The remaining pronator teres and the biceps brachii provide some active rotation of the forearm. When the tumor demands amputation of the proximal third of the forearm, rotation is lost. Elbow flexion and extension are preserved, and rotation of the forearm is replaced by manipulation at the terminal end of the prosthesis. A Muenster-type prosthesis with epicondylar support is often needed with proximal transforearm amputations. Disarticulation at the elbow is functionally superior to a very proximal transforearm amputation, because flexion contracture can be problematic. Myoelectric prostheses are functional at this level of amputation but tend to respond slowly and are heavy to wear. Researchers recently reported a prosthesis with independent finger movement that is still in development.[10] The more conventional sling harness prostheses with either active opening or active closing terminal devices tend to be more widely accepted and used. They are extremely durable and therefore spend more time being worn and less time in the repair shop. Many individuals who have undergone transforearm amputation use their residual forearm as a post and their elbow as a vise grip and elect not to wear a prosthesis. As long as elbow flexion is maintained, these individuals can be quite facile at carrying objects in this manner (**Figure 2**).

Elbow Disarticulation

Elbow disarticulation is a simple, relatively bloodless upper extremity amputation. Triceps-based or anterior skin flaps are durable and heal nicely. Prosthetic considerations are the same as those for a transhumeral amputation, accepting a limb length inequality at the elbow. This result is not usually seen as a significant cosmetic deformity.

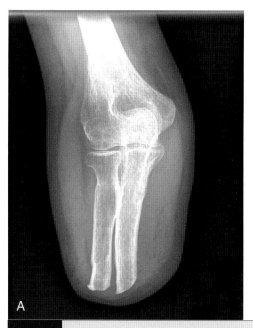
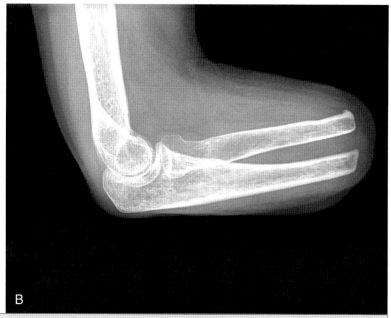

Figure 2 AP (**A**) and lateral (**B**) radiographs after proximal transforearm amputation are shown. This patient prefers not to use a prosthesis. The patient works in the healthcare profession and is extremely functional.

Humerus

Tumors of the elbow or distal arm can be managed with transhumeral amputation. Anterior (elbow flexor) and posterior (elbow extensor) muscle groups can undergo myodesis, and shoulder function is retained. Longer anterior or posterior flaps can be designed to accommodate tumor resection. Function is significantly better in patients whose deltoid insertion is preserved. Amputations of the proximal third of the humerus result in very limited independent function and are functionally shoulder disarticulations. They result in muscle contractures secondary to functional muscle imbalance. Prostheses for patients with transhumeral amputation are problematic largely because of gravity. Intimate fit of the residual humerus within the prosthesis is difficult to accomplish, but without it, the ability to move two articulating joints is very challenging. Many prostheses have elbow positions that are set manually, and only the terminal device is active. Myoelectric prostheses are in various stages of development but still have weight and stability problems. Direct endoskeletal attachment with osseointegration has been performed and shows great promise[11] but is still experimental.

Shoulder Disarticulation and Forequarter Amputation

When the shoulder girdle is involved with a process requiring amputation, a decision must be made between shoulder disarticulation and forequarter amputation. If the deltoid can be preserved as a flap and the glenohumeral joint is not directly involved, shoulder disarticulation is the procedure of choice. The deltoid is elevated, preserving its posterior neurovascular bundle, and the skin of the axilla is cut transversely, creating

superior and inferior flaps. A lymph node dissection can be done at this time as well, provided the vascular supply to the deltoid is not sacrificed. If the humeral head is not involved, transecting the surgical neck and leaving the head in situ is preferable. This method leaves a more cosmetic shoulder such that wearing a shirt or blouse is easier, more comfortable, and more natural appearing (**Figure 3**). Flap closure is not compromised by this preservation. Functional prostheses at this level are cumbersome, but many patients find a cosmetic arm to be of benefit.

Forequarter amputation is the ablation of the entire upper extremity. Clavicle, scapula, and arm all are resected en bloc. The deep plane of dissection is the chest wall. Anteriorly based flaps use the pectoralis major as the primary muscle for closure, whereas posteriorly the trapezius is used. The type of flap is often dictated by the location of the tumor. The resection of the involved ribs and chest wall can be combined with this amputation.[12] The cosmetic result is a severe slope from the neck to the abdomen (**Figure 4**). This result makes wearing clothes difficult, and a static, cosmetic shoulder pad is usually fabricated and worn by the patient to assist with cosmesis.

Flaps

Free and pedicled soft-tissue flaps have the potential to modify the level and functionality of upper extremity amputations.[13,14] Soft-tissue tumors may not require bone resection, but higher levels of amputation are often dictated by the lack of soft tissue for closure. If a microvascular surgeon is available, it may be feasible to manipulate soft-tissue flaps to achieve a more functional level of amputation. For several forequarter am-

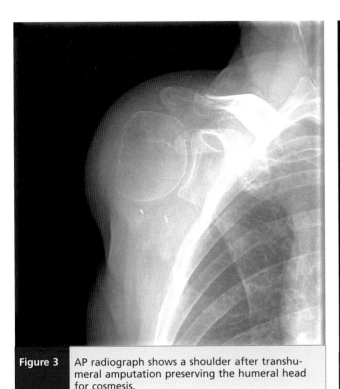

Figure 3 AP radiograph shows a shoulder after transhumeral amputation preserving the humeral head for cosmesis.

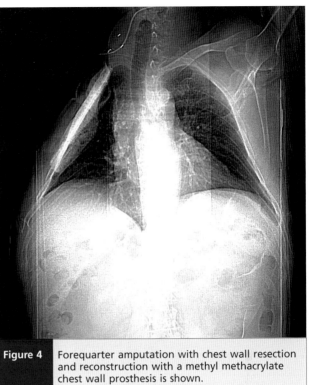

Figure 4 Forequarter amputation with chest wall resection and reconstruction with a methyl methacrylate chest wall prosthesis is shown.

putations, the authors of this chapter have used the uninvolved forearm of the ipsilateral side for a free muscle and skin transfer in the manner described by the authors of a 1998 article[15] and have found this ingenious "fillet flap" technique to be of great benefit.

Lower Extremity Amputations

Lower extremity amputations are commonly performed for malignancy, and amputation remains an important procedure in this setting.[16] In general, postoperative functional deficits are directly proportional to the volume of tissue removed, and the energy expenditure of ambulation increases incrementally from distal amputations (phalanges) to more proximal levels (hip disarticulation or hemipelvectomy). Amputations distal to the midfoot do not substantially increase the metabolic requirement of ambulation. Hindfoot amputations increase this cost by approximately 15%, transtibial amputations increase it by approximately 25%, transfemoral amputations increase it by approximately 75%, and hip disarticulations or hemipelvectomies increase it by approximately 200%.[17,18]

Phalanges
Toe amputations in musculoskeletal oncology are unusual, and most literature on this subject consists of case reports. Toe amputations are generally well tolerated without functional deficit or the need for shoe modification. The notable exception to this trend is the great toe, which is important in push-off strength in

quick walking and running. If oncologically feasible, it is preferable from a functional standpoint to amputate distal to the base of the proximal phalanx, because this procedure will preserve the flexor hallucis brevis insertion and improve stability. If the entire hallux must be removed, a shoe insert and rigid foot plate may be required for ambulation and shoe comfort.[5,6,18]

Ray Resection
Malignancies that involve the metatarsus can necessitate resection of an entire ray. This procedure entails resection of the metatarsal bones and phalanx to the level of the tarsometatarsal joint (Lisfranc joint) as well as the associated musculotendinous structures. Like phalangeal resections, single ray resections are well tolerated with excellent cosmetic and functional results. Shoe modification is not necessarily required, although some patients derive benefit from simple measures such as an extra sock or a foam insert. Also reminiscent of phalangeal resections, amputation of the first ray requires special mention. Resection of the entire first ray from the medial cuneiform distally causes abnormal gait, medial foot instability, and loss of push-off strength. In this instance, reconstruction with allograft or autograft may be desirable if a segmental resection is possible. Otherwise, a shoe insert and rigid foot plate can improve function.[5,6,19]

Transmetatarsal
If a malignancy of the distal midfoot involves more than two rays, a transmetatarsal amputation may be

6: Special Considerations in Tumor Management

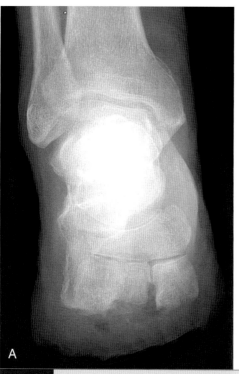
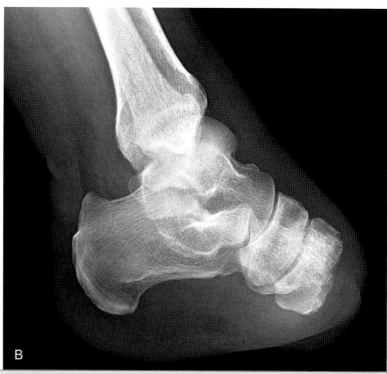

Figure 5 AP (**A**) and lateral (**B**) views of a tarsometatarsal (Lisfranc) joint amputation are shown. The patient is an 86-year-old farmer who had extensive, poorly differentiated squamous cell carcinoma of the foot. With the use of a shoe filler, the patient remains very active.

warranted. This amputation involves transection of all five metatarsal bones distal to the Lisfranc joint. If oncologically possible, bone resections should mimic the anatomic cascade of the foot, and border metatarsals should be osteotomized slightly proximal to the middle three metatarsals.[5,6] This technique will assist with closure. Metatarsal amputation closure can be particularly challenging because there is not always adequate soft tissue following oncologic resection, and free flaps to this area are tenuous. Careful preoperative planning is therefore essential for this amputation. Transmetatarsal amputation provides a functional, end-bearing residual limb, but shoe wear and stable ambulation require a shoe insert.

Midfoot

Amputations of the midfoot can be performed through the tarsometatarsal joint (Lisfranc amputation) or the transverse tarsal joint (Chopart amputation). Both of these amputations provide end-bearing residual limbs. Both procedures are also plagued by the problem of unbalanced pull of the Achilles tendon, which results in equinus contracture. To counteract this common complication, several authors advocate Achilles tendon lengthening at the time of amputation, followed by application of a rigid dressing. Transfer of the tibialis anterior tendon insertion to the talus has also been described. Patients with Lisfranc or Chopart amputation

may require additional support with an orthosis, a shoe filler, or a combination of these[6,18,19] (**Figure 5**).

Hindfoot/Ankle

Pirogoff and Syme amputations are similar and are performed at the level of the ankle joint. Both amputations transect the bone just proximal to the tibial plafond, and both malleoli are transected at the same level. These amputations provide an end-bearing residual limb that relies on the tough, durable tissue of the heel pad. In a Syme amputation, the heel pad is subperiosteally dissected from the calcaneus and secured to the distal tibia, usually through drill holes with nonabsorbable sutures. A Pirogoff amputation, in contrast, does not dissect the heel pad from the calcaneal tuberosity. Rather, the tuberosity is osteotomized perpendicular to the long axis of the calcaneus and osteosynthesized directly to the tibial osteotomy. Proponents of the Pirogoff amputation claim that osteosynthesis diminishes heel pad migration.

Prosthetic fitting and wear can be challenging in these amputations. The long residual limb limits options of prosthetic foot and ankle components, and may necessitate a shoe lift on the contralateral side to balance limb lengths.[4-6,18] End bearing on the residual limb without a prosthesis is possible for short distances, which confers some benefit in selected patients when compared with a transtibial amputation.

Tibia

Transtibial amputation is a durable, predictable solution for malignancies of the distal tibia, ankle, or foot. Postoperative function can be quite high, and patients with transtibial amputation readily participate in recreational and sporting activities. Probably the greatest concern after adequate oncologic margins is length of the residual limb. A longer residual limb will allow the patient to exert more torque and control through the prosthesis, but if the residual limb is too long, soft-tissue closure can be compromised and prosthetic options may be limited. Many authors have reported that 12.5 to 17.5 cm of residual tibia is the "sweet spot" that maximizes length, ensures adequate soft-tissue closure, and offers prosthetic options. The fibula should be transected slightly proximal to the tibial osteotomy. This technique will facilitate comfort, closure, and prosthetic fitting.

Flap creation is largely dictated by oncologic margins. Standard fish-mouth incisions and posterior flap incisions are both popular. In some instances, atypical skew flaps are required. Although tension-free closure is important, excessive tissue at the end of the residual limb will diminish prosthetic control and should be avoided. Deep closure can be obtained with myoplasty of opposing muscle groups or with tension myodesis, which attaches muscle directly to the tibia through drill holes. Proponents of myodesis claim that attaching muscle groups to bone under physiologic tension provides a replacement insertion for the muscles and is a superior option in younger, more active patients. Both options can yield excellent oncologic and functional results.[4-6]

Knee Disarticulation

Knee disarticulation is performed less commonly than transtibial and transfemoral amputation. The main advantages of knee disarticulation are that it provides an end-bearing residual limb, all the adductor attachments are maintained, and prosthetic design does not require ischial contact or containment as is the case with transfemoral amputations. One recent study claimed that patients with knee disarticulations experienced less phantom pain and phantom limb sensation than patients with transtibial or transfemoral amputation.[20] The main disadvantage of this amputation level is that because the entire length of the femur is maintained, the center of rotation of the amputated side is necessarily distal to the uninvolved side. This results in gait abnormality and cosmetic concerns.[5,6]

Femur

The consequence of the loss of the knee joint is reflected by the dramatic increase in the metabolic cost of ambulation from a transtibial amputation to a transfemoral amputation. As with transtibial amputation, the length of the residual limb is a major concern with transfemoral amputation. Residual limbs shorter than 5 cm behave functionally as hip disarticulations. To achieve optimal function without limiting prosthetic knee options, 50% to 75% of the femur should be retained. The fish-mouth incision is typically used, and adherence to standard amputation guidelines with regard to the handling of neural and vascular structures is of the utmost importance. The use of adductor myodesis is controversial. Proponents claim that myodesis of the adductor tendon to the lateral femur results in significantly greater adduction power and prevents lateral drift of the femur in the prosthetic socket. There is not always sufficient myotendinous tissue to perform an adductor myodesis, but it is suggested that if this tissue is sufficient, a myodesis should be performed. The standard myoplasty of the hamstrings to the quadriceps can then be performed superficial to the adductor myoplasty. Special postoperative considerations specific to transfemoral amputations are discussed at the end of this chapter.

Hip Disarticulation

Hip disarticulation is performed for tumors of the proximal femur or surrounding soft tissues that (1) do not involve the hip joint and (2) are too proximal for a transfemoral amputation but do not require a hemipelvectomy. After ligation of the femoral vessels and transection of the femoral and sciatic nerves, the gluteal musculature is dissected from the proximal femur and brought anteriorly and medially to close the defect. Hip disarticulation prostheses are cumbersome, difficult to maneuver, and costly in terms of energy expenditure.[5,6]

Hindquarter

Variously termed pelvic amputation, hindquarter amputation, or external hemipelvectomy, the removal of the lower extremity along with some or all of the hemipelvis is fortunately a rare occurrence. Its use has largely been supplanted by the internal hemipelvectomy, where the involved pelvis is removed and the lower limb is left attached.

A traditional hemipelvectomy involves no osteotomies: the pubic symphysis and sacroiliac joints are divided and the entire innominate bone is removed with the subjacent limb. If oncologically possible, a portion of the innominate bone can be left intact. This procedure is termed a modified external hemipelvectomy. Although it is technically more difficult, a modified external hemipelvectomy provides some functional advantages for the patient. Leaving a portion of the pubis intact creates less of a defect in the pelvic floor and decreases the risk of hernia formation. Likewise, the ischium also provides pelvic floor attachments and has the additional advantage of enabling easier and more level sitting for the patient. Leaving the iliac crest or wing simplifies clothing wear, because the patient maintains more of a buttock curvature and has an easier time with pants and belts. Maintaining these bony structures also leaves more tissue in place should the patient wish to ambulate with a prosthesis.

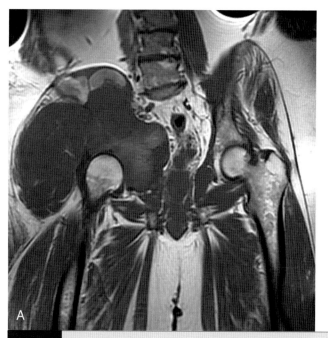
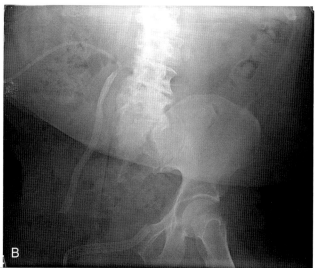

| Figure 6 | **A,** Preoperative coronal T1-weighted MRI of a patient with a chondrosarcoma involving the entire right hemipelvis and sacral ala is shown. **B,** Radiograph showing an extended external hemipelvectomy. |

An extended hemipelvectomy is performed through the sacrum. A longitudinal osteotomy of the sacrum, taking as much as half of the sacral bodies, is performed instead of sacroiliac joint division (**Figure 6**). All nerve roots on the ipsilateral side are divided, so bowel, bladder, and sexual dysfunction are possible.[21]

Vascular involvement, especially of the external iliac vessels, is one of the most common indications for this procedure because extensive vascular reconstruction may not be possible. Tumor extent can force amputation, because extreme tumor bulk can preclude pelvic resection with limb retention. Progression of disease from the pelvis into the limb may also render limb salvage inadvisable or impossible. One of the more common indications for hemipelvectomy is palliation. Neglected tumors can invade either or both of the sciatic and femoral systems, causing unremitting pain that may be untreatable with medical or interventional means and thus require amputation.[22]

Hindquarter Flaps

Once the decision to perform a hindquarter amputation has been made, the most important consideration is the type of flap to be used. This decision depends on the vascular involvement and where viable tissue will remain. The choices are one of three rotational flaps or one of two free flaps. If the tumor involves the posterior pelvis and sciatic notch, an anterior flap hemipelvectomy is performed. The entire quadriceps muscle is dissected from the femur, the superficial femoral artery is ligated near the Hunter canal, and a flap consisting of the femoral vessels, entire quadriceps mechanism, and anterior thigh skin is elevated. The external iliac

vessel is freed to the common iliac, and the internal iliac/hypogastric system is ligated. The pelvis and leg are then removed, and the anterior thigh is rotated into the resultant defect.[23] If the tumor involves the anterior pelvis and the external iliac vessels, a posterior flap is used. This flap is dependent on the gluteal vessels. The myocutaneous flap is developed by extending an iliofemoral incision around and into the buttock crease. This method allows the abductors to be removed from the iliac wing and greater trochanter and rotated backward upon the gluteal pedicle as it exits the greater sciatic notch. The external iliac vessels are then ligated, the pelvis is removed, and the buttock is rotated forward to close the resultant defect.[24] If the inferior obturator ring can be maintained, an obturator rotational flap can be used. This is a small myocutaneous flap from the medial thigh. Although it is not generally large enough to cover an entire hemipelvectomy defect, this flap can cover the anterior portion, an area often at risk with a posterior flap hemipelvectomy. The obturator flap can be rotated into the groin region, allowing the posterior flap to be shortened and maintain better viability.

If the tumor extent involves both the internal and external iliac systems, the common iliac vessels must be divided. In this case, a rotational flap is not possible, and a free flap must be used. All relevant anatomic structures should be identified, and all osteotomies at least visualized before the vessels are ligated. As in an anterior flap hemipelvectomy, the quadriceps myocutaneous flap can also be used as a free flap. In this method, the quadriceps flap is raised from the femur in an identical manner, but the femoral vessels are divided at the appropriate time, the pelvis is removed, and a free thigh flap is used. If the proximal thigh is involved, a fillet of leg flap also can be used. In this procedure, a guillotine amputation is performed proximal to the knee, similar to a long transfemoral amputation. The superficial and deep posterior compartments are removed as a myocutaneous flap, which is then used to fill the hemipelvectomy defect, with a vascular anastomosis at the iliac level.[24]

Although hindquarter amputation can be a lifesaving procedure,[25] and the oncologic results can be excellent, the functional results are generally poor.[26] Hemipelvic prostheses can be fashioned but are rarely functional beyond ambulation. Older patients generally do not ambulate and are wheelchair dependent. Younger individuals may ambulate functionally, but ambulation typically decreases with age. Results of hemipelvectomy for sarcoma have generally been better than those for carcinoma, because carcinoma requiring hemipelvectomy often is the result of extensive disease.[27]

Rotationplasty

Rotationplasties are a series of procedures designed to preserve limb length. The goal of rotationplasty is to convert a hip disarticulation or transfemoral amputation into a transtibial amputation. The foot is left intact, and, via 180° rotation of the limb, acts as a short tibia. Rotationplasty thus converts the ankle into a functional knee and uses either the native hip or a substitute, depending on the type of procedure performed. Rotationplasty was popularized as a treatment of proximal femoral focal deficiency and is often called van Nes rotationplasty. It is used primarily in the pediatric population but can be considered in adults whose lifestyle or occupational demands are not compatible with an endoprosthesis.

Types of Rotationplasties

Different types of rotationplasties to address the reconstructive needs of various skeletal deficiencies were described in 1988.[28] In broad terms, either knee rotationplasty (type A) or hip rotationplasty (type B) is performed. Type A rotationplasties rely on osteosynthesis between the tibia and femur. The native hip is left intact, and after appropriate tumor resection, the limb is rotated 180° and the tibia and femur are plated together. Type B rotationplasties remove the proximal femur. In a type BI rotationplasty, the proximal femur is removed and the distal femur is fixed into the remaining acetabulum. The rotated knee then acts as a hip. Type BII rotationplasties remove the lower pelvis as well, requiring osteosynthesis between the distal femur and the remaining iliac wing. In type BIII rotationplasties, the entire femur must be removed. In children with open physes, the soft tissues around the acetabulum are reconstructed to the native proximal tibia. With skeletal growth, the proximal tibia remodels and reshapes to form a pseudofemoral head, with resultant skeletal stability.[29]

Two conditions are mandatory for a successful rotationplasty: a functional sciatic nerve and a functional foot and ankle. If tumor resection mandates sciatic sacrifice, rotationplasty is contraindicated. Likewise, foot deformities and other conditions affecting the foot will lead to a dysfunctional reconstruction. Vascular supply to the remaining limb is also critical, and the presence or history of a deep vein thrombosis must be considered another contraindication.

Rotationplasty is technically demanding. Consideration must be made for osteosynthesis, skin flaps, and vascular reconstruction. Problems with any of these can cause the procedure to fail, resulting in a transfemoral amputation or hip disarticulation. Choosing appropriate skin and muscular flaps is important. In all types of rotationplasty, most of the quadriceps is removed and myodesis of the gastrocnemius-soleus complex to the remaining quadriceps is performed. Skin flaps should therefore parallel the muscular flaps with most of the anterior thigh skin being excised, and the posterior skin of the calf being used to fill this defect. Clearly, in most individuals there is a discrepancy between the size of the proximal thigh and the proximal leg. A novel incision technique was recently suggested to account for this mismatch.[30] Rotationplasty disrupts the lymphatic backflow from the remaining limb, and wound complications are therefore common. This lymphatic flow tends to reconstitute over time, but edema management is important, and great care should be taken in skin handling to minimize flap necrosis and infection. The authors of a 2008 study reviewed 25 rotationplasties at their institution in an attempt to identify risk factors for failure.[31] In addition to the considerations listed previously, they found that large tumors, poor response to chemotherapy, and pathologic fracture also predict the failure of rotationplasty surgery.

In the skeletal reconstruction, consideration should be given to limb length. In children, the growth remaining from the remaining physes can be calculated, and the limb can be made an appropriate length to yield equivalent "knee" lengths when growth is complete. In adults, limb lengths should facilitate prosthetic fitting, posture, and gait. Correct rotation is of the utmost importance. Initial rotation should be marked before osteotomies are performed, because determining limb rotation for reconstruction while rotating the distal segment on a neurovascular pedicle is extremely difficult. Rotational malalignment has substantial consequences, and care should be taken to ensure that the foot points directly posteriorly after osteosynthesis has occurred.

Two methods for dealing with the femoral vessels have been described: coiling the vessels with the sciatic nerve, or vascular resection and reanastomosis. Although coiling is seemingly simpler, it requires substantially more vascular dissection and could compromise oncologic margins. Resection and reanastomosis requires a vascular surgeon but has the advantages that both vessels are the correct length at the conclusion of

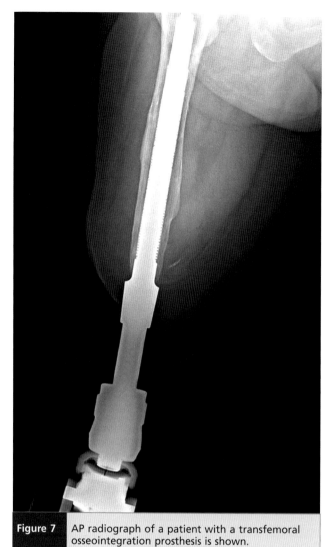

Figure 7 AP radiograph of a patient with a transfemoral osseointegration prosthesis is shown.

the treatment and that the vein is not kinked by coiling.

Although the procedure is rife with complications and technical difficulties, the functional result of a successful rotationplasty is excellent. Most patients function at the level of a transtibial amputation.[32] Oxygen consumption, duration of prosthetic use, and walking speed have generally paralleled the results seen in transtibial amputations in healthy individuals.

Recent Advances: Osseointegration

Although the term osseointegration prosthesis could apply to any metallic prosthesis that achieves stable ingrowth into the surrounding bone, in this setting it describes an intraosseous, transcutaneous prosthesis that is used for reconstruction after amputation. In this system, a metallic prosthesis is stably integrated into a bone (most commonly the femur after transfemoral amputation) and exits through the terminal end of the residual limb. A modified coupling is then used to attach this piece to whatever exoprosthesis the patient is

using. This method provides a stable anchor between the residual limb and the exoprosthesis, without use of a socket (**Figure 7**). Although the notion of a metallic prosthesis exiting through the skin is foreign to most orthopaedic concepts, this device is analogous to a well-fixed external fixator pin: if the pin is stable and the surrounding skin is not irritated by the metal, it can be maintained for weeks to months to complete treatment. Osseointegration prostheses can be maintained for years to decades, and if the device is stable in the bone, infection and osteomyelitis will not occur.

Although they are not FDA-approved in the United States, these devices are increasing in popularity in Europe. Three systems are available, each with a slightly different design for osseointegration. Each deals with the skin penetration (or stoma) in a different manner.[33] Essential to all three systems is stable, permanent osseointegration.[34] If this is not achieved, instability in both the skin and bony envelope will occur, with resultant failure.

The primary advantage of osseointegration is that a prosthetic socket is not used. This technique provides a host of benefits including increased comfort (when sitting, standing, and in hot weather), elimination of common socket pressure phenomena and dermatitis, elimination of the need to fabricate a new socket should the patient gain or lose weight, increased ease and speed of donning the prosthesis, and the allowance of thigh muscle hypertrophy. All of these advantages result in increased prosthetic use, greater acceptance of the amputation, and higher function. Ambulation is improved by eliminating socket discomfort and enhancing proprioception. This improvement encourages confidence in ambulation on uneven surfaces and a more normal gait pattern.[35] Finally, osseointegration provides an excellent option for patients whose residual limbs are too short or misshapen to accommodate a conventional socket.

Active infection is a contraindication to this procedure. Severe osteoporosis is a relative contraindication, because a stable press-fit construct must be achieved for osseointegration to occur.

The most serious complication of this procedure is infection, and it is of paramount importance to distinguish infection from colonization.[36] Colonization is universal. Like the presence of oral or nasal flora, skin flora will colonize the stoma, and will exist down to the zone of skin integration. Colonization can extend to the bone-implant interface. As long as no symptoms are present, it should not be considered osteomyelitis and should not be treated.

The functional results of osseointegration prostheses have been encouraging. Gait, energy expenditure, and balance all have been studied. Force plate and video analyses demonstrate a more normal gait than is achieved by patients with conventional amputation of the same level.[34,37] Although the overall complication rate with osseointegration has been high, so has patient satisfaction.[34,37] Even in the face of major complications, such as periprosthetic fracture or osteomyelitis, most patients have not wished to return to socket use.[35]

Postoperative Dressings

Postoperative wound dressings can be a source of discomfort and frustration for both patients and orthopaedic surgeons. Initial dressings of both upper and lower extremity amputations should provide gentle compression of the residual limb. This compression is accomplished very well with elastic bandages.[6,18,38] Bandages should be gently anchored to the proximal residual limb without forming a tourniquet, which would be counterproductive. The elastic wrap should then proceed in a figure-of-8 or spica pattern such that gentle compression is delivered to the entire residual limb in a distal-to-proximal fashion. This approach can be most difficult with short residual humeri or femora. In these instances, anchoring the elastic bandage around the chest or pelvis, respectively, is recommended. These dressings, if carefully applied, do not require frequent daily revisions and are very comfortable for the postoperative patient. After about 2 weeks, the residual limb should be healed enough to allow use of a "shrinker sock." These are also elastic, and several varieties are commercially available.

Additional considerations specific to lower extremity amputation include the patient's sleeping habits in the early postoperative period. Contractures of the knee and hip, once established, are very difficult to overcome and complicate prosthetic fitting and use. Therefore, patients with transtibial or transfemoral amputation should be discouraged from placing pillows or bolsters under their knees or residual femora, respectively. When comfortable, patients with transfemoral amputation should be encouraged to sleep in the prone position. Use of this sleeping position is a very good technique for actively avoiding hip flexion contracture.

Phantom Pain

Neuropathic pain or phantom pain can be a difficult problem in both the short and long term for patients with amputation. Multiple studies show that a high percentage of patients encounter these difficulties.[18,20,39,40] The subtle difference between phantom limb sensation and phantom pain must be appreciated. Phantom limb sensation is the experience that one's amputated extremity has "fallen asleep" or has "pins and needles." Phantom pain, in contrast, is a sharp, intense, temporary debilitating pain experienced in the amputated part. This unique subset of neuropathic pain is the subject of ongoing research. Multiple pharmacologic agents and nerve treatments have been tried with varying levels of success.[41-43] Because phantom pain and phantom limb sensation are incompletely understood, consultation with a neurologist or pain specialist may be beneficial for patients with recent amputation and should be considered. It is the anecdotal experience of this chapter's authors, along with that of colleagues in physical medicine and rehabilitation, that prosthetic use and training can be of benefit and can decrease the patient's frequency of phantom pain, but this experience has not been borne out in the literature.

Patients should also be encouraged to perform residual limb desensitization exercises in the early postoperative period.[18] This exercise entails gentle tapping at the end of the residual limb once the incision is healed. Tapping gradually increases in intensity and pressure, which prepares both the limb and the patient for the eventual sensation of prosthesis wear. This exercise probably has a psychological benefit to patients with recent amputation as well.

Summary

The evolution of limb salvage techniques have decreased the incidence of amputations performed by orthopaedic oncologists. Modern orthopaedic oncologists must still be facile with the indications, technical demands, and rehabilitative potentials of amputations for those situations when limb salvage is not possible because of anatomic or oncologic concerns. Rather than a perceived failure of treatment, amputation should be viewed as a viable reconstructive option. As prosthetic advances and new technologies come to light, the functional capacities of amputations will be continually enhanced and improved. Amputation remains an important tool in the surgical treatment of malignancy.

Annotated References

1. Ayerza MA, Farfalli GL, Aponte-Tinao L, Muscolo DL: Does increased rate of limb-sparing surgery affect survival in osteosarcoma? *Clin Orthop Relat Res* 2010;468(11):2854-2859.

   The authors asked whether limb-sparing procedures in high-grade osteosarcoma increased over the past three decades, and whether this increase affected survival and ultimate amputation rates. They concluded that patients with osteosarcoma treated in the most recent two decades had higher rates of limb salvage treatment and survival and lower rates of secondary amputation.

2. Gailey R, Allen K, Castles J, Kucharik J, Roeder M: Review of secondary physical conditions associated with lower-limb amputation and long-term prosthesis use. *J Rehabil Res Dev* 2008;45(1):15-29.

   The authors reviewed the literature on secondary complications among people with lower-limb amputation who are long-term prosthesis wearers. Level of evidence: II.

3. Simon MA: Limb salvage for osteosarcoma in the 1980s. *Clin Orthop Relat Res* 1991;270:264-270.

4. Menendez LR, ed: *Orthopaedic Knowledge Update: Musculoskeletal Tumors*. Rosemont, IL, American Academy of Orthopaedic Surgeons, 2002.

5. Schwartz HS, ed: *Orthopaedic Knowledge Update: Musculoskeletal Tumors 2*. Rosemont, IL, American Academy of Orthopaedic Surgeons, 2007.

6. Canale ST, ed: *Campbell's Operative Orthopaedics*, ed 10. St. Louis, MO, Mosby, 2003.

7. Green H, Pederson W, eds: *Green's Operative Hand Surgery*, ed 5. Philadelphia, PA, Elsevier, 2005.

8. Motta A, López C, Acosta A, Peñaranda C: Subungual melanoma in situ in a Hispanic girl treated with functional resection and reconstruction with onychocutaneous toe free flap. *Arch Dermatol* 2007;143(12): 1600-1602.

    The authors presented a case report of a successful partial toe-to-thumb transplant in a young patient with malignancy. Level of evidence: IV.

9. Puhaindran ME, Athanasian EA: Double ray amputation for tumors of the hand. *Clin Orthop Relat Res* 2010;468(11):2976-2979.

    The authors reported a series of five double ray resections in musculoskeletal oncology patients. Although double ray amputation results in worse functional outcome than single ray amputation, good key pinch, tip pinch, and tripod pinch can be preserved when the deep motor branch of the ulnar nerve is preserved, and the hand can still assist in bimanual activities. Level of evidence: IV.

10. Yang P, Abdel-Malek K, Patrick A, Lindkvist L: A multi-fingered hand prosthesis. *Mech Mach Theory* 2004;39:555-581.

11. Jönsson S, Caine-Winterberger K, Brånemark R: Osseointegration amputation prostheses on the upper limbs: Methods, prosthetics and rehabilitation. *Prosthet Orthot Int* 2011;35(2):190-200.

    The authors described their two-stage osseointegration technique in 37 patients with upper limb amputations. There were 10 thumb, 1 partial hand, 10 transradial, and 16 transhumeral amputations. Of these, 30 patients actively used their prosthesis and had improved function and quality of life. Level of evidence: IV.

12. Malawer M, Sugarbaker P: *Musculoskeletal Cancer Surgery: Treatment of Sarcomas and Related Diseases*. Dordrecht, The Netherlands, Kluwer, 2001.

13. Jones NF, Jarrahy R, Kaufman MR: Pedicled and free radial forearm flaps for reconstruction of the elbow, wrist, and hand. *Plast Reconstr Surg* 2008;121(3):887-898.

    The authors presented a retrospectively analyzed series of 67 pedicled and free radial forearm flaps for reconstruction of the elbow, wrist, and hand. The authors suggested that the antegrade pedicled radial forearm flap is the optimal flap for coverage of defects around the elbow, and the reverse radial forearm flap is the optimal choice for coverage of moderate-sized defects of the wrist and hand. Level of evidence: IV.

14. Moreira-Gonzalez A, Djohan R, Lohman R: Considerations surrounding reconstruction after resection of musculoskeletal sarcomas. *Cleve Clin J Med* 2010; 77(suppl 1):S18-S22.

    The defects left by resection of bone and soft-tissue sarcomas often require reconstructive surgery to provide adequate wound coverage, preserve limb function, and optimize cosmetic results. Immediate reconstruction should always be considered after resection with a negative margin, and should be attempted whenever possible. Level of evidence: V.

15. Cordeiro PG, Cohen S, Burt M, Brennan MF: The total volar forearm musculocutaneous free flap for reconstruction of extended forequarter amputations. *Ann Plast Surg* 1998;40(4):388-396.

16. Marulanda GA, Henderson ER, Johnson DA, Letson GD, Cheong D: Orthopedic surgery options for the treatment of primary osteosarcoma. *Cancer Control* 2008;15(1):13-20.

    The surgical management of patients with osteosarcoma is challenging. No difference in survival has been shown between amputations and adequately performed limb-sparing procedures. Optimal tumor resection and a functional residual limb with increased patient survival are the goals of modern orthopaedic oncology. Level of evidence: V.

17. Beck LA, Einertson MJ, Winemiller MH, DePompolo RW, Hoppe KM, Sim FF: Functional outcomes and quality of life after tumor-related hemipelvectomy. *Phys Ther* 2008;88(8):916-927.

    Hemipelvectomy is a life-changing treatment for pelvic malignancies. The authors compared functional outcomes and quality of life of patients following internal or external hemipelvectomies, and found that patients with external hemipelvectomy had more bladder problems and were less independent. Level of evidence: II.

18. Vaccaro AR, ed: *Orthopaedic Knowledge Update 8*. Rosemont, IL, American Academy of Orthopaedic Surgeons, 2005.

19. Simon MA, Dempsey S, eds: *Surgery for Bone and Soft-Tissue Tumors*. Philadelphia, PA, Lippincott-Raven, 1998.

20. Behr J, Friedly J, Molton I, Morgenroth D, Jensen MP, Smith DG: Pain and pain-related interference in adults with lower-limb amputation: Comparison of knee-disarticulation, transtibial, and transfemoral surgical sites. *J Rehabil Res Dev* 2009;46(7):963-972.

    This study demonstrated that patients with knee disarticulation amputation used prostheses significantly less than did patients with transtibial amputation. However, no evidence was found that patients with knee disarticulation amputation have worse outcomes in terms of pain and pain-related interference with physical function; in fact, they may have more favorable long-term outcomes. Level of evidence: II.

21. Todd LT Jr, Yaszemski MJ, Currier BL, Fuchs B, Kim CW, Sim FH: Bowel and bladder function after major sacral resection. *Clin Orthop Relat Res* 2002;397:36-39.

22. Parsons CM, Pimiento JM, Cheong D, et al: The role of radical amputations for extremity tumors: A single institution experience and review of the literature. *J Surg Oncol* 2012;105(2):149-155.

    The authors evaluated 40 patients who underwent forequarter or hindquarter amputation. They concluded that in the absence of conservative options, major amputations are indicated for the management of advanced tumors. These operations can be performed safely, resulting in effective palliation of debilitating symptoms. Although recurrence rates remain high, some patients have prolonged survival. Level of evidence: IV.

23. Kulaylat MN, Froix A, Karakousis CP: Blood supply of hemipelvectomy flaps: The anterior flap hemipelvectomy. *Arch Surg* 2001;136(7):828-831.

24. Senchenkov A, Moran SL, Petty PM, et al: Soft-tissue reconstruction of external hemipelvectomy defects. *Plast Reconstr Surg* 2009;124(1):144-155.

    This study reviewed most of the soft-tissue flap options after hemipelvectomy. Technical considerations and complications are well described. Level of evidence: IV.

25. Carter SR, Eastwood DM, Grimer RJ, Sneath RS: Hindquarter amputation for tumours of the musculoskeletal system. *J Bone Joint Surg Br* 1990;72(3):490-493.

26. Griesser MJ, Gillette B, Crist M, et al: Internal and external hemipelvectomy or flail hip in patients with sarcomas: Quality-of-life and functional outcomes. *Am J Phys Med Rehabil* 2012;91(1):24-32.

    This study used multiple outcome measures to investigate quality of life in patients after internal or external hemipelvectomy. All outcome measures demonstrated significantly reduced quality of life for all patients. No differences between the amputation and limb salvage procedures could be determined. Level of evidence: III.

27. Baliski CR, Schachar NS, McKinnon JG, Stuart GC, Temple WJ: Hemipelvectomy: A changing perspective for a rare procedure. *Can J Surg* 2004;47(2):99-103.

28. Winkelmann W: Rotationplasty in the local treatment of osteosarcoma. *Semin Orthod* 1988;3:40-47.

29. Hardes J, Gosheger G, Vachtsevanos L, Hoffmann C, Ahrens H, Winkelmann W: Rotationplasty type BI versus type BIIIa in children under the age of ten years: Should the knee be preserved? *J Bone Joint Surg Br* 2005;87(3):395-400.

30. Ossendorf C, Exner GU, Fuchs B: A new incision technique to reduce tibiofemoral mismatch in rotationplasty. *Clin Orthop Relat Res* 2010;468(5):1264-1268.

    The authors presented a new incision technique for rotationplasty about the knee. This technique was used in eight patients. The wounds healed uneventfully in all of the patients. Level of evidence: IV.

31. Sawamura C, Hornicek FJ, Gebhardt MC: Complications and risk factors for failure of rotationplasty: Review of 25 patients. *Clin Orthop Relat Res* 2008;466(6):1302-1308.

    Rotationplasty is only rarely indicated, and the surgical complications or risk factors for failure of the procedure have not been well described. The authors reviewed 25 patients who underwent rotationplasty, focusing on risk factors for failure and postoperative complications. Level of evidence: IV.

32. Fuchs B, Kotajarvi BR, Kaufman KR, Sim FH: Functional outcome of patients with rotationplasty about the knee. *Clin Orthop Relat Res* 2003;415:52-58.

33. Chimutengwende-Gordon M, Pendegrass C, Blunn G: Enhancing the soft tissue seal around intraosseous transcutaneous amputation prostheses using silanized fibronectin titanium alloy. *Biomed Mater* 2011;6(2):025008.

    A specialized silanized fibronectin coating applied to a metallic surface enabled increased fibroblast binding to the prosthesis. This technique may improve the seal at the stomal interface. Level of evidence: III.

34. Hagberg K, Brånemark R: One hundred patients treated with osseointegrated transfemoral amputation prostheses—rehabilitation perspective. *J Rehabil Res Dev* 2009;46(3):331-344.

    One hundred patients with 106 prostheses were followed for an 18-year period. Eleven patients had treatment failure. An integrated process of rehabilitation designed to stimulate osseointegration is described. Level of evidence: IV.

35. Aschoff HH, Clausen A, Tsoumpris K, Hoffmeister T: Implantation of the endo-exo femur prosthesis to improve the mobility of amputees [in German]. *Oper Orthop Traumatol* 2011;23(5):462-472.

    Thirty-nine patients who underwent implantation of an osseointegration prosthesis were studied. Four prostheses failed because of soft-tissue or bone infection, or device fracture. Two failures were replaced. Multiple soft-tissue infections occurred as a result of a poor early design and responded to design modification. Thirty-seven patients would repeat the procedure. Level of evidence: IV.

36. Tillander J, Hagberg K, Hagberg L, Brånemark R: Osseointegrated titanium implants for limb prostheses attachments: Infectious complications. *Clin Orthop Relat Res* 2010;468(10):2781-2788.

    This study investigated stomal flora in osseointegration implants. An infection rate of 5% to 18% was determined, and resulted in 1 of 39 implants requiring removal. Colonization without infection was common, with *Staphylococcus aureus* and coagulase-negative staphylococcus being the most common organisms found. Level of evidence: II.

6: Special Considerations in Tumor Management

37. Hagberg K, Brånemark R, Gunterberg B, Rydevik B: Osseointegrated transfemoral amputation prostheses: Prospective results of general and condition-specific quality of life in 18 patients at 2-year follow-up. *Prosthet Orthot Int* 2008;32(1):29-41.

    This article describes the first prospective study of osseointegration prostheses. Of 18 patients, 17 successfully used the device; one device failed as a result of loosening. All patients with successful devices demonstrated improvement in all quality-of-life and functional scores, with fewer prosthesis-related problems. Level of evidence: IV.

38. Alsancak S, Köse SK, Altınkaynak H: Effect of elastic bandaging and prosthesis on the decrease in stump volume. *Acta Orthop Traumatol Turc* 2011;45(1):14-22.

    The authors compared the effects of elastic bandaging, pneumatic prosthesis, and temporary prosthesis on postoperative residual limb management. Level of evidence: II.

39. Byrne KP: Survey of phantom limb pain, phantom sensation and stump pain in Cambodian and New Zealand amputees. *Pain Med* 2011;12(5):794-798.

    The primary objective of this study was to compare the prevalence of phantom limb pain in patients with amputation in New Zealand and Cambodia and to assess the demographics of a sample of patients from these two countries. Despite very different environments, no difference in the phantom limb pain was found between the groups. Level of evidence: II.

40. Daigeler A, Lehnhardt M, Khadra A, et al: Proximal major limb amputations: A retrospective analysis of 45 oncological cases. *World J Surg Oncol* 2009;7:15.

    Proximal major limb amputations severely interfere with patients' body function and are a valuable option in the treatment of extremity malignancies or severe infections. Despite short survival, high complication rates, and postoperative pain, patients' quality of life can be improved for the time they have remaining. Level of evidence: IV.

41. Lefaucheur JP, Drouot X, Cunin P, et al: Motor cortex stimulation for the treatment of refractory peripheral neuropathic pain. *Brain* 2009;132(pt 6):1463-1471.

    Epidural motor cortex stimulation has been proposed as a treatment of chronic, drug-resistant neuropathic pain of various origins. Regarding pain syndromes caused by peripheral nerve lesions, only case series have previously been reported. The authors presented the results of the first randomized controlled trial using chronic motor cortex stimulation in these patients. Level of evidence: I.

42. Tognù A, Borghi B, Gullotta S, White PF: Ultrasound-guided posterior approach to brachial plexus for the treatment of upper phantom limb syndrome. *Minerva Anestesiol* 2012;78(1):105-108.

    Ultrasound guidance can be successful at localizing the brachial plexus for the purpose of placing a continuous pain infusion. Level of evidence: IV.

43. Neumann V, O'Connor RJ, Bush D: Cryoprobe treatment: An alternative to phenol injections for painful neuromas after amputation. *AJR Am J Roentgenol* 2008;191(6):W313, author reply W314.

    The authors concluded that cryotherapy in combination with high-resolution sonography may have a useful role as a highly controllable and minimally invasive method of treating neuroma-related pain, which may reduce the risk of local tissue necrosis compared with phenol injections. Level of evidence: IV.

Index

Index

Bisphosphonates
  metastatic bone disease and, 365
  myeloma, 212
  pathologic fracture prevention in
    metastatic bone disease and, 332
  PDB, 42
Bone
  angiosarcoma of, 198–199
  chondrosarcoma of, 181–189
  hemangioma of, 93, 94f
  leiomyosarcoma of, 198
Bone banking, 420–421
Bone-forming tumors, benign
  enostosis, 115–116
  melorheostosis, 116–117
  osteoblastoma, 111–114
  osteoid osteoma, 107–111
  osteoma, 114–115
  osteopathia striata, 117–118
  osteopoikilosis, 116
Bone grafting
  biology, 420
  bone banks, 420–421
  concepts in, 419–424
  definitions, 419
  fibular, 393–394
  substitutes, 423–424, 423t
Bone infarcts, as pseudotumor, 46
Bone island. See Enostosis
Bone lesions
  benign cystic, 87–92
  benign fibrous, 123–130
  benign histiocytic, 123–130
  lytic, 42
  malignant, 6-7, 7F, 8F, 9-10
  radiolucent, 87
Bone metastases
  biology, 319–320, 320f
  breast cancer, 321f, 322–324
  kidney cancer, 326
  lung cancer, 324, 324f
  lymphoma, 326–327
  multiple myeloma, 324–326, 325f
  pathophysiology of, 319–327
    disease-specific, 321–327
  physiology, 320–321, 321f, 322f
  prostate cancer, 321–322
  thyroid cancer, 326
  upper extremity
    forearm, wrist, and hand, 343–344,
      343f
    humerus, 339–343
    surgical management of, treatment
      algorithm for, 339–344, 340f
Bone sarcomas. See also Sarcomas
  AJCC staging system for, 9, 9t
  targeted agents for, 67–72
    adoptive immunotherapy and, 72
    CDK4 and, 71
    Hh inhibitors and, 72
    histone deacetylase inhibitors and,
      71
    HSP90 inhibitors and, 71

  IGF1R inhibitors and, 70–71
  MDM2 inhibitors and, 71
  mTOR inhibitors and, 71
  oncolytic viruses and, 72
  RANKL and, 71–72
  γ-secretase inhibitors and, 72
  tyrosine kinase inhibitors and,
    67–70, 68t
  VEGF inhibitors and, 70
  targeted therapy for, 65–72
    historical perspective on, 65–66
Bone tumors
  chemotherapy, 53–54
  clinical presentation of, 3–11
  diagnoses of, by age, 5t
  diagnoses of, by location, 4, 4t
  GCTB, 133–142
  malignant lesions
    clinical presentation of, 6–7, 7f, 8f
    staging of, 9–10
  malignant primary, 195–200
  staging of, 7–10
Bone tumors, benign
  clinical presentation, 3–6, 3f, 4f
  endosteal thinning and, 4, 5f
  observation, 147
  pain and, 4–6
  radiographic appearance, 4
  staging, 8–9, 8t
  surgical treatment, 147–152
    embolization, 149–150, 149f
    open curettage, 147–149
    RFA and, 150–151
    UBCs and, 150
Bortezomib, 212
Breast cancer
  bone metastasis pathophysiology and,
    321f, 322–324
  metastatic bone disease and, 365–366,
    366f
Buschke-Ollendorff syndrome, 116

C

CABIN1 gene. See Calcineurin-binding
    protein 1 gene
Café-au-lait areas, fibrous dysplasia and,
    123t
Calcaneal bone cysts
  histology, 92
  imaging, 91–92, 91f
  treatment, 92
Calcineurin-binding protein 1
  (CABIN1) gene, 266
Calcium phosphate biomaterials, 423
Calcium sulfate, 423
Campanacci disease, 126
Cancer cells, hallmarks of, 31–32
Cancer diagnosis, 31–32
Carbon ions, radiation therapy with, 81
Cardiomyopathy, 56–57
Cartilage tumors, benign
  chondroblastoma, 102–103

  chondromyxoid fibroma (CMF),
    103-104
  enchondroma, 99–102
  enchondromatosis, 102
  multiple osteochondromatosis, 99
  osteochondroma, 97–99
  periosteal chondroma, 102
Cediranib, 70
Cellular schwannoma, 265
Cervical spine, spinal metastases surgery
  and, 358–359, 359f
Chemosensitivities by subtype, 56, 57t
Chemotherapy. See also specific agents
  angiosarcoma, 54–55
  bone tumor, 53–54
  chondrosarcoma, 54
  Ewing sarcoma, 54
  GIST, 56
  HAART and, 55–56
  liposarcoma, 55
  LMS, 55
  NRSTS, 54–56, 56f
  osteosarcoma, 53–54, 162–164, 166
  pediatric patients and effects of,
    431–432
  physis and effects of, 431–432
  RMS, 54
  sarcoma, late effects of, 56–58, 57t
  skeletally immature patients and
    effects of, 429
  on skeletally immature patients and
    effects of, 429
  soft-tissue sarcoma, 54–56, 309–310,
    310t
  systemic, osteosarcoma, 162–164
Chemotherapy-resistant sarcomas, 55.
  See also Sarcomas
Children's Oncology Group (COG), 55
Chondroblastomas
  benign cartilage tumors, 102–103
  clinical features, 102–103
  genetics, 103
  pathology, 103
  radiographic findings, 102–103, 103f
  treatment, 103
Chondroid lipoma, 260
Chondromyxoid fibroma (CMF)
  clinical features, 103-104
  genetics, 104
  pathology, 104
  radiographic findings, 104
  treatment, 104
Chondrosarcomas
  of bone, 181–189
  chemotherapy, 54
  clear cell, 182
    histologic characteristics, 185–186
  dedifferentiated, 182
    histologic characteristics, 186
    radiographic characteristics, 184
  extraskeletal myxoid, 182, 301–303
  grade 1, 181–182
    histologic characteristics of, 185

M
